Contents

Preface

Passing specialist examinations in internal medicine is a difficult milestone for many doctors, but is a mandatory requirement for career progression. Pass rates in these examinations are generally low due to 'high standards' and 'stiff competition'. Thorough preparation is essential and requires a broad knowledge of internal medicine. The pressures of a busy clinical job and nights 'on call' make it almost impossible for doctors to wade through heaps of large text books to acquire all the knowledge that is required to pass the examinations.

The aim of this book is to provide the busy doctor with a comprehensive review of questions featured most frequently in the MRCP (II) examination in internal medicine. The MRCP (II) examination has a best of 5/n from many answer format. The vast majority of the questions in the book follow the same pattern; however, we have chosen to include several scenarios with open ended questions to stimulate the medical thought process. The level of difficulty of each question is of the same standard as MRCP (II) examination. However, some cases are deliberately more difficult for teaching purposes.

A broad range of subjects is covered in over 400 questions ranging from metabolic medicine to infectious diseases. Precise answers and detailed discussion follow each question. Where appropriate, important differential diagnoses, diagnostic algorithms and up-to-date medical lists are presented. Many questions comprise illustrated material in the form of radiographic material, electrocardiograms, echocardiograms, blood films, audiograms, respiratory flow loops, histological material, and slides in ophthalmology, dermatology and infectious diseases. Over 200 commonly examined illustrations are included.

Tutorials are included at the end of the book to aid the interpretation of illustrated material as well as important, and sometimes difficult, clinical data, such as respiratory function tests, cardiac catheter data and dynamic endocrine tests.

The book will prove invaluable to all those studying for higher examinations in internal medicine, and to their instructors.

Sanjay Sharma
Consultant Cardiologist
Lecturer for Medipass Intensive Courses
for the MRCP Part 2

Rashmi Kaushal
Consultant Physician and Endocrinologist

Classification of Cases

Cardiology
1, 10, 11, 13, 22, 25, 32, 40, 52, 53, 54, 62, 63, 66, 68, 74, 78, 80, 94, 95, 100, 121, 123, 125, 130–132, 138, 144, 150, 160, 167, 178, 180, 184, 193, 197, 199, 202, 203, 207, 208, 223, 226, 229, 232, 235, 237, 243, 246, 259, 266, 270, 285, 287, 291, 296, 301, 305, 307, 309, 318, 323, 324, 327, 331, 332, 335, 342, 350, 353, 362, 368, 377, 387, 389, 391

Dermatology
116, 154, 173, 316

Endocrinology and diabetes
5, 9, 23, 39, 46, 76, 82, 89, 92, 101, 106, 107, 127, 134, 146, 159, 164, 168, 173, 181, 199, 218, 220, 238, 242, 254, 260, 261, 273, 281, 328, 334, 372, 373, 379, 397, 401

Environmental medicine
140

Gastroenterology
3, 6, 19, 24, 33, 64, 72, 75, 104, 127, 133, 143, 148, 162, 169, 182, 188, 201, 231, 276, 293, 306, 338, 339, 347, 367, 369, 371, 383, 393, 394, 400

Genetics
47, 85, 151, 170, 194, 195, 269, 315, 361

Haematology
12, 38, 49, 69, 70, 73, 86, 87, 102, 114, 115, 117, 120, 122, 142, 156, 163, 175, 191, 204, 211, 216, 219, 233, 258, 263, 265, 295, 297, 299, 308, 313, 336, 346, 351, 352, 358, 376, 385, 392, 394

Immunology
15, 155, 374

Infectious diseases
16, 18, 26, 41, 51, 83, 88, 93, 110, 128, 142, 143, 149, 152, 154, 158, 166, 176, 212, 221, 225, 234, 262, 267, 277, 280, 319, 322, 325, 337, 345, 351, 383, 386, 388

Metabolic medicine
9, 29, 34, 38, 50, 71, 74, 81, 82, 84, 90, 129, 134, 136, 147, 153, 161, 179, 189, 214, 215, 230, 248, 257, 271, 275, 283, 310, 321, 326, 329, 333, 334, 398

Nephrology
4, 17, 24, 29, 44, 53, 59, 60, 85, 92, 118, 119, 126, 135, 137, 141, 152, 185, 198, 228, 244, 245, 249, 250, 251, 278, 289, 294, 303, 304, 317, 328, 344, 354, 381, 382

Neurology
30, 65, 67, 93, 98, 103, 105, 108, 112, 128, 139, 145, 190, 192, 200, 239–241, 247, 253, 255, 256, 268, 274, 288, 290, 292, 307, 314, 330, 345, 365, 390, 395, 399

Obstetric medicine
130–132, 190, 193, 348

Oncology
117, 216, 258, 358, 359

Ophthalmology
282, 345

Radiology
2, 18, 64, 88, 97, 99, 124, 183, 187, 222, 227, 252, 280, 300, 302, 311, 343, 349, 355, 357, 360, 363

Respiratory medicine
8, 14, 21, 35, 36, 37, 43, 45, 55, 56, 58, 61, 72, 79, 91, 99, 111, 113, 157, 164, 196, 217, 225, 272, 279, 298, 304, 327, 341, 349, 356, 370, 380, 384, 396

Rheumatology
4, 15, 17, 31, 42, 71, 77, 87, 96, 109, 141, 171, 174, 177, 196, 198, 200, 210, 236, 264, 320, 324, 340, 364, 375, 401, 402

Therapeutics/toxicology
7, 8, 20, 27, 28, 36, 48, 57, 68, 77, 116, 118, 119, 165, 172, 175, 186, 205, 206, 209, 213, 224, 251, 284, 286, 312, 316, 317, 332, 339, 366, 378

Rapid Review of

Clinical Medicine
for MRCP Part 2

Second Edition

Sanjay Sharma
BSc (Hons) FRCP (UK) MD
Consultant Cardiologist
University Hospital Lewisham
and Kings College Hospital
London, UK

Rashmi Kaushal
BSc (Hons) MRCP (UK)
Consultant Physician and Endocrinologist
West Middlesex Hospital
Kingston, UK

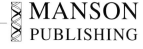
MANSON
PUBLISHING

Dedication

For Ravi, Ashna, Anushka, Ishan, Shivani and Milan

Acknowledgements

We are grateful for the help of several colleagues who helped provide slides for the book:

Dr L Wilkinson, Ms S Gowrinath, Ms H Derry, Mr P Radomskij, Dr J Waktare, Ms A O'Donoghue, Dr S Rosen, Dr A Mehta, Dr L Shapiro, Professor M E Hodson, Dr G Rai, Dr A Ghuran, Professor C Oakley, Ms F Goulder, Dr J Axford, Dr S Jain, Dr M Stodell, Dr B Harold, Dr D Seigler, Dr C Travill, Dr G Barrison, Dr D Hackett, Dr J Bayliss, Dr R Lancaster, Dr R Foale, Dr W Davies, Professor D Sheridan, Professor W McKenna, Professor G MacGregor, Dr A Belli, Dr Adams, Dr J Joseph, Dr M Impallomeni, Dr D Banerjee, Dr N Essex, Dr S Nussey, Dr S Hyer, Dr A Rodin, Dr M Prentice, Dr N Mir, Mrs K Patel and Dr J Jacomb-Hood.

We are also grateful for the assistance of the Audiovisual Departments at Luton and Dunstable Hospital, St Mary's (Paddington) Hospital and St George's Hospital Medical School and the ECG, Echocardiography and Radiology Department at St George's Hospital Medical School and University Hospital Lewisham.

Second impression 2007

Copyright © 2006 Manson Publishing Ltd

ISBN 10: 1–84076–070–2
ISBN 13: 978-1-84076-070-5

A CIP catalogue record for this book is available from the British Library.

For full details of all Manson Publishing titles, please write to:
Manson Publishing Ltd
73 Corringham Road
London NW11 7DL, UK
Tel: +44 (0)20 8905 5150
Fax: +44 (0)20 8201 9233
Website: www.mansonpublishing.com

Printed in Spain

Abbreviations

5-HIAA   5'-hydroxyindole acetic acid
AIIRB   angiotensin II receptor blocker
AAFB   acid–alcohol fast bacilli
ACE   angiotensin-converting enzyme
ACTH   adrenocorticotrophic hormone
ADH   antidiuretic hormone
AF   atrial fibrillation
AIDS   acquired immune-deficiency syndrome
AIN   acute interstitial nephritis
AIP   acute intermittent porphyria
ALA   aminolaevulinic acid
ALT   alanine transaminase (SGPT)
AML   acute myeloid leukaemia
AMP   adenosine 5'-monophosphate
ANA   antinuclear antibody
ANCA   antineutrophil cytoplasmic antibodies
ANF   antinuclear factor
APCKD   adult polycystic kidney disease
APTT   activated partial thromboplastin time
AR   aortic regurgitation
ARDS   adult respiratory distress syndrome
ARVC   arrhythmogenic right ventricular cardiomyopathy
AS   aortic stenosis
ASD   atrial septal defect
ASO   antistreptolysin
AST   aspartate transaminase (SGOT)
ATN   acute tubular necrosis
AZT   zidovudine
BCG   bacille Calmette–Guérin
BIH   benign intracranial hypertension
BP   blood pressure
BT   bleeding time
BTS   British Thoracic Society
CAH   chronic active hepatitis
CAP   community acquired pneumonia
CCF   congestive cardiac failure
CFA   cryptogenic fibrosing alveolitis

CFTR   cystic fibrosis transmembrane regulator (protein)
CML   chronic myeloid leukaemia
CMV   cytomegalovirus
COPD   chronic obstructive pulmonary disease
CPAP   continuous positive airway pressure
CREST   calcinosis, Raynaud's syndrome, oesophageal problems, scleroderma, telangiectasia
CRF   chronic renal failure
CRP   C-reactive protein
CSF   cerebrospinal fluid
CSS   Churg–Strauss syndrome
CT   computed tomography
CVA   cerebrovascular accident
CVP   central venous pressure
CXR   chest X-ray
DBP   diastolic blood pressure
DC   direct current
DHCC   dihydroxy-cholecalciferol
DIC   disseminated intravascular coagulation
DIDMOAD   diabetes insipidus, diabetes mellitus, optic atrophy and deafness
DM   diabetes mellitus
DT   delerium tremens
DVT   deep-vein thrombosis
EAA   extrinsic allergic alveolitis
EBV   Epstein–Barr virus
ECG   electrocardiogram
EEG   electroencephalogram
ELISA   enzyme-linked immunosorbent assay
EMF   endomyocardial fibrosis
EMG   electromyogram
ENT   ear, nose and throat
EPO   erythropoietin
ERCP   endoscopic retrograde cholangiopancreatogram
ESR   erythrocyte sedimentation rate
FBC   full blood count
FDP   fibrinogen degradation product
FES   fat embolism syndrome
FEV1   fixed expiration volume in 1 second
FFP   fresh-frozen plasma
FNA   fine-needle aspiration

FSH   follicle stimulating hormone
FTA   fluorescent treponemal antibody
FVC   forced vital capacity
GBM   glomerular basement membrane
GCT   giant cell tumour
GFR   glomerular filtration rate
GH   growth hormone
GHRH   growth hormone releasing hormone
GI   gastrointestinal
GP   general practitioner
GPI   glucophosphatidylinositol
GT   glutamyltransferase
GTN   glyceryl trinitrate
Hb   haemoglobin
HbSS   sickle cell anaemia
HC   Hereditary Copro porphyria
HCC   hydroxy-cholecalciferol
HCM   hypertrophic cardiomyopathy
HCV   hepatitis C virus
HCG   human chorionic gonadotrophin
HELLP   haemolysis, elevated liver enzymes and low platelets
HHT   hereditary haemorrhagic telangiectasia
HIT   heparin-induced thrombocytopenia
HIV   human immunodeficiency virus
HONK   hypersimilar non-ketotic diabetic coma
HR   heart rate
HRT   hormone replacement therapy
HS   hereditary spherocytosis
HSMN   hereditary sensorimotor neuropathy
HUS   haemolytic uraemic syndrome
ICD   implantable cardioverter defibrillator
ICP   intracranial pressure
INR   International Normalized Ratio
IVP   intravenous pyelogram
IVU   intravenous urogram
JVP   jugular venous pressure
KCO   corrected carbon monoxide transfer factor

LBBB	left bundle branch block	NASH	non-alcoholic steatohepatitis	SMA	smooth muscle antibody
LDH	lactate dehydrogenase	NIPPV	non-invasive positive pressure ventilation	SPECT	single photon emission computed tomography
LFT	liver function tests			SROS	Steele–Richardson–Olszewski syndrome
LH	luteinizing hormone	NSAID	non-steroidal anti-inflammatory drug		
LHON	Leber's hereditary optic neuropathy	NSTEMI	non-ST elevation myocardial infarction	STEMI	ST elevation myocardial infarction
LHRH	luteinizing hormone releasing hormone	NYHA	New York Heart Association	SVT	supraventricular tachycardia
LMWH	low-molecular weight heparin	OSA	obstructive sleep apnoea	TB	tuberculosis
LQTS	long QT-syndrome	PAN	polyarteritis nodosa	TCAD	tricyclic antidepressant overdose
LVEDP	left ventricular end-diastolic pressure	PAS	periodic acid-Schiff	TIA	transient ischaemic attack
LVH	left ventricular hypertrophy	PBC	primary biliary cirrhosis	TIBC	total iron-binding capacity
MAHA	microangiopathic haemolytic anaemia	PBG	porphobilinogen	TIPSS	transjugular intrahepatic portosystemic shunt
		PCOS	polycystic ovary syndrome		
MAOI	monoamine oxidase inhibitor	PCR	polymerase chain reaction	TLC	total lung capacity
		PCT	porphyria cutanea tarda	TLCO	total lung carbon monoxide transfer factor
MCH	mean cell haemoglobin	PCV	packed cell volume		
MCHC	mean cell haemoglobin content	PCWP	pulmonary capillary wedge pressure	TOE	transoesophageal echocardiography
MCV	mean cell volume	PE	pulmonary embolism	TPA	tissue plasminogen activator
MELAS	mitochondrial encephalopathy, lactic acidosis, stroke-like syndrome	PEFR	peak expiratory flow rate	TPHA	treponema pallidum haemagglutination test
		PFO	patent foramen ovale		
		PKD	polycystic kidney disease	TRH	thyrotrophin releasing hormone
		PMLE	progressive multifocal leucoencephalopathy		
MEN	multiple endocrine neoplasia			TSAT	transferrin saturation
		PMR	polymyalgia rheumatica	TSH	thyroid stimulating hormone
MERRF	myoclonic epilepsy and red ragged fibres	PNH	paroxysmal nocturnal haemoglobinuria		
				TT	thrombin time
MGUS	monoclonal gammopathy of undetermined significance	PRL	prolactin	TTP	thrombotic thrombocytopenic purpura
		PRV	polycythaemia rubra vera		
		PSC	primary sclerosing cholangitis	U&E	urea and electrolytes
MPO	myeloperoxidase			URTI	upper respiratory tract infection
MR	mitral regurgitation	PT	prothrombin time		
MRA	magnetic resonance angiography	PTH	parathormone or parathyroid hormone	US	ultrasound
				UTI	urinary tract infection
MRCP	magnetic resonance cholangiopancreatogram	PVE	prosthetic valve endocarditis	VDRL	Venereal Diseases Research Laboratory test
MRI	magnetic resonance imaging	RA	rheumatoid arthritis	VF	ventricular fibrillation
		RBBB	right bundle branch block	VIP	vasointestinal polypeptide
MRSA	methicillin resistant *Staphylococcus aureus*	REM	rapid eye movement	VMA	vanilyl mandelic acid
		RMAT	rapid macroagglutination test	VP	variegate porphyria
MRV	magnetic resonance venography			VR	ventricular rate
		RTA	renal tubular acidosis	VSD	ventricular septal defect
MSH	melanocyte stimulating hormone	RV	residual volume	VT	ventricular tachycardia
		SADS	sudden adult death syndrome	WCC	white cell count
NADPH	nicotinamide adenine dinucleotide phosphate (reduced)			WPW	Wolff–Parkinson–White (syndrome)
		SAM	systolic anterior motion of the mitral valve		
NAPQI	N-acetyl-p-benzoquinoneimine	SAP	serum amyloid protein		
		SIADH	syndrome of inappropriate antidiuretic hormone		
NARP	neuropathy, ataxia, retinitis pigmentosa	SLE	systemic lupus erythematosus		

Question 1

A 49-year-old male presented to the Accident and Emergency Department with a one-hour history of severe central chest pain. He smoked 30 cigarettes per day. Physical examination was normal. The 12-lead ECG revealed ST segment elevation in leads V1–V4. There were no contraindications to thrombolysis.

What is the best treatment to improve coronary perfusion?
a. IV Streptokinase.
b. IV Tenectoplase.
c. IV Alteplase.
d. Half-dose tenectoplase and half-dose abciximab.
e. Primary coronary angioplasty.

Question 2

A 68-year-old woman presented with pain and tingling in the left arm when she raised her hands for prolonged periods. On examination both pulses were palpable in the upper limbs. The chest X-ray was abnormal. Aortography was performed with the arms down (**2a**) and with the arms up (**2b**).

What was the abnormality on the chest X-ray?
a. Left-sided bronchogenic carcinoma.
b. Left cervical rib.
c. Retrosternal thyroid.
d. Notching of the ribs.
e. Widened mediastinum.

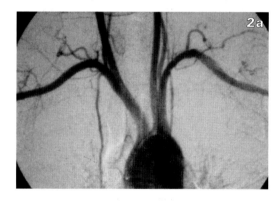 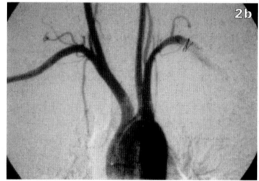

Question 3

A 28-year-old male presented with a six-month history of weight loss of 8 kg, generalized abdominal discomfort and diarrhoea. On examination he was pale and slim, but there were no other significant abnormalities.

Investigations are shown.

What is the diagnosis?
a. Crohn's disease.
b. Intestinal lymphangiectasia.
c. Coeliac disease.
d. Small bowel lymphoma.
e. Hypogammaglobulinaemia.

Hb	9 g/dl
WCC	4.6×10^9/l
Platelets	200×10^9/l
MCV	76 fl
ESR	38 mm/h
Sodium	141 mmol/l
Potassium	4 mmol/l
Urea	3 mmol/l
Creatinine	68 μmol/l
Corrected calcium	2.02 mmol/l
phosphate	0.8 mmol/l
Alkaline phosphatase	190 iu/l
Albumin	38 g/l
IgA	<0.1 g/l (NR 0.8–4.0 g/l)
IgG	9.0 g/l (NR 7.0–18.0 g/l)
IgM	0.6 g/l (NR 0.4–2.5 g/l)
IgA anti-endomyosial antibody	Absent

Answer 1

> e. Primary coronary angioplasty.

Coronary reperfusion may be achieved with thrombolytic agents (which promote fibrinolysis) or by coronary angioplasty. In the UK patients with ST elevation myocardial infarction are conventionally treated with thrombolytic agents. Early treatment is crucial to salvage myocardium and reduce the risk of sudden death and severe left ventricular dysfunction. Current goals for the speed of treating with a thrombolytic agent include a door-to-needle time of 20 minutes or a call-to-needle time of 60 minutes.

Thrombolytic agents used commonly include streptokinase, alteplase, tenectoplase and reteplase. Streptokinase is less favoured compared with the other thrombolytic agents because it is less effective at restoring coronary perfusion and is associated with slightly worse outcomes. The GUSTO I study compared front-loaded alteplase therapy with streptokinase in patients with ST EMI. Alteplase was superior to streptokinase in reducing mortality (1% absolute reduction in mortality at 30 days with alteplase) and was associated with greater coronary patency rates. In the GUSTO trial the benefit was greatest in patients aged under 75 years and those with anterior myocardial infarction. However, streptokinase is still used extensively in developing countries and in many hospitals in the UK. Alteplase, tenectoplase and reteplase appear to be equally effective. Tenectoplase and reteplase are easier to administer (as a single bolus).

There have been trials evaluating the role of combined half-dose thrombolytic therapy and half-dose platelet glycoprotein IIb/IIIa receptor blockers, e.g. tenectoplase plus abciximab (ASSENT 3) and reteplase plus abciximab (GUSTO IV). These trials suggest that the combination may be associated with slightly higher coronary patency rates and fewer ischaemic events but they have not demonstrated a mortality benefit. These trials have also demonstrated higher rates of intracranial bleeding in the elderly, hence combination therapy is not recommended at present.

Although thrombolytic treatment is associated with a significant reduction in mortality from myocardial infarction, it does have important limitations. Firstly, greatest benefit from thrombolysis is achieved in patients treated within 4 hours of the onset of symptoms. Even with thrombolysis normalization of blood flow is seen in only 50–60% of cases. Recurrent ischaemia occurs in 30% of cases and frank thrombotic coronary occlusion in 5–15%. Re-infarction occurs in up to 5% of cases while in hospital. Also major bleeding is recognized in 2–3% of cases. For these reasons several trials were set up comparing primary angioplasty with thrombolysis in STEMI.

Primary angioplasty is superior to thrombolysis. It is associated with lower mortality and lower re-infarction rates. The likelihood of a pre-discharge positive exercise test is also reduced by primary angioplasty. In hospitals where facilities for primary angioplasty are available, primary angioplasty should be considered over thrombolysis. Best results occur when the door-to-balloon time is less than 2 hours.

Answer 2

> b. Left cervical rib.

There is mechanical occlusion of the left subclavian artery on raising the left arm due to a left cervical rib. Cervical ribs are common in the normal population and are usually asymptomatic. In rare circumstances a cervical rib may cause pressure on the subclavian vessels and the brachial plexus causing transient vascular insufficiency or paraesthesiae in the upper limb.

Answer 3

> c. Coeliac disease.

Diarrhoea, weight loss, abdominal discomfort and isolated IgA deficiency are highly suggestive of coeliac disease. Anti-endomyosial antibodies are highly sensitive and specific for the diagnosis of coeliac disease. Anti-endomyosial antibodies are IgA antibodies, therefore they will not be detected in patients with low IgA antibody levels. Since coeliac disease is also associated with IgA deficiency it is important to be aware of serum IgA levels before interpreting anti-endomyosial antibodies in patients with malabsorption. (See Question 276.)

Question 4

A 53-year-old male was admitted to hospital with a two-week history of coughing and breathlessness. Apart from a longstanding history of mild asthma he had been relatively well with respect to the respiratory tract. He had been on a skiing trip six weeks previously, without any respiratory problems.

He had a past history of depression, for which he took lithium five years ago, and suffered from occasional tension headaches, for which he took simple analgesia.

On examination he appeared pale and unwell. His heart rate was 90 beats/min and regular. His blood pressure measured 160/94 mmHg. The JVP was not raised. Both heart sounds were normal and the chest was clear. Abdominal examination did not reveal any abnormality. Urinalysis demonstrated blood ++ and protein ++.

Investigations performed in hospital are shown.

Hb	7 g/dl
WCC	$11 \times 10^9/1$
	(neutrophils $8 \times 10^9/l$,
	lymphocytes $2 \times 10^9/l$,
	eosinophils $1 \times 10^9/l$)
ESR	38 mm/h
Sodium	134 mmol/l
Potassium	4.6 mmol/l
Urea	48 mmol/l
Creatinine	798 mmol /l
Renal ultrasound	
Both kidneys measured 12 cm: there was no evidence of ureteric obstruction.	

What is the most likely diagnosis?
  a. Rapidly progressive glomerulonephritis. ✓
  b. Analgesic nephropathy.
  c. Renal amyloidosis.
  d. Churg–Strauss syndrome.
  e. IgA nephritis.

Question 5

A 52-year-old male presented with impotence. He had a four-year history of insulin-dependent diabetes mellitus. There was no history of headaches or vomiting. The patient was a non-smoker and did not consume alcohol. Apart from insulin he took simple analgesia for joint pains.

Investigations are shown.

FBC	Normal
Sodium	135 mmol/l
Potassium	4 mmol/l
Urea	6 mmol/l
Creatinine	100 mmol/l
Bilirubin	12 mmol/l
AST	200 iu/l
ALT	220 iu/l
Alkaline phosphatase	128 iu/l
Albumin	8 g/l
Thyroxine	100 nmol/l
TSH	2.6 mu/l
Testosterone	7 nmol/l (NR 10–35 nmol/l)
LH	1.5 iu/l (NR 1–10 iu/l)
FSH	1 iu/l NR 1–7 iu/l)

LHRH test:	20 min:	60 min:
LH	3 iu/l	2 iu/l
FSH	2 iu/l	2 iu/l

What test would you perform to confirm the diagnosis?
  a. MRI scan of the brain.
  b. Serum prolactin level.
  c. Serum ferritin.
  d. Dynamic pituitary function tests.
  e. Liver ultrasound.

Answer 4

> d. Churg–Strauss syndrome.

The patient has a past history of asthma, eosinophilia and rapidly progressive glomerulonephritis. The most probable diagnosis is Churg–Strauss syndrome. The assumption that he probably has rapidly progressive glomerulonephritis is based on the fact that he was well enough to ski six weeks ago, which would be highly unlikely in a patient with end-stage renal disease. The identification of normal-sized kidneys during renal ultrasonography supports acute rather than chronic renal failure (*Table A*).

Churg–Strauss syndrome is a small-vessel multi-system vasculitis characterized by cutaneous vasculitic lesions, eosinophilia (usually $<2.0 \times 10^9/l$), asthma (usually mild), mononeuritis or polyneuropathy and rarely glomerulonephritis (10% of cases). Gastrointestinal and cardiac involvement is recognized.

Pulmonary findings dominate the clinical presentation with paroxysmal asthma attacks and presence of fleeting pulmonary infiltrates. Asthma is the cardinal feature and may be present for years before overt features of a multi-system vasculitis become apparent. Skin lesions, which include purpura and cutaneous and subcutaneous nodules, occur in up to 70% of patients. Gastrointestinal complications include mesenteric ischaemia or gastrointestinal haemorrhage. Cardiac involvement is characterized by myo-pericarditis.

The diagnosis is usually clinical and supported by the presence of a necrotizing granulomatous vasculitis with extravascular eosinophilic infiltration on lung, renal or sural biopsy. The American College or Rheumatology criteria for the diagnosis of Churg–Strauss syndrome are tabulated (*Table B*). Serum ANCA (MPO subset) are elevated but this finding is also present in microscopic polyangitis.

The prognosis of untreated CSS is poor, with a reported five-year survival rate of only 25%. Corticosteroid therapy has been reported to increase the five-year survival rate to more than 50%. In patients with acute vasculitis the combination of cyclophosphamide and prednisone is superior to prednisolone alone.

Although rapidly progressive glomerulonephritis also features in the answer options section, the presence of asthma and eosinophilia make Churg–Strauss syndrome the best answer. It is worth noting however, that rapidly progressive glomerulonephritis may also rarely be

associated with eosinophilia. Causes of renal failure and eosinophilia are tabulated (*Table C*).

The history of analgesia for headaches raises the possibility of analgesic nephropathy as the cause of his presentation; however, analgesic nephropathy is usually insidious and many patients present for the first time with renal failure. The majority have abnormalities on renal ultrasound scans. Analgesic nephropathy alone does not explain asthma or eosinophilia.

Table A Phases of Churg–Strauss syndrome:

1. The *prodromal* phase, which may be present for years and comprises of rhinitis, nasal polyposis and frequently asthma.
2. The *eosinophilic* phase, which can remit and recur for years. It is characterized by the onset of peripheral blood and tissue eosinophilia, resembling Loeffler's syndrome, chronic eosinophilic pneumonia or eosinophilic gastroenteritis.
3. The *vasculitic* phase, which usually occurs in the third or fourth decades of life and is characterized by a life-threatening systemic vasculitis of small and occasionally medium-sized vessels. This phase is associated with constitutional symptoms and signs, fever and weight loss.

Table B American College of Rheumatology 1990 criteria for Churg–Strauss syndrome

The presence of four or more of the manifestations below is highly indicative of Churg–Strauss syndrome:
- Asthma
- Eosinophilia (10% on WCC differential)
- Mononeuropathy or polyneuropathy
- Migratory or transient pulmonary infiltrates
- Systemic vasculitis (cardiac, renal, hepatic)
- Extravascular eosinophils on a biopsy including artery, arteriole or venule

---

Table C Causes of renal failure and eosinophilia

- Rapidly progressive glomerulonephritis
- Churg–Strauss syndrome
- Acute tubulo-interstitial nephritis
- Cholesterol micro-emboli

Answer 5

> c. Serum ferritin.

The clinical features and the data are consistent with the diagnosis of idiopathic haemochromatosis. The insulin-dependent diabetes mellitus suggests pancreatic

involvement, and abnormal liver function is consistent with hepatic infiltration.

The patient has a low testosterone level with an inappropriately low gonadotrophin response indicating secondary hypogonadism due to excessive iron deposition in the pituitary. Secondary hypogonadism is the most common endocrine deficiency in hereditary haemochromatosis. Primary hypogonadism due to testicular iron deposition may occur with this disorder but is much less common than secondary hypogonadism.

In the context of the question, a serum ferritin level >500 mg/l would be diagnostic of primary haemochromatosis. Alcohol-related liver disease, chronic viral hepatitis, non-alcoholic steatohepatitis and porphyria cutanea tarda also cause liver disease and increased serum ferritin concentrations even in the absence of iron overload.

Hepatic iron overload in haemochromatosis is associated with an increased risk of hepatocellular carcinoma. Patients with haemochromatosis are also at increased risk of hypothyroidism and are susceptible to certain infections from siderophoric (iron-loving) organisms such as *Listeria* spp., *Yersinia enterocolitica* and *Vibrio vulnificus*, which are picked up from eating uncooked seafood.

Question 6

A 38-year-old English male was investigated after he was found to have an abnormal liver function test during a health insurance medical check. He worked in an information technology firm. Apart from occasional fatigue he was well. He consumed less than 20 units of alcohol per week. The patient had only travelled out of Europe twice and on both occasions he had been to North America. He took very infrequent paracetamol for aches and pains in his ankles and knees. There was no history of hepatitis or transfusion or blood products. He had been married for 5 years. Systemic enquiry revealed infrequent episodes of loose stool for almost 4 years.

On examination he appeared well. There were no stigmata of chronic liver disease. Abdominal examination revealed a palpable liver edge 3 cm below the costal margin. There were no other masses. Examination of the central nervous system was normal.

Investigations were as shown.

Hb	12.6 g/dl
WCC	8×10^9/l
Platelets	210×10^9/l
MCV	90 fl
Sodium	136 mmol/l
Potassium	4.1 mmol/l
Urea	6 mmol/l
Creatinine	100 mmol/l
AST	60 iu/l (NR 10–40 iu/l)
ALT	78 iu/l (NR 5–30 iu/l)
Alkaline phosphatase	350 iu/l (NR 25–100 iu/l) ↑
Bilirubin	22 mmol/l (NR 2–17 µmol/l)
Albumin	38 g/l (NR 34–48 g/l)
Total cholesterol	5.2 mmol/l
Triglyceride	3.1 mmol/l
Blood glucose	6 mmol/l
Ferritin	256 mg/l (NR 15–250 mg/l)
Serum Fe	28 mmol/l (NR 14–32 mmol/l)
TIBC	50 mmol/l (NR 40–80 mmol/l)
Serum caeruloplasmin	Slightly reduced
24-hr urine copper	Slightly elevated
IgG	19 g/l (NR 7–18 g/l)
IgA	4.2 g/l (NR 0.8–4.0 g/l)
IgM	5.0 g/l (NR 0.4–2.5 g/l)
Anti-nuclear antibodies	Positive 1/32
Smooth muscle antibodies	Not detected
Antimitochondrial antibodies	Not detected
Hep B sAg	Not detected
Hep C virus antibodies	Not detected
Abdominal ultrasound	Normal

What is the most probable diagnosis?
a. Autoimmune hepatitis.
b. Primary sclerosing cholangitis.
c. Primary biliary cirrhosis.
d. Haemochromatosis.
e. Wilson's disease.

Question 7

A 17-year-old girl presented with jaundice three days after having taken a paracetamol and alcohol overdose during an argument with her boyfriend.

What is the best marker of prognosis?
a. Serum aspartase transaminase.
b. Serum alkaline phosphatase.
c. Serum bilirubin.
d. Prothrombin time.
e. Paracetamol level.

Answer 6

> b. Primary sclerosing cholangitis.

This is a relatively difficult question. The history of loose stool is crucial in making the diagnosis in this particular case in the absence of data from the ERCP. Diarrhoea and biochemical evidence of cholestasis (alkaline phosphatase greater than transaminases) should lead to the clinical suspicion of primary sclerosing cholangitis (PSC). The aetiology of PSC is unknown but immunological destruction of intra- and extra-hepatic bile ducts is the main pathological feature. 90% of PSC is associated with inflammatory bowel disease, particularly ulcerative colitis, and hence the importance of the intermittent diarrhoea. Ulcerative colitis is the most frequent association with primary sclerosing cholangitis. A raised alkaline phosphatase level in a patient with ulcerative colitis (in the absence of bone disease) should raise the possibility of PSC. The frequency of PSC is inversely proportional to the severity of ulcerative colitis. Other associations of PSC include coeliac disease.

Patients with PSC may be asymptomatic at presentation but can present with advanced liver disease. Fatigue and pruritis are common complaints as with the other cholestatic disorders. Approximately one-fifth of the patients also complain of right upper quadrant pain.

The diagnosis is confirmed with ERCP that shows strictures within biliary ducts. Complications are those of chronic cholestasis, notably statorrhoea, fat-soluble vitamin malabsorption, large biliary strictures, cholangitis, cholangiocarcinoma and colonic carcinoma. There are no effective pharmacological agents that greatly retard the progression of the disorder. Patients are treated with cholestyramine to reduce pruritis. Fat-soluble vitamin supplementation is necessary owing to steatorrhoea. Antibiotic prophylaxis during instrumentation of the biliary tree is mandatory to reduce the risk of bacterial cholangitis. Ciprofloxacin is the prophylactic antibiotic drug of choice prior to ERCP. Biliary stenting may improve biochemistry and symptoms; however, the definitive treatment for PSC is hepatic transplantation.

Although a cholestatic picture is also recognized in primary biliary cirrhosis, alcohol abuse and viral hepatitis there is nothing in the history or investigations to indicate these conditions as the cause of his illness. Primary biliary cirrhosis affects mainly females in the fifth decade onwards. Furthermore, the absence of anti-mitochondrial antibodies is against the diagnosis. The ferritin is modestly raised but not high enough to suggest hereditary haemochromatosis. High ferritin levels are also a feature of chronic viral hepatitis, alcohol-related hepatitis and non-alcoholic steato-hepatitis. Hypergamma-globulinaemia and raised autoantibody titres are features of primary sclerosing cholangitis but also occur in other immunological liver disorders such as chronic active viral hepatitis, auto-immune hepatitis and biliary cirrhosis.

Patients with cholestasis also have lowish caerulo-plasmin levels and increased blood and urine copper levels. The abnormal copper metabolism in this case should not lead to the candidate diagnosing Wilson's disease, since there are many features above to indicate PSC. Furthermore, patients with Wilson's disease usually have a hepatitic biochemistry picture and often have co-existing neuro-psychiatric disease.

Answer 7

> d. Prothrombin time.

Important risk markers for severe hepatic injury after paracetamol overdose include a PT >20 seconds 24 h after ingestion, pH <7.3 and creatinine >300 μmol/l. (See Questions 27 and 206.)

Question 8

A 16-year-old girl presented with an 18-month history of progressive breathlessness on exertion. On admission she was breathless at rest. She had a past history of acute myeloid leukaemia, for which she had been treated with six courses of chemotherapy, followed by bone marrow transplantation supplemented with radiotherapy and cyclophosphamide treatment five years ago. She was regularly followed up in the haematology clinic. Lung function tests three years ago revealed an FEV1/FVC ratio of 80%. On examination she was breathless at rest, and cyanosed. There was no evidence of clubbing. Auscultation of the lung fields revealed fine inspiratory crackles in the mid and lower zones. Repeat lung function tests revealed an FEV1/FVC ratio of 86% and a transfer factor of 60% predicted.

What is the cause of her symptoms?
  a. Previous radiotherapy.
  b. CMV pneumonitis.
  c. *Pneumocystis carinii* pneumonia.
  d. Cyclophosphamide-induced lung fibrosis.
  e. Severe anaemia.

Question 9

A 21-year-old man was admitted to the intensive care unit after a road traffic accident during which he suffered a severe head injury. He required ventilation.
  Investigations are shown.

Sodium	↓ 128 mmol/l
Potassium	3.6 mmol/l
Creatinine	81 mmol/l
Urea	↓ 4 mmol/l
Thyroxine	30 nmol/l
TSH	2 mu/l
Serum cortisol	1000 nmol/l
	(NR 170–700 nmol/l)

What is the cause of the hyponatraemia?
  a. Hypopituitarism.
  b. Addison's disease.
  c. Syndrome of inappropriate ADH secretion.
  d. Hypothyroidism.
  e. Cushing's syndrome.

Question 10

A 40-year-old woman with dilated cardiomyopathy is seen in the heart failure clinic complaining of a persistent dry cough. Her exercise capacity is 1 mile while walking on the flat. She can climb two flights of stairs without difficulty. Her medication consists of ramipril 10 mg daily, aspirin 75 mg daily, carvedilol 6.25 mg twice daily and frusemide 40 mg daily. On examination her heart rate is 70 beats/min and her blood pressure is 100/60 mmHg. Both heart sounds are normal and the chest is clear.

How would you alter her treatment?
  a. Add spironolactone.
  b. Substitute ramipril with losartan.
  c. Reduce carvedilol to 3.125 mg twice daily.
  d. Double the dose of furosemide.
  e. Add digoxin.

Answer 8

> d. Cyclophosphamide-induced lung fibrosis.

The patient presents with progressive symptoms associated with a restrictive lung defect and a low transfer factor. The findings are most consistent with cyclophosphamide-induced pulmonary fibrosis.

Cyclophosphamide-induced lung fibrosis is rare and is most likely to occur in patients who have had concomitant pulmonary radiation therapy or have taken other drugs associated with pulmonary toxicity. The disorder usually occurs in patients who have been taking low doses for relatively prolonged periods (over six months) and presents several years after cessation of the drug and hence the deterioration of symptoms with time. The disorder has a relentless progression and inevitably results in terminal respiratory failure. It is minimally responsive to corticosteroids. Fine end-inspiratory crackles and clubbing do not usually form part of the clinical spectrum.

The diagnosis is clinical. Chest X-ray reveals reticulo-nodular shadowing of the upper zones. Lung function tests demonstrate a restrictive lung defect. Lung biopsy is not helpful.

Cyclophosphamide *per se* is not toxic to the lungs; however, it is metabolized in the liver to toxic metabolites such as hydroxycyclophosphamide, acrolein and phosphoramide mustard, which are responsible for pulmonary damage. Genetic factors may play a role in determining which individuals develop pulmonary fibrosis after exposure to the drug.

Cyclophosphamide therapy can also result in an acute pneumonitis during treatment with the drug that causes cough, dyspnoea, hypoxia and bilateral nodular opacities in the upper zones of the lung. Acute cyclophosphamide-induced pneumonitis responds to cessation of the drug and corticosteroid therapy.

The differential diagnosis in this case is radiation-induced fibrosis. Radiotherapy to the pulmonary area usually causes a pneumonitis that presents with cough, dyspnoea, a restrictive lung defect and low transfer factor. It is more common in patients also taking cyclo-phosphamide or bleomycin. Unlike cyclophosphamide-induced pulmonary fibrosis the condition is not associated with an inexorable decline. Indeed many patients show improvement in symptoms and objective pulmonary function testing within 18 months of stopping radiotherapy.

Causes of drug-induced pulmonary fibrosis

- Cyclophosphamide
- Busulphan
- Methysergide
- Methotrexate
- Amiodarone
- Nitrofurantoin
- Minocycline
- Ethambutol
- Penicillamine

Answer 9

> c. Syndrome of inappropriate ADH secretion.

The patient has a low sodium concentration in the context of a head injury. The thyroid function tests suggest the possibility of a secondary hypothyroidism, i.e. a low TSH and a low thyroxine concentration, and hence the possibility of damage to the pituitary. However, the very high cortisol level indicates that pituitary function is probably normal (high ACTH production secondary to stress) and therefore the abnormal thyroid function tests represent sick euthyroid syndrome. Low T4, T3 and TSH levels are recognized in critically ill patients with non-thyroid illnesses. Originally such patients were thought to be euthyroid, therefore the term sick euthyroid syndrome was used to describe these biochemical abnormalities. There is evidence now that these abnormalities represent genuine acquired transient central hypothyroidism. Treatment with thyroxine in these situations is not helpful and may be harmful. It is thought that these changes in thyroid function during severe illness may be protective by preventing excessive tissue catabolism. Thyroid function tests should be repeated after at least six weeks following recovery.

Critical illness may also reduce T4 by reducing thyroid binding globulin levels, and T3 is rapidly reduced owing to inhibition of peripheral de-iodination of T4.

Answer 10

> b. Substitute ramipril with losartan.

The patient is in NYHA functional class II with respect to her symptoms. She is on the correct dose of ramipril and is appropriately being treated with a beta-blocker. The dry cough that the patient is experiencing is almost certainly the side-effect of ramipril. Angiotensin-converting enzyme inhibitors are associated with a dry cough in 15–20% of patients owing to increases in circulating bradykinin levels. In such patients the ACE inhibitor should be stopped and substituted with an angiotensin receptor blocker such as losartan. The efficacy of losartan compared with an ACE inhibitor (captopril) was fully evaluated in the ELITE II study.

The study revealed similar mortality rates and similar rates of progression of heart failure when comparing patients on losartan 50 mg daily with those prescribed captopril 50 mg three times daily. The study suggests that losartan is as effective as ACE inhibitors in the management of heart failure. However, the use of losartan in heart failure is still currently reserved for patients who develop side-effects to ACE inhibitors. A recent study evaluating the role of angiotensin receptor blockers (CHARM study; evaluated candesartan) in patients with heart failure showed reduced hospitalization rates and mortality in heart failure patients who were on candesartan instead of an ACE inhibitor, or candesartan as additional therapy to an ACE inhibitor.

Question 11

A 60-year-old male was admitted to the coronary care unit with central chest pain. Physical examination was normal. The blood pressure measured 110/68 mmHg. The 12-lead ECG was normal and the troponin T level was not raised. The blood sugar was normal. The cholesterol level on admission was 6.3 mmol/l. The patient underwent an exercise stress test that was positive. A subsequent coronary angiogram revealed an 80% stenosis in the proximal aspect of the left anterior descending artery that was successfully treated with a coronary artery stent. Echocardiography revealed a normal-sized left ventricle with good systolic function. The patient was discharged home on aspirin 75 mg daily, clopidogrel 75 mg daily and simvastatin 40 mg daily. He had been completely pain free after the procedure, and an exercise stress test performed four weeks after the procedure was negative for myocardial ischaemia for 10 minutes.

> What other medication should the patient receive to improve his cardiovascular prognosis?
> a. Atenolol.
> b. Ramipril.
> c. Candesartan.
> d. No further treatment required.
> e. Isosorbide dinitrate.

Question 12

A 62-year-old obese male with a known medical history of hypertension presented with generalized headaches and lethargy. He was taking bendroflumethiazide, 2.5 mg once daily for hypertension. The only other past medical history included a left-sided deep vein thrombosis six months previously. There was no history of alcohol abuse or smoking.

> What is the cause of his symptoms?
> a. Obstructive sleep apnoea.
> b. Gaissbock's syndrome.
> c. Polycythaemia rubra vera.
> d. Renal cell carcinoma.
> e. Chronic hypoxaemia.

On examination he was obese. His chest was clear and examination of the abdomen did not reveal any abnormality.

Investigations are shown.

Hb	20 g/dl
MCV	88 fl
WCC	15 × 10⁹/l
Platelets	500 × 10⁹/l
PCV	0.66 l/l
Sodium	141 mmol/l
Potassium	4.2 mmol/l
Urea	8 mmol/l
Creatinine	110 μmol/l
Urate	0.44 mmol/l

Answer 11

> b. Ramipril.

The Heart Outcomes Prevention Evaluation Study (HOPE) evaluated the role of angiotensin-converting enzyme inhibitors (ramipril) in populations at high risk of cardiovascular events without any evidence of left ventricular dysfunction. The study assessed 9297 high-risk patients, defined as (1) aged >55 years; (2) history of coronary artery disease, stroke or peripheral vascular disease; or (3) diabetes mellitus and at least one risk factor for coronary artery disease including hypertension, increased total cholesterol, smoking and micro-albuminuria. The patients were randomized to ramipril 10 mg daily or placebo. The primary outcome was a combined endpoint of myocardial infarction, stroke or cardiovascular death. The mean follow up was five years.

Patients treated with ramipril had a 14% event rate of the combined morbidity and mortality endpoint whereas placebo-treated patients had a 17.8% event rate. The 21% decrease in events was seen in all pre-specified groups, indicating that ACE inhibitor therapy with ramipril significantly reduces morbidity and mortality in a high-risk population with normal left ventricular function. Based on this study all patients with coronary artery disease, cerebrovascular disease, peripheral vascular disease and diabetes mellitus plus one other risk factor for coronary artery disease should be prescribed an ACE inhibitor, specifically ramipril.

The patient should remain on aspirin for life and take clopidogrel for a year following deployment of a stent. The CURE study showed that aspirin and clopidogrel together were associated with a lower incidence of myocardial infarction and death in patients with unstable angina and non-ST elevation myocardial infarction compared with aspirin alone for up to a year.

The patient no longer has subjective or objective evidence of myocardial ischaemia, and in the absence of hypertension or left ventricular dysfunction there is no indication for a beta-blocker.

Nitrates do not alter prognosis in coronary artery disease. There is no evidence as yet that angiotensin receptor blockers improve cardiovascular prognosis in patients with coronary artery disease in the absence of hypertension or left ventricular dysfunction.

Answer 12

> c. Polycythaemia rubra vera.

The high Hb is suggestive of polycythaemia. There is nothing in the history to indicate a secondary cause, e.g. hypoxia, renal carcinoma, adrenal tumour. Although he was obese, there was nothing else in the history to allow the diagnosis of obstructive sleep apnoea.

The high white cell count and platelet count favour primary polycythaemia (polycythaemia rubra vera). Headache and lethargy are common symptoms of polycythaemia rubra vera. Polycythaemia rubra vera causes lethargy due to hyperviscosity and raised interleukin-6 levels. Other classic features include visual disturbance, abdominal pain and pruritis.

Many patients with polycythaemia rubra vera have splenomegaly; however, a palpable spleen is absent in approximately one third of patients.

> **Criteria for the diagnosis of polycythaemia rubra vera**
>
> Raised red cell mass and normal pO_2 with either splenomegaly or two of the following:
> - WCC >12 × 10^9/l
> - Platelets >400 × 10^9/l
> - Raised B_{12} binding protein
> - Low neutrophil alkaline phosphatase concentration
>
> (See Questions 39, 73 and 211.)

Question 13

The ECG below was taken from a young boy who experienced syncope. On examination he had a systolic murmur.

What is the most probable underlying diagnosis?
 a. Coarctation of the aorta.
 b. Dextrocardia.
 c. Pulmonary stenosis.
 d. Wolff–Parkinson–White syndrome.
 e. Hypertrophic cardiomyopathy.

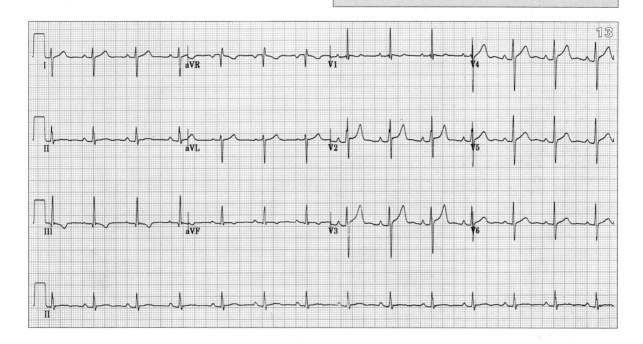

Question 14

An 18-year-old male was admitted with sudden sharp pain in the left infrascapular area. He was not breathless on mild exertion. He was usually fit and well. He was an occasional smoker. There was no history of respiratory problems. On examination there was reduced air entry at the left lung base. The oxygen saturation on air was 96%. The CXR revealed a left-sided pneumothorax. There was less than 2 cm rim of air between the edge of the lung and the ribs.

What is the management?
 a. Admit and observe for 24 hours.
 b. Attempt aspiration of pneumothorax.
 c. Prescribe 100% oxygen for a few hours.
 d. Insert chest drain.
 e. Allow home and repeat CXR after a week.

Answer 13

> c. Pulmonary stenosis.

The patient has a systolic murmur. The ECG shows right axis deviation, a dominant R wave in V1 and relatively prominent S waves in V5 and V6. The sum of the R in V1 and in V6 is > 1.25 mV which indicates right ventricular hypertrophy. The answer that would fit with all the information is pulmonary stenosis. Coarctation of the aorta and hypertophic cardiomyopathy are associated with left ventricular hypertrophy. The absence of a short PR interval and delta waves are against the diagnosis of WPW syndrome.

Answer 14

> e. Allow home and repeat CXR after a week.

The question tests knowledge of the guidelines for the management of pneumothorax set by the British Thoracic Society.

The patient has a relatively small pneumothorax (<2 cm rim of air between lung and ribs) with minimal symptoms and can walk slowly without becoming breathless. There is no history to suggest chronic lung disease. In such a case no treatment is recommended and the patient may be discharged. Patients are advised not to over-exert themselves and to return if they develop breathlessness. A repeat CXR is recommended after a week to ensure that the pneumothorax has resolved.

If the patient has a pneumothorax >2 cm rim of air between the lung and the chest wall on the CXR, or has pain or dyspnoea at rest or on minimal exertion then aspiration is recommended. If aspiration is successful the patient is allowed home and reviewed with repeat CXR in one week. If aspiration is unsuccessful a second attempt is made at aspiration. If the lung still remains deflated then insertion of a chest drain is recommended.

In patients with chronic lung disease the following criteria should be used to decide whether aspiration or insertion of a chest drain is the first procedure of choice. Patients aged <50 years, who are relatively asymptomatic and have a small pneumothorax, should be aspirated and observed in hospital for 24 hours (assuming aspiration is successful). If aspiration is unsuccessful in this group of patients then insertion of a chest drain is advised. In patients aged >50 years, with symptoms and with larger pneumothoraces (>2 cm air between lung and chest wall) a chest drain is necessary.

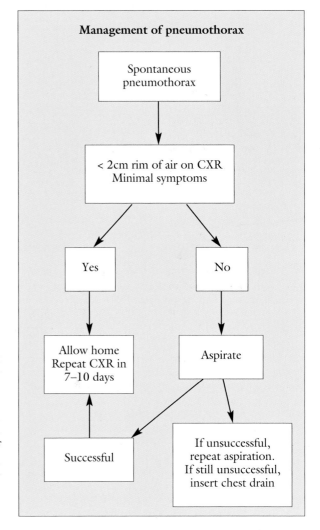

Management of pneumothorax

Spontaneous pneumothorax → < 2cm rim of air on CXR Minimal symptoms → Yes / No

Yes → Allow home Repeat CXR in 7–10 days

No → Aspirate → Successful → Allow home Repeat CXR in 7–10 days

Aspirate → If unsuccessful, repeat aspiration. If still unsuccessful, insert chest drain

Question 15

A 44-year-old was seen in the rheumatology clinic in December complaining of malaise, joint pains and tingling in the hands and feet. She had been diagnosed as having Raynaud's phenomenon several years ago. The patient had consulted several doctors for intermittent malaise and joint pains. There was no history of night sweats, dyspnoea, or problems with swallowing. The patient took paracetamol on a PRN basis for joint pains.

On examination she had palpable purpura on the thighs and arms. There was no obvious evidence of joint swelling. Abdominal examination revealed hepatomegaly palpable 3 cm below the costal margin. Neurological examination revealed decreased sensation in the hands and feet. The blood pressure was 110/80 mmHg.

Investigations are shown.

Hb	10 g/dl
WCC	9×10^9/l
Platelets	490×10^9/l
ESR	90 mm/h
Sodium	139 mmol/l
Potassium	4.2 mmol/l
Urea	9 mol/l
Creatinine	140 μmol/l
Bilirubin	15 mmol/l
AST	90 iu/l
Alkaline phosphatase	122 iu/l
Albumin	33 g/l
Rheumatoid factor	IgM Positive (titre 1/640)
C3	0.2 g/l (NR 0.55–1.2 g/l)
C4	0.09 g/l (NR 0.2–0.5 g/l)
Hep C Virus AB	Positive
Hep B sAg	Negative
Urinalysis	Blood +
	Protein ++

What is the best management of the patient's illness?
  a. Prednisolone.
  b. Cyclophosphamide.
  c. Chlorambucil.
  d. Pegylated interferon-α plus ribavarin.
  e. Plasmapharesis.

Question 16

A 30-year-old businessman developed sudden onset of fever, sore throat, diarrhoea and myalgia. Over the next three days he noticed a widespread rash affecting his face, trunk, palms and soles. He was usually fit and well and had only consulted his GP once in the past 10 years for a typhoid vaccine before travelling to India. Over the past four months he had established business links with a company in Thailand and had visited the country on three occasions. His last visit to Thailand was eight weeks previously. He was married with two young children. He was not taking any medications and had no history of drug allergy.

On examination his temperature was 38.6°C. There was cervical lymphadenopathy. Inspection of the oral cavity revealed several painful ulcers affecting the tongue. The pharynx was oedematous and red with minimal tonsillar exudates. The chest was clear. Abdominal examination was normal.

Investigations are shown.

Hb	13 g/dl
WCC	11×10^9/l
	(neutrophils 6×10^9/l,
	lymphocytes 4×10^9/l)
Platelets	130×10^9/l
Monspot test	Negative
Sodium	135 mmol/l
Potassium	3.8 mmol/l
Urea	6 mmol/l
Creatinine	80 μmol/l
Bilirubin	23 μmol/l
ALT	45 iu/l
AST	49 iu/l

What is the diagnosis?
  a. Acute HIV infection.
  b. Secondary syphilis.
  c. Acute hepatitis infection.
  d. Infectious mononucleosis.
  e. Acute CMV infection.

Answer 15

> d. Pegylated interferon-α plus ribavarin.

This is a difficult question; however, the clue lies in the fact that the patient has evidence of current or previous infection with hepatitis virus and has Raynaud's phenomenon, palpable purpura (vasculitis), neuropathy and hypocomplementaemia. The diagnosis is consistent with mixed essential cryoglobulinaemia. Cryoglobulins are immunoglobulins that precipitate in the cold. They are associated with auto-immune haemolysis, Raynaud's disease (in severe cases they can cause acronecrosis), vasculitis, peripheral neuropathy, glomerulonephritis and hepatosplenomegaly. Complement is reduced. HCV is thought to play an aetiological role in the development in type II and type III cryoglobulinaemia.

Types of cryoglobulinaemia

Type	Immunoglobulins	Associated condition(s)
I	Monoclonal immunoglobulin	Multiple myeloma Waldenstrom's macroglobulinaemia
II	Polyclonal IgG and monoclonal rheumatoid factor IgM	Hepatitis C and hepatitis B
III	Mixed IgG and polyclonal rheumatoid factor	Chronic inflammation Hepatitis C Lymphoproliferative disease

The diagnosis is based upon history, skin biopsy (if purpura present), hypocomplementaemia and presence of cryoglobulins. Investigation for cryoglobulinaemia should always include serology for hepatitis C infection. Treatment for acute cryoglobulinaemia causing severe renal impairment or acronecrosis is plasmapharesis, though in less acute situations prednisolone and cyclophosphamide are effective. Chlorambucil has also been used with success. When cryoglobulinaemia is secondary to HCV infection, the treatment of choice includes the combination of pegylated interferon-a and ribavarin. Ribavarin should be used with caution in patients with renal failure.

Answer 16

> a. Acute HIV infection.

The main differential diagnosis is between infectious mononucleosis, CMV infection and acute HIV infection. All three are associated with sore throat, rash, fever and atypical lymphocytes. Mouth ulcers are usually absent in EBV and CMV infection. Furthermore the rash in infectious mononucleosis is usually an idiosyncratic reaction to ampicillin whereas it is part of HIV seroconverson. The main clinical features differentiating infectious mononucleosis from acute HIV infection are tabulated below. The rash in CMV infection usually spares the palms and soles. (See Question 325.)

Differentiation between infectious mononucleosis and acute HIV infection

Parameter	Infections mononucleosis	HIV infection
Onset of symptoms	Over a few days	Abrupt
Mouth ulcers	Absent usually	Often present
Rash	Usually secondary to ampicillin	Part of HIV seroconversion
Diarrhoea	Unusual	Common
Tonsillar exudates	Prominent	Mild
White cell count	May be elevated	Elevated or suppressed
Atypical lymphocytes	Frequent (90%) and numerous	Present in 50%
Transaminitis	Common	Common
Thrombocytopenia	Common	Common

Question 17

A 69-year-old woman with rheumatoid arthritis presented with swollen ankles. She was diagnosed as having rheumatoid arthritis over 18 years ago and had been relatively well controlled on non-steroidal anti-inflammatory drugs until six months ago, when her joint pains and swelling required the addition of penicillamine to control her symptoms. The patient had a past history of hypertension, for which she took bendroflumethiazide.

On examination she had symmetrical joint deformities consistent with rheumatoid arthritis. The heart rate was 90 beats/min and irregular. Her blood pressure measured 140/90 mmHg. The JVP was not raised. Both heart sounds were normal and the chest was clear. Abdominal examination was normal. Inspection of the lower limbs revealed pitting oedema.

Investigations are shown.

Hb	11 g/dl
WCC	5×10^9/l
Platelets	190×10^9/l
Sodium	134 mmol/l
Potassium	4.5 mmol/l
Urea	6 mmol/l
Creatinine	70 µmol/l
Bilirubin	11 µmol/l
Alkaline phosphatase	100 iu/l
Albumin	26 g/l
Urinalysis	Protein +++

What is the management?
- a. Stop penicillamine.
- b. Start prednisolone.
- c. Start ACE inhibitor therapy.
- d. Arrange renal biopsy.
- e. Arrange IVU.

Question 18

A 59-year-old female presented with weakness of both legs. An MRI scan of the spine is shown (**18**).

What is the cause of her symptoms?
- a. Syringomyelia.
- b. Paravertebral abscess.
- c. Thoracic disc prolapse.
- d. Metastatic spinal cord compression.
- e. Extradural meningioma.

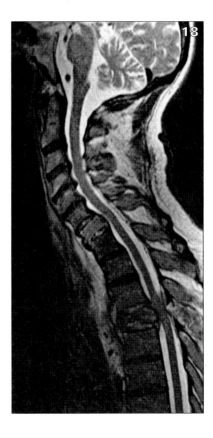

Answer 17

> a. Stop penicillamine.

The patient has heavy proteinuria and gives a relatively recent history of onset of swollen ankles shortly after starting penicillamine. The most likely diagnosis is penicillamine-induced membranous nephropathy, which usually occurs within 6–12 months of the initiation of drug therapy. Proteinuria resolves in virtually all cases after stopping the drug but this may take several months. Other causes of heavy proteinuria secondary to membranous nephropathy in rheumatoid arthritis include gold therapy.

Renal amyloidosis is a recognized cause of heavy proteinuria complicating chronic rheumatoid arthritis. While it is possible that the patient may have renal amyloidosis, the relationship of the proteinuria to the initiation of penicillamine points to a drug-induced membranous nephropathy.

Other causes of renal disease in rheumatoid arthritis include analgesic nephropathy, focal segmental glomerulonephritis and rheumatoid vasculitis. All are characterized by blood in the urine. Analgesic nephropathy is usually secondary to non-steroidal anti-inflammatory drugs and paracetamol. The proteinuria is rarely severe enough to cause nephrotic syndrome. Focal segmental glomerulonephritis is rare and is excluded by the absence of red cells in the urine. Rheumatoid vasculitis has a predilection for skin and the peripheral nervous system but in very rare circumstances may affect the kidneys. It is more likely in patients with severe disease, nodule formation, high titres of rheumatoid factor and hypocomplementaemia. (See Question 320.)

Answer 18

> d. Metastatic spinal cord compression.

This is a T2 weighted image that shows evidence of cord compression from a collapsed thoracic vertebra. The vertebra in question is infiltrated by tumour and appears white. The vertebra above are also infiltrated with tumour (appear white). The vertebra below the collapsed vertebra appear normal (black).

Interpretation of MRI Scans		
Substance	**T1 weighted**	**T2 weighted**
Water/vitreous/CSF	black	light grey or white
Fat	white	light grey
Muscle	grey	grey
Air	black	black
Fatty bone marrow	white	light grey
Brain white matter	light grey	grey
Brain grey matter	grey	very light grey

T1 Weighted Imaging

Provides anatomical information

Low signal – Black
- Cortical bone
- Air
- Rapidly flowing blood
- CSF

Intermediate signal – Grey
- Grey matter is darker than white matter

High signal – White
- Fat in bone, scalp and orbit

T2 Weighted Imaging

Provides pathological information

Low signal – Black
- Cortical bone
- Air
- Rapidly flowing blood
- Haemosiderin

Intermediate signal – Grey
- White matter is darker than grey matter

High signal – White
- CSF or water

Question 19

A 16-year-old girl presented with intermittent episodes of lower colicky abdominal pain for six months. In the interim she had lost almost 6.4 kg in weight. Her appetite was not impaired. There was no history of diarrhoea, although the patient had complained of intermittent constipation and abdominal bloating. The patient was English in origin. She had no family history of note. She had last travelled abroad to Barbados on holiday a year ago. The only other past medical history included a short episode of painful ankles associated with circular erythematous skin lesions.

On examination she was thin and mildly clubbed. The heart rate was 90 beats/min and regular. The blood pressure measured 100/55 mmHg. There was evidence of a BCG scar on inspection of the left upper arm. Both heart sounds were normal and the chest was clear. Abdominal examination revealed vague tenderness affecting the hypogastrum and right iliac fossa.

Investigations are shown.

Hb	10 g/dl
WCC	11×10^9/l
Platelets	498×10^9/l
ESR	55 mm/h
U&E	Normal
AST	20 iu/l
ALT	22 iu/l
Bilirubin	12 μmol/l
Albumin	33 g/l
Stool culture	Negative
Chest X-ray	Minor calcification, a few perihilar nodes

What is the diagnosis?
  a. Sarcoidosis.
  b. Intestinal lymphoma.
  c. Intestinal tuberculosis.
  d. Crohn's disease.
  e. Irritable bowel syndrome.

Question 20

A 24-year-old patient was admitted to hospital with acute asthma for the fourth time in the past six years. The asthma was usually precipitated by a coryzal illness or exposure to allergens. There was no other past medical history of note. The patient usually inhaled ventolin as required, salmeterol inhaler twice daily, becotide inhaler twice daily and had recently been prescribed aminophylline 450 mg twice daily.

On admission she had a bilateral wheeze. The PEFR was 200 l/min. The oxygen saturation on air was 86% and on 28% oxygen it was 94%. The chest X-ray revealed hyperinflated lungs. The patient was commenced on nebulized bronchodilators, prednisolone 30 mg daily and amoxycillin. The following day she developed a rash therefore the amoxycillin was substituted with erythromycin.

The patient improved significantly over the next 48 hours but then suffered three successive grand mal seizures, which necessitated ventilation.

What was the most likely cause of the epileptic seizures?
  a. Hypoxia.
  b. Meningitis.
  c. Benign intracranial hypertension.
  d. Theophylline toxicity.
  e. Herpes encephalitis.

Answer 19

> d. Crohn's disease.

Abdominal cramps, weight loss, erythema nodosum (raised circular skin lesions) and raised inflammatory markers are highly suggestive of inflammatory bowel disease. Tenderness in the right iliac fossa points to the possibility of terminal ileal disease and hence Crohn's disease, although this is a non-specific feature since many conditions may cause right iliac fossa tenderness. Diarrhoea is not always a prominent feature in Crohn's disease.

Although ileo-caecal TB may present in a similar fashion, her race and the presence of a BCG scar is against the diagnosis. Sarcoidosis enteropathy has been reported but this is very rare and usually in association with other features of this multi-system disorder. Small bowel lymphoma may present in a similar fashion; however, diarrhoea is a prominent feature. Raised inflammatory markers are against the diagnosis of irritable bowel disease, which is a functional rather than inflammatory disorder. (See Answers 31, 394.)

Answer 20

> d. Theophylline toxicity.

The question tests the candidate's knowledge about drugs interacting with aminophylline and inhibiting its metabolism. With respect to the treatment of lower respiratory tract infections, both quinolone and macrolide antibiotics (e.g. ciprofloxacin, erythromycin respectively) inhibit aminophylline metabolism.

Features of theophylline toxicity include nausea, vomiting, hypotension, cardiac arrhythmias and seizures. Other drugs that inhibit the metabolism of theophylline include cimetidine, propranolol, allopurinol, thiobendazole and the contraceptive pill. In the context of asthma, hypokalaemia (sometimes a consequence of nebulized salbutamol) is also associated with theophylline toxicity.

Symptoms do not usually occur until plasma theophylline concentrations exceed 20 mg/l. The most adverse effects of theophylline toxicity, such as cardiac arrhythmias and seizures, generally occur at plasma theophylline levels >40 mg/l.

The management of theophylline toxicity is usually supportive. In patients who have taken an overdose, the aim is to prevent absorption in the stomach. There are three main strategies in the management of theophylline toxicity (shown below):

Strategy 1 (if patient is stable)
- Gastric lavage followed by oral activated charcoal administration is effective.

Strategy 2
- Treat arrhythmias with beta-blockers; unfortunately many patients taking theophylline for therapeutic reasons have contraindications to beta-blockers. In these patients lignocaine may be used for ventricular arrhythmias and verapamil for supraventricular arrhythmias including atrial fibrillation.
- Treat seizures with diazepam or barbiturates; phenytoin is not very effective.

Strategy 3 (rarely required)
- Haemodialysis is very effective in treating life-threatening toxicity, i.e. patients with a plasma theophylline level of >100 mg/l who have profound hypotension, fatal cardiac arrhythmias and seizures. Age and concomitant hepatic disease are important factors in relation to prognosis with theophylline toxicity. Patients aged >60 years with liver disease may be dialysed at theophylline levels of around 60 mg/l.

Question 21

A 64-year-old Asian man presented with a six-week history of dyspnoea and wheeze. For two weeks he had also developed a cough productive of yellow sputum and fever. There was no history of night sweats. The patient had not travelled abroad for over 20 years.

Investigations are shown.

Hb	13 g/dl
WCC	11 × 10^9/l
	(neutrophils 8 × 10^9/l,
	lymphocytes 1 × 10^9/l
	eosinophils 2 × 10^9/l)
Platelets	258 × 10^9/l
ESR	30 mm/h
Biochemistry	Normal
Chest X-ray	Diffuse perihilar infiltrates
Sputum culture	Negative

What is the most probable diagnosis?
  a. Churg–Strauss syndrome.
  b. Tuberculosis.
  c. Allergic bronchopulmonary aspergillosis.
  d. Tropical pulmonary eosinophilia.
  e. Asthma.

Question 22

A 78-year-old patient presented with sudden onset of severe breathlessness. He had a history of ischaemic heart disease and had suffered two myocardial infarctions in the past three years. He had an 11-year history of hypertension that had been well controlled. He was a non-smoker. His medication consisted of aspirin, ramipril, atenolol, bendroflumethiazide and simvastatin.

On examination he had a heart rate of 146 beats/min. The pulse was irregular. The blood pressure was 100/68 mmHg. Both heart sounds were quiet. Auscultation of the lungs revealed widespread inspiratory crackle and expiratory wheeze. The ECG showed atrial fibrillation with a rapid ventricular rate and q waves in the anterior leads.

What is the safest drug for restoring sinus rhythm?
  a. IV digoxin.
  b. IV amiodarone.
  c. IV flecanide.
  d. IV esmolol.
  e. IV dofetolide.

Question 23

An 81-year-old man with non-insulin-dependent diabetes mellitus was found unconscious by his carer. Blood tests performed on admission to hospital are shown.

Sodium	153 mmol/l
Potassium	5.4 mmol/l
Urea	40 mmol/l
Creatinine	310 μmol/l
Glucose	60 mmol/l

What is the best combination of infusions in the management of the patient?
  a. IV saline (0.45%), IV insulin and subcutaneous heparin.
  b. IV saline (0.9%), IV insulin and subcutaneous heparin.
  c. IV sodium bicarbonate, IV insulin and subcutaneous heparin.
  d. IV dextrose saline, IV insulin and subcutaneous heparin.
  e. IV dextrose (5%), IV insulin and subcutaneous heparin.

Answer 21

> c. Allergic bronchopulmonary aspergillosis.

The history of cough sputum, eosinophilia and perihilar infiltrates is most consistent with allergic broncho-pulmonary aspergillosis in the context of the history given. There is no drug history to indicate an eosinophilic pneumonitis, nor a history of travel to the tropics to suggest tropical pulmonary eosinophilia. Churg–Strauss syndrome is unlikely in the absence of vasculitis, neuropathy or renal involvement. Asthma does not cause pulmonary infiltrates. Tuberculosis does not usually cause eosinophilia.

The diagnosis of allergic bronchopulmonary eosinophilia is made in patients with asthma, proximal bronchiectasis and parenchymal infiltrates in the perihilar area. The presence of high titres of IgE and IgG antibodies and a positive hypersensitivity skin test to *Aspergillus fumigatus* testing confirm the diagnosis. Treatment is with a prolonged course of itriconazole.

Tropical pulmonary eosinophila is an immune reaction to infection with the human filarial parasites *Wucheria bancrofti* and *Brugia malayi*. It is characterized by a non-productive cough, wheeze, fever, weight loss, lymphadenopathy, eosinophilia and patchy infiltrates on the chest X-ray. The condition occurs in patients infected in the tropics. The worm is rarely identified but the condition responds to diethycarbamazine, the drug normally used to treat filariasis. (See Question 396.)

Answer 22

> b. IV amiodarone.

The patient has rapid atrial fibrillation in the context of ischaemic heart disease and has evidence of pulmonary oedema. One has to assume that left ventricular function is impaired to answer this question since it is highly unlikely that a heart rate of 146 beats/min would cause left ventricular failure in a patient with normal left ventricular function. Amiodarone, dofetolide and flecainide are capable of restoring sinus rhythm. Of these amiodarone is the least negatively inotropic.

Flecainide is relatively contraindicated in patients with known coronary artery disease. Dofetolide is a class III anti-arrhythmic agent that is effective at restoring sinus rhythm in patients with persistent AF (up to seven days) or more permanent AF. Dofetolide is less negatively inotropic than many other drugs that may be effective in restoring sinus rhythm such as propafenone (class IC), quinidine, disopyramide (class IA) and sotalol (class III), but experience regarding its use in the UK is relatively limited. Digoxin is effective in controlling ventricular rate in AF but does not restore sinus rhythm. Esmolol is a very short-acting beta-blocker (class II antiarrhythmic agent) that is not useful at restoring sinus rhythm.

Answer 23

> b. IV saline (0.9%), IV insulin and subcutaneous heparin.

The patient has a hyperosmolar non-ketotic diabetic coma (HONK). The fluid of choice is saline. The strength of saline used initially is always 0.9% since it is effective at restoring volume and has a lower risk of causing large drops in plasma osmolality, a risk factor for the development of cerebral oedema. If despite adequate hydration, the sodium remains >150 mmol/l some authorities advocate switching to half-strength saline (0.45%). The patient has severe dehydration creating a hyperviscosity state that may predispose him to arterial and venous thromboses. Heparin therapy is mandatory to prevent such complications during the management of HONK. (See Question 84.)

Question 24

A 13-year-old girl was admitted with a two-day history of lower abdominal pain and blood-stained diarrhoea. Three days later, she developed pains in her ankles and right elbow and felt nauseous. Positive findings on examination were a purpuric rash affecting the arms and legs, periorbital oedema and a blood pressure of 150/95 mmHg.

Investigations are shown.

Hb	10 g/dl
WCC	$12 \times 10^9/l$
Platelets	$136 \times 10^9/l$
MCV	70 fl
ESR	35 mm/h
PT	13 s (control 13 s)
APTT	34 s (control 36 s)
Sodium	138 mmol/l
Potassium	5.9 mmol/l
Creatinine	130 μmol/l
Urinalysis	Blood ++
	Protein ++

1: What is the most probable diagnosis?
   a. Haemolytic–uraemic syndrome.
   b. IgA nephritis.
   c. Henoch–Schönlein purpura.
   d. Systemic lupus erythematosus.
   e. Polyarteritis nodosa.

2: List two investigations that would be most useful in confirming the diagnosis.
   a. Skin biopsy.
   b. Renal biopsy.
   c. Blood cultures.
   d. TT.
   e. Serum fibrinogen level.
   f. Serum IgA level.
   g. Serum ANF level.
   h. Serum ANCA.
   i. Blood film.
   j. 24-hour urine collection for protein.

Question 25

A 39-year-old African male was referred to the blood pressure unit with persistent blood pressure readings of 140–150/90–95 mmHg over the past six months. He was a non-smoker and consumed 4 units of alcohol per week. The patient weighed 89 kg and measured 1.7 m. Physical examination was normal with the exception of a blood pressure reading of 150/92 mmHg.

Investigations are shown.

Sodium	136 mmol/l	
Potassium	4.2 mmol/l	
Urea	5 mmol/l	
Glucose	4.1 mmol/l	
Total cholesterol	4.1 mmol/l	
Triglycerides	1.2 mmol/l	
12-lead ECG	Sinus rhythm	
	Right axis deviation	
Urinalysis	Protein	0
	Blood	0
	Cells	0

What is the best initial management for the raised blood pressure?
   a. Beta-blocker.
   b. Angiotensin-converting enzyme inhibitor.
   c. Low-salt diet, regular exercise.
   d. Calcium channel antagonist.
   e. Thiazide diuretic.

Answer 24

> 1: c. Henoch–Schönlein purpura.
> 2: a. Skin biopsy.
>   b. Renal biopsy.

The combination of lower abdominal pain, bloody diarrhoea, purpuric rash and nephritis in a young girl are highly suggestive of Henoch–Schönlein purpura. The condition is a small-vessel vasculitis that occurs most commonly in children aged 4–15 years. It is characterized by gastrointestinal symptoms which comprise abdominal pain, diarrhoea, and rectal bleeding, flitting arthralgia affecting large joints, a purpuric rash characteristically affecting the lower limbs and buttocks and an acute nephritis. Complications include intestinal perforation, haemorrhage and intussusception and acute renal failure.

The diagnosis is usually clinical; however, tissue diagnosis is possible with skin or renal biopsy. Skin biopsy demonstrates a leucoclastic vasculitis with IgA deposition. Renal biopsy reveals mesangial IgA deposition associated with a glomerulonephritis. Renal histology is indistinguishable from IgA nephropathy. In this case, more marks are given to skin biopsy because it is safer and more practical than renal biopsy. Serum IgA levels are depressed in approximately 50% of cases. The management is usually supportive, although there may be a role for methylprednisolone in cases of acute crescentic nephritis.

The condition must not be confused with the haemolytic uraemic syndrome (discussed in Answer 152), which is also characterized by diarrhoea and renal failure.

Answer 25

> c. Low-salt diet, regular exercise.

The patient is young and has mild hypertension on presentation. He does not have any other risk factors for cardiovascular disease or evidence of secondary end-organ damage as a result of the raised blood pressure. In this particular case the initial management plan should include a low-salt diet, regular exercise and weight loss. The patient should be observed carefully for up to a year and should only be commenced on pharmacological therapy if the blood pressure remains above 140/85 mmHg.

If treatment is indicated after a year, the drugs of choice are thiazide diuretics or calcium channel blockers. Angiotensin-converting enzyme inhibitors and beta-blockers are not particularly effective as monotherapy because both drugs act by suppressing renin levels, which are already relatively low in Afro-Caribbean patients. However, these patients may respond to ACE inhibitors and beta-blockers when prescribed with drugs that activate the renin–angiotensin–aldosterone system, i.e. thiazide diuretics and calcium channel blockers.

Both lifestyle modification and pharmacological therapy would be indicated if the patient had a blood pressure ≥160/100 mmHg, or evidence of secondary end-organ damage, or other risk factors for coronary artery disease at presentation.

There is a high prevalence of hypertension in individuals of Afro-Caribbean origin, with almost 50% of patients over the age of 40 years being affected. This particular group of patients generally develop hypertension at a younger age and are at higher risk of hypertensive complications such as stroke, heart failure and renal failure than Caucasian patients. Hypertension in Afro-Caribbean patients is salt sensitive and responds well to a low-salt diet.

Question 26

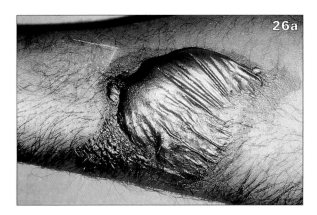

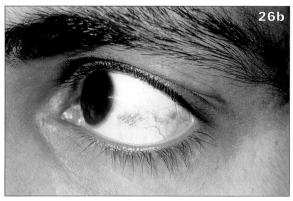

A 41-year-old male was admitted to hospital with acute confusion. He had been generally unwell for two days. A worried neighbour looked through his letter box when he failed to answer the doorbell, and found him lying on the floor. There was no other history of note.

Hb	11 g/dl
WCC	24 × 10⁹/l
Platelets	30 × 10⁹/l
Sodium	135 mmol/l
Potassium	5 mmol/l
Creatinine	156 µmol/l
PT	48 s (control 13 s)
Fibrinogen degradation products	>25,000

On examination, he was confused. He had a widespread rash (**26a**). His left eye is shown (**26b**). The heart rate was 120 beats/min; the blood pressure was unrecordable. There was no evidence of nuchal rigidity, and Kernig's sign was negative. There was no focal neurological deficit. Examination of the cardiovascular, respiratory and gastrointestinal tract was normal.

Investigations are shown.

Which single investigation would you perform next?
a. Blood cultures.
b. CT scan brain.
c. CSF for microscopy and culture.
d. Chest X-ray.
e. Throat swab for culture.

Question 27

A 36-year-old woman is seen in the Accident and Emergency Department after having taken 40 paracetamol tablets with a quarter-bottle of vodka six hours earlier, following an argument with her husband. She was nauseous, but had not vomited. There was no past medical history of note. A physical examination was normal.

1. List two immediate management steps from the following list:
a. Gastric lavage.
b. IV dextrose 5%.
c. Oral activated charcoal.
d. Fresh-frozen plasma.
e. IV sodium bicarbonate.
f. IV N-acetyl cysteine.
g. IV flumazenil.
h. IV vitamin K.
i. IV saline (0.9%).
j. IV prochlorperazine.

Investigations are shown.

Sodium	138 mmol/l
Potassium	3.9 mmol/l
Urea	5.1 mmol/l
Bicarbonate	18 mmol/l
PT	15 s (control 15 s)
Serum paracetamol level	200 mg/l

2. Which one of the following investigations would you perform the next day to assess her prognosis?
a. Serum potassium.
b. Serum magnesium.
c. Arterial pH.
d. Serum paracetamol concentration.
e. Serum aspartate transaminase.

Answer 26

> a. Blood cultures.

The eye demonstrates a conjunctival haemorrhage. The rash is a necrotic purpuric rash, which is typical of meningococcal septicaemia. The patient has septic shock and requires immediate therapy. The recognition that he has meningococcal septicaemia is important for the choice of antibiotics that you will use. In medical emergencies, the reader must be familiar with the drugs that are used in that particular emergency, but not necessarily the dosage, as this can be found in the British National Formulary or the equivalent. Although most *Neisseria meningitidis* strains are sensitive to benzyl penicillin, it is prudent to cover the patient with additional cephalosporin or aminoglycoside antibiotic therapy until the sensitivities of the organism are known. The circulation must be restored to prevent hypoperfusion of vital organs, particularly the kidneys. The presence of low platelets, high fibrinogen degradation products and abnormal clotting is suggestive of DIC, which should be treated with fresh-frozen plasma to prevent haemorrhage.

Neisseria meningitidis, the causal Gram-negative diplococcus, can be cultured from the CSF in over 80% of cases with evidence of neurological involvement. However, the presence of very low levels of platelets and DIC is contraindicated because of the dangers of bleeding into the spinal canal, particularly because the yield is just as high from nasal swabs. It is also possible to isolate the meningococcal antigen from blood before blood culture results are available. This test is particularly useful if antibiotics have been given before the patient is brought to hospital (negative blood cultures).

Meningococcal meningitis and septicaemia are caused by serogroups B and C. Septicaemia is associated with widespread petechial haemorrhage. Conjunctival haemorrhage may be the first physical manifestation. Shock is common owing to the production of a circulating endotoxin. DIC is a commonly recognized complication that may result in adrenal haemorrhage (Waterhouse–Friderichsen syndrome). Meningitis is often characterized by a myalgia, headache, photophobia, neck stiffness, nausea and vomiting. In the absence of DIC, the diagnosis is made rapidly by performing a Gram stain on the CSF. Blood cultures are positive in the majority of patients with meningitis. Focal neurological signs are less common than in pneumococcal meningitis.

Note: individuals in contact with affected patients must receive rifampicin chemoprophylaxis.

Answer 27

> 1. c. Oral activated charcoal.
>   f. IV N-acetyl cysteine.
> 2. c. Arterial pH.

The drug should be given within 8–10 hours of ingestion of the overdose, and continued while the liver function is abnormal. It is useful because it replenishes cellular glutathione stores and reduces oxidative damage caused by the toxic metabolite, NAPQI. An alternative to this is methionine. Gastric lavage is useful if performed within 1 hour of the overdose.

The patient has taken 20 g of paracetamol. An ingestion of 15 g is considered potentially serious in most patients. The toxicity of paracetamol is related to the production of a toxic metabolite of paracetamol. This is NAPQI, which usually is immediately conjugated with glutathione and excreted. In paracetamol overdose, the toxic metabolite is produced in excess and depletes cellular glutathione. The liver is unable to deactivate NAPQI, which is responsible for massive hepatic necrosis and hepatic failure. Patients may have nausea, anorexia or vomiting on the first day. After 72 hours, features of liver and renal failure may ensue.

The three most important prognostic markers in paracetamol overdose are serum creatinine concentration, arterial pH and prothrombin time. A rise in serum creatinine level due to renal failure is a bad prognostic sign. A level of over 300 mmol/l is associated with over 70% mortality. Systemic acidosis (due to the failure of clearance of lactate by the liver) more than 24 hours after the overdose is associated with a poor prognosis. A pH of below 7.3 is associated with only a 15% chance of survival. The PT is usually the first liver test to become abnormal. A PT of >20 s at 24 hours after overdose is suggestive of significant hepatic damage, and a peak PT of >180 s is associated with a 90% mortality.

Question 28

A 52-year-old female was brought into the Accident and Emergency Department after being found collapsed outside a public house. There was no one accompanying her, and there was no information regarding her next of kin.

On examination, she was very drowsy and had a Glasgow coma score of 6 out of 15. Her pupils were 10 mm each and reacted very sluggishly to light. On attempting to examine her fundi, she was noted to have coarse nystagmus, but a clear view of her fundi did not demonstrate any abnormalities. The tone in all her limbs was increased and her reflexes were brisk. The plantars were both upgoing. The heart rate was 135 beats/min, and regular. The blood pressure was 105/60 mmHg. The respiratory rate was 20/min. Examination of the precordium and lung fields was normal, but examination of the abdomen revealed a firm palpable mass 4 cm above the symphysis pubis. The patient was catheterized and drained of 2 litres of urine. Investigations are shown.

Shortly after the lumbar puncture, the patient had a generalized seizure which lasted 30 s. The attending nurse raised concerns about an arrhythmia on the cardiac monitor, and a 12-lead ECG was performed (**28**).

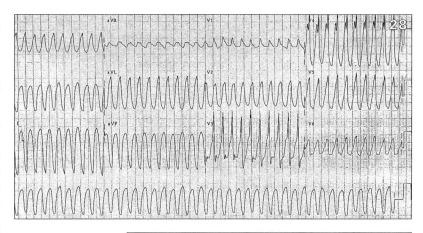

1. Calculate the plasma osmolality.
2. Explain the discrepancy between the calculated plasma osmolality and the measured plasma osmolality.
3. Give two possible explanations for the low urine osmolality.
4. What is shown on the ECG?
5. What diagnosis best fits all the information given above?
6. What three investigations would you perform to help in this patient's management?

Hb	14 g/dl
WCC	12×10^9/l
Platelets	221×10^9/l
MCV	88 fl
Sodium	144 mmol/l
Potassium	4.0 mmol/l
Urea	13 mmol/l
Creatinine	100 μmol/l
Bicarbonate	20 mmol/l
Chloride	108 mmol/l
Calcium	2.4 mmol/l
Phosphate	1.3 mmol/l
Bilirubin	12 μmol/l
AST	33 iu/l
Gamma GT	28 iu/l
Alkaline phosphatase	120 iu/l
Plasma osmolality	333 mOsm/l
Urine osmolality	120 mOsm/l
Blood glucose	6 mmol/l
Chest X-ray	Normal-sized heart and clear lung fields
Skull X-ray	Normal; no fractures seen
Brain CT scan	Normal
Lumbar puncture:	
CSF pressure	100 cmH$_2$O
Cells	3/mm^3
Protein	0.35 g/l
Glucose	3 mmol/l
ECG	Sinus tachycardia; right axis deviation

Answer 28

1. The plasma osmolality is calculated by the formula 2 ([Na] + [K]) + [Urea] + [Glucose]. In this case, the calculated plasma osmolality is 315 mOsm/l.
2. The measured plasma osmolality is higher than the calculated one, suggesting that the patient has ingested something which has not been measured, but has the effect of increasing the plasma osmolality. The most likely possibility in this case is alcohol ingestion. Although lithium contributes to plasma osmolality, it would be very unusual for the lithium concentration to be high enough to increase the plasma osmolality by 18 mOsm/l, considering that a serum lithium concentration of 2.5 mmol/l causes dangerous toxicity.
3. Nephrogenic diabetes insipidus from lithium therapy or inhibition of ADH secretion as a result of alcohol ingestion.
4. There is a broad-complex tachycardia with extreme axis deviation and concordance of the QRS complexes in the chest leads. These findings are suggestive of ventricular tachycardia.
5. Tricyclic antidepressant drug overdose with alcohol.
6. i. Arterial blood gases.
   ii. Serum lithium level.
   iii. Blood alcohol level.

Arrhythmias usually settle on correction of hypoxia and acidosis. Administration of class I antiarrhythmic agents may paradoxically worsen arrhythmias, with the exception of phenytoin. Status epilepticus should be corrected with intravenous diazepam.

Epileptic seizures and ventricular arrhythmias in a patient found collapsed should raise the suspicion of tricyclic antidepressant drug overdose. The low urine osmolality suggests that the patient has probably taken the overdose together with alcohol, and it is possible that she may have also taken lithium. The normal CT scan of the brain and normal CSF are against pathology in the central nervous system. She has dilated pupils, which is against narcotic abuse. Indeed, the combination of dilated pupils, tachycardia and urinary retention are all suggestive of the anticholinergic side-effects of tricyclic antidepressants. Severe lithium toxicity is associated with seizures, coma and ventricular arrhythmias, but anticholinergic effects are not a feature. In addition, lithium toxicity is associated with ataxia and dysarthria. Chronic lithium ingestion may cause hypothyroidism. Sodium-depleting drugs such as diuretics lead to excess absorption of lithium by the kidney, and predispose to toxicity.

The arterial blood gases are an important investigation because they will identify hypoxia and acidosis, both of which precipitate ventricular arrhythmias in patients with tricyclic antidepressant overdose. The serum lithium level will be useful to determine whether lithium has been ingested, and will help decide whether the patient should have forced diuresis. In general, patients with a serum lithium of >3 mmol/l should have forced diuresis. Haemodialysis is recommended if serum lithium exceeds 4 mmol/l.

The management of the patient is outlined below.

The management of tricyclic antidepressant overdose

- Protect the airway, and give oxygen via a mask
- Gastric lavage under anaesthetic supervision (within 12 hours of ingestion) followed by activated charcoal via a nasogastric tube
- Monitor on a high-dependency unit
- Correct hypoxia
- Correct acidosis with IV sodium bicarbonate
- Intravenous fluids to improve blood pressure
- Epileptic seizures should be corrected with IV lorazepam or diazepam. Phenytoin is contra-indicated
- Ventricular arrhythmias respond to correction of acidosis and hypoxia. IV sodium bicarbonate is the mainstay of prevention and treatment of ventricular arrhythmias and should be administered in all patients with ventricular tachycardia or acidosis or in patients with a QRS duration >110 msec

Question 29

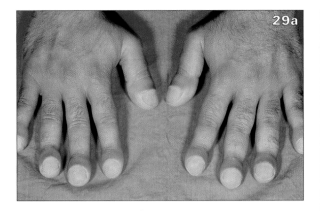

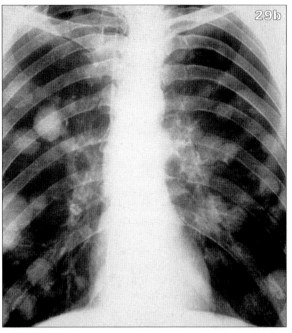

A 76-year-old male presented with a three-month history of anorexia, weight loss and fever. Apart from sweating excessively at night and feeling very thirsty, he did not have any other symptoms. He was a non-smoker and had been a schoolteacher for 40 years before retiring.

On examination, he was thin. The finding on inspection of his hands is shown (**29a**). The heart rate was 100 beats/min and the blood pressure 180/105 mmHg. His temperature was 37.8°C (100°F). Examination of the cardiovascular system and the respiratory system was normal. Abdominal examination revealed minimal tenderness and some fullness in the right loin. Examination of the genitalia revealed some oedema of the scrotum. The lower limbs were oedematous.

Investigations are shown.

Hb	18 g/dl
WCC	10 × 10⁹/l
Platelets	300 × 10⁹/l
ESR	110 mm/h
Sodium	140 mmol/l
Potassium	3.1 mmol/l
Creatinine	120 µmol/l
Calcium	2.6 mmol/l
Albumin	36 g/l
Chest X-ray (**29b**)	
CT scan of abdomen (**29c**)	
Urinalysis	Blood +++
	Protein +
	Bilirubin 0

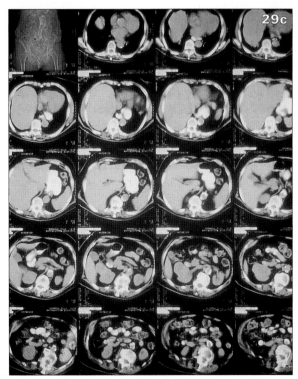

1. Give two explanations for the serum calcium level.
2. What is the most probable diagnosis?
3. List three important tests you would perform to help achieve a diagnosis.
4. What is the management?

Answer 29

1. i. Bone metastases.
   ii. PTH-related peptide secretion from a right-sided renal carcinoma.
2. Right-sided renal carcinoma.
3. i. Renal angiography.
   ii. Renal venography and inferior vena cavogram.
   iii. Bone scan to detect bony metastases.
4. Surgical removal of the right kidney if his general health will allow.

This patient presents with anorexia, weight loss, and a fever that may represent sepsis or malignancy. The right loin tenderness and haematuria are suggestive of renal involvement. The chest X-ray reveals multiple opacities in both lungs which represents a cannon-ball metastases from the right kidney. CT scan of the abdomen reveals a carcinoma of the right kidney which is invading the inferior vena cava; hence the scrotal and lower-limb oedema. Hypernephroma characteristically presents with a triad of haematuria, loin pain and swelling. Haematuria is present in 50% of cases, but pain and swelling are less frequent. Non-specific symptoms such as anorexia, weight loss and fatigue may be present for several months before the diagnosis is made. The neoplastic cells often produce peptide hormones such as erythropoietin, renin, ADH and PTH-related peptide. This patient has a relative polycythaemia, hypercalcaemia, hypokalaemia and hypertension, which reflect erythropoietin, PTH-related peptide and renin secretion, respectively. Fever is present in approximately 20% of patients and is probably secondary to the secretion of a pyrogen by the tumour. Hypertension is present in approximately 30% of patients. Metastases usually occur via the bloodstream, although direct invasion of the renal veins or the inferior vena cava is relatively common. Some 10% of hypernephromas are bilateral, so close attention is given to the contralateral kidney when reviewing the CT scan. Venography and arteriography allow assessment of invasion of the veins and the vascularity of the tumour, respectively. Urine cytology may reveal malignant cells but the diagnostic yield is low. Removal of the hypernephroma (even when distant metastases are present) improves survival and causes regression of the metastases in many, but not all, patients. Radiotherapy and chemotherapy have been used in the treatment of this tumour, but the results are not very encouraging. The overall survival rate is 30–50%.

Question 30

An 84-year-old female was referred to clinic with increasing forgetfulness. Her GP had commenced her on a small dose of haloperidol for agitation eight months ago. According to the staff at the nursing home where she resided, she had become increasingly confused over the past few months and more recently had developed odd movements affecting her face, arms and legs. Her GP had reviewed her two weeks previously and stopped the haloperidol; however, she remained confused and the movement disorder had become much more pronounced. She was not taking any other medication.

On examination, she had a mental test score of 4/10. Her vital parameters were normal. She exhibited intermittent yawning motions of the mouth, with occasional tongue protrusion. There were semi-purposeful movements of her arms and legs. There was also clinical evidence of increased tone and cogwheel rigidity on neurological examination of her limbs.

A CT scan of the brain revealed generalized cerebral atrophy and calcification of the basal ganglia.

What is the cause of her movement disorder?
 a. Multi-infarct dementia.
 b. Lewy body dementia.
 c. Extrapyramidal side-effects of haloperidol.
 d. Pseudohypoparathyroidism.
 e. Hypoparathyroidism.

Question 31

A 33-year-old Iranian male was investigated for a six-month history of general malaise, weight loss, fever, pain in his knees, ankles and wrists and a sore mouth. On systematic enquiry, he gave a two-year history of a recurrent sore mouth that made it difficult for him to eat. Just before the onset of all his symptoms he had experienced an attack of abdominal pain and bloody diarrhoea which resolved after a week. He was seen by a gastroenterologist shortly afterwards, who diagnosed an inflammatory colitis, possibly secondary to infection. A rectal biopsy was performed by the gastroenterologist, and this was reported as a non-specific colitis. The patient had never experienced any abdominal symptoms after this, but had several episodes of soreness affecting the mouth. In addition, he developed painful eyes and pain on intercourse and on voiding urine. There was no history of urethral discharge. Shortly afterwards he was admitted to hospital with a femoral vein thrombosis, which was treated with anticoagulants and thought to be secondary to dehydration and immobility from his diarrhoeal illness. During the past six weeks his health had deteriorated. He had arthralgia and a fever. He had been married for five years. He denied extramarital sex. His wife was well, and had not experienced any similar symptoms.

On examination, the patient appeared unwell.

Examination of his oral cavity revealed an abnormality (**31a**). His eyes were sore (**31b**). He had submandibular lymphadenopathy. His ankle, wrist and knee joints were tender, and joint movements were restricted. In addition, he had painful lesions on his legs (**31c**). Examination of his genitalia and anal areas are shown (**31d, e**). He also pointed out an erythematous lesion approximately 2 cm in diameter that had developed at the site of venepuncture during a blood test performed by his GP two days earlier. All other aspects of the physical examination were normal. Investigations are shown.

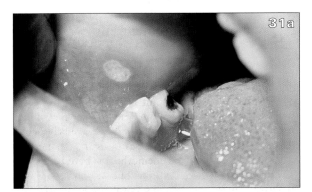

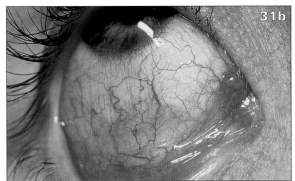

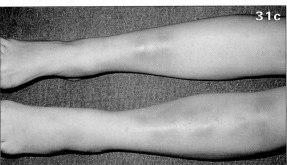

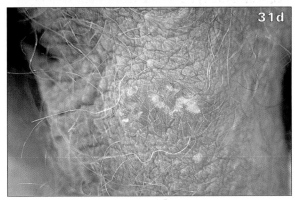

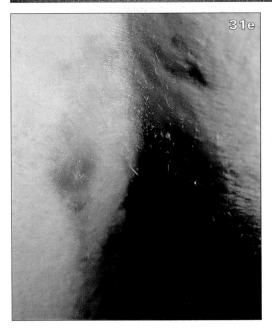

Hb	9.8 g/dl
WCC	13 × 10⁹/l
Platelets	450 × 10⁹/l
MCV	82 fl
CRP	200 g/l
Rheumatoid factor	Absent
Antinuclear antibody	Absent
Radiology of painful joints	Normal

What is the most probable diagnosis?
  a. Crohn's disease.
  b. Ulcerative colitis.
  c. Reiter's syndrome.
  d. Behçet's syndrome.
  e. Gonococcal septicaemia.

Answer 30

c. Extrapyramidal side-effects of haloperidol.

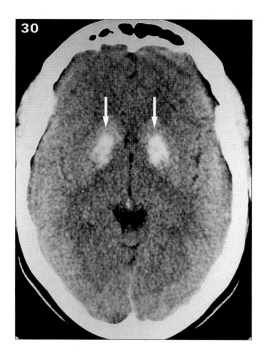

The woman has clinical evidence of dyskinesia and parkinsonism. The most common cause of her neurological signs is drug-induced extrapyramidal disease. Neuroleptic drugs which include haloperidol are extensively used in treating agitation in the elderly. By blocking dopamine receptors in the basal ganglia, these drugs can offset extrapyramidal side-effects which include tremor, dystonia, akathisia, parkinsonism and tardive dyskinesia. Acute dystonic reactions appear within the first few hours or days, and consist of oculogyric crises, torticollis or trismus. Fortunately, they are uncommon, and resolve as soon as the drug is withdrawn. Chronic tardive dyskinesias are the most serious complication and affect 20% of patients on chronic neuroleptic therapy. They usually occur after a patient has been on treatment for at least three months, and can be made worse in the first few weeks after stopping the offending drug. In 60% of cases the dyskinesia resolves over three years after drug withdrawal; however, in the remainder of patients the movement disorder persists and is very difficult to treat. Characteristic features involve lip smacking, tongue protrusion, orofacial mouthing, trunk rocking and distal chorea of the hands and feet. A combination of any of these features may be present.

Cerebral calcification is an incidental finding in 0.5% of CT scans in the elderly. About 20–30% of patients with widespread calcification of the basal ganglia exhibit neurological signs which include parkinsonism, chorea, epilepsy, ataxia and dementia. There is an association between calcification of the basal ganglia and hypoparathyroidism or pseudohypoparathyroidism. Rare causes of basal ganglia calcification (**30**, arrowed) are cerebral irradiation and mitochondrial diseases.

Answer 31

d. Behçet's syndrome.

The patient has oral, genital and anal ulcers (**31a**, **d** and **e**, respectively), conjunctivitis (**31b**), arthritis, erythema nodosum (**31c**) and features of a systemic illness. There has been a single episode of bloody diarrhoea and a previous femoral vein thrombosis. The differential diagnoses include Crohn's disease, Reiter's syndrome and Behçet's syndrome (*Table A*). Reiter's syndrome is classically a triad of conjunctivitis, urethritis and arthritis 1–4 weeks after an episode of bacterial dysentery or a sexually transmitted urethritis. Other features include plantar fasciitis, Achilles tendinitis, keratoderma blennorrhagica, circinate balanitis, stomatitis, hepatitis, cardiac and neurological involvement, and occasionally amyloidosis. It is possible that the diarrhoeal illness may have been dysenteric and offset the reactive features of Reiter's disease. There is no history of promiscuity or urethral discharge. Venous thrombosis affects about 4% of patients with Reiter's disease and occurs early in the disease. Mouth ulcers are common in Reiter's disease and are painless. Erythema nodosum is not a feature of Reiter's syndrome. Arthritis is asymmetrical and usually affects the knee and ankle joints. The most common joint to be affected in the upper limb is the wrist, as in this case; however, joint involvement occurs early, whereas in this case the disease has been present for two years.

Crohn's disease is a chronic granulomatous inflammatory disease of the gastrointestinal tract of unknown cause, and is a strong possibility in this case. Bloody diarrhoea is a recognized feature of Crohn's colitis. Colonic disease is associated with perianal disease in just over 30% of patients. A seronegative reactive arthritis is a recognized complication of Crohn's disease. Erythema nodosum occurs in some cases. Genital ulcers are rare, as is deep-vein thrombosis. Urethral involvement and dysuria only occur when an inflammatory fistula develops between the colon and the ureter. Recurrent urinary tract infections due to faecaluria can cause urethral stricture.

Behçet's syndrome is the most probable diagnosis. Behçet's syndrome is a recurrent multifocal disorder that persists over many years. It is characterized by recurrent mouth and genital ulcers, ocular lesions, and skin, joint and neurological involvement. The incidence is high in Japan and in countries bordering the Mediterranean. Oral and genital ulcers are present in most patients.

Ulcers can affect the pharynx and cause dysphagia. Genital ulcers can cause dysuria and dyspareunia. Ocular lesions are the most serious development. Recurrent uveitis and iridocyclitis, retinal vascular lesions and optic atrophy can lead to loss of vision in 50% of patients with ocular involvement. Erythema nodosum is a recognized feature. Other skin manifestations include a diffuse pustular rash affecting the face, erythema multiforme. The pathergy is a useful diagnostic sign. Pricking the skin can lead to erythema around the affected part within 24–48 hours, which is a relevant feature in our patient.

A seronegative arthritis affects about 40% of patients and commonly involves knees, ankles and wrists. Recurrent thrombophlebitis of the legs is a significant feature of Behçet's syndrome, leading to venous thrombosis. Less often, superior or inferior cava thrombosis may occur. Abdominal pain and bloody diarrhoea have also been documented. Asymptomatic proteinuria is a recognized feature, but on a few occasions may reflect renal amyloidosis. Neurological complications occur in 20% of patients. Organic confusional states, meningoencephalitis, transient or persistent brainstem syndromes, multiple sclerosis and parkinsonian-type disorders are all recognized.

Behçet's syndrome is a clinical diagnosis. There is no specific diagnostic test. HLA-B51, B_{12}, DR2, DR7 and Drw52 are associated with the syndrome. Acute-phase proteins are elevated and immune complexes are present. The pathergy test is a simple useful test. Genital ulcers and oral complications are treated with topical steroids. In severe cases, systemic steroids become necessary, together with azathioprine, which acts as a steroid-sparing agent. Colchicine, cyclosporin and levamisole have also been used in the management of this condition. The causes of orogenital ulceration are given in *Table B*.

Table A Causes of orogenital ulcers

Behçet's syndrome	Syphilis
Crohn's disease	Gonococcal infection
Herpes simplex virus	HIV
Ulcerative colitis	Pemphigus pemphigoid
Reiter's syndrome	Stevens–Johnson
Lichen planus	syndrome

Table B Causes of orogenital ulcers and venous thromboses

Behçet's syndrome	Ulcerative colitis
Crohn's disease	Reiter's syndrome

Question 32

A 16-year-old female was admitted with a six-month history of myalgia, loss of weight and night sweats. Over the past six weeks she had started to become breathless on exertion. On admission to hospital she had a temperature of 38.1°C (100.6°F). On auscultation of the precordium, there was an early diastolic murmur at the left lower sternal edge. Examination of the chest, abdomen and central nervous system was normal, with the exception of her fundi, one of which is shown (**32a**). An echocardiogram was performed to investigate the murmur (**32b**).

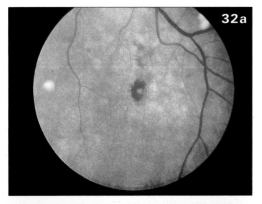

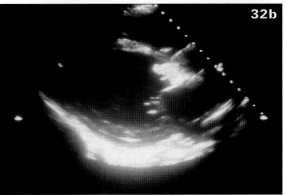

1. What is the diagnosis?
   a. Systemic lupus erythematosus.
   b. Polyarteritis nodosa.
   c. Infective endocarditis.
   d. Marantic endocarditis.
   e. Libmann–Sacks endocarditis.

2. What investigation would you perform to confirm the diagnosis?
   a. Autoantibody screen.
   b. Serum ANCA.
   c. Serum complement.
   d. Blood cultures.
   e. Serology for atypical bacteria.

Answer 32

> 1. c. Infective endocarditis.
> 2. d. Blood cultures.

Fever, diastolic murmur, presence of echogenic mass on the aortic valve and a Roth's spot in the retina (haemorrhagic areas with a pale centre) are consistent with the diagnosis of infective endocarditis. Clinical features of infective endocarditis are tabulated (*Table A*). Blood cultures are the single most important investigation in the diagnosis of infective endocarditis, and are positive in 90% of cases. Serial blood cultures should be performed, because a single set of blood cultures may not necessarily reveal the culprit organism. Although transthoracic echocardiography is extremely useful in confirming the presence of vegetations, the absence of vegetations does not exclude endocarditis, as vegetations <3 mm will not be seen on a transthoracic echocardiogram. A transoesophageal echocardiogram has a much higher sensitivity in identifying bacterial vegetations compared to transthoracic echocardiography. In approximately 10% of cases an organism is not identified despite repeated blood cultures. The two most common reasons for this are prior treatment with antibiotics before culturing the blood, or that the endocarditis is due to a fastidious organism with respect to conventional blood culture media. In patients who are immunosuppressed, endocarditis may be due to fungi that may be difficult to culture, and in very rare circumstances endocarditis may be a manifestation of SLE (Libmann–Sacks endocarditis) or a manifestation of malignancy, when it is termed marantic endocarditis (*Tables B* and *C*).

Table A Causes of Roth spots and other stigmata of endocarditis

Causes of Roth spots	*Clinical features of endocarditis*
Infective endocarditis	Pyrexia
SLE	Cardiac murmur
Polyarteritis nodosa	Splinter haemorrhages
Severe anaemia	Osler's nodes: small; painful
Leukaemia	Janeway lesions: macular; painless
	Roth spots
	Splenomegaly
	Microscopic haematuria/nephritis

Table B Causes of culture-negative endocarditis

Infective	*Non-infective*
• *Brucella* spp.	• SLE (Libmann–Sacs)
• *Coxiella burnetti*	• Marantic endocarditis
• *Chlamydia spp.*	
• *Mycoplasma* spp.	
• *Legionella* spp.	
• Histoplasmosis	
• *Tropherema whipelli*	
• Fungi	

Table C Common causes of culture-positive endocarditis

- *Streptococcus viridans*
- *Staphyloccus aureus*
- *Streptococcus faecalis* (associated with carcinoma of the colon)
- Enterococci

Question 33

A 51-year-old accountant presented with a six-month history of persistent dull right upper quadrant pain and fever. The pain did not radiate elsewhere, but was exacerbated on lying on her right side. During this period she had intermittent pale bulky stool which was difficult to flush, and episodic dark urine. More recently, her appetite was reduced and she had lost approximately 1 kg in weight during the past month. Over the past week she had difficulty sleeping due to itching all over her body, and her colleague at work commented on a yellowish pigmentation in her eyes. Six months before this, she had been relatively well. She had a past history of a cholecystectomy for cholesterol stones at the age of 32 and subsequently had an ERCP and removal of sludge from the common bile duct six years ago. She consumed 10 units of alcohol per week. She was married with two sons, aged 20 and 18. Three months ago she had been on holiday in Scotland. She was not taking any regular medication.

On examination, she was slightly icteric. Inspection of her hands is shown (**33**).

There were spider naevi on her arms neck and face and scratch marks around her trunk and lower limbs. She had a temperature of 39°C (102.2°F). Her heart rate was 120 beats/min and blood pressure 140/80 mmHg. There were a few inspiratory crackles on auscultation of the right lung base. Abdominal examination demonstrated firm, slightly tender hepatomegaly 4 cm below the costal margin, and a moderately enlarged spleen. There were no other abdominal masses, and there was no evidence of shifting dullness. Rectal examination was normal.

Investigations are shown.

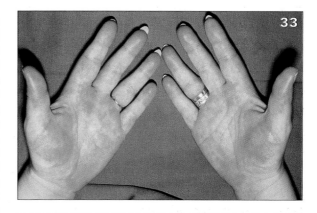

AST	60 iu/l
Alkaline phosphatase	360 iu/l
Bilirubin	82 μmol/l
Albumin	25 g/l
Total protein	93 g/l
INR	1.49
Chest X-ray	Normal

1. What investigation would you perform to ascertain the cause of her illness?
   a. Blood cultures.
   b. Liver biopsy.
   c. ERCP.
   d. Ultrasound of the biliary tract.
   e. Alpha-fetoprotein level.

2. What is the cause of her current presentation?
   a. Sclerosing cholangitis.
   b. Secondary biliary cirrhosis.
   c. Primary biliary cirrhosis.
   d. Cholangiocarcinoma.
   e. Recurrent cholangitis.

Question 34

A 75-year-old male was seen by his GP with a five-day history of wheeze and ankle swelling. He was prescribed some medication, but continued to deteriorate and was admitted to hospital.

Investigations are shown.

1. What is the acid-base disturbance?
2. Suggest two possible causes for this metabolic picture.

Arterial blood gases:	
pH	7.33
PaO$_2$	7 kPa
PaCO$_2$	6.5 kPa
Bicarbonate	20 mmol/l
Sodium	133 mmol/l
Potassium	5 mmol/l
Urea	28 mmol/l
Creatinine	200 μmol/l

Answer 33

1. a. Blood cultures.
2. e. Recurrent cholangitis.

The key in this question is a prior history of cholelithiasis affecting the gallbladder and the biliary tree. Stones in the bile duct are a nidus for infections, particularly when there has been instrumentation, as in this case. Cholangitis is characterized by the triad of right upper quadrant pain, jaundice and fever. This patient has had previous episodes suggestive of cholangitis, and the best answer for the presenting complaint is recurrent cholangitis. She also has evidence of cirrhosis, which is almost certainly secondary to chronic cholestasis. Although cholangiocarcinoma may rarely complicate biliary cholestasis, this is unlikely given the mode of presentation. Cholangiocarcinoma characteristically presents with intermittent jaundice, and causes duct obstruction before the onset of biliary cirrhosis. Primary sclerosing cholangitis is very uncommon. The aetiology is thought to be auto-immune, but the trigger factor is unknown. More usually, it is associated with ulcerative colitis, but may occur in patients with HIV either as a direct insult from HIV or due to opportunistic CMV, cryptosporidial and *Entamoeba* infection. Although it may lead to secondary biliary cirrhosis, it is unlikely in this case, given the history of chronic cholestasis. Primary biliary cirrhosis (PBC) is usually insidious. It is much more common in females and usually presents with pruritis and jaundice. Stones are not a recognized feature of PBC.

The investigation of choice is blood cultures, which have high positive yield in cholangitis. The most common organism isolated is *Escherichia coli*. Hepatic ultrasonography should be performed in all cases to exclude a secondary hepatic abscess, and to assess the common bile duct. ERCP and sphincterotomy may be therapeutic. There is no role for α-fetoprotein and liver biopsy in this case. α-Fetoprotein is often modestly elevated in cirrhosis of the liver, but grossly elevated in hepatocellular carcinoma. The presentation here is of cholangitis. A liver biopsy should never be the first line of investigation in a jaundiced patient with a fever.

Answer 34

1. Combined respiratory and metabolic acidosis.
2.i. Acute cardiac failure.
   ii. Severe exacerbation of obstructive airways disease and pre-renal failure from diuretics.

The patient has a respiratory acidosis that is characterized by a $PaCO_2$ of 6.5 kPa or more, and a pH below 7.35, and is hypoxic. In the acute situation, respiratory acidosis is not compensated by the kidney, but after 3–5 days the kidneys retain bicarbonate ions to compensate, which results in normalization of the pH at the expense of a relative metabolic alkalosis. In this patient the bicarbonate is slightly low, suggesting a metabolic acidosis. This may be due to coexistent renal disease that prevents adequate compensation, or to another factor causing metabolic acidosis. The serum urea and creatinine levels are elevated, but there is a relatively larger increase in the serum urea, suggesting dehydration in this case. It is possible that he was prescribed a diuretic for symptoms of chronic obstructive airways disease, which have precipitated renal failure by causing dehydration.

An alternative suggestion is that he has developed severe cardiac failure leading to pulmonary oedema causing hypoxia and respiratory acidosis and hypoperfusion of the kidneys, resulting in metabolic acidosis from renal failure. Other causes of combined respiratory and metabolic disorders are shown (*Table*).

Other causes of combined respiratory and metabolic acidosis

- Aspirin poisoning
- Severe pneumonia with renal failure due to septicaemia or interstitial nephritis (Legionnaire's disease)
- Septicaemia from any cause complicated by ARDS
- Malaria complicated by pneumonia
- Acute renal failure and fluid overload
- Renal pulmonary syndromes: anti-GBM disease, Wegener's granulomatosis, microscopic polyarteritis nodosa
- Acute massive pulmonary embolism
- Cardiac arrest (before ventilation)

Question 35

A 14-year-old male presented with joint pains, polydipsia and polyuria.

Respiratory function tests are shown.

	Actual	Predicted
FEV$_1$ (l)	2.0	4.5
FVC (l)	4.0	5.6
FEV$_1$/FVC	50%	80%
TLC (l)	4.9	7.0
Residual volume (l)	1.7	2.2
KCO (mmol/l/kPa)	5.0	10

1. What is demonstrated by the respiratory function tests?
2. In the context of the history, what is the diagnosis?
3. How would you confirm the diagnosis?
4. If these were the respiratory function tests of a young male with recurrent respiratory tract infections, what diagnosis would you consider?

Question 36

A 64-year-old patient who had been attending the cardiology clinic for 15 years presented with increasing breathlessness on exertion and a reduced appetite. Examination of the face is shown (**36a, b**).

Investigations are shown.

Hb	13 g/dl
WCC	7 × 10^9/l
Platelets	190 × 10^9/l
MCV	80 fl
Sodium	135 mmol/l
Potassium	4.1 mmol/l
Urea	8 mmol/l
Creatinine	100 µmol/l
Bilirubin	48 µmol/l
AST	160 iu/l
Alkaline phosphatase	180 iu/l
Albumin	39 g/l
Thyroxine	190 nmol/l
TSH	<0.1 mu/l
ECG	Atrial fibrillation
	Ventricular rate 80/min
Echocardiogram	Enlarged left atrium
	Normal-sized left ventricle with good function
	Normal valves

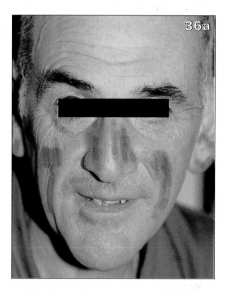

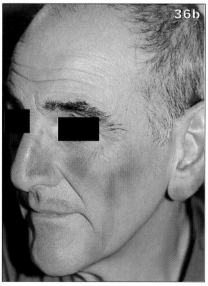

1. Give one possible explanation for the breathlessness and all the abnormalities on the blood tests.
2. What investigation would you perform to investigate the breathlessness further?

Answer 35

> 1. A mixed obstructive and restrictive defect with a reduced KCO. The low FEV1/FVC ratio is in keeping with an obstructive defect; however, the low residual volume also suggests a restrictive pattern.
> 2. The combination of polydipsia and polyuria with respiratory involvement is suggestive of diabetes insipidus. In a young patient with a mixed restrictive and obstructive defect the most likely diagnosis is histiocytosis X.
> 3. Transbronchial lung biopsy/liver biopsy/trephine aspirate may all show histiocytes and small round cells.
> 4. Cystic fibrosis.

Histiocytosis X is a benign disorder of unknown aetiology. It generally affects many systems, but in up to 25% of cases only one system may be involved. The peak age of presentation is between 2 and 4 years, and the condition affects males more than females. The skin, bones, ears, lungs, eyes, and the reticuloendothelial and central nervous systems are most often affected. A skin rash is common. Individual histiocytomas are pinkish-brown papules of 1–5 mm in diameter. Respiratory manifestations include lung fibrosis, bullae and large airway obstruction by histiocytomas. Therefore, both restrictive and/or obstructive respiratory function patterns may occur. Bone involvement with marrow infiltration may be associated with pancytopenia. Any bone may be involved, but there appears to be a special predilection to the skull bones, where it manifests as large radiolucent lesions. Otitis externa and a troublesome aural discharge occur in some patients. Ocular involvement is usually characterized by a retro-orbital mass, resulting in proptosis. Hepatosplenomegaly and lymphadenopathy may be present. Occasionally, lymphadenopathy may be massive. One-third of patients develop diabetes insipidus due to histiocytic infiltration of the pituitary stalk. Spinal cord compression may occur in exceptional cases.

The diagnosis is based on the demonstration of histiocytes and small round cells in histological specimens of affected tissues. Management is with steroids, but in some cases cytotoxic drugs such as vincristine or etoposide may be useful. In some cases spontaneous regression may occur.

Answer 36

> 1. Amiodarone toxicity.
> 2. Formal lung function tests including a KCO estimation.

The patient has biochemical evidence of hepatitis and hyperthyroidism. In a patient who has been attending the cardiology clinic for several years, and has underlying atrial fibrillation, it is highly likely that these abnormalities are due to the toxicity of amiodarone which was prescribed to control the AF. Amiodarone is a class III anti-arrhythmic agent which is very effective in the management of ventricular and supraventricular arrhythmias; however, it is associated with several side-effects and complications (*Table*). Lung fibrosis is an important complication and almost certainly accounts for the patient's breathlessness. Early interstitial fibrosis may not be apparent on chest X-ray, but is suggested by a low KCO on respiratory function tests. Both hyperthyroidism and hypothyroidism are recognized due to the iodine content of the drug. Asymptomatic biochemical hepatitis may occur and some patients may progress to cirrhosis of the liver. Patients on amiodarone should have an annual thyroid test, an LFT and a KCO estimation. Photosensitivity is common, and long-term use is associated with slate-grey skin pigmentation (**36a, b**). Corneal microdeposits are universal and may cause night glare; however, these resolve on withdrawal of the drug.

Side-effects and complications of amiodarone

Side-effects	Complications
Nausea	Optic neuritis
Metallic taste in the mouth	Peripheral neuropathy
	Myopathy
Nightmares	Hepatitis/cirrhosis
Tremor	Alveolitis
Headaches	Hyper/hypothyroidism
Rashes including phototoxicity	Epididymitis
	Conduction tissue disturbances

Question 37

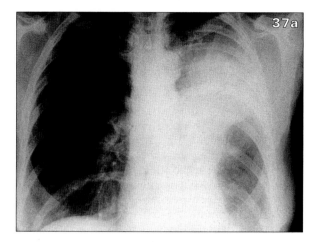

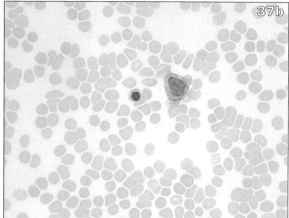

A 66-year-old retired plumber was seen in the Accident and Emergency Department with progressively increasing dyspnoea and left-sided chest discomfort, which was worse on inspiration. He had been seen by his GP one week previously, and treated with antibiotics for a chest infection. According to his wife, his appetite had been reduced and he had lost at least 6.5 kg in weight over six weeks. He stopped smoking five years previously, but before this was smoking 30 cigarettes per day for over 40 years.

On examination, he appeared thin and tachypnoeic. There was no clinical evidence of cyanosis, but he had early clubbing. His voice was hoarse. Respiratory examination revealed reduced chest expansion of the left hemithorax and dullness to percussion with reduced air entry affecting the left anterior hemithorax. A chest radiograph taken is shown (**37a**).

The patient was given oral amoxycillin and erythromycin for one week, and asked to return for repeat chest X-ray in two weeks. However, only four days later he was admitted as an emergency with increasing confusion. According to his wife, he had been extremely thirsty and was waking several times each night to pass large volumes of urine!

Investigations on this occasion are shown.

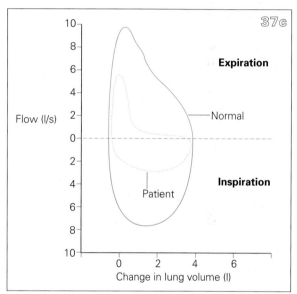

Hb	10.8 g/dl
WCC	14.2 × 10⁹/l
Platelets	80 × 10⁹/l
MCV	91 fl
Sodium	133 mmol/l
Potassium	3.9 mmol/l
Urea	18 mmol/l
Creatinine	179 µmol/l
Glucose	8.1 mmol/l
Urinalysis	Glucose 0
	Ketones +

Blood film (**37b**)
Flow loop curve (**37c**)

1. What is the probable underlying diagnosis?
2. What are the two abnormalities on the flow loop curve?
3. Give five possible reasons for his confusion.
4. What are the most likely reasons for his polydipsia and polyuria?
5. Give two reasons why this man is incurable.

Answer 37

1. Bronchial carcinoma affecting the left lung.
2. i. Severely reduced expiratory flow consistent with obstructive airways disease.
   ii. Reduced inspiratory flow limb consistent with upper airways obstruction. In this case it is probably due to a laryngeal nerve palsy causing vocal cord paralysis. (See 'Interpretation of Respiratory Flow Loop Curves', page 420.)
3. i. Hypercalcaemia.
   ii. Cerebral metastases.
   iii. Hypoxia.
   iv. Concurrent respiratory tract infection.
   v. Dehydration.
4. i. Hypercalcaemia.
   ii. Cranial diabetes insipidus.
5. i. Local and distant metastases (recurrent laryngeal nerve, bone and brain).
   ii. Poor respiratory reserve.

The chest X-ray (**37a**) demonstrates a large mass arising from the left hilum, which is complicated by left upper lobe collapse. The risks for developing bronchial carcinoma are smoking and the possibility of asbestos exposure during his occupation as a plumber.

The excessive thirst and polyuria reflect diabetes insipidus. Cerebral metastases may infiltrate the hypothalamus or posterior pituitary to cause cranial diabetes insipidus by affecting the production and release of ADH, respectively. Hypercalcaemia may render the distal renal tubules refractory to the action of ADH and produce a nephrogenic diabetes insipidus. In this case, the hypercalcaemia is probably due to bony metastases because the blood film demonstrates a leuco-erythroblastic picture suggesting marrow infiltration (**37b**); however, in squamous cell bronchial carcinoma the hypercalcaemia may also be due to ectopic secretion of a PTH-related peptide.

The main contraindications to surgery include local and distant metastases and poor respiratory reserve.

Question 38

A 76-year-old Polish male was found collapsed in the toilet by the home help. He had been generally unwell for the past five months and was easily fatigued. His appetite was reduced because he felt constantly nauseous. He was seen in the Accident and Emergency Department one month ago with abdominal pain, and was diagnosed as having constipation, for which he was prescribed senna. He had not been out of bed for four days. He had a past history of hypertension and osteoarthritis. He lived alone and was becoming increasingly dependent on the social services as his health deteriorated. He smoked ten cigarettes per day.

On examination, he was confused and agitated, and appeared pale. He was malnourished and clinically dehydrated. There was no evidence of cyanosis or lymphadenopathy. His temperature was 39°C (102.2°F). The heart rate was 110 beats/min and blood pressure 105/50 mmHg. The JVP was not raised. Examination of his tongue is shown (**38a**). On examination of the cardiovascular system, he had a fourth heart sound. Respiratory examination revealed a respiratory rate of 30/min. Movement of the right hemithorax was reduced. Percussion note was dull from the right mid-zone to the base. The abdomen was thin. A liver edge was palpable

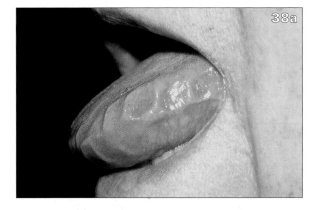

3 cm below the costal margin. Examination of the central nervous system was difficult owing to his confusion and agitation, but there was no evidence of paralysis. He was clutching his right forearm and seemed to be in severe pain on the slightest movement of his right arm. The knee and ankle jerks were absent, but the plantar response was normal. Examination of the left fundus revealed an abnormality (**38b**). Inspection of his legs is shown (**38c**).

Investigations are shown.

Hb	8 g/dl
WCC	25×10^9/l
Platelets	90×10^9/l
Blood film (**38d**)	
ESR	148 mm/h
Sodium	130 mmol/l
Potassium	4 mmol/l
Urea	16 mmol/l
Total protein	50 g/l
Albumin	18 g/l
Alkaline phosphatase	220 iu/l
AST	26 iu/l
Bilirubin	13 μmol/l
Arterial blood gases (40% O_2):	
pH	7.4
PaO_2	9 kPa
$PaCO_2$	5 kPa
Bicarbonate	18 mmol/l
Chest X-ray (**38e**)	
X-ray, right arm (**38f**)	
Bone marrow aspirate	Dry tap
Urinalysis	Protein +++
	No organisms

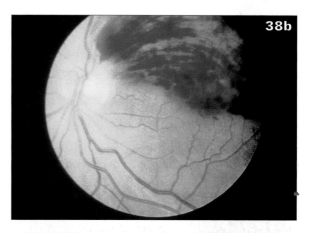

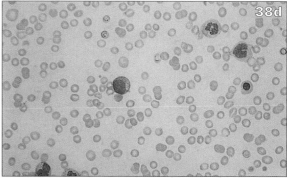

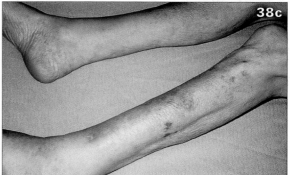

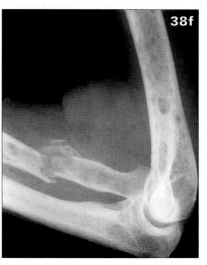

1. What is the diagnosis?
2. What is the cause of the abnormality in the left fundus?
3. Why does the patient have a painful right arm?
4. Comment on two abnormalities seen on his legs and give an explanation for each one.
5. List five complications of the disease that are evident in this patient.

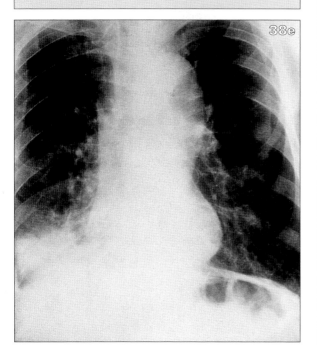

Answer 38

1. Multiple myeloma.
2. Branch retinal vein occlusion.
3. He has a pathological fracture affecting his right radius.
4. i. Oedema due to nephrotic syndrome.
   ii. Bruising secondary to thrombocytopenia or amyloid related capillary fragility.
5. i. Sepsis affecting the right lung as a result of immunoparesis. Bronchopneumonia and renal failure are the most common causes of death in multiple myeloma.
   ii. Amyloidosis. The tongue is enlarged owing to amyloid infiltration. The patient is oedematous and hypoalbuminaemic and has marked proteinuria, suggesting nephrotic syndrome, which is a manifestation of renal amyloid. Amyloid often affects the heart in myeloma, and is an important cause of death. Skin deposits, a peripheral neuropathy and massive hepatic infiltration are all recognized features of amyloidosis associated with multiple myeloma.
   iii. Bony involvement. There are numerous lytic lesions affecting the right humerus and a pathological fracture. The blood picture (**38d**) reflects a leuco-erythroblastic picture which, in this case, is probably due to marrow infiltration of myeloma cells, although severe sepsis is also a recognized cause. The typical appearance of plasma cells is shown in the marrow (**38g**). The cell nuclei sit at the edge of the cytoplasm and are well defined.
   iv. Hyperviscosity leading to venous thrombosis in the retinal vein. Hyperviscosity occurs when the paraprotein level is very high. Venous and arterial thrombosis can occur almost anywhere.
   v. Renal failure. The raised urea suggests renal failure. There are several recognized causes of renal failure in myeloma, which are shown (*Table*). Myeloma is also a recognized cause of proximal RTA; however, this does not cause renal failure *per se*.

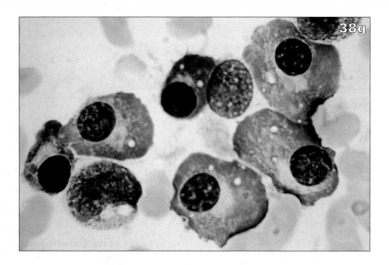

Recognized causes of renal failure in myeloma

- Tubular obstruction by light chain deposits
- Infiltration of plasma cells in the kidney ('myeloma kidney')
- Hypercalcaemia
- Hyperuricaemic nephropathy
- Amyloidosis
- Recurrent pyelonephritis secondary to immunoparesis
- Renal vein thrombosis secondary to hyperviscosity
- Renal failure secondary to analgesics, such as non-steroidal anti-inflammatory drugs
- Renal failure secondary to contrast agents, e.g. for an IVP

Question 39

A 60-year-old female presented with a four-month history of headaches and general malaise. Over the past three weeks she had developed nausea and epigastric pain after meals. She was restless at night and had noticed occasional palpitations, but attributed these symptoms to fear of illness. She also had of episodic diarrhoea. On examination, she appeared anxious. She had an irregular swelling in her neck, which moved vertically with swallowing. Her heart rate was 120 beats/min, and regular; blood pressure was 180/105 mmHg. Examination of all the major systems was normal. Investigations are shown.

Hb	17 g/dl
WCC	9×10^9/l
Platelets	300×10^9/l
Sodium	135 mmol/l
Potassium	3.4 mmol/l
Urea	10 mmol/l
Creatinine	120 µmol/l
Calcium	2.8 mmol/l
Phosphate	0.6 mmol/l
Blood glucose	10 mmol/l
TSH	3 mu/l

1. What is the cause of this patient's epigastric pain?
2. Give two explanations for the diarrhoea.
3. What is the most likely cause for the hypertension?
4. How would you explain her haemoglobin level?
5. What is the complete diagnosis?
6. List two tests you would perform to investigate the thyroid swelling.

Question 40

M-mode echocardiograms of two women (A and B), who were investigated for breathlessness in a busy cardiology clinic, are shown (40a, b).

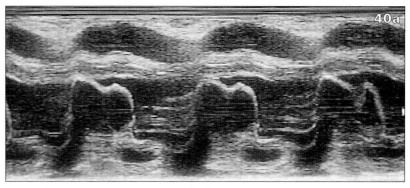

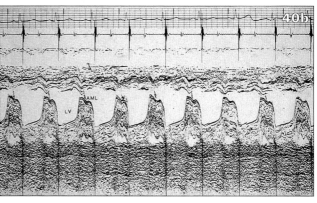

1. What is the diagnosis in female A?
   a. Mitral valve prolapse.
   b. Hypertrophic cardiomyopathy.
   c. Mitral valve endocarditis.
   d. Rheumatic mitral stenosis.
   e. Aortic regurgitation.

2. What is the diagnosis in female B?
   a. Hypertrophic cardiomyopathy.
   b. Atrial myxoma.
   c. Mitral valve endocarditis.
   d. Pericardial effusion.
   e. Rheumatic mitral stenosis.

Answer 39

1. Hypercalcaemia (peptic ulcer disease, pancreatitis).
2. i. Raised calcitonin levels.
   ii. Phaeochromocytoma.
3. Phaeochromocytoma.
4. Secondary polycythaemia in association with phaeochromocytoma.
5. Multiple endocrine neoplasia type 2 (MEN 2).
6. i. Fine-needle aspiration of the thyroid.
   ii. Serum calcitonin.

The patient has hypercalcaemia and hypertension associated with palpitations. She has an irregular swelling in the neck, which is consistent with a thyroid goitre. The TSH is normal, indicating that she is euthyroid. The low serum phosphate and high calcium levels indicate that primary hyperparathyroidism is the most likely cause of the raised calcium. Although primary hyperparathyroidism by itself is a recognized cause of hypertension, it does not account for the palpitations and restlessness, which are best explained by a coexisting phaeochromocytoma. The combination of primary hyperparathyroidism and phaeochromocytoma should lead one to consider the possibility of MEN 2. In the context of this question it is very probable that the thyroid goitre represents a medullary cell carcinoma.

MEN 2 consists of tumours arising from thyroid C cell carcinoma, the parathyroid gland and the adrenal medulla; the latter is the most common expression of the disorder. It is rare below the age of 20, and becomes more common from there onwards. One-third of cases occur in patients aged over 70 years. The genetic abnormality is within the RET proto-oncogene on chromosome 10. The gene encodes a transmembrane glycoprotein receptor tyrosine kinase.

Medullary cell carcinoma develops in 80% of cases and is usually the first presentation; however, MEN 2 accounts for only 10–20% of all medullary cell carcinomas. Management is with surgery. Persistently elevated calcitonin levels after surgery suggest that the patient is not cured. Phaeochromocytomas occur in 50% of cases and are usually bilateral and may be asymptomatic; therefore, annual screening with urinary catecholamine measurements is advised. Hyperparathyroidism occurs in only 5–10% and is restricted to certain families.

Screening in families with known disease is by genetic testing. Patients who are gene-positive should have a prophylactic thyroidectomy at a young age, and should then be screened annually with serum PTH, and urinary catecholamine estimation. In those families in whom a genetic abnormality has not been demonstrated, annual serum calcitonin should also be performed, and fine-needle aspiration of the thyroid is indicated if a goitre appears, or if the calcitonin becomes elevated.

Answer 40

1. a. Mitral valve prolapse.
2. b. Atrial myxoma.

Female A (40a): the mitral valve has a normal appearance in diastole. In systole, both the anterior and posterior leaflets appose normally in the beginning; however, in mid systole there is posterior movement (prolapse) of both leaflets, but predominantly the posterior leaflet. This is characteristic of mitral valve prolapse and is responsible for the mid-systolic clicks and/or the mid-systolic murmur of mitral regurgitation. Mitral valve prolapse is present in 2–5% of the general population. It is generally benign but may be associated with symptoms of sharp inframammary chest pain, breathlessness even with normal ventricular function, palpitation and odd neurological symptoms. There is a risk of infective endocarditis in patients with consequent mitral regurgitation, in whom prophylactic antibiotics during dental work are recommended, and supraventricular arrhythmias. Mitral valve prolapse has been implicated as a cause of sudden cardiac death in highly trained athletes, but its significance as the only finding at post-mortem is controversial because the high prevalence of the condition may mean the finding is coincidental, rather than causal. It is more likely that death may have been caused by the association of mitral valve prolapse with the Wolff–Parkinson–White syndrome causing atrial fibrillation which degenerates to ventricular fibrillation, or the LQTS, which causes polymorphic ventricular tachycardia.

Female B (40b): there is echogenic shadowing in the mitral valve orifice that is typical of atrial myxoma. The condition is discussed in Answer 178. (See also Echocardiography, page 421.)

Question 41

A 45-year-old woman presented with a three-week history of fever, persistent dry cough, headache and photophobia. She lived with her son, who owned two greyhounds and several racing pigeons. The patient had not travelled abroad.

On examination she had a temperature of 38.2°C (100.8°F) and was slightly confused. She had a generalized macular rash but there was no obvious evidence of lymphadenopathy.

Examination of the respiratory system was normal, with the exception of a respiratory rate of 18 per min. Both heart sounds were normal; there were no added heart sounds or murmurs. Abdominal examination revealed hepatomegaly palpable three finger-breadths from the costal margin and a palpable spleen 2 cm below the costal margin.

Investigations are shown.

Hb	11 g/dl
WCC	12 × 10⁹/l
Platelets	380 × 10⁹/l
Sodium	130 mmol/l
Potassium	3.7 mmol/l
Urea	8 mmol/l
Creatinine	70 μmol/l
Bilirubin	12 μmol/l
AST	46 iu/l
ALT	52 iu/l
Alkaline phosphatase	100 iu/l
Albumin	34 g/l

What is the first-line antibiotic of choice in her management?
   a. Ciprofloxacin.
   b. Tetracycline.
   c. Erythromycin.
   d. Benzyl penicillin.
   e. Rifampicin.

Question 42

A 42-year-old woman with a past medical history of systemic lupus erythematosus that was well-controlled on methotrexate, presented with a four-day history of right lower chest pain that was sharp in character and worse on inspiration, along with chest wall tenderness. There was no history of cough, breathlessness, haemoptysis or fever.

Investigations are shown.

Hb	11.2 g/dl
WCC	6 × 10⁹/l
Platelets	260 × 10⁹/l
ESR	23 mm/h
CRP	3 g/l
Sodium	134 mmol/l
Potassium	4.1 mmol/l
Urea	9 mmol/l
Creatinine	130 μmol/l
C3	0.35 g/l (NR 0.55–1.20 g/l)
C4	0.26 g/l (NR 0.2–0.5 g/l)
Chest X-ray	Normal
Oxygen saturation on air	98%

What is the diagnosis?
   a. Costochondritis.
   b. Pulmonary embolism.
   c. Relapse of systemic lupus erythematosus.
   d. Right lower lobe pneumonia.
   e. *Pneumocystis carinii* infection.

Answer 41

> b. Tetracycline.

A history of dry cough, fever, headache and photophobia in a patient who is in contact with racing pigeons is consistent with the diagnosis of psittacosis, which is caused by the Gram-negative bacterium *Chlamydia psittaci*. Psittacine birds are the primary reservoir and man is an incidental host. The organism is transmitted to man via aerosol inhalation of faecal and urinary products on bird feathers. *Chlamydia psittaci* infection is an occupational hazard in pet-shop employees, veterinary doctors and nurses, zoo personnel and workers in poultry processing plants. *Chlamydia psittaci* infection is rare and accounts for 1% of all atypical pneumonias.

Clinical presentation includes a dry cough and fever, which may be abrupt in onset. Headache is a prominent feature and may be accompanied by photophobia; however, genuine meningitis is a rare complication of the infection. Malaise, night sweats, anorexia, diarrhoea and delirium are recognized. The respiratory features may be mild but fulminant respiratory failure may occur in a few cases.

Extrapulmonary complications do occur but with a much lower frequency than in *Mycoplasma pneumonia* infection (*Table A*). Jaundice is rare.

Respiratory examination reveals evidence of pleurisy, consolidation or effusion. Splenomegaly and hepatomegaly are present in 10% of cases.

Rapid diagnosis is not possible. The diagnostic investigation of choice is the complement fixation test. First-line therapy is tetracycline or doxycycline. Erythromycin is a second-line drug.

Other chlamydial infections (*Table B*)
Infection due to *Chlamydia pneumoniae* causes pneumonia that is indistinguishable from pneumonia secondary to *Streptococcus pneumoniae* infection. Unlike *Mycoplasma* infection, which affects young individuals, *Chlamydia pneumoniae* infection affects patients in the seventh and eighth decades. Hoarseness, pharyngitis and sinusitis are common. The white cell count is normal and the chest X-ray usually shows patchy subsegmental consolidation.

Extrapulmonary complications as seen in *Mycoplasma pneumonia* and psittacosis are recognized but rare. Of interest is the fact that infection has been associated with atherosclerosis. Diagnosis and treatment are the same as for *Chlamydia psittaci* infection.

Table A Extrapulmonary complications of *Chlamydia psittaci* infection (psittacosis)

Cardiac	Endocarditis, pericarditis and myocarditis
Neurological	Encephalitis, transverse myelitis, Guillain–Barré syndrome
Glomerulonephritis	
Pancreatitis	
Haemolysis	
Thyroiditis	
Dermatological	Erythema nodosum

Table B Infections causes by *Chlamydia* species

Chlamydia trachomatis	
	Males
	Non-gonococcal urethritis
	Lymphogranuloma venerum
	Epididymitis
	Prostatitis
	Proctitis (homosexuals)
	Reactive arthritis (Reiter syndrome)
	Females
	Non-gonococcal urethritis
	Cervicitis
	Pelvic inflammatory disease
	Peri-hepatitis (Fitzhugh–Curtis syndrome)
	Newborns (born to infected mothers)
	Conjunctivitis
	Pneumonia
Chlamydia pneumoniae	Pneumonia
Chlamydia psittaci	Psittacosis

Answer 42

> c. Relapse of systemic lupus erythematosus.

This is a difficult question since there is a very limited amount of data provided. However, the combination of serositis, myalgia, low ESR relative to CRP, and complement at the lower limits of normal in a patient with SLE is suggestive of recurrence of lupus rather than any of the other options provided. (See Question 264.)

Question 43

A 72-year-old male with a known history of chronic obstructive airway disease had eight admissions to hospital with a cough and breathlessness over a 12-month period. He had stopped smoking two years previously. His normal exercise capacity was limited to 27.5 metres on the flat before stopping. He was taking salmeterol, pulmicort and oxivent inhalers, and had received several courses of steroids in the past year.

On examination he was cyanosed. His heart rate was 100 beats/min and regular. His blood pressure measured 110/70 mmHg. The JVP was raised 4 cm above the costal margin at 45°. The trachea was central. Chest expansion was generally reduced. Percussion note was hyper-resonant and on auscultation of the lungs there was generalized reduction of air entry throughout. Both heart sounds were soft but there were no added heart sounds or murmurs.

Investigations are shown.

Hb	19 g/dl
PCV	0.56 l/l
WCC	8×10^9/l
Platelets	340×10^9/l
MCV	82 fl
Chest X-ray	Hyper-inflated lung fields
Arterial blood gases:	
pH	7.35
PaO_2	7.5 kPa
$PaCO_2$	6.1 kPa
Bicarbonate	34 mmol/l
Echocardiography	Normal left ventricle.
	Right ventricular hypertrophy and dilatation
	Pulmonary artery pressure of 42 mmHg

Which treatment is most useful for long-term survival?
   a. Oral aminophylline.
   b. Diuretic therapy.
   c. Regular venesection.
   d. High-dose steroids.
   e. Long-term oxygen therapy.

Question 44

A 35-year-old type 1 diabetic presented eight months following a renal transplant with fever, night sweats and malaise. He had experienced two episodes of transplant rejection, which were successfully reversed with corticosteroids. He was currently maintained on prednisolone and ciclosporin. On examination he had a temperature of 39°C (102.2°F). The heart rate was 120 beats/min and blood pressure was 140/60 mmHg. The respiratory rate was 40/min. Precordial examination revealed an early diastolic murmur at the left lower sternal edge. The chest was clear. The abdomen including the graft was non-tender.

Investigations are shown.

What is the most likely diagnosis?
   a. Acute renal transplant rejection.
   b. CMV infection.
   c. Infective endocarditis.
   d. Gram-negative sepsis.
   e. Ciclosporin nephrotoxicity.

Hb	10 g/dl
WCC	10×10^9/l
Neutrophils	7×10^9/l
Lymphocytes	2.5×10^9/l
Eosinophils	0.04×10^9/l
Basophils	0.1×10^9/l
Monocytes	0.4×10^9/l
Platelets	300×10^9/l
ESR	100
Sodium	130 mmol/l
Potassium	5.5 mmol/l
Chloride	87 mmol/l
Bicarbonate	22 mmol/l
Urea	9 mmol/l
Creatinine	130 μmol/l
Glucose	6 mmol/l
Urine output	45 ml/hr
Urinary microscopy	Red blood cells and no white cell casts
ECG	Sinus tachycardia

Answer 43

> e. Long-term oxygen therapy.

Indications for long-term oxygen therapy are a PO$_2$ of 7.3–8 kPa once stable and either secondary polycythaemia, nocturnal hypoxaemia, peripheral oedema or pulmonary hypertension. The patient in question fulfils the criteria. Other patients for whom long-term oxygen therapy may be considered include those who have normal oxygen saturation at rest but desaturate on exercise, and those in whom exercise capacity is improved with oxygen therapy.

Answer 44

> c. Infective endocarditis.

Infection is the commonest life-threatening complication of long-term immunosuppressive therapy (*Table*). More than 6 months post-transplant most patients have stable allografts and are maintained on minimal immunosuppressive therapy. Infection in the majority of these patients is usually similar to that seen in the general population. The patient in question has a murmur of aortic regurgitation and a high fever, raising the possibility of infective endocarditis.

The overall incidence of bacterial endocarditis is much greater in renal transplant recipients than in the general population. Independent risk factors for bacterial endocarditis include a history of hospitalization for valvular heart disease, graft loss and increased duration of dialysis before transplantation. The mean time from transplantation to diagnosis of endocarditis is estimated to be three and a half years (range two months to 15 years), with an overall mortality of 50%.

The increased susceptibility of renal transplant recipients to infective endocarditis can probably be explained by a combination of necessary invasive procedures (e.g. intravascular line placement) during the immediate post-transplant period as well as immunosuppression for prevention of organ rejection. Pre-existing valvular abnormality in renal transplant patients may also be conducive to endocarditis similar to that in non-transplant patients. Immunosuppression plays an important role in the development of fungal endocarditis, but may also be important in the clearance of streptococci from the blood in this patient population. In contrast to the frequent pre-existing valve abnormality associated with bacterial endocarditis, the great majority of solid organ transplant recipients with *Aspergillus* endocarditis have no pre-existing valvular abnormalities. Myocardial abscesses have been commonly reported with *Aspergillus* endocarditis.

The most common causes of endocarditis among renal transplant recipients are fungi (particularly *Aspergillus* species) and *S. aureus*. Less common causes include *Corynebacterium* species, viridans streptococci, vancomycin-resistant *Enterococcus* species, *Brucella* species, *Clostridium* species, *Nocardia* species and *Erysipelothrix* species.

Skin manifestations of endocarditis and/or splenomegaly seem to be uncommon in transplant patients, while septic emboli and mycotic aneurysms are more frequent. The most common clinical signs and symptoms at the time of presentation are fever and embolic phenomena. The mitral valve is thought to be the most frequently involved cardiac valve, followed by the intramural cardiac surface and the aortic valve. Even in the absence of immunosuppression the leucocyte count is elevated in only 20–30% of cases and may be normal.

Most episodes of acute rejection occur in the first six months after surgery. However, the absence of a rise in serum creatinine, fall in urine output and graft pain/tenderness make rejection unlikely.

Ciclosporin nephrotoxicty is a recognized complication in transplant patients and is characterized by a falling glomerular filtration rate, hyperkalaemia, hyperuricaemia and a hyperchloraemic acidosis.

Infection in immunosuppressive therapy	
Time	*Infection*
Month 1	Usual post-surgical infections (as seen in immunocompetent patients)
Months 2–6	CMV and other opportunistic infections
Month 6 onwards	Community acquired infections (viral and bacterial) and recurrence of inadequately treated opportunistic infections

Question 45

A 52-year-old woman was referred to a chest physician with a six-month history of dyspnoea associated with a non-productive cough, intermittent fever and night sweats. At the onset of the illness her symptoms were intermittent, usually worse in the evenings, but over the past few weeks they had become more persistent. The patient also complained of reduced appetite and loss of weight. She had worked on a farm with her husband for the past four years. She smoked ten cigarettes per day. There was no previous history of breathlessness.

On examination she was thin. There was evidence of peripheral cyanosis but no clubbing. Auscultation of the lungs was normal. The chest X-ray showed reticulo-nodular shadowing affecting the upper and mid zones.

What is the most probable diagnosis?
   a. Cryptogenic fibrosing alveolitis.
   b. Chronic bronchitis.
   c. Tuberculosis.
   d. Extrinsic allergic alveolitis.
   e. Allergic bronchopulmonary aspergillosis.

Question 46

A 19-year-old man was admitted for further investigation for a six-month history of lethargy and depression. 11 months previously he had collapsed while on holiday in San Francisco when walking on a very hot day and was treated for dehydration. The patient had a history of epilepsy that was confined to the winter months! He was one of three siblings. His sisters, aged 17 and 20, were fit and well.

On examination he was 1.52 m tall. He had a short neck and a left-sided divergent squint. There was no pallor. His heart rate was 68 beats/min and his blood pressure was 110/70 mmHg. There was a palpable thyroid goitre. Neurological examination was normal as was examination of all other systems.

Blood tests performed by the GP are shown.

Hb	13 g/dl
WCC	4.5×10^9/l
Platelets	259×10^9/l
Sodium	137 mmol/l
Potassium	3.9 mmol/l
Urea	4 mmol/l
Creatinine	70 μmol/l
Calcium	1.8 mmol/l
Phosphate	1.9 mmol/l
Albumin	42 g/l
Alkaline phosphatase	100 iu/l
Bicarbonate	24 mmol/l
TSH	18 iu/l
Thyroxine	40 iu/l
24-h urinary calcium excretion	Increased
Chest X-ray	Normal

What is the most probable unifying diagnosis?
   a. Hypoparathyroidism.
   b. Hypothyroidism.
   c. Pseudohypoparathyroidism.
   d. Polyglandular endocrine deficiency type II.
   e. Polyglandular endocrine deficiency type I.

Question 47

A 28-year-old woman who is eight weeks pregnant attends a genetic counselling service with her husband, who is a lawyer. His brother is heterozygous for the Δ508 mutation for cystic fibrosis. The husband agrees to be screened and is also found to be heterozygous for the mutation. The pregnant woman in question declines the screening test.

Assuming that the Δ508 mutation has a prevalence of 1:20 in the British population, what is the chance of her having a child with the condition?
   a. 1 in 20.
   b. 1 in 80.
   c. 1 in 400.
   d. 1 in 160.
   e. 1 in 4.

Answer 45

> d. Extrinsic allergic alveolitis.

The patient is a farmer's wife and her original symptoms were consistent with an allergic (hypersensitivity) pneumonitis; however, more recently she has developed persistent breathlessness, suggesting advanced parenchymal lung disease. Repeated episodes of pneumonitis progress to pulmonary fibrosis. The CXR in the acute and subacute forms of the disorder may reveal fleeting micronodular interstitial shadows affecting the upper, mid and lower zones. It is important to note that the CXR may be normal in a few cases. In more chronic cases the CXR is similar to that seen in cryptogenic fibrosing alveolitis except that in EAA fibrosis is usually more pronounced in the upper zones.

Diagnostic features of EAA:

1. Evidence of exposure to a recognized antigen
2. Compatible clinical radiographic and physiological features (i.e. cough, wheeze, fever, micronodular shadows in upper, mid or lower zones, restrictive lung defect)
3. Bronchoalveolar lavage with lymphocytosis (with low CD4 to CD8 ratio)
4. Positive inhalation challenge test
5. Compatible histopathological changes

The diagnosis is possible without histological confirmation on lung biopsy if criteria 1–3 are met.

Farm workers have a higher risk of developing chronic obstructive airways disease than the general population; however, the history and chest X-ray findings mean that EAA is a better answer. Cryptogenic pulmonary fibrosis is unlikely in the presence of an obvious precipitating factor such as *Micropolyspora faenii* in this case and should only be considered once EAA has been excluded. Allergic bronchopulmonary aspergillosis is characterized by wheeze, raised eosinophil count, and proximal bronchiectasis on the chest X-ray. (See Question 272.)

Answer 46

> c. Pseudohypoparathyroidism.

The patient has low calcium and high phosphate levels in the absence of abnormal renal function. The differential diagnosis is between hypoparathyroidism and pseudohypoparathyroidism. Pseudohypoparathyroidism is due to the end-organ resistance to the effects of PTH, which are mediated via adenylate cyclase. The morphological features in this patient (short stature, squint) are more common in pseudohypoparathyroidism. Furthermore, the patient has biochemical hypothyroidism, which is a more common association with pseudohypoparathyroidism and is due to end-organ resistance to the actions of TSH, which also mediates its effects via adenylate cyclase. (See Question 159.)

Answer 47

> b. 1 in 80.

The gene frequency of the mutation in question is 1/20, hence the chances of the pregnant woman carrying the mutation is 1 in 20. Her husband has been screened and is a definite carrier. Therefore, the chances of them both having a heterozygous genetic mutation is

$$1/20 \times 1/1 = 1/20.$$

If both partners are heterozygous for an autosomal recessive disorder such as cystic fibrosis, the chances of a child being affected is 1 in 4. Therefore the overall chances of the couple having a child with cystic fibrosis is $1/20 \times 1/4 = 1/80$. (See Genetics page 415.)

Question 48

An alcoholic vagrant was admitted to the Accident and Emergency Department after being found collapsed on the street. Four hours previously he had been spotted wandering outside the hospital and appeared well.

On examination he had a Glasgow coma scale of 5. His heart rate was 120 beats/min and regular. The blood pressure measured 80/50 mmHg. The respiratory rate was 24/min. The patient was apyrexial. The pupils were dilated. Neurological examination revealed blurred disk margins and depressed reflexes.

Investigations are shown.

Sodium	131 mmol/l
Potassium	5.4 mmol/l
Urea	5 mmol/l
Creatinine	110 μmol/l
Bicarbonate	12 mmol/l
Chloride	96 mmol/l
Glucose	6 mmo/l
Amylase	120 iu/l
	(NR <220 iu/l)
Plasma osmolality	320 mOsm/l
ECG	Sinus tachycardia, left axis deviation
Arterial blood gases:	
pH	7.21
PaO_2	9 kPa
$PaCO_2$	2.1 kPa
Bicarbonate	12 mmol/l
Blood lactate	6 mmol/l
Urinalysis	Protein 0
	Glucose 0
	Ketones +

What is the diagnosis?
a. Euglycaemic ketoacidosis.
b. Methanol toxicity.
c. Ethylene glycol poisoning.
d. Tricyclic antidepressant overdose.
e. Hepatic encephalopathy.

Question 49

A 29-year-old woman presented with sudden onset of weakness affecting the left side of the body. There was no history of headaches or head injury. She had previously been well with the exception of having mild Raynaud's disease. The patient had a history of two previous miscarriages four years ago but had had a successful pregnancy six months previously that was complicated by a below-knee deep vein thrombosis. She worked as a clerk in a large business firm prior to her pregnancy. Her appetite was good and her weight was stable.

On examination she had a left facial palsy and obvious left-sided weakness. Her heart rate was 80 beats/min and regular. The blood pressure was 150/88 mmHg. The temperature was 36.8°C (98.2°F). Both heart sounds were normal; there was a soft systolic murmur in the pulmonary area. The chest was clear. Investigations are shown.

Hb	11 g/dl
WCC	$11 \times 10^9/l$
Platelets	$152 \times 10^9/l$
ESR	11 mm/h
CT scan brain	Infarct in right middle cerebral artery territory
Trans-thoracic echocardiogram	Normal.

What is the most probable cause of the stroke?
a. Atrial septal defect complicated by paradoxical embolus.
b. Atrial myxoma.
c. Saggital vein thrombosis complicating recent pregnancy.
d. Lupus anticoagulant syndrome.
e. Cerebral abscess.

Answer 48

> b. Methanol toxicity.

The main differential diagnoses of severe metabolic acidosis and collapse specific to an individual who abuses alcohol includes methanol toxicity, ethylene glycol poisoning, acute severe pancreatitis and acute hepatic failure. The patient has a normal amylase therefore acute pancreatitis is unlikely. The actual plasma osmolality is higher than the calculated plasma osmolality (approximately 284 mOsm/l) suggesting the presence of a large concentration of an osmotically active substance. The most probable candidates include methanol or ethylene glycol (anti-freeze). Both conditions present with drunkenness, acidosis and coma and in untreated cases the mortality is high. Methanol and ethylene glycol are relatively toxic; however, once ingested they are metabolized to formic acid (methanoic acid) and glycolic acid, respectively, by the enzyme alcohol dehydrogenase, both of which are very toxic.

Patients with methanol toxicity may complain of headache, nausea, fatigue or reduced visual acuity if not comatosed. Reduced visual acuity is due to optic nerve damage resulting from increased concentrations of formic acid, the oxidized metabolite of methanol. Mydriasis, reduced visual reflexes to light and hyperaemia of the optic disc are early features of methanol toxicity. Untreated patients may develop blindness. Patients with ethylene glycol poisoning may present in a similar fashion; however, reduced visual acuity is not a classical feature whereas flank pain and renal failure due to crystallization of oxalic acid in the renal tubules is common. Urinalysis under Wood's light in patients with ethylene glycol poisoning may reveal oxalate crystals in the urine but an absence does not exclude the diagnosis. Patients with ethylene glycol poisoning also develop severe cardiac failure if untreated. The presence of visual symptoms favour methanol intoxication in this case.

The management of methanol toxicity and ethylene glycol toxicity is the same, as tabulated below. Tricyclic anti-depressant overdose can also present with acidosis and dilated pupils; however, one would have expected brisk reflexes and possible wide QRS complexes on the 12-lead ECG. (See Question 28.)

The management of methanol toxicity and ethylene glycol toxicity

Step 1	Gastric decontamination within the first 4 hours of ingestion
Step 2	Intravenous bicarbonate in the presence of acidosis (100 ml of 8.4% sodium bicarbonate)
Step 3	Intravenous fomepizole (specific alcohol dehydrogenase inhibitor) should be used early, starting with a bolus of 15 mg/kg in dextrose 5% in 100 ml followed by an infusion of 10 mg/kg every 12 hours for the next 48 hours and then 15 mg/kg every 12 hours until the concentration of methanol or ethylene glycol has fallen below 20 mg/dl
Step 4	Haemodialysis in patients with refractory acidosis despite bicarbonate and fomepizole therapy or as first line in patients with a methanol level of >15 mmol/l (50 mg/dl) or an ethylene glycol level of >20 mg/dl
Step 5	Folic acid in methanol toxicity promotes the metabolism of formic acid to carbon dioxide and water. Pyridoxine and thiamine in ethylene glycol poisoning promote metabolism of ethylene glycol to less toxic metabolites such as glycine

Answer 49

> d. Lupus anticoagulant syndrome.

The patient has a predisposition to arterial and venous thromboses. She has had miscarriages in the second trimester. She also has Raynaud's phenomenon and thrombocytopenia, all of which are characteristic of lupus anticoagulant syndrome. The normal echocardiogram in this context rules out an atrial septal defect and hence a paradoxical embolus as a cause of the stroke. Echocardiography may show evidence of verrucous (Libmann–Sack) endocarditis. The manifestations of antiphospholipid syndrome are tabulated.

Manifestations of antiphospholipid syndrome

- Predisposition to arterial and venous thromboses
- Mid-trimester miscarriages in females
- Migraines
- Depression
- Chorea
- Epilepsy
- Livedo reticularis
- Thrombocytopenia
- Haemolysis
- Avascular necrosis of head of femur
- Pulmonary hypertension
- Libmann–Sack endocarditis

Question 50

A 70-year-old male presented with a one-week history of increasing confusion. According to his wife his general health had been deteriorating for about three months. His appetite was reduced. He complained of abdominal discomfort and felt excessively thirsty. He had been a heavy smoker since the age of 16.

On examination he had reduced skin turgor. The heart rate was 110 beats/min. Heart sounds were normal. The chest was clear. Abdominal examination revealed a palpable colon with hard faeces.

Investigations are shown.

Hb	11 g/dl
WCC	11 × 10⁹/l
Platelets	100 × 10⁹/l
Sodium	139 mmol/l
Potassium	5 mmol/l
Urea	20 mmol/l
Creatinine	190 μmol/l
Calcium	3.2 mmol/l
Phosphate	1.4 mmol/l
Albumin	32 g/l

What is the immediate step in his management?
  a. IV pamidronate.
  b. IV furosemide.
  c. IV saline (0.9%).
  d. IV hydrocortisone.
  e. IV calcitonin.

Question 51

A 40-year-old woman presented at the Accident and Emergency Department with a 48-hour history of headache and neck stiffness. She had returned from a holiday in the south of France just one week previously. On examination she had a temperature of 37.8°C (100.0°F). Her blood pressure measured 120/70 mmHg. There was no rash. Neurological examination was normal, with the exception of mild nuchal rigidity. Investigations are shown.

CT scan of brain	Normal
CSF analysis:	Appearance – clear
WCC	20 per mm³
	(80% lymphocytes)
Protein	0.48 g/l
Glucose	2.3 mmol/l (simultaneous blood glucose 4.5 mmol/l)
Gram stain	No organism identified

What is the diagnosist?
  a. *Herpes* simplex encephalitis.
  b. Listeria meningitis.
  c. Viral meningitis.
  d. Lyme disease.
  e. Bacterial meningitis.

Question 52

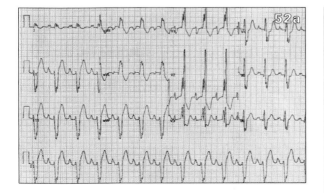

Which five statements about this 12-lead ECG (**52a**) are correct?
  a. Ventricular tachycardia.
  b. Left axis deviation.
  c. Voltage for left atrial enlargement.
  d. LBBB.
  e. Right axis deviation.
  f. Voltage criteria for right ventricular hypertrophy.
  g. RBBB.
  h. Voltage criteria for right atrial enlargement.
  i. Voltage criteria for left ventricular hypertrophy.
  j. Dissociated P-waves.
  k. Capture beats.
  l. Delta waves.

Answer 50

> c. IV saline (0.9%).

The patient has symptomatic hypercalcaemia. In general patients with hypercalcaemia rarely exhibit symptoms if the serum calcium is below 3 mmol/l. Treatment of symptomatic hypercalcaemia has to be instituted before the underlying cause is identified (*Table*). The most important aspect of management is vigorous rehydration. Most patients are dehydrated owing to fluid loss from the kidneys resulting from nephrogenic diabetes insipidus. Fluid loss may also occur from the gastrointestinal tract owing to vomiting. The general recommendation is to treat with 4 litres of saline over 24 hours and review hydration status. Some guidelines recommend the concomitant use of furosemide, as this promotes hyper-calcuria; however, in diuresis it may worsen dehydration and is best reserved for patients who exhibit fluid overload after rehydration.

All patients should receive intravenous bisphosphonates after rehydration. Most patients respond rapidly to bisphosphonate therapy. The drug can cause a bone pain, transient pyrexia, flu-like illness, rashes or iritis. Patients who do not respond to bisphosphonates may benefit from intramuscular calcitonin but the hormone is usually poorly tolerated owing to flushing, nausea and diarrhoea. Some cases of resistant hypercalcaemia respond to high-dose corticosteroid therapy. Following the acute treatment of hypercalcaemia the aim is to identify and treat the underlying cause.

Management of symptomatic hypercalcaemia

Step 1	Rehydration with intravenous saline
Step 2	Intravenous bisophosphonate therapy
Step 3	Identify and treat underlying cause if possible

Answer 51

> c. Viral meningitis.

The patient has a lymphocytic meningitis with a normal CSF protein and a very slight reduction in CSF glucose (*Table*). The differential diagnosis is between viral meningitis (and some cases of viral meningitis do cause a very slight reduction in glucose) or meningitis due to brucellosis, lyme disease, listeria monocytogenes, and partially treated bacterial meningitis. The patient has been to the south of France and one could infer that she may have indulged in soft cheeses and developed listerosis; however, listerosis usually affects immunocompromised patients including neonates and pregnant women. The patient has none of the pointers for diagnoses other than viral meningitis. (See Question 267.)

Normal CSF values

Opening pressure	60–150 mmH$_2$O
Protein content	0.2–0.4 g/l
Glucose	<2/3 blood glucose
White cell count	<5/mm^3
Red cells	0
IgG	15% of total CSF protein

Answer 52

> b. Left axis deviation.
> c. Voltage for left atrial enlargement.
> f. Voltage criteria for right ventricular hypertrophy.
> g. RBBB.
> h. Voltage criteria for right atrial enlargement.

The criteria for left and right atrial and ventricular hypertrophy are discussed in Answer 259. Bundle branch block is characterized by a wider QRS complex (more than 120 ms; three small squares on the ECG). In RBBB the QRS complex in lead VI has an rsR pattern and in LBBB the QRS complex in lead VI has a qS pattern (**52b**)

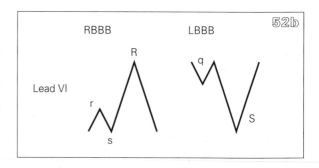

Question 53

A 63-year-old male with a known history of myocardial infarction, hypertension and peripheral vascular disease is admitted with breathlessness. The blood pressure measured 158/96 mmHg. Blood results are shown.

He was treated with diuretics and then commenced on an ACE inhibitor but after 72 hours the urea was 20 mmol/l and creatinine was 250 mmol/l. Echocardiography revealed mild impairment of left ventricular function.

Sodium	137 mmol/l
Potassium	4.5 mmol/l
Urea	11 mmol/l
Creatinine	130 mmol/l
Troponin T	<0.1ng/l (NR <0.1 ng/l)
Arterial gases (room air):	
pH	7.31
$PaCO_2$	6.4 kPa
PaO_2	7.1 kPa
Bicarbonate	16 mmol/l
Chest X-ray	Severe pulmonary oedema
ECG	LBBB
Urinalysis	Protein 0
	Blood 0

What is the most probable cause for his presentation?
a. Myocardial infarction.
b. Hypertensive cardiomyopathy.
c. Renal artery stenosis.
d. Cardiac tachycarrhythmia.
e. Myocardial dysfunction secondary to acidosis.

Question 54

A 74-year-old woman presented with a transient syncopal episode. There was a previous history of paroxysmal atrial fibrillation and congestive cardiac failure. Medications on admission included amiodarone 200 mg od, furosemide 40 mg od, enalapril 20 mg od and warfarin. The ECG on admission is shown (**54a**). Electrolytes were as follows:

While on the ward the patient complained of feeling unwell. A repeat ECG is shown (**54b**). The patient was fully conscious. The blood pressure was 160/60 mmHg.

Sodium	138 mmol/l
Potassium	4.2 mmol/l
Urea	11 mmol/l
Creatinine	128 μmol/l
Magnesium	0.8 mmol/l (NR)

What is the immediate treatment of the arrhythmia shown on **54b**?
a. IV amiodarone 300 mg.
b. IV metoprolol 5 mg.
c. IV isoprenaline infusion.
d. IV magnesium bolus (8 mmol/l).
e. IV lignocaine 100 mg.

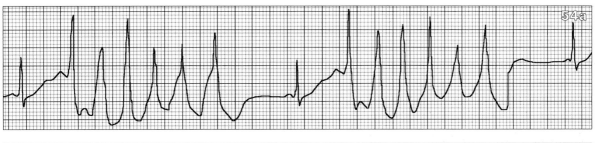

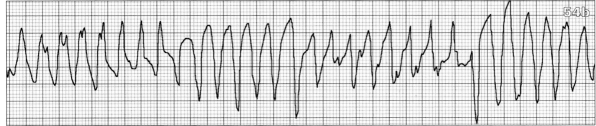

Answer 53

> c. Renal artery stenosis.

The patient presents with acute pulmonary oedema. He has a background history of ischaemic heart disease, peripheral vascular disease and hypertension. The differential diagnosis is between heart failure secondary to hypertensive heart disease, myocardial infarction or flash pulmonary oedema secondary to renal artery stenosis. The possibility of renal artery stenosis should always be considered in a patient with peripheral vascular disease and impaired renal function. The serum cardiac troponin is not raised, excluding myocardial infarction. The left ventricular function is only mildly impaired and should not cause such severe pulmonary oedema unless the patient suffered an episode of myocardial stunning due to severe ischaemia resulting from major atheromatous disease in the proximal left coronary artery, or a very rapid tachyarrhythmia. The diagnosis of renal artery stenosis is evident by the doubling of serum creatinine within three days of starting an ACE inhibitor.

Flash pulmonary oedema is a recognized complication of renal artery stenosis due to diastolic dysfunction from chronic hypertension. Presumably labile hypertension and salt and water retention through activation of the renin–angiotensin–aldosterone system are responsible. Flash pulmonary oedema is usually a feature of bilateral renal rather than unilateral renal artery stenosis. The diagnosis can be made using low-contrast CT scan of the kidneys or magnetic resonance angiography of the renal arteries.

The causes of simultaneous cardiac and renal failure are tabulated below.

Causes of simultaneous cardiac and renal failure

- Chronic hypertension
- Diabetes mellitus
- Generalized atherosclerosis (coronary and reno-vascular disease)
- Polyarteritis nodosa and other vasculitides
- Systemic sclerosis
- Antiphospholipid syndrome
- Infective endocarditis
- Amyloidosis
- Ethylene glycol poisoning

Answer 54

> d. IV magnesium bolus (8 mmol/l).

The initial ECG shows a nodal bradycardia with marked prolongation of the QT interval and U waves. The serum potassium and magnesium are normal. The most probable cause of the bradyarrhythmia and the prolongation of the QT is amiodarone toxicity. Prolonged QT is usually associated with polymorphic VT (torsades de pointes) but monomorphic ventricular tachycardia is also recognized. The most effective urgent treatment to terminate the VT is IV magnesium even in the presence of a normal serum magnesium level. The amiodarone should be stopped immediately. The patient will be at risk of further ventricular tachycardia while the QT remains prolonged. The QT interval may be shortened by an isoprenaline infusion or by temporary cardiac pacing at a ventricular rate >60/min. It may take several days before the effects of amiodarone are reversed.

Questions 55 and 56

A 69-year-old male consulted his GP with pleuritic chest pain and had reduced air entry at the left lung base. He had experienced a dry cough, fever and myalgia for 48 hours prior to the onset of the chest pain. He was a non-smoker. On examination he was alert and orientated with a mini-mental score test of 10/10. The blood pressure was 100/66 mmHg. The respiratory rate was 32/min.

Investigations are shown.

Hb	14 g/dl
WCC	$9 \times 10^9/l$
Platelets	$480 \times 10^9/l$
CRP	60 g/l
Sodium	133 mmol/l
Potassium	4.1 mmol/l
Urea	7.5 mmol/l
Creatinine	110 μmol/l
Chest X-ray	Left lower lobe consolidation
Oxygen saturation on air	94%

The patient received seven days of appropriate antibiotic therapy but remains unwell with intermittent pyrexia and anorexia. A repeat chest X-ray revealed findings consistent with a pleural effusion. A diagnostic aspiration was performed and analysis of the effusion is shown below.

Aspiration:	
Appearance	Purulent
Gram stain	Negative
Culture	Sterile
pH	7.1
Pleural fluid LDH	1000 iu/l (Plasma LDH 200 iu/l)
Pleural fluid protein	40 g/l (Total plasma protein 72 g/l)

Question 55

What is the management of this patient?
 a. Treat in the community with amoxycillin.
 b. Treat in the community with amoxycillin and clarythromycin.
 c. Admit to hospital and treat with oral amoxycillin and clarythromycin.
 d. Admit to hospital and treat with IV cefuroxime and oral clarythromycin.
 e. Admit to hospital and treat with ciprofloxacin.

Question 56

What is the ongoing management of this patient?
 a. Continue with current antibiotic therapy for another week and repeat CXR.
 b. Initiate anti-tuberculous therapy.
 c. Organize CT scan thorax.
 d. Perform pleural biopsy.
 e. Drain effusion using an intercostal drain and continue with aggressive antibiotic therapy.

Question 57

A 19-year-old girl was seen by her GP complaining of a 24-hour history of nausea and vomiting. She was prescribed some medication. Later that evening her boyfriend brought her into the Accident and Emergency Department stating that she had been unable to speak and had a very stiff neck.

On examination she appeared well. She was alert and orientated without any difficulty with her speech. She was unable to account for the episode encountered by her boyfriend but denied any previous similar 'attacks'. While being examined she was seen to become rigid. Her jaw was fixed open and her eyes were deviated up and to the left.

Which single step would you take in the management of this patient?
 a. Intravenous diazepam.
 b. Intravenous procyclidine.
 c. Intramuscular haloperidol.
 d. Reassure strongly.
 e. Guanidine hydrochloride.

Answers 55 and 56

Answer 55

d. Admit to hospital and treat with IV cefuroxime and oral clarithromycin.

The patient has a community-acquired pneumonia (CAP) as evidenced by symptoms and signs of a lower respiratory tract infection and consolidation on the chest X-ray.

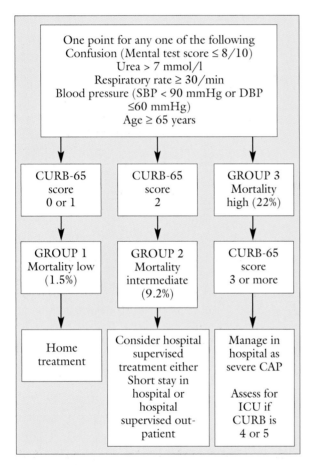

Streptococcus pneumoniae is the most frequently isolated organism in CAP, followed by *Haemophilus influenzae* and then *Mycoplasma pneumoniae*. Accurate assessment of the severity of pneumonia is necessary to guide the need for hospitalization and/or intravenous antibiotic therapy. In the UK, the CURB-65 score has been adopted for assessing the severity of pneumonia and stratifying patients into prognostic groups and management pathways (algorithm). Patients with a CURB-65 score of 3 or more have severe CAP and require hospitalization and treatment with intravenous antibiotics (*Table*). Other markers of poor prognosis in relation to pneumonia include a white cell count <4 or >20 ×10^9/l and an albumin concentration <30 g/l.

Recommended antibiotic therapy for severe CAP is a beta-lactam based antibiotic in combination with a macrolide (*Table*). In this particular case, where the CURB-65 score is 3, the patient should be admitted to hospital and receive intravenous cefuroxime and oral clarithromycin.

Antibiotic recommendations for CAP

	Preferred	*Alternative*
Home treated	Oral amoxicillin	Oral erythromycin or Oral clarithromycin
Hospital treated (not severe)	Oral amoxicillin + Oral erythromycin or Oral clarithromycin	Oral levofloxacin or Oral moxifloxacin
Hospital treated (severe)	IV co-amoxiclav or IV cefuroxime or IV cefotaxime + Oral erythromycin or Oral clarithromycin	Oral levofloxacin + IV benzylpenicillin

Answer 56

e. Drain effusion using an intercostal drain and continue with aggressive antibiotic therapy.

The pneumonia has been complicated by an empyema, which is characterized by frank pus in the pleural space. Organisms may be seen on Gram stain or isolated during culture. Biochemical investigation of the purulent fluid will reveal high protein and LDH concentrations and low pH and glucose concentration. The treatment of empyema involves drainage with an intercostal drain followed by a prolonged course of antibiotic therapy, including anaerobic cover.

Parapneumonic effusions complicate approximately 50% of all pneumonias. Most effusions are sterile and resolve with conventional antibiotic therapy. A small proportion become infected (complicated parapneumonic effusion or empyema) and require drainage. Features of complicated parapneumonic effusions include high protein and LDH concentration (patients with empyema characteristically have an LDH concentration >1000 iu) and low pH (<7.3) The presence of frank pus, organisms on pleural fluid Gram stain or culture and low pleural fluid pH are indications for prompt drainage using an intercostal drain.

Answer 57

> b. Intravenous procyclidine.

The description is typical of acute dystonia following treatment for vomiting. The culprit agent is a neuroleptic agent used to treat vomiting, classically metoclopramide or prochlorperazine. Both drugs work by blocking dopaminergic type 2 receptors in the mid-brain. Side-effects include acute dystonia. Chronic use is associated with tardive dyskinesia. Treatment is with intravenous procyclidine or benzotropine, which are both anti-cholinergic agents, or intramuscular diphenhydramine, which is an anti-histamine.

Question 58

A 72-year-old male presented with a two-month history of right-sided chest discomfort and weight loss. The symptoms were present most of the day and relieved partly by paracetamol. He was a heavy smoker and had a six-year history of chronic obstructive pulmonary disease requiring three hospital admissions. He had just finished a two-week course of high-dose prednisolone two weeks before developing chest discomfort. He had been treated for pulmonary tuberculosis at the age of 34 years.

On examination he was afebrile. He did not have finger clubbing. The percussion note at the base of the right lung was dull. Auscultation of the lungs revealed reduced air entry at the right lung base.

Investigations are shown.

Hb	11 g/dl
WCC	12×10^9/l
Platelets	300×10^9/l
Sodium	131 mmol/l
Potassium	3.6 mmol/l
Urea	7 mmol/l
Glucose	4.8 mmol/l
Protein	60 g/l
LDH	180 iu/l
Chest X-ray	Hyperinflated left lung Moderate pleural effusion right lung
Pleural fluid:	
Protein	29 g/l
LDH	180 iu/l
Glucose	3 mmol/l
Gram stain	Negative
Cytology	Mesothelial cells only

What investigation is required next?
  a. Bronchoscopy.
  b. Contrast enhanced thoracic CT scan.
  c. Ventilation/perfusion scan.
  d. Echocardiogram.
  e. Pleural biopsy.

Question 59

A 10-year-old boy presented with a three-week history of swollen ankles. On examination his blood pressure measured 100/60 mmHg. The JVP was not raised. Both heart sounds were normal and his chest was clear.

Investigations are shown.

Hb	12 g/dl
WCC	5×10^9/l
Platelets	200×10^9/l
Blood film	Normal
Sodium	134 mmol/l
Potassium	3.7 mmol/l
Urea	6 mmol/l
Creatinine	90 μmol/l
Albumin	21g/l
24-hour urine protein	3.6 g/l

What is the first-line management step?
  a. Oral high-dose prednisolone therapy.
  b. No therapy (mere observation).
  c. Intravenous furosemide infusion.
  d. Perform renal biopsy before instituting treatment.
  e. Cyclophosphamide.

Answer 58

> b. Contrast enhanced thoracic CT scan.

The patient is a smoker and presents with right-sided chest discomfort and has a pleural effusion. The pleural fluid protein concentration is <30 g/l. Sole reliance on the pleural fluid protein content would result in an erroneous misinterpretation of a transudative effusion. However, pleural fluid protein measurements should be interpreted in the context of the serum protein concentration. In patients with abnormal serum protein or pleural fluid protein concentrations close to 30 g/l more stringent criteria are required to differentiate a pleural transudate from an exudate (*Table A*).

According to the Light's criteria, the effusion has the biochemical features of an exudate. The pleural glucose concentration is also low (*Table B*). The differential diagnosis is between malignant pleural involvement, complicated parapneumonic effusion, and tuberculous effusion. There is no obvious evidence of an infection and in the context of a long history of smoking, the prospect of malignancy has to be considered. Indeed malignancy is the commonest cause of an exudative pleural effusion in patients aged >60 years. Cytological analysis reveals malignant cells in <25% of cases with malignant pleural effusions. The patient should have a contrast enhanced CT scan followed by a CT guided or thoracoscopic pleural biopsy. Contrast enhanced CT scan should precede pleural biopsy in most cases of undiagnosed effusion. Bronchoscopy is not helpful unless there are specific features to suggest an underlying bronchial malignancy such as haemoptysis.

Table A Light's criteria for pleural fluid exudates

- Pleural fluid protein to serum protein ratio >0.5
- Pleural fluid LDH to serum LDH ratio >0.6
- Pleural fluid LDH >$^2/_3$ the upper limit of normal serum LDH

Table B Causes of low pH and low glucose effusions

- Complicated parapneumonic effusion or empyema
- Malignant pleural effusion
- Rheumatoid pleuritis
- Lupus pleuritis
- Tuberculous pleural effusion
- Oesophageal rupture (also has high amylase)

Answer 59

> a. Oral high dose prednisolone therapy.

The patient has nephrotic syndrome. The commonest cause of nephrotic syndrome in children is minimal change glomerulonephritis, accounting for 90% of all cases of nephrotic syndrome in children aged below 10 years, and 50% of children aged above 10 years. The causes of nephrotic syndrome are tabulated below (*Table A*).

A trial of high-dose prednisolone (1 mg/kg per day) is the first-line management step in children presenting with pure heavy proteinuria and peripheral oedema. Most children achieve remission within two weeks and almost all children are in remission within eight weeks. Patients refractory to high-dose steroids are treated with cyclophosphamide, ciclosporin or chlorambucil. Furosemide infusion is rarely indicated unless the patient has marked peripheral oedema.

Adults presenting with heavy proteinuria have minimal change glomerulonpehritis in 20% of cases and generally respond more slowly to, and relapse more frequently on, steroid therapy. Therefore a renal biopsy is generally advocated to help elucidate the exact cause before instituting therapy. In contrast renal biopsy in children is only indicated in rare circumstances (*Table B*). (See Question 137.)

Table A Causes of minimal change glomerulonephritis

- Immune
- Non-steroidal anti-inflammatory drugs
- Hodgkin's lumphoma
- Food allergy (cow's milk)
- Bee-sting reaction
- Lithium
- Pamidronate

Table B Indications for renal biopsy in children with heavy proteinuria

- Presence of red cells/casts in the urine
- Obvious evidence of a multi-system vasculitis
- Patients with frequent relapses
- Patients refractory to conventional therapy

Question 60

A 68-year-old man presented with a cholestatic blood picture, and hepatobiliary ultrasound revealed dilated extra-hepatic ducts. He underwent an ERCP which was complicated by *E. coli* septicaemia. One week following the procedure the renal function was as follows:

Sodium	131 mmol/l
Potassium	4.9 mmol/l
Urea	28 mmol/l
Creatinine	430 μmol/l

The urea and electrolytes prior to ERCP were normal. On examination he was clinically euvolaemic. His heart rate was 80 beats/min and regular, and his blood pressure measured 130/80 mmHg. A urinary catheter was placed in the bladder and he was passing 40 ml of urine per hour.

Which of the following agents are of proven benefit in improving renal function in a situation such as this?
   a. High-dose steroids.
   b. Intravenous dopamine.
   c. High-dose furosemide infusion.
   d. Intravenous mannitol.
   e. None of the above.

Question 61

A 50-year-old shipyard worker presented with a single episode of haemoptysis comprising approximately one egg cup-full of fresh blood. He gave a two-year history of progressively increasing breathlessness and a persistent cough. He had never experienced any chest pain. He stopped smoking two months previously after a chest infection which took several weeks to resolve, but before that was smoking 20–30 cigarettes/day. He kept pigeons in his teenage years, but had not had any direct contact with birds since. The only other past medical history of note was a four-year history of mild hypertension, for which he was taking propranolol 80 mg three times daily.

On examination, he was centrally cyanosed and had early finger clubbing. The respiratory rate was 23/min. On examination of the respiratory system the chest expansion was symmetrical, but generally reduced. The trachea was central. On auscultation of the lung fields there were fine end-inspiratory crackles at both lung bases. Precordial examination was normal, with the exception of a loud pulmonary component to the second heart sound.

Investigations are shown.

Hb	14 g/dl
WCC	9×10^9/l
Platelets	190×10^9/l
MCV	91 fl
ESR	64 mm/h
Sodium	132 mmol/l
Potassium	3.7 mmol/l
Urea	7 mmol/l
Creatinine	91 μmol/l
Arterial blood gases:	
pH	7.44
PaO_2	7.1
$PaCO_2$	3.4
Bicarbonate	21
O_2 saturation	75%
Chest X-ray	Irregular, linear shadowing at both lung bases
Sputum microscopy	No abnormalities
Flow loop (**61**)	

1: What is the cause of the haemoptysis?
   a. Mesothelioma.
   b. Carcinoma of the bronchus.
   c. Extrinsic allergic alveolitis.
   d. TB.
   e. Pulmonary embolus.

2: What is the cause of his breathlessness?
   a. Chronic obstructive airways disease.
   b. Therapy with propranolol.
   c. Extrinsic allergic alveolitis.
   d. Cryptogenic fibrosing alveolitis/diffuse pulmonary fibrosis.
   e. Asbestosis.

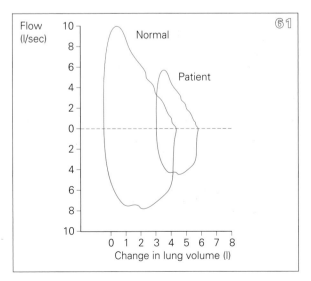

Answer 60

> e. None of the above.

The patient has probably developed renal failure secondary to acute tubular necrosis arising from *E. coli* septicaemia. Acute tubular necrosis generally lasts between one and three weeks. Most patients make a recovery and return to their normal or near normal renal function. The management of acute renal failure due to acute tubular necrosis is supportive.

Nephrotoxic agents are stopped or avoided. Hypovolaemia is corrected with intravenous saline whilst monitoring central venous pressure. Urine output is monitored with a urinary catheter *in situ*. Once the patient is euvolaemic, the quantitative daily fluid replacement is equal to the volume of urine output plus an additional 500 ml to allow for insensible losses. The patient is carefully monitored for signs of fluid overload or uraemic encephalopathy. The serum urea, electrolyte and arterial pH are monitored closely.

Acute haemodialysis is recommended in patients with renal failure associated with fluid overload causing pulmonary oedema, uraemic encephalopathy, dangerous hyperkalaemia (≥ 7 mmol/l) or a low arterial pH.

There is no proven therapy to help expedite recovery. Although dopamine has been advocated in the past, prospective controlled studies have failed to show any improvement in renal function in acute renal failure patients treated with dopamine. Furosemide has been conventionally used to convert oliguric acute tubular necrosis to non-oliguric tubular necrosis, however, studies suggest that the use of high-dose diuretics may be associated with death and retard recovery of renal function. Steroids have no role in the management of acute tubular necrosis but are helpful in the management of acute glomerulonephritis.

Answer 61

> 1: a. Mesothelioma
> 2: e. Asbestosis.

The main features of this case are a long-term smoker who presents with haemoptysis. He has worked in the shipyard, an occupation which was historically associated with asbestos exposure. He has objective evidence of lung fibrosis; he is hypoxic, his chest X-ray shows linear shadowing in the lower zones and the flow loop is consistent with shrunken lungs. In the context of this case the most likely cause for lung fibrosis and breathlessness is asbestosis. The history of keeping pigeons may implicate extrinsic allergic alveolitis as a possible cause; however, it has been a long time since he was exposed to avian antigens. Furthermore, EAA classically causes upper zone reticulo-nodular shadowing on the chest X-ray, whereas asbestosis is associated with shadowing in the lower zones.

While there are several causes of haemoptysis, the most probable cause in this case is bronchial carcinoma. Both bronchial carcinoma and mesothelioma malignancies are associated with asbestos exposure. However, the chest X-ray does not mention obvious pleural thickening or pleural effusion, which are classic features of mesothelioma; therefore an underlying bronchial carcinoma would need to be excluded. Smoking and asbestos exposure together increase the risk of bronchial carcinoma several fold. With the exception of EAA, all the possibilities mentioned may also cause haemoptysis; however, the history is atypical for pulmonary embolus and tuberculosis would be lower down in the differential diagnosis than lung malignancy.

Questions 62 and 63

A 62-year-old male presented with fever and breathlessness four weeks after a prosthetic aortic valve replacement for aortic stenosis. On examination he appeared pale and had a temperature of 38°C (100.4°F). Auscultation of the heart revealed a prosthetic second heart sound and a long early diastolic murmur. Auscultation of the lungs revealed inspiratory crackles at both lung bases.

Initial investigations are shown.

Hb	11 g/dl
WCC	15×10^9/l
Platelets	400×10^9/l
ESR	70 mm/h
Sodium	140 mmol/l
Potassium	4.2 mmol/l
Urea	8 mmol/l
Creatinine	130 μmol/l
12-lead ECG	Left bundle branch block (old)
Chest X-ray	Cardiomegaly and pulmonary oedema

Question 62

Which two of the following investigations will provide the most diagnostic information?
- a. C-reactive protein.
- b. Renal ultrasound.
- c. ASO titres.
- d. Serial blood cultures.
- e. Transthoracic echocardiography.
- f. Urinalysis for blood.
- g. Complement fixation tests for *Coxiella burnetii*.
- h. Transoesophageal echocardiography.

Question 63

Which organism is most likely to be present in the blood culture?
- a. *Streptococcus viridans*.
- b. *Staphylococcus aureus*.
- c. *Staphylococcus epidermidis*.
- d. Organism from the HACEK group.
- e. *Enterococci*.

Question 64

A 38-year-old male was investigated for abnormal liver function tests following investigation of intermittent episodes of diarrhoea. He was generally fit and well. He consumed no more than 10 units of alcohol per week. He did not take any medications. He had a past history of jaundice after a visit to India 8 years previously, which had resolved spontaneously.

Investigations are shown.

Hb	11 g/dl
WCC	7×10^9/l
Platelets	190×10^9/l
CRP	12 g/l
Bilirubin	19 μmol/l
ALT	32 iu/l
Alkaline phosphatase	178 iu/l
Albumin	33 g/l
Thyroxine	102 nmol/l
TSH	1.2 nmol/l
Hepatobiliary ultrasound	Normal
ERCP (**64**)	

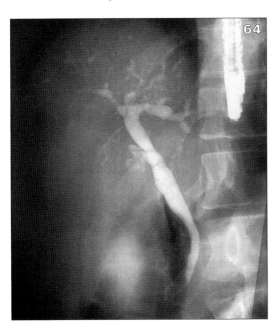

What is the cause of the raised alkaline phosphatase?
- a. Primary sclerosing cholangitis.
- b. Primary biliary cirrhosis.
- c. Stones in the common bile duct.
- d. Amoebic liver abscess.
- e. Hepatic vein thrombosis.

Answers 62 and 63

Answer 62

d. Serial blood cultures.

h. Transoesophageal echocardiography.

Answer 63

c. *Staphylococcus epidermidis.*

The patient has developed a fever and murmur of aortic regurgitation only four weeks after a prosthetic aortic valve replacement, indicating early prosthetic valve endocarditis. In early PVE, micro-organisms usually reach the prosthesis by direct contamination during the intra-operative period or via haematogenous spread several days or weeks after surgery. The consequences of early PVE are grave as the organisms have direct access to the prosthesis annulus-interface and to perivalvular tissue around the sutures lines since the valve is not endothelialized. Patients with early PVE commonly develop valve dehiscence and annular abscesses. The risk of embolic phenomena is also greater with PVE. The clinical features are similar to native valve endocarditis.

Diagnosis relies on culturing the organisms from the blood. Three sets of blood cultures should be taken at intervals of >1 hour within the first 24 hours if the diagnosis is highly likely in a sick patient. If the patient is not acutely ill or when the diagnosis is not obvious, six sets of blood cultures should be taken within the first 24 to 48 hours. The commonest organisms cultured in early PVE are *Staphylococcus epidermidis* followed by *Staphylococcus aureus* and then fungi. In contrast, organisms cultured in late PVE are similar to those causing infection on native valves.

Transoesophageal echocardiography is the investigation of choice and is advocated as the first-line echocardiographic modality in the investigation of PVE. TOE is much more sensitive than transthoracic echocardiography at identifying vegetations on the prosthetic valve. It is also superior at identifying complications such as paravalvular abscesses and fistula formation.

The treatment comprises high-dose intravenous antibiotics for six weeks. The need for surgical intervention is much higher than with native valve endocarditis. Indications for surgery in PVE and native valve endocarditis are tabulated (*Table*).

Indications for surgery in valve endocarditis

Prosthetic valve endocarditis
- Early PVE in first 2 months or less after surgery
- Murmurs suggestive of valve dysfunction
- Moderate to severe heart failure
- Annular or aortic root abscess or new cardiac conduction abnormalities on ECG
- Persistent fever for 10 or more days despite appropriate antibiotic therapy
- *Staphylococcus aureus* or fungi cultured from the blood

Native valve endocarditis
- Acute AR or MR with heart failure
- Annular or aortic root abscess
- Fungal endocarditis
- Evidence of persistent infection despite appropriate antibiotic therapy for 10 days (fever, leucocytosis and bacteraemia)

Answer 64

---

a. Primary sclerosing cholangitis.

The ERCP shows multiple strictures and dilatations in the intrahepatic ducts and in the left and right hepatic ducts. The finding is characteristic of primary sclerosing cholangitis, which is a chronic progressive inflammatory disorder of medium and small-sized bile ducts. The history of intermittent loose stool in the patient is particularly relevant in this question because over 90% of cases are associated with ulcerative colitis. The most useful diagnostic test is an ERCP or a MRCP (magnetic resonance cholangiopancreatogram). A liver biopsy is rarely diagnostic. (See Questions 6 and 104.)

Question 65

A 52-year-old man was admitted to the intensive care unit with difficulty in breathing after a coryzal illness. He had a six-week history of rapidly progressive muscular fatigue which was worse at the end of the day. More recently he had had difficulty with speech and chewing food while eating.

On examination he had bilateral ptosis and marked facial muscle weakness. Power in all four limbs was diminished. The heart rate was 90 beats/min and regular. The respiratory rate was 30/min but respiration was shallow. Investigations are shown.

His condition deteriorated and he was transferred to the intensive care unit for invasive ventilation.

Hb	15 g/dl
WCC	9×10^9/l
Platelets	200×10^9/l
Electrolytes	Normal
Chest X-ray	Elevation of both hemi-diaphragms
	Lungs normal
Arterial blood gases:	
pH	7.1
$PaCO_2$	9 kPa
PaO_2	7 kPa
FVC (baseline)	0.8 l
FVC (after 2 mg edrophonium)	1.2 l

What is the ideal therapeutic strategy in his immediate management?
a. Emergency thymectomy.
b. Intravenous neostigmine.
c. Intravenous methylprednisolone.
d. Plasmapheresis.
e. Azathioprine.

Question 66

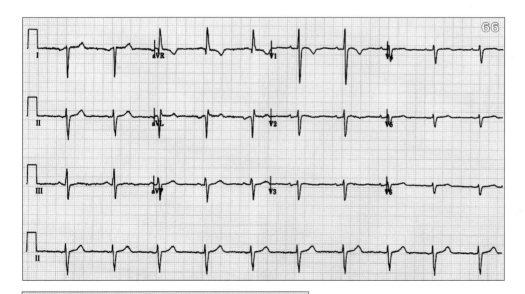

What is the ECG diagnosis (**66**)?
a. Right ventricular hypertrophy.
b. Dextrocardia.
c. Wolff–Parkinson–White syndrome.
d. Left ventricular hypertrophy.
e. Right bundle branch block.

Answer 65

> d. Plasmapheresis.

The patient presents with acute generalized muscle weakness and respiratory failure. There is a six-week history of muscle fatigue, which is a cardinal feature of myasthenia gravis. Response to edrophonium (Tensilon), a short-acting anti-cholinesterase agent, supports the diagnosis of myasthenia gravis, although false-positive results are common.

Patients with myasthenia gravis may present with myasthenic crises, which comprise severe muscle weakness including respiratory and bulbar muscles. Such crises may be precipitated by intercurrent illness as in this case, or they may be spontaneous events. The treatment for myasthenic crisis is shown in *Table A*.

Plasmapheresis directly removes anti-cholinergic receptor antibodies from the circulation. Treatment is given for up to 2 weeks and is effective for 1–2 months. Plasmapheresis is reserved for acute situations or preparation for thymectomy. Intravenous immunoglobulin is as effective as plasmapheresis in acute myasthenic crises. The mode of action of intravenous immunoglobulin is uncertain. Anti-cholinesterase drug therapy may cause a cholinergic crisis that is also characterized by muscle weakness. The differentiation between a cholinergic crisis and a myasthenic crisis is based upon the presence of abdominal cramps, excessive sweating and bradycardia in the former. However, a history is not always available during a crisis, therefore anti-cholinesterase drugs are withdrawn in patients with myasthenia gravis who present with features of severe generalized muscle weakness.

The management of patients with chronic myasthenia gravis is summarized in *Table B*.

Table A Management of myasthenic crisis

Step 1   Elective ventilation
Step 2   Withdrawal of anti-cholinesterase drugs
             (if applicable)
Step 3   Plasmapheresis or intravenous
             immunoglobulin

Table B Management of chronic myasthenia gravis

Treatment regime	*Indications*
Oral anti-cholinesterase therapy	Mild symptoms Ocular myasthenia
Immunosuppressive drugs	
Corticosteroids	To attempt remission in patients with moderate or severe symptoms
Azathioprine	Failure to remit on steroid therapy
Cyclosporin	
Thymectomy*	Patients with thymoma

* Some neurologists recommend thymectomy even in the absence of thymoma in all patients between puberty and 60 years of age since most patients have abnormalities of the thymus gland.

Answer 66

> b. Dextrocardia.

The patient has a dominant R wave in V1 which would be consistent with all five choices provided in the question. There is a rightward QRS and P wave axis, a deep S wave in lead I and dominant R wave in aVr which are highly unusual and should raise the suspicion of either erroneous upper limb lead transposition or dextrocardia. The progressive dimunition of the R waves on transition from lead V1 to V6 indicates dextrocardia. In pure upper limb lead transposition the R wave transition in V1 to V6 is normal.

Question 67

An 18-year-old girl presented with a six-month history of daytime somnolence that was causing embarrassment during lecture theatres and while talking to friends. She was apprehensive about driving because she did not have any recollection about how she had driven from one destination to another and felt that she may have fallen asleep while driving on a few occasions. She had vivid frightening dreams just as she fell asleep, which would wake her frequently. On waking she was unable to move for a few minutes. Three months previously the patient underwent cardiac investigations for intermittent episodes of sudden collapse that occurred when she laughed out loud. The episodes were not associated with loss of consciousness.

The patient had a past history of insulin-dependent diabetes mellitus since the age of 7 years that was very well controlled. She had recently commenced the oral contraceptive pill but was not on any other medication. There was no family history of note. Investigations are shown.

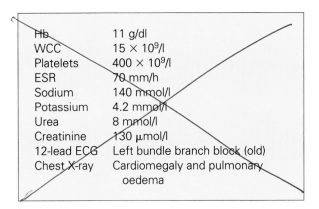

Hb	11 g/dl
WCC	$15 \times 10^9/l$
Platelets	$400 \times 10^9/l$
ESR	70 mm/h
Sodium	140 mmol/l
Potassium	4.2 mmol/l
Urea	8 mmol/l
Creatinine	130 μmol/l
12-lead ECG	Left bundle branch block (old)
Chest X-ray	Cardiomegaly and pulmonary oedema

What is the diagnosis?
 a. Acute intermittent porphyria.
 b. Episodic hypoglycaemia.
 c. Epilepsy.
 d. Narcolepsy.
 e. Long QT syndrome.

Question 68

A 70-year-old man with a known history of ischaemic heart disease and congestive cardiac failure presented with nausea and abdominal discomfort. He was taking digoxin 250 μg , frusemide 40 mg and lisinopril 20 mg. The patient had been recently commenced on amiodarone for atrial fibrillation. On examination the JVP was raised 4 cm above the sternal angle. There was a third heart sound. The liver edge was palpable 3 cm below the costal margin and there was mild ankle oedema. The digoxin level was 3 iu (NR 1–2 iu).

What is the best action to improve his symptoms without compromising cardiac function?
 a. Stop digoxin.
 b. Stop amiodarone.
 c. Stop enalapril.
 d. Halve the dose of digoxin.
 e. Halve the dose of amiodarone.

Answer 67

> d. Narcolepsy.

The patient has excessive daytime somnolence, hypnagogic hallucinations, cataplexy and sleep paralysis. This combination is consistent with the diagnosis of narcolepsy. Spontaneous recovery of the events is inconsistent with hypoglycaemic episodes. Torsades de pointes due to long QT syndrome may present with episodic collapse during intense emotion; however, consciousness is impaired in collapse associated with long QT syndrome. (See Question 266.)

Excessive daytime somnolence is a cardinal feature of narcolepsy. The symptoms are improved after a brief nap.

Hypnagogic hallucinations are vivid and often frightening hallucinations just after falling asleep or just before waking. They are effectively a mixture of REM sleep and wakefulness.

Cataplexy is defined as sudden episodes of bilateral muscle weakness leading to partial or complete collapse. It is usually triggered by strong emotions such as anger, laughter or intense excitement. Weakness is present for 1–2 minutes. Consciousness is not impaired. Almost two-thirds of patients with narcolepsy go on to develop cataplexy.

Sleep paralysis is a complete inability to move 1 or 2 minutes after waking and is often accompanied by hypnagogic hallucinations.

Narcolepsy is caused by the loss of the hypothalamic neuropeptide orexin. Orexins are released from synaptic terminals during wakefulness and increase the activity of brain regions associated with wakefulness. Narcolepsy has strong association with the HLA antigens DR2 and DQ1 (HLA DR2 [99%]).

The diagnosis is clinical but an overnight polysomonogram and a multiple sleep latency test are performed to exclude other causes of hypersomnolence. Overnight polysomonography may be normal in patients with narcolepsy but may demonstrate spontaneous wakenings and REM sleep within 20 minutes of falling asleep. Normal patients do not go into REM sleep for 80–100 minutes after the onset of sleep since orexin inhibits REM sleep. The following day a multiple sleep latency test is performed in which a patient is allowed to nap every 2 hours on four or five occasions. Patients with narcolepsy fall asleep within 5 minutes whereas most normal patients take 10–15 minutes to fall asleep. The naps in narcolepsy patients induce REM sleep, and the presence of sleep-onset REM in two or more naps is highly suggestive of narcolepsy.

Treatment is with modafinil, a non-amphetamine wake-inducing drug. The alternative is methylphenidate, an amphetamine drug.

Answer 68

> d. Halve the dose of digoxin.

The patient has abdominal discomfort and nausea. The differential diagnosis for his symptoms includes hepatic congestion secondary to heart failure, digoxin toxicity or gastro-intestinal side-effects of amiodarone (usually occur within a few days of starting the drug). In this particular situation the plasma digoxin level is raised and hence digoxin toxicity is the most likely cause (*Tables A* and *B*). Amiodarone may promote digoxin toxicity by competing for digoxin binding sites hence increasing plasma digoxin

levels. The dose of digoxin should be halved when amiodarone is initiated. The patient had clinical evidence of cardiac decompensation; therefore, the best management step would be halve the dose of digoxin rather than stop it altogether. Digoxin is cleared fairly quickly by the kidneys (one-third of the body content per day) and the symptoms should settle. Remember that digoxin toxicity can cause fatal rhythm disturbances (both tachy- and bradyarrhythmias).

Table A Features of digoxin toxicity

- Gastro-intestinal effects
  Anorexia, nausea, vomiting, abdominal pain and diarrhoea
- Xanthopsia
- Neuralgia
- Cardiac rhythm disturbances
- Headache
- Dizziness
- Epileptic seizures

Table B Causes of digoxin toxicity

- Electrolyte disturbances
  Hypokalaemia
  Hypomagnesaemia
  Hypercalcaemia
- Hypothyroidism
- Renal impairment
- Drugs
  Amiodarone   Increases plasma levels by displacing it from binding proteins
  Calcium antagonists
  Ciclosporin
  Quinidine
  ACE inhibitors   May reduce renal clearance

Question 69

A 15-year-old Nigerian female was admitted with right upper quadrant abdominal pain. She had a history of sickle cell anaemia, and had several admissions with hand and foot crises. During the last two admissions she complained of abdominal pain. She was born in England. She was the only child of a middle-class family.

On examination, she was distressed with pain. The temperature was 37.6°C (99.7°F). She was mildly jaundiced. The pulse was 105 beats/min, and blood pressure 100/75 mmHg. On examination of the respiratory system there was dullness to percussion on the anterior aspect of the right lung. Abdominal examination revealed tenderness in the right upper quadrant. The liver was palpable 3 cm below the costal margin.

Investigations are shown.

Hb	6 g/dl
WCC	12 × 10⁹/l
Platelets	200 × 10⁹/l
U&E	Normal
AST	50 iu/l
Alkaline phosphatase	150 iu/l
Albumin	34 g/l
Urine osmolality	120 mOsm/kg
Urinalysis	Urobilinogen +++
	Blood 0
	Protein 0
	Bilirubin 0
Chest X-ray	Opacification in the right upper zone

1. What is the cause of the abdominal pain?
2. What investigation would you request next?
3. What is the cause of the girl's respiratory and chest X-ray findings?
4. Explain the urine osmolality.

Question 70

A 25-year-old female presented with a right calf deep-vein thrombosis.

Blood results are shown.

Hb	12 g/dl
WCC	7 × 10⁹/l
Platelets	140 × 10⁹/l
PT	13 s (control 12 s)
APTT	59 s (control 40 s)
Antinuclear antibody factor	Not detected
Double-stranded DNA	Not detected

1. What is the diagnosis?
2. List three tests you would perform to confirm the diagnosis.
3. Apart from thrombotic tendencies, list other manifestations of this condition.

Answer 69

1. Acute cholecystitis.
2. Ultrasound examination of the liver.
3. Right upper lobe pneumonia.
4. Chronic tubulo-interstitial nephritis or renal papillary necrosis leading to impaired concentrating ability.

Sickle cell anaemia is discussed in detail in Answer 263. This question tests the reader's knowledge of complications secondary to sickle cell anaemia.

The story is typical of cholecystitis which, in this case, is secondary to pigment gallstones. Hepatic infarction due to a sickling crisis in the liver is unlikely because it would be associated with a higher AST. Sequestration is unlikely because it is very rare in older patients with sickle cell anaemia. The shadowing on the chest X-ray is probably secondary to streptococcal pneumonia. Patients with sickle cell anaemia are hyposplenic as a result of autosplenic infarction. As a result, they are predisposed to bacterial infections by capsulated organisms such as *Streptococcus pneumoniae*, *Neisseria meningitidis* and *Haemophilus influenzae*. Pulmonary infarction may also cause pulmonary shadowing on the chest X-ray – but is less likely in the absence of pleurisy – and severe breathlessness.

Sickle cell anaemia is inherited as an autosomal recessive condition. A point mutation in the β-globin gene leads to the substitution of glutamine by valine at position 6. In the deoxygenated state, this leads to sickling of cells. Chronic low-grade haemolysis is common and predisposes to pigment gallstones. Painful sickle cell crises are due to occlusion of small vessels, producing severe pain from affected organs. The bones are most commonly involved, particularly those of the hands and feet. Other crises include haemolytic, aplastic and sequestration crises (*Table*). An aplastic crisis may complicate infection with parvovirus B17. Sequestration crises are fatal and usually occur in young patients. Precipitating factors for sickling include hypoxia, infection, dehydration and pain.

Sickle cell crises

- Thrombotic (hand foot syndrome, abdominal pain, pulmonary infarction and strokes)
- Haemolytic
- Aplastic
- Sequestration

Answer 70

1. Antiphospholipid syndrome.
2 . i. Antiphospholipid antibodies (these may result in a false positive VDRL test).
 ii. Failure of APTT to improve after addition of normal plasma.
 iii. Lupus anticoagulant.
3. Any of the following:
 i. Recurrent abortions.
 ii. Livedo reticularis.
 iii. Pulmonary hypertension.
 iv. Transient ischaemic attacks.
 v. Chorea.
 vi. Migraines.
 vii. Valvular heart disease.
 viii. Thrombocytopenia.

The antiphospholipid syndrome usually affects young women and is characterized by arterial and venous thromboses and recurrent abortions (*Table*). There may be evidence of thrombocytopenia. It is caused by circulating antiphospholipid antibodies, which are IgG and IgM immunoglobulins directed against phospholipid molecules. They were first described in SLE, but may be present in a wide variety of autoimmune conditions and have been associated with multiple sclerosis, acquired immunodeficiency syndrome (AIDS) and carcinomatosis.

Antiphospholipid antibodies can be present in patients taking medications such as phenytoin, procainamide and hydralazine. The antibodies may occur in isolation – the antiphospholipid syndrome. Cross-reaction with other antiphospholipid antibodies produces a false-positive Wassermann (VDRL) test. Some antibodies have an anticoagulant effect on coagulation tests *in vitro*, characterized by a prolonged APTT (with or without a minor prolongation of the PT time) which fails to correct after addition of normal plasma, suggesting the presence of a coagulation inhibitor. These antibodies are termed the 'lupus anticoagulant'. Despite the *in vitro* effect, the presence of the lupus anticoagulant has the opposite effect *in vivo*, and predisposes affected individuals to recurrent thrombotic events. Recurrent abortions are thought to be due to placental infarction. Other associations of the antiphospholipid syndrome have been mentioned (see Answer 49, 53). The diagnosis is made

Causes of arterial and venous thromboses

- Paroxysmal nocturnal haemoglobinuria
- Paradoxical emboli
- Myeloproliferative disorders
- Homocystinuria
- Sickle cell anaemia

by detection of antiphospholipid antibodies in the serum. Specific tests for the detection of the lupus anticoagulant antibodies are available. A negative VDRL and absence of circulating lupus anticoagulant does not exclude the presence of antiphospholipid antibodies. Management is with prophylactic anticoagulant therapy.

Question 71

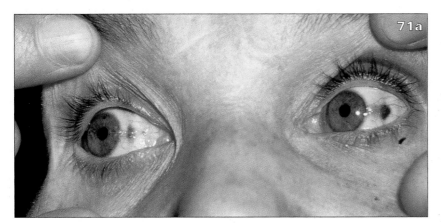
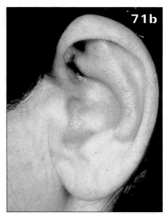

A 35-year-old male was seen in clinic with a 12-year history of backache. He was a keen football player, but for over 11 years had not participated in sport owing to the disabling pain. He had been seeing an osteopath for almost 10 years. His back pain was originally controlled, but had now become unbearable. He had pain in his lower and upper back that was worsened by movement of the spine. Over the past two years he had noticed intermittent pain and swelling in both his knees, which had responded to ibuprofen. There was no history of diarrhoea, skin rashes or mouth ulcers. He experienced transient dysuria after a trip to Amsterdam at the age of 21, but this cleared after a course of penicillin from his doctor. There was no family history of back pain.

On examination, he was in pain. He had lost his lumbar lordosis. Examination of his eyes and ear are shown (**71a, b**). His knee joints were swollen, with bilateral effusions; examination of the rest of his joints was normal. Cardiovascular, respiratory, abdominal and neurological examinations were all normal.

Investigations are shown.

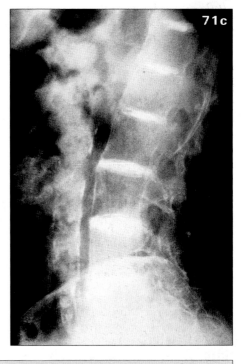

Hb	15 g/dl
WCC	10×10^9/l
Platelets	230×10^9/l
ESR	30 mm/h
Calcium	2.3 mmol/l
Phosphate	0.8 mmol/l
Alkaline phosphatase	90 iu/l
Albumin	40 g/l
X-ray of spine (**71c**)	
Urinalysis	Glucose ++
	Protein 0

1. What is the diagnosis?
2. How would you confirm the diagnosis?
3. How would you account for the result of urinalysis?

Answer 71

1. Alkaptonuria.
2. Urinary homogentisic acid level. Urine becomes dark on standing.
3. Homogentisic acid is a reducing substance and therefore gives a positive reaction to glucostix (Clinistix). Other substances that produce a false-positive glucostix test are shown *(Table)*. Glucose oxidase (Clinitest) sticks do not give this false-positive reaction.

Alkaptonuria is inherited as an autosomal recessive trait. There is a deficiency in the enzyme homogentisic acid oxidase, leading to accumulation of homogentisic acid in the urine and increased pigmentation (ochronosis) in cartilage and connective tissue. Urine becomes dark on standing owing to oxidation and polymerization of homogentisic acid. Freshly voided urine appears normal in colour, so these patients do not often report dark urine. Abnormal pigmentation is found in the ear and sclerae (**71a, b**) as well as articular cartilage (at surgery). Premature arthritis predominantly affecting the back, and later the large joints, is the most serious manifestation of the disorder. Intervertebral disc calcification is characteristic of alkaptonuria and is seen on the spinal X-ray (**71c**). The knees are commonly affected. The sacro-iliac joints are spared. Calcification of the aorta is often seen on the chest X-ray.

A low-protein diet is recommended to reduce the amount of homogentisic acid, which is a breakdown product of tyrosine; however, this does not prove very effective.

Causes of a false-positive Clinistix test

- Fructose
- Pentose
- Lactose
- Salicylates
- Ascorbic acid
- Homogentisic acid

Question 72

An 18-year-old male was referred to the respiratory out-patient clinic with a three-year history of progressively increasing breathlessness. Until the age of 15 years he was able to participate in school sports, but since then he had noticed increasing fatigue and breathlessness on exertion. He was diagnosed as having exercise-induced asthma and was prescribed salbutamol and beclomethasone inhalers, with initial relief of his symptoms until he was 16 years of age, when his symptoms started to deteriorate. At this stage he was seen by a hospital specialist, who felt that he had resistant asthma and started him on a two-week trial of oral steroids, which proved to be successful. Subsequently, the dose of inhaled steroid was increased. Three months before coming to clinic his symptoms had deteriorated considerably. He was breathless on walking less than 200 metres on the flat at a slow pace. His appetite was reduced, and he had noticed that his ankles were swollen towards the end of the day. He was a non-smoker, and had never consumed alcohol. He was currently at a college attempting to do his GCSE examinations, but was having considerable difficulty because of his illness. He was an only child. Both parents were well and had a shared business. They were non-smokers. The family had a pet budgerigar.

On examination, the patient was thin. He was below the 10th centile for weight, and on the 50th centile for height. He appeared very slightly jaundiced, but was not cyanosed or clubbed. His heart rate was 120 beats/min and regular. The blood pressure was 110/65 mmHg. The JVP was not elevated. The respiratory rate was 28/min. Chest expansion was symmetrical, but moderately reduced. The percussion note was resonant and auscultation revealed reduced breath sounds in the lungs, particularly at both bases. On examination of the abdomen, the liver edge was palpable 3 cm below the costal margin. In addition, the tip of the spleen was just palpable. There was no clinical evidence of ascites; however, there was pitting ankle oedema to the shins.

Investigations are shown.

Hb	17 g/dl
WCC	9×10^9/l
Platelets	130×10^9/l
MCV	100 fl
Sodium	135 mmol/l
Potassium	4.1 mmol/l
Urea	3 mmol/l
Creatinine	60 µmol/l
Calcium	2.1 mmol/l
Phosphate	1.0 mmol/l
Total protein	66 g/l
Albumin	31 g/l
Bilirubin	58 µmol/l
AST	49 iu/l
Alkaline phosphatase	600 u/l

Chest X-ray (**72**)
Lung function:

PEFR	200/min (predicted 550/min)
FEV$_1$	2.0 l (predicted 4.2 l)
FVC	4.1 l (predicted 5.6 l)
TLC	7.5 l (predicted 6.4 l)
KCO	0.7 mmol/l/kPa (predicted 1.6 mmol/l/kPa)

Arterial blood gases:

pH	7.34
PaO$_2$	8.4 kPa
PaCO$_2$	5.6 kPa
Bicarbonate	32 mmol/l
Base excess	+10

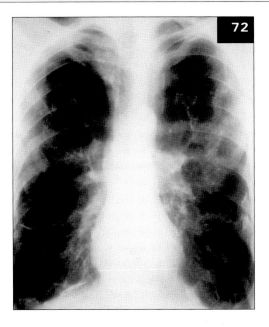

72

What single test would you request to confirm the diagnosis?
  a. Sweat sodium concentration.
  b. Liver biopsy.
  c. Transbronchial lung biopsy.
  d. Serum immunoglobulins.
  e. Measurement of serum α-1 antitrypsin and its electrophoretic mobility.

Question 73

A 48-year-old baker presented with a right deep-vein thrombosis affecting the right calf. Apart from a swollen right calf, physical examination did not demonstrate any other abnormality.

Investigations are shown.

Hb	18 g/dl
PCV	0.57 l/l
MCV	89 fl
WCC	9×10^9/l
Neutrophils	92%
Lymphocytes	8%
Monocytes	4%
Platelets	388×10^9/l
Blood film	Normal

1. What is the haematological abnormality?
    a. Pseudopolycythaemia.
    b. Secondary polycythaemia.
    c. Primary polycythaemia.
    d. Myelofibrosis.
    e. Essential thrombocythaemia.
2. List at least three investigations you would perform to determine the underlying cause.

Answer 72

> e. Measurement of the serum α-1 antitrypsin and its electrophoretic mobility.

The patient has hyperinflated lung fields, an obstructive lung defect with reduced transfer factor and evidence of cirrhosis of the liver. The combination of chronic lung disease and cirrhosis of the liver in a young patient should raise suspicion of two important diagnoses: α-1 antitrypsin deficiency; and cystic fibrosis. In this case, the chest X-ray is against the diagnosis of cystic fibrosis (**72**). Patients with cystic fibrosis often have cystic bronchiectasis, patchy consolidation and fibrotic changes. Furthermore, the absence of cough productive of sputum is also against the diagnosis of cystic fibrosis.

α-1 antitrypsin deficiency is a rare autosomal recessive disorder due to a genetic abnormality on chromosome 14. The absence or reduced levels of this protease inhibitor leads to alveolar and liver damage. There are several different abnormal alleles for the gene. 'M' is the normal allele, and 'Z' and 'S' are the most frequently encountered abnormal alleles. The expression of each phenotype is suffixed by the letters 'Pi', which stand for protease inhibitor. PiZZ and Pi null null are associated with a high risk of premature emphysema, but only the PiZZ genotype is associated with cirrhosis (*Table*).

The majority of patients with α-1 antitrypsin levels of less than 20% present with emphysema in the fifth decade. Cirrhosis usually occurs at a young age, and patients with the PiZZ genotype may present with neonatal jaundice. The diagnosis is confirmed by measuring the levels of α-1 antitrypsin.

The respiratory manifestations are treated with some success by using synthetic α-1 antitrypsin, but the hepatic manifestation of this condition requires liver transplantation.

Genotype	α-1 antitrypsin levels
PiMM	Normal
PiSS	>50%
PiZZ	<10%
PiSZ	20%
Pi null null	Nil

Answer 73

> 1. b. Secondary polycythaemia.
> 2. i. Red cell mass estimation.
>   ii. Arterial blood gases.
>   iii. Abdominal ultrasound scan with particular reference to the kidneys and the liver.
>   iv. α-fetoprotein.
>   v. Erythropoietin level.

The patient has an elevated haemoglobin and a raised PCV. The differential diagnosis is between pseudopolycythaemia, primary polycythaemia (polycythaemia rubra vera) or a secondary polycythaemia. In pseudopolycythaemia, the Hb and the PCV are raised owing to haemoconcentration resulting from any cause of reduced extracellular volume (dehydration, diuretics). Pseudopolycythaemia can be differentiated from true polycythaemia by red cell mass estimation, which will reveal a normal red cell volume to extracellular fluid volume ratio in pseudopolycythaemia, and a raised ratio in true polycythaemia. A popular cause of pseudopolycythaemia in the MRCP and similar examinations is Gaissbock's syndrome, which occurs in middle-aged men who are usually obese and have a smoking history. In this case, the red cell volume is normal, but the plasma volume is reduced. True polycythaemia is divided into primary polycythaemia and secondary polycythaemia. The former is a result of a myeloproliferative disorder causing erythroid hyperplasia independent of raised circulating erythropoietin, and is better known as polycythaemia rubra vera. In addition to a raised Hb and red cell count, the white cells are also increased in 70% and the platelets in 50% of cases, and physical examination may demonstrate a palpable spleen. In contrast, secondary polycythaemia is due to raised levels of circulating erythropoietin, either owing to a physiological reason, for example, living at high altitude, chronic lung disease, or cyanotic heart disease or owing to inappropriate secretion of erythropoietin from various sources (*Table*). In this condition, the white cells and platelets are unaffected, and the spleen is not palpable.

When faced with a patient with raised Hb and PCV who also has raised white cells, platelets and a palpable spleen, the diagnosis is polycythaemia rubra vera. The investigation required to confirm the diagnosis is a bone marrow aspirate, which will show erythroid hyperplasia and increased megakaryocytes. The leucocyte alkaline phosphatase concentration is also increased. When the white cell and platelet counts are normal, and there is no evidence of splenomegaly, then secondary causes must be sought. The investigation of secondary causes is shown (**73**).

Important note: in polycythaemia rubra vera there is a tendency to bleed. Many patients have occult bleeding from the gastrointestinal tract, and have normal Hb and a high red cell count, but microcytic red cell indices. In these patients, the clue that they may have polycythaemia rubra vera comes from the elevated white cell and platelet counts (see Answer 211).

Causes of polycythaemia

Pseudopolycythaemia
- Dehydration
- Gaissbock's syndrome

Primary
- Polycythaemia rubra vera

Secondary
1. Physiological increase in erythropoietin (due to chronic hypoxaemia):
    - Chronic lung disease
    - Living at high altitudes
    - Cyanotic heart disease
    - Smoking (carboxyhaemoglobin)
    - Familial (HbM)

2. Inappropriate increase in erythropoietin:
    - Renal cell carcinoma, polycystic kidneys, transplant kidney
    - Adrenal tumours (phaeochromocytoma)
    - Hepatocellular carcinoma
    - Ovarian fibroma
    - Cerebellar haemangioblastoma (part of Von Hippel–Lindau)

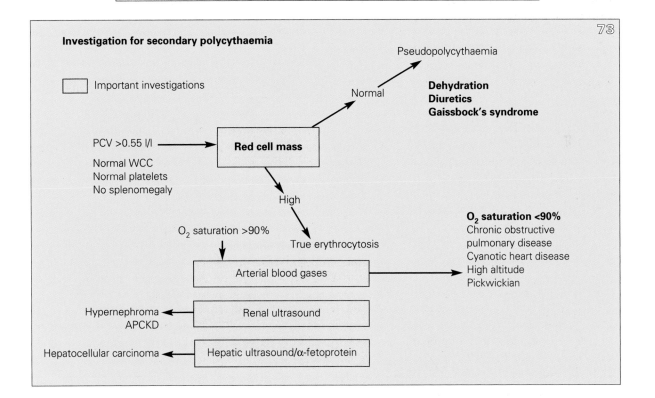

Investigation for secondary polycythaemia

73

Important investigations

PCV >0.55 l/l → **Red cell mass**

Normal WCC
Normal platelets
No splenomegaly

Normal → Pseudopolycythaemia

Dehydration
Diuretics
Gaissbock's syndrome

High → True erythrocytosis

O_2 saturation >90% → Arterial blood gases

O_2 saturation <90%
Chronic obstructive
pulmonary disease
Cyanotic heart disease
High altitude
Pickwickian

Hypernephroma ← Renal ultrasound
APCKD

Hepatocellular carcinoma ← Hepatic ultrasound/α-fetoprotein

Question 74

A 62-year-old former insurance broker presented to the cardiology out-patient clinic with a five-week history of increasing breathlessness and ankle swelling that started while on a three-week holiday in Spain. Over the past three days he had become breathless at rest, and was having to sleep propped up on four pillows to help his symptoms. His GP had commenced him on a small dose of diuretic, which had not made any difference. There was no history of chest pain and no coryzal illness over the past few months. Eight months previously he was diagnosed as having diabetes mellitus, which was not well controlled on oral hypoglycaemic agents, and he had recently started insulin injections. The only other past medical history of note was intermittent pain and swelling in both knees that was helped by taking an NSAID. He was married and had three sons. He had never smoked, and consumed a very occasional glass of wine. There was a strong family history of diabetes and ischaemic heart disease. His father had died from 'heart failure'.

On examination, he was slightly tanned. He was breathless on mild exertion. His heart rate was 110 beats/min and regular. His blood pressure was 100/60 mmHg. Examination of the neck is shown (74a). The apex was displaced in the 6th intercostal space and anterior axillary line. On auscultation of the precordium there was a loud third heart sound, and a soft systolic murmur in the mitral area. Auscultation of the lung fields demonstrated basal inspiratory crackles bilaterally. The ankles were swollen. Abdominal examination revealed a palpable liver edge 4 cm below the costal margin, but there was no other palpable organomegaly.

Initial investigations are shown below.

The patient was treated with intravenous diuretics and made a good recovery. He underwent invasive investigation (74f, g), and was discharged on an ACE inhibitor, furosemide and digoxin. He was reviewed in the cardiology clinic three months later when he complained of some right upper quadrant discomfort and that he had experienced three hypoglycaemic episodes following discharge. The examining cardiologist detected a palpable liver edge, but there was no obvious evidence of cardiac failure. Plans were made for him to have a liver ultrasound scan and to be reviewed again in three months. However, one week before his clinic appointment he was admitted with increasing right upper quadrant pain, abdominal distension and ankle oedema.

On examination he had a heart rate of 100 beats/min and a blood pressure of 100/65 mmHg. The JVP was not raised and the heart sounds were normal. The abdomen was distended from ascites, and the ankles were swollen. Urinalysis was normal. The dose of his diuretics was increased and his ascites started to resolve. An abdominal ultrasound scan was performed. The ultrasound appearance, with the probe in the left lower costal margin, is shown (74h). A liver biopsy was also performed (74i).

Hb	14 g/dl
WCC	$10 \times 10^9/l$
Platelets	$158 \times 10^9/l$
MCV	90 fl
Sodium	134 mmol/l
Potassium	3.5 mmol/l
Urea	11 mmol/l
Creatinine	110 µmol/l
AST	100 iu/l
ALT	110 iu/l
Alkaline phosphatase	130 u/l
Albumin	38 g/l
Blood glucose	6 mmol/l
ECG (74b)	
Chest X-ray (74c)	
Echocardiogram	Parasternal long-axis view (74d); four-chamber view (74e)

1. What was the original cause of this patient's admission?
2. What is shown on the chest X-ray?
3. What is the abnormality on the 12-lead ECG?
4. What does the echocardiogram demonstrate?
5. What invasive investigation was performed during the initial hospital admission, and what did it demonstrate?
6. What is the most probable cause for the pain in his knees?
7. What was the cause of his second admission?
8. What is demonstrated on the abdominal ultrasound scan?
9. What is the stain used on the liver biopsy, and what is its significance?
10. What is the unifying diagnosis?
11. Suggest one therapeutic management step.
12. Suggest one non-therapeutic management step.

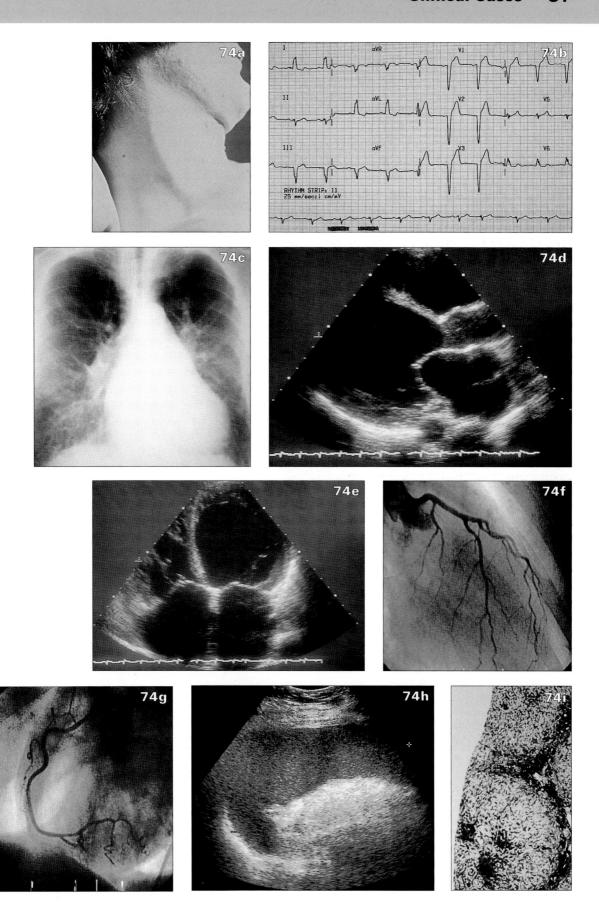

Answer 74

1. Congestive cardiac failure.
2. Cardiomegaly and pulmonary oedema.
3. LBBB (*Table A*).
4. Dilated left ventricle. The upper limit of normal size for the left ventricular end-diastolic dimension is 54 mm. Each white line on the scan represents 10 mm.
5. Coronary angiography, which demonstrates a normal left and right coronary artery. See diagrammatic representation of the coronary anatomy (**74J**).
6. Chondrocalcinosis (*Table B*).
7. Cirrhosis of the liver complicated by portal hypertension.
8. Enlarged spleen which, in the presence of ascites, would be consistent with the diagnosis of portal hypertension in the context of this history.
9. Perl's stain, which is used to demonstrate the presence of iron. In the presence of iron, Perl's stain produces a dark blue/black colour.
10. Idiopathic haemochromatosis.
11. Weekly venesection until the serum ferritin is normal.
12. Screen his sons for the genetic disorder. This could be done genetically, or with iron studies. Affected asymptomatic relatives can thus be treated before there is any tissue damage.

Table A Causes of LBBB

- Ischaemic heart disease
- Cardiomyopathy
- Aortic stenosis
- Hypertensive heart disease
- Cardiac conduction tissue disease
- Following insertion of a pacemaker

Table B Causes of chondrocalcinosis

- Calcium pyrophosphate arthropathy (pseudo gout)
- Gout
- Hyperparathyroidism
- Haemochromatosis
- Hypophosphatasia
- Hypothyroidism
- Wilson's disease
- Alkaptonuria
- Lead poisoning

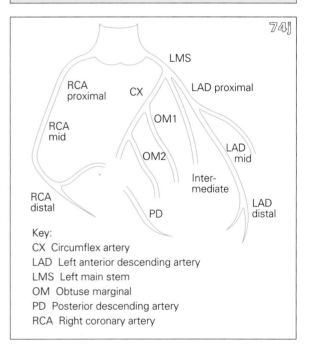

Key:
CX Circumflex artery
LAD Left anterior descending artery
LMS Left main stem
OM Obtuse marginal
PD Posterior descending artery
RCA Right coronary artery

In the absence of alcohol abuse, the combination of a dilated cardiomyopathy with normal coronary arteries, diabetes mellitus, arthropathy, and cirrhosis of the liver in a pigmented individual can all be explained by idiopathic haemochromatosis, an autosomal recessive genetic disorder characterized by increased iron absorption from the gastrointestinal tract with subsequent deposition in the skin, liver, heart, pancreas, gonads and the pituitary gland. The genetic defect is a point mutation on the gene HLA FE, which is the short arm of chromosome 6. The mutation results in the substitution of the amino acid cysteine by tyrosine at position 282. The actual function of the gene is unknown. There is also an association with HLA-A3, B7 and HLA-A3, B14. The most common presentation in homozygotes is with lethargy and malaise, although joint pains, particularly in the knee, symptoms of diabetes mellitus and skin pigmentation may also be the initial presenting complaints. Males are more susceptible than females who are protected by menstruation. Alcohol abuse may cause the same clinical picture in heterozygotes. Cardiac involvement leads to dilated or restrictive cardiomyopathy and an abnormal ECG, but haemochromatosis is a rare cause of cardiomyopathy. Deposition of excess iron in the liver leads to cirrhosis and an increased predisposition to hepatocellular carcinoma. Chondrocalcinosis is a recognized complication, most commonly affecting the metacarpophalangeal and knee joints. Hypogonadism results from direct infiltration into the gonads and into the pituitary.

The diagnosis can be made genetically, but this is currently expensive and iron studies continue to remain the 'gold standard' test. The serum iron is high, the total iron-binding capacity is low, and the serum ferritin is usually in the thousands. The transferrin saturation and

Table C Differential diagnosis of conditions causing simultaneous cardiac and liver disease

	Liver	*Heart*
Alcohol abuse	Cirrhosis	Dilated cardiomyopathy
Haemochromatosis	Cirrhosis	Dilated cardiomyopathy
Pericardial constriction	Cirrhosis	Cardiac failure
Chronic tricuspid regurgitation	Hepatic congestion	Cardiac failure
Carcinoid tumour with hepatic metastases	Metastases	Pulmonary/tricuspid stenosis
Sarcoidosis	Granulomas	Restrictive cardiomyopathy
HIV	Hepatitis	Myopericarditis
Neoplasia	Metastases	Pericardial effusion
Storage disorders	Hepatic dysfunction	Cardiomyopathy

the iron-binding saturation index ([Fe]/[TIBC]) are very sensitive and are typically above 90% in patients with homozygous haemochromatosis. A liver biopsy demonstrates iron overload in the presence or absence of micronodular cirrhosis. There is deposition of iron in the liver parenchyma and the bile duct canaliculi, but the Kupffer cells are spared. A dry iron content of over 180 mg is highly suggestive of the diagnosis.

In some cases, idiopathic haemochromatosis is difficult to differentiate from alcoholic liver disease, which is also associated with raised serum ferritin levels and increased iron deposition in the liver (*Table C*). The liver biopsy is very helpful in this respect because it demonstrates coexisting changes of alcohol-related liver disease such as Mallory's hyaline and, in contrast to idiopathic haemochromatosis, iron deposition occurs in the Kupffer cells.

Question 75

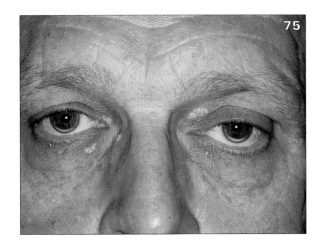

75

disease. A barium meal and ultrasound scan of the hepatobiliary system were normal.

On examination, he was thin. The external appearance of his eyes is shown (**75**). There was no pallor, clubbing or lymphadenopathy. His heart rate was 98 beats/min and blood pressure 140/90 mmHg. The heart sounds were normal and his chest was clear. He had a soft left carotid bruit. On examination of his abdomen he was tender in the epigastrum and umbilical area. There were no abdominal bruits. Neurological examination was normal.

A 55-year-old male was admitted with a three-month history of abdominal pain that was dull in nature and often radiated to his back. The pain was precipitated by meals and started 2 hours after eating. The patient had intermittent diarrhoea productive of foul, bulky stool, and had lost almost 3 kg in weight in three months. He had been diagnosed as having non-insulin-dependent diabetes mellitus six years ago, and had an inferior myocardial infarction two years later. He smoked 20 cigarettes per day and had never consumed alcohol. There was a strong family history of ischaemic heart

1. What is the diagnosis?
   a. Cholelithiasis.
   b. Mesenteric ischaemia.
   c. Carcinoma of the head of pancreas.
   d. Chronic pancreatitis.
   e. Non-alcoholic steatohepatitis.

2. How would you confirm the diagnosis?
   a. Hepatobiliary ultrasonography.
   b. CT scan abdomen.
   c. ERCP.
   d. Mesenteric angiography.
   e. Liver biopsy.

Answer 75

> 1. b. Mesenteric ischaemia. The differential diagnosis includes carcinoma of the pancreas or chronic pancreatitis.
> 2. d. Mesenteric angiography.

The patient has chronic abdominal pain after meals, steatorrhoea and weight loss. All three differential diagnoses could account for this picture. He has stigmata of hyperlipidaemia (the eyes reveal xanthelasma and corneal arcus) and peripheral vascular disease (carotid bruit). He is diabetic, and a long-term smoker. All these factors favour atherosclerosis, making the diagnosis of intestinal ischaemia more likely in the examination situation, although there is no reason why a patient with generalized arteriosclerosis should not develop carcinoma of the pancreas or chronic pancreatitis, which is idiopathic in almost 50% of cases. Severe atheroma affecting the coeliac axis would account for the symptoms. Increased intestinal motility after a meal exacerbates ischaemia, causing pain. The ischaemic small bowel loses functional capacity and therefore a malabsorption syndrome develops. The combination of fear of pain from eating and malabsorption is responsible for weight loss. Zollinger–Ellison syndrome can present with abdominal pain following meals and steatorrhoea; however, in this case the barium meal is invariably abnormal, revealing multiple gastric, duodenal or jejunal ulcers. The possibility of cholelithiasis is excluded by the normal hepatobiliary ultrasound scan.

Mesenteric ischaemia is essentially a diagnosis of exclusion. In this situation the patient would have a CT scan of the abdomen and an ERCP to check for carcinoma of the pancreas and chronic pancreatitis. If these tests are negative, mesenteric angiography would help validate the clinical suspicion of mesenteric ischaemia. Some patients can have severe atherosclerosis of the mesenteric arteries and be completely asymptomatic; therefore, this finding does not necessarily diagnose mesenteric ischaemia as the cause of his symptoms unless other potential causes have been excluded. Non-alcoholic steatohepatitis is not usually associated with abdominal pain.

Question 76

A 34-year-old female presented with a six-week history of epigastric pain that radiated to her back and that was precipitated by meals. There was no accompanying nausea or vomiting. Her GP prescribed ranitidine and antacid solution, which relieved the discomfort to some extent. Just one month previously she had requested a blood sugar check because she had developed nocturia, but the test was normal. According to her husband, she had started to become miserable and spoke very little. She attributed this to fear of having an abdominal malignancy because her maternal aunt had just died from carcinoma of the stomach. The only other family history of significance was that her father had undergone an operation on his neck 20 years ago to treat kidney stones. She did not consume alcohol and was a non-smoker. She worked in a confectioner's shop near the house. She had two daughters, aged eight and six.

On examination, the patient had mild tenderness on palpation of the epigastrum, but all other physical examination was normal.

Investigations are shown.

The patient underwent surgery shortly afterwards, which improved all her symptoms, and she remained well for six years; following this, the abdominal pain returned. The pain was associated with dyspepsia. She also complained of intermittent episodes of foul-smelling diarrhoea. She was prescribed ranitidine once again; however, on this occasion it proved to be ineffective. She was advised to stay on ranitidine and referred to a gastroenterologist, who performed upper gastrointestinal endoscopy and demonstrated many small ulcers in the antrum of the stomach and the first and second part of the duodenum. A serum gastrin level was also performed and it was 500 pg/ml (NR <100 pg/ml). He commenced the patient on 40 mg of omeprazole, after

Hb	12 g/dl
WCC	7×10^9/l
Platelets	380×10^9/l
MCV	88 fl
ESR	11 mm/h
Sodium	135 mmol/l
Potassium	4 mmol/l
Urea	7.1 mmol/l
Creatinine	89 µmol/l
Chloride	118 mmol/l
Bicarbonate	19 mmol/l
Calcium	3.0 mmol/l
Phosphate	0.7 mmol/l
Alkaline phosphatase	345 iu/l
Blood glucose	4.6 mmol/l
Abdominal X-ray	Faecal loading, but no bowel obstruction
Urinary calcium	20 mmol/l

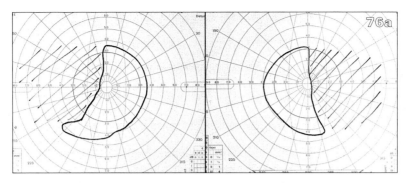

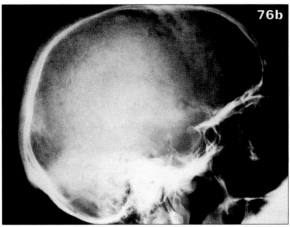

which her symptoms improved. Her GP had tried to reduce the dose to 20 mg after six weeks, but she started developing abdominal pain and the dose was raised back up to 40 mg.

The patient remained well for a further two years, after which she presented with increasing lethargy and headaches. She had stopped menstruating, and had reduced libido. Her appetite was reduced, but she had not lost any weight.

On examination, she was pale and had very scanty axillary and pubic hair. Her skin was dry. Her pulse was 62 beats/min and blood pressure 105/65 mmHg. Examination of her fundi showed slightly pale discs. Her visual fields are shown (**76a**). Neurological examination of her arms and legs and examination of the other systems was normal.

Further investigations are shown.

Hb	10 g/dl
WCC	6×10^9/l
Platelets	300×10^9/l
MCV	81 fl
ESR	25 mm/h
Sodium	129 mmol/l
Potassium	4 mmol/l
Urea	4 mmol/l
Creatinine	89 µmol/l
Calcium	2.1 mmol/l
Phosphate	1.2 mmol/l
Alkaline phosphatase	92 iu/l
Thyroxine	4 nmol/l
TSH	0.1 mu/l
FSH	0.3 iu/l
LH	0.3 iu/l
PRL	4,500 mu/l
Skull X-ray (**76b**)	

1. What was the initial diagnosis?
2. Which surgical procedure had her father undergone?
3. What was the cause of the pain six years later?
4. Which investigation would you have performed to confirm the diagnosis six years later?
5. What is the abnormality on the visual fields?
6. What is demonstrated on the skull X-ray?
7. What was the cause of her headaches?
8. Which single diagnosis accounts for all her presentations?
9. Should anyone else be investigated?

Answer 76

1. Hyperparathyroidism.
2. Parathyroidectomy.
3. Peptic ulceration resulting from a gastrinoma.
4. Assessment of serum gastrin after intravenous secretin or measurement of gastric acid output after the administration of pentagastrin. In normal individuals, secretin causes suppression of serum gastrin levels; however, in patients with gastrinomas, gastrin secretion is not suppressed and may even demonstrate a paradoxical rise. Pentagastrin reduces gastric acid production in normal individuals, but not in patients with gastrinomas.
5. The patient has a bitemporal hemianopia, suggesting a lesion compressing the optic chiasm. This could be a meningioma, an aneurysm, a pituitary tumour or a cerebral metastasis.
6. There is enlargement of the pituitary fossa, a double floor to the sella turcica and erosion of the posterior clinoid process. The findings are consistent with a pituitary tumour.
7. Raised intracranial pressure resulting from a large prolactinoma. A prolactinoma is the most common pituitary tumour associated with multiple endocrine neoplasia (MEN) 1. Prolactinomas are associated with amenorrhoea, galactorrhoea, hirsutism and infertility in females. In males prolactinomas cause impotence, oligospermia, infertility and galactorrhoea. Note: hyperprolactinaemia does not cause gynaecomastia. There are several causes of raised PRL (*Table*), but a PRL of over 3,000 mu/l is highly suggestive of prolactinoma. Treatment is with bromocriptine for small tumours and surgery for larger ones.
8. Multiple endocrine neoplasia type 1.
9. The condition is autosomal dominant, so there is a 50% chance of her offspring inheriting the condition. Therefore, both daughters should be screened for the condition.

MEN 1 is characterized by tumours of the parathyroid gland (95%), islet cells (50%) and the pituitary gland (33%). Abnormality within a gene termed the menin gene on chromosome 11 is responsible, but the function of the gene is yet to be elucidated. Hypercalcaemia is the first presentation, usually from the third decade onwards. Islet cell tumours (usually gastrinomas or insulinomas) occur in the fourth or fifth decade, and pituitary tumours (usually prolactinomas) occur in the fifth or sixth decade.

Screening is with yearly calcium/PTH and PRL, and a two-yearly pituitary MRI. Patients are made aware of symptoms of islet cell tumours so that they present early.

Causes of hyperprolactinaemia

- Prolactinoma
- Hypothalamic or pituitary stalk lesions
- Hypothyroidism
- Coitus
- Pregnancy
- Nipple suckling
- Stress
- Oral contraceptive pill
- Dopamine antagonist drugs, e.g. phenothiazines
- PCOS
- Chronic renal failure
- Chest wall damage/trauma

Question 77

A 48-year-old male with rheumatoid arthritis presented with a cough, high fever and painless jaundice. He had a seven-year history of rheumatoid arthritis affecting his shoulders, elbows, wrists, hands and feet, and which was refractory to therapy with NSAIDs. Over the past 16 months his symptoms had progressed, and he had been switched to immunosuppressant drugs, which had controlled his symptoms. He was a non-smoker and consumed less than 2 units of alcohol per week.

On examination he was unwell, jaundiced and had a temperature of 39°C (102.2°F). Examination of the oral cavity revealed candidal infection and palatal petechiae. On auscultation of the lung fields there were coarse crackles at the right lung base. On abdominal examination there was evidence of a palpable spleen 3 cm below the costal margin.

Investigations are shown.

Hb	7.1 g/dl
WCC	1.4 × 10⁹/l
Platelets	33 × 10⁹/l
MCV	103 fl
Reticulocyte count	<1%
INR	1.9
ESR	70 mm/h
CRP	190 g/l
Sodium	136 mmol/l
Potassium	4 mmol/l
Urea	6 mmol/l
Creatinine	110 µmol/l
Bilirubin	180 µmol/l
AST	180 iu/l
Alkaline phosphatase	450 iu/l
Albumin	29 g/l

1. Give three possible causes for this patient's presentation.
2. Which six investigations would you perform on admission?
3. Give three explanations for the raised MCV.
4. List two immediate management steps.

Question 78

The following cardiac catheter data is from a 10-year-old male after a murmur was heard during a school medical.

1. What are the two main abnormalities?
2. What is the diagnosis?

Chamber	Pressure (mmHg)	Oxygen saturation(%)
Right atrium	5	74
Right ventricle	20/6	74
Pulmonary artery	32/12	92
PCWP	3	
Left ventricle	100/8	96
Aorta	90/65	96

Answer 77

1. i. Septicaemia secondary to respiratory infection precipitated by methotrexate-induced neutropenia.
   ii. Septicaemia secondary to respiratory infection precipitated by azathioprine-induced neutropenia.
   iii. Septicaemia secondary to respiratory tract infection due to Felty's syndrome.
2. i. Chest X-ray.
   ii. Oxygen saturation.
   iii. Blood cultures.
   iv. Urine culture.
   v. Throat swab for culture.
   vi. Hepatobiliary ultrasound scan.
3. i. Megaloblastic anaemia due to methotrexate or azathioprine.
   ii. Megaloblastic anaemia due to folate deficiency (methotrexate inhibits dihydrofolate reductase).
   iii. Liver cirrhosis.
4. i. Stop immunosuppressant drug.
   ii. Broad-spectrum intravenous antibiotics following a septic screen. Usually the combination of a penicillin and aminoglycoside or a third-line cephalosporin is used.

This patient with rheumatoid arthritis presents with a respiratory tract infection and high fever. The blood tests reveal a profound neutropenia, which has almost certainly predisposed him to the respiratory and oral *Candida* infection. In the context of rheumatoid arthritis, the neutropenia is either drug-induced or secondary to hypersplenism (part of Felty's syndrome). Felty's syndrome alone cannot explain the abnormal bilirubin and alkaline phosphatase which, in the absence of abdominal pain, suggest either a cholestatic hepatitis or cirrhosis of the liver. Both methotrexate and azathioprine, which are sometimes used as immunosuppressants in rheumatoid arthritis, may also cause hepatitis and cirrhosis. The mode of action of these drugs is to interfere with purine nucleotide synthesis required for nucleic acid generation. All cells in the body with a rapid turnover time are affected, particularly the cells in the marrow – hence the pancytopenia. The raised MCV is probably due to a megaloblastic anaemia, but may be due to chronic liver disease.

Methotrexate-induced liver cirrhosis only complicates 1% of all patients taking the drug. Liver disease is more common in patients consuming over 10 units of alcohol per week, patients with diabetes and patients taking the drug frequently. In the early stages the symptoms are non-specific and comprise anorexia and nausea; however, late disease presents with portal hypertension, varices or hepatocellular failure. Azathioprine-induced hepatitis is rare but may occur early in patients taking allopurinol, as the latter drug potentiates the effects of azathioprine.

The immediate management of this patient is a septic screen (blood cultures, urine culture, throat and nasal swabs) followed by broad-spectrum antibiotics. Be careful when performing blood gases in a patient with low platelets and abnormal clotting. Oxygen saturation using a pulse oximeter is the safest method of determining arterial oxygenation in this case. An ultrasound scan of the biliary system should be requested to exclude biliary obstruction.

Answer 78

1. i. Elevated pulmonary artery pressure.
   ii. Step up in oxygen saturation in the pulmonary artery.
2. The findings are consistent with a patent ductus arteriosus with a left-to-right shunt.

Question 79

A 25-year-old male presented to the Accident and Emergency Department with a three-day history of pleuritic, left-sided chest pain and increasing breathlessness. The symptoms started suddenly while he was playing football. He denied any chest trauma. Until then he had been fit and well, and there was no past medical history of note. His father died suddenly at the age of 32 years.

On examination he was thin and tall and distressed with pain. There was no pallor or cyanosis. He had a wide arm span. The heart rate was 100 beats/min and blood pressure 150/80 mmHg. The respiratory rate was 32/min. The trachea was deviated to the right. Percussion appeared to be reduced on the right side and was loud on the left side. The left lung base was dull to percussion. On auscultation of the lung fields breath sounds were absent on the left side and normal on the right side. Auscultation of the precordium demonstrated quiet heart sounds and a soft mid-systolic murmur. The femoral pulses were easily palpable. The left calf was bruised and slightly tender. He attributed this to an injury sustained during the football match. The ECG revealed normal sinus rhythm. The ECG complexes were small, but there were no other abnormalities.

1. Which test would you perform to reach a diagnosis?
2. What is the cause of his respiratory symptoms?
3. What is the management?
4. What is the unifying diagnosis?

Question 80

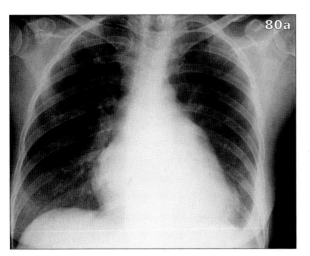

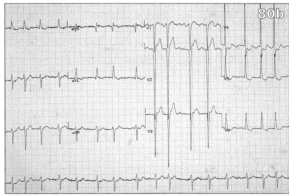

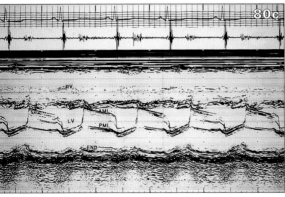

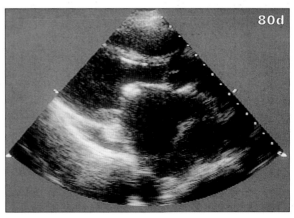

A 66-year-old female was investigated for a six-month history of increasing breathlessness and palpitation. She had a long history of hypertension. A chest X-ray (**80a**), ECG (**80b**), M-mode and 2-D echocardiograms (**80c, d**, respectively) are shown.

1. What does the chest X-ray reveal?
2. What is the abnormality on the ECG?
3. List two abnormalities on the 2-D echocardiogram.
4. List four abnormalities on the M-mode echocardiogram.
5. Which three pharmacological agents would you prescribe for this patient?

Answer 79

1. Chest radiography.
2. A large, left-sided pneumothorax.
3. Insertion of a chest drain.
4. Marfan's syndrome.

A large pneumothorax in a symptomatic patient receives relief with chest drain insertion rather than simple needle aspiration. Pleuritic chest pain and increasing breathlessness occur in pleurisy with or without pleural effusion, pneumonia, pulmonary embolism and lung malignancy. The physical signs are suggestive of a large left pleural effusion. The trachea is deviated to the right, and there are no breath sounds on auscultation of the left lung. The right lung sounds comparatively dull to percussion when compared with the left lung, which is hyper-resonant. There also appears to be a small effusion at the base of the left lung, which is not uncommon with pneumothoraces and represents either blood or an inflammatory exudate.

Causes of pneumothorax include asthma, emphysema, stab wound to the lung or following a fractured rib, fibrotic lung disease, suppurative lung disease (rupture of a lung abscess into a bronchus, staphylococcal pneumonia), pneumoconiosis, neurofibromatosis, tuberose sclerosis, Marfan's syndrome, Ehlers–Danlos syndrome and lymphangioleiomyomatosis. Most cases are idiopathic and occur in tall, thin men. A rare form, usually left-sided, occurs in women during menstruation (catamenial pneumothorax). It is possibly due to pulmonary endometriosis.

The underlying diagnosis and the cause of the pnemothorax in this case is Marfan's syndrome. This is suggested by his tall height, cardiac mumur consistent with mitral valve prolapse and a possible family history of the condition, i.e. his father died prematurely. The syndrome is caused by a mutation in the gene encoding the connective tissue protein fibrillin on chromosome 15. The condition is inherited as an autosomal dominant trait. Affected individuals are tall, have a wide arm span, arachnodactyly and skeletal deformities which include kyphoscoliosis, high arched palate, and pectus excavatum. The joints are hyperextensile. Other associations include lens dislocation and retinal detachment. Mitral valve prolapse and aortic dilatation are recognised cardiac manifestations. Aortic dissection or rupture are the commonest cause of death. Patients with Marfan's syndrome have a higher incidence of pneumothorax than the general population.

Answer 80

1. An enlarged cardiothoracic ratio and evidence of an enlarged left atrium. Features of an enlarged left atrium include a prominent left heart border, a double shadow behind the heart and splaying of the carinae, with elevation of the left hilum.
2. Atrial fibrillation (for causes, see *Table*, Answer 138). There is a complete absence of P-waves and a beat-to-beat variation of the RR-interval. This patient also has voltage criteria for left ventricular hypertrophy, presumably secondary to the hypertension or coexisting mitral regurgitation.
3. i. Enlarged left atrium.
   ii. A thickened dome-shaped appearance of the mitral valve in diastole, which is consistent with mitral stenosis.
4. i. Thickening of the anterior mitral valve leaflet, which is characterized by loss of its normal 'M'-shape in diastole.
   ii. Multiple echoes on the anterior mitral valve leaflet that suggest fibrosis.
   iii. Reduced mitral valve excursion.
   iv. Anterior movement of the posterior leaflet in diastole (in normal individuals the posterior leaflet moves backwards in diastole). (See Echocardiography, page 421.)
5. i. Digoxin to control ventricular rate.
   ii. Furosemide to help improve breathlessness from pulmonary congestion.
   iii. Warfarin as prophylaxis to thromboembolism. Patients with mitral stenosis and atrial fibrillation have a 35% chance of having an embolic CVA per annum.

Question 81

A 47-year-old businessman was referred to the dermatology clinic with a rash over his hands, scalp and face. He had been generally well. He smoked 20 cigarettes per day and drank 8–10 units of alcohol on a daily basis. There was no other significant medical history of note. The patient had not taken any medication, with the exception of occasional chlorpheniramine to help relieve his symptoms. On examination he had vesicular lesions affecting his face, forearms, hands (**81**) and scalp. All other physical examination was essentially normal.

Investigations are shown.

Hb	18.5 g/dl
WCC	7×10^9/l
Platelets	149×10^9/l
MCV	101 fl
Sodium	135 mmol/l
Potassium	3.9 mmol/l
Urea	4 mmol/l
Creatinine	80 µmol/l
Blood glucose	10 mmol/l
Bilirubin	25 µmol/l
AST	52 iu/l
Alkaline phosphatase	450 iu/l
Albumin	37 g/l
Globulins	30 g/l
Gamma GT	52 iu/l
Serum ferritin	550 µg/l
Skin biopsy	Subepidermal blisters with perivascular deposition of PAS-staining material

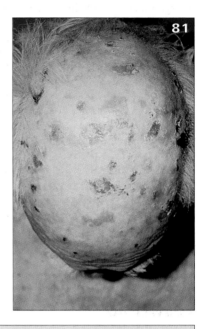

1. What is the most probable diagnosis?
2. State two tests to confirm the diagnosis.
3. What two factors should this patient avoid?
4. Apart from avoidance, give two other therapeutic measures.

Question 82

A 13-year-old female was admitted under the surgeons with acute abdominal pain. The blood pressure was 100/60 mmHg.

Investigations are shown.

Sodium	131 mmol/l
Potassium	7.2 mmol/l
Urea	13 mmol/l
Creatinine	121 µmol/l
Bicarbonate	8 mmol/l
Chloride	96 mmol/l
Abdominal X-ray	Normal
Urinalysis	Glucose +++

1. What is the acid-base disturbance?
2. What is the most likely cause for the abnormality?
3. List three therapeutic management steps.

Answer 81

1. PCT.
2. i. Urinary uroporphyrin level.
   ii. Uroporphyrin decarboxylase assay on red blood cells.
3. i. Sunlight.
   ii. Alcohol.
4. i. Venesection.
   ii. Chloroquine.

The blistering skin rash in a patient with a history of excess alcohol consumption and biochemical evidence of liver disease is suggestive of the diagnosis of PCT.

PCT is a rare disorder of haem synthesis that is inherited as an autosomal dominant trait. It is one of the most commonly tested porphyrias in higher medical examinations, and is caused by a reduced activity or complete absence of the enzyme uroporphyrin decarboxylase, which catalyses the conversion of uroporphyrin to coproporphyrin. This leads to an excess of uroporphyrins in the blood and urine. The result is a pruritic photosensitive blistering rash that affects areas exposed to sunlight, and cirrhosis of the liver. Blisters on the skin lesion contain PAS-positive material. The clinical effect of this deficiency becomes most apparent in genetically predisposed patients who consume excess alcohol or other drugs that are enzyme-inducers for haem synthesis (most commonly anticonvulsants and oestrogens). Hepatic involvement is common and is predominantly due to the effects of excess alcohol. The liver biopsy demonstrates macronodular cirrhosis and Mallory's hyaline. A proportion of patients with liver disease also have evidence of iron overload in the blood and liver, resulting in a raised serum ferritin and a positive Perl's stain on liver biopsy, respectively; in addition, approximately 20% develop diabetes mellitus. The condition may be confused with haemochromatosis (iron overload, cirrhosis and diabetes); however, haemochromatosis is not associated with a blistering rash. A secondary polycythaemia may also occur and appears to compound the condition.

Treatment is by abstaining from alcohol and avoiding sunlight. In patients with a high Hb, weekly venesection (not more than 1 unit) until the Hb is less than 12 g/dl helps to alleviate the skin manifestations. Chloroquine, which binds uroporphyrin and helps urinary clearance, is commonly used in the management of PCT.

Answer 82

1. Metabolic acidosis with a high anion gap.

2. Diabetic ketoacidosis.

3. i. Intravenous calcium gluconate to prevent hyperkalaemic cardiac arrest.
   ii. Intravenous insulin infusion to halt further ketoacidosis.
   iii. Intravenous saline to rehydrate patient and correct acidosis.

The patient has a very low serum bicarbonate, which is indicative of a metabolic acidosis. The heavy glycosuria is the clue to the cause of the acidosis. Diabetic ketoacidosis is the result of insulin deficiency. It may occur in previously undiagnosed insulin-dependent diabetes mellitus, established insulin-dependent diabetics who are on suboptimal insulin doses or who have interrupted insulin therapy, and insulin-dependent diabetics who have intercurrent illness resulting in increases in hormones which antagonize the effects of insulin. In the absence of insulin, hepatic gluconeogenesis is increased, but peripheral glucose uptake is decreased; the result is an osmotic diuresis and dehydration. Peripheral oxidation of free fatty acids is increased, which results in an increase in ketones, leading to a metabolic acidosis. Both the acidosis and hypoperfusion of the kidneys due to hypovolaemia contribute to the hyperkalaemia (reduced potassium excretion). Treatment involves rehydration and insulin replacement. If the serum potassium is above 6.8 mmol/l, calcium gluconate is advised to prevent hyperkalaemia-induced cardiac arrest. Intravenous bicarbonate should only be given if the arterial pH is <7. (See Acid–base Disturbance, page 426.)

Question 83

A 14-year-old male was admitted with a headache and drowsiness. Three days previously he had complained of a sore throat.

Investigations are shown.

CT scan of brain	Normal
CSF:	
Opening pressure	160 cmH$_2$O
Cells	200 neutrophils/mm^3
	20 red cells/mm^3
Protein	1.2 g/l
Glucose	2.4 mmol/l
Gram stain (**83a**)	

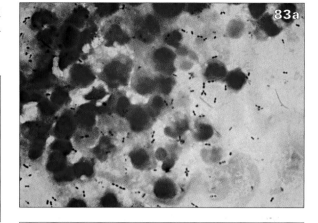

1. What is the diagnosis?
    a. Streptococcal meningitis.
    b. Meningococcal meningitis.
    c. Haemophilus influenzae meningitis.
    d. Tuberculous meningitis.
    e. Cryptococcal meningitis.
2. What is the management?

Question 84

A 64-year-old West Indian male was admitted after his daughter noted that he had become increasingly drowsy over the past 48 hours. He had a 10-year history of diabetes mellitus for which he was taking chlorpropamide. Before the deterioration, he had complained of increasing urinary frequency and excessive thirst. He recently saw his GP, and was noted to have a blood pressure of 170/100 mmHg for which he had been commenced on a thiazide diuretic.

On examination he was drowsy and apyrexial, but answered questions appropriately. There was reduced skin turgor. The heart rate was 110 beats/min and regular, and the blood pressure was 115/60 mmHg. The heart sounds were normal, and the chest was clear. Examination of the abdomen did not reveal any abnormality, and there was no focal neurological deficit.

Investigations are shown.

Hb	15 g/dl
WCC	13 × 10^9/l
Platelets	179 × 10^9/l
Sodium	151 mmol/l
Potassium	5 mmol/
Urea	17 mmol/l
Creatinine	140 µmol/l
Urinalysis	Glucose +++
	Protein +

1. What is the diagnosis?
2. List six investigations which should be performed on this patient.
3. List four steps in your management.

Answer 83

> 1. **a.** Streptococcal meningitis.
> 2. Intravenous cefotaxime on admission. The antibiotic can be switched to benzylpenicillin if the organism is sensitive to penicillin.

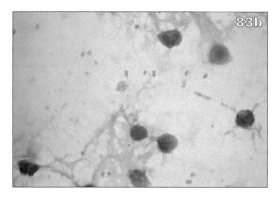

The CSF neutrophil count is consistent with a bacterial meningitis (see Answer 267). The three commonest bacterial meningitides worldwide include those due to *Streptococcus pneumoniae*, *Neisseria meningitidis*, and *Haemophilus influenzae*. The Gram stain reveals Gram-positive (stain blue–purple) cocci, therefore the most likely diagnosis is *S. pneumoniae*.

N. menigitidis is a Gram-negative (stains pink) diploccocus (**83b**). *H. influenzae* is a Gram-negative bacillus (pink rods in **83c**).

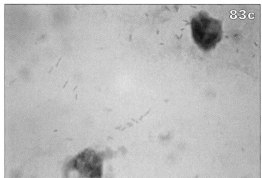

All three present with fever, headache, neck stiffness and photophobia. A necrotic purpuric rash is characteristic of menigitis due to *N. meningitidis*, but may occur with all three types.

Answer 84

> 1. Hyperosmolar non-ketotic diabetic coma (HONK).
>
> 2. i. Plasma osmolality.
>   ii. Blood glucose.
>   iii. Blood cultures.
>   iv. Urine culture.
>   v. Chest X-ray.
>   vi. ECG.
>
> 3. i. Rehydration with 0.9% saline.
>   ii. Insulin infusion of 1–3 units/h.
>   iii. Anticoagulation.
>   iv. Treat underlying cause.

Hyperosmolar non-ketotic diabetic coma usually complicates middle-aged or elderly patients with non-insulin-dependent diabetes mellitus and is characterized by a marked increase in blood glucose (usually higher than 50 mmol/l) and a consequent increase in plasma osmolality. Ketonuria is absent and acidosis is mild or absent. The actual pathogenesis of the condition is unclear, but possible triggers include consumption of large amounts of sugary drinks, infection, recent prescription of thiazide diuretics or steroids and myocardial infarction. Patients present with thirst, polyuria, impaired level of consciousness and sometimes evidence of the precipitating disorder.

Investigations reveal a high blood glucose and plasma osmolality. The plasma sodium is usually elevated owing to pure water loss from osmotic diuresis; however, it may be falsely low (pseudohyponatraemia) owing to the presence of excess lipids. The serum pH is usually normal, but the patient may have a mild acidosis. Other investigations that should be performed are an infection screen and an ECG (beware of silent myocardial infarction in a diabetic patient!).

Management includes rehydration with normal saline. In patients with persisting severe hypernatraemia despite treatment with normal saline (sodium >150 mmol/l), half-strength saline is used. Insulin is infused carefully as HONK is more sensitive to insulin than diabetic ketoacidosis. The patient is given 4 units immediately followed by an infusion of 1–3 units/h. The aim is to reduce the plasma osmolality by approximately 3 mOsm/h. A rapid reduction in plasma osmolality is dangerous because it may precipitate cerebral oedema. Bicarbonate infusion is not required. Prophylactic anticoagulation with heparin is recommended because the high glucose concentration and dehydration result in hyperviscosity. After treatment of the acute state the patient should be recommenced on an oral hypoglycaemic agent.

Question 85

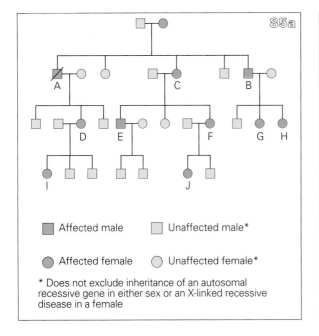

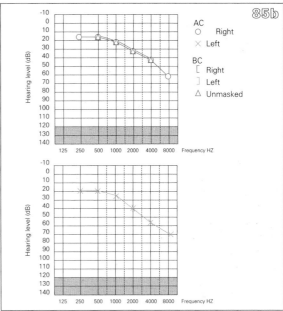

Affected male ■ Unaffected male* ☐

Affected female ● Unaffected female* ○

* Does not exclude inheritance of an autosomal recessive gene in either sex or an X-linked recessive disease in a female

The chart above (**85a**) is the pedigree of a family with a rare condition. All members are affected by the same condition. Patient A is dead, but he had a history of progressive renal failure, and had a renal transplant which was affected by a separate renal disease causing haematuria and rapid deterioration of renal function. An audiogram and a picture of his fundus have been removed from his case notes and are shown (**85b, c**). His sister (patient C), aged 70 years, was deaf and had intermittent haematuria, but her creatinine was 89 µmol/l. His brother (patient B), aged 65 years, had a renal transplant 14 years previously and was also deaf. Patients D, F, G, H, I and J all had a history of intermittent haematuria, but serum creatinine was within the normal range in each case. Patients D and H had premature cataracts, and patient J was blind, but did not have cataracts. Patient E was aged 38 and was on the transplant list for renal failure. He had been fitted with a hearing aid aged 26 years, and had had intermittent haematuria since he was aged 7 years.

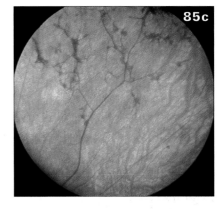

1. What is the mode of transmission of the disorder?
2. What is shown on the audiogram?
3. Why may patient J have been blind?
4. What is the underlying condition in the affected members of this family?
5. Which renal disease did patient A develop in his transplanted kidney?

Question 86

A 45-year-old male attended to become a blood donor. Blood results were as follows (0 = no agglutination, + = agglutination):

1. What is the patient's blood group?
2. Give at least two possible underlying diagnoses.

Patient's cells against anti-A = 0
Patient's cells against anti-B = 0
Patient's cells against anti-A and anti-B = 0
Patient's serum against red cells with antigen A = 0
Patient's serum against red cells with antigen B = 0
Patient's cells against anti-D = +
Immunoglobulins: IgM 0.2 g/l; IgG 1.5 g/l; IgA 0.1 g/l

Answer 85

> 1. The mode of inheritance is X-linked dominant.
> 2. There is progressive and severe hearing loss at higher frequencies which is typical of sensorineuronal deafness. (See Audiograms, page 416.)
> 3. It is possible that she had retinitis pigmentosa just like her great uncle (patient A).
> 4. The condition is Alport's syndrome.
> 5. Anti-GBM disease.

There is no male-to-male transmission which is characteristic of X-linked conditions. Affected males transmit the disease to all female offspring in conditions inherited by an X-linked dominant trait, whereas affected females pass the disease to 50% of all their offspring.

Alports's syndrome is an X-linked hereditary nephritis characterized by progressive glomerular disease, ocular and auditory abnormalities. The renal manifestations begin early in childhood, comprising asymptomatic haematuria and proteinuria. Progressive renal deterioration has a bimodal age distribution, presenting between 16–35 years and 45–60 years. Only males develop progressive renal failure. Affected females develop asymptomatic haematuria, but progression to renal failure does not occur. Sensorineuronal loss occurs in 30–50% of patients, and many patients have ocular abnormalities which include myopia, retinitis pigmentosa (**85c**) and cataracts. Renal biopsy reveals thinning of the GBM, but as the disease progresses the membranes become thin and start to split. The genetic defect is in the α-5 chain of type IV collagen which is located on the X chromosome, but collagen defects in the α-3 and α-4 chains of type IV collagen on chromosome 2 have also been described in some families. All three types of α chains combine to form the collagen network in the GBM. Some patients with Alport's syndrome develop anti-GBM antibodies after renal transplantation. The risk is greatest in patients with a large deletion in the gene encoding the α-3 chain of type IV collagen, in which case the Goodpasture antigen is not expressed and therefore the Goodpasture antigen in the transplanted organ is recognized as foreign. Some 5% of patients with transplants for Alport's syndrome will develop anti-GBM disease.

Answer 86

> 1. Blood group O rhesus-positive (absent anti-A and anti-B).
> 2. Hypogammaglobulinaemia due to:
>   i. Thymoma.
>   ii. Chronic lymphatic leukaemia.
>   iii. Myeloma.
>   iv. Lymphoma.
>   v. Drugs.
>   vi. Common variable hypogammaglobulinaemia.
>   vii. HIV infection.

The patient's red cells fail to agglutinate with sera containing anti-A and anti-B, suggesting that the patient is blood group O, i.e. the cells do not express the antigens A or B on the cell surface. His cells agglutinate with serum containing anti-D, indicating that his cells express the rhesus D antigen. Patients with blood group O have anti-A and anti-B antibodies which are of the IgG, IgM and the IgA class. The serum from an O-positive individual should normally agglutinate blood cells expressing antigens A and B, unless the antibodies are present in very low titre. Failure of the appropriate agglutination may arise in conditions predisposing to hypogammaglobulinaemia and with paraproteinaemias. In generalized hypogammaglobulinaemia the low levels of IgG, IgM and IgA are responsible for the poor response. With paraproteinaemias, one of the immunoglobulin subset levels may be elevated (usually IgG) due to autonomous production. These antibodies are monoclonal and are not directed towards any specific antigen. They are generally ineffective. Autonomous production of a monoclonal antibody also leads to paraparesis of the other immunoglobulin subtypes, causing further immunosuppression.

This man has evidence of hypogammaglobulinaemia. He is 40 years of age and is unlikely to have an inherited hypogammaglobulinaemia because one would associate this with a previous history of infections. An acquired hypogammaglobulinaemia is more likely, and examples include chronic lymphatic leukaemia, lymphoma, myeloma and thymoma.

Question 87

A 35-year-old woman presented with an epileptic seizure five days after having a baby by Caesarean section. There was no previous history of epilepsy. She had been well throughout her pregnancy. She had had two normal pregnancies without any complication.

On examination her heart rate was 90 beats/min and regular and her temperature was 37.9°C (100.2°F). The blood pressure was 180/102 mmHg. She had a Glasgow coma score of 13/15. There was no evidence of a focal neurological deficit. Investigations are shown.

What is the immediate management?
  a. Intravenous high-dose steroids.
  b. Platelet transfusion.
  c. Vitamin K.
  d. Plasma exchange with fresh-frozen plasma.
  e. Warfarin.

Hb	10 g/dl	Sodium	137 mmol/l
WCC	11 × 10⁹/l	Potassium	4.6 mmol/l
Platelets	45 × 10⁹/l	Urea	10 mmol/l
Blood film	Normochromic normocytic anaemia	Creatinine	130 μmol/l
	Fragmented red cells;	Bilirubin	11 μmol/l
	microspherocytes	AST	34 iu/l
PT	14 s (control 14 s)	LDH	1530 iu/l (NR 252–525 iu/l)
APTT	45 s (control 44 s)	Alkaline phosphatase	80 iu/l
Factor V level	Normal	Albumin	30 g/l
Factor VII level	Normal	Urinalysis	Protein ++
		CT scan brain	Normal

Question 88

A 68-year-old Sri Lankan woman presented with a three-week history of lower back pain and progressive weakness of the lower limbs. She had a temperature of 37.9°C (100.2°F). Investigationsare shown.

Hb	10 g/dl
WCC	13 × 10⁹/l
Platelets	460 × 10⁹/l
ESR	120 mm/h
CRP	200 g/l
Blood cultures	Sterile
Lumbar spine X-ray	(**88a**)
MRI scan lumbar spine	(**88b**)

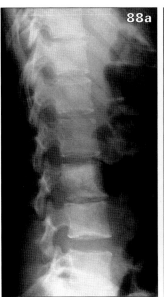 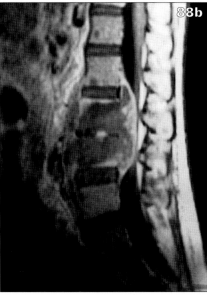

What would be the next management step?
  a. Start IV flucloxacillin and IV gentamicin.
  b. Start conventional anti-tuberculous treatment.
  c. Arrange bone scan.
  d. Organize CT-guided aspiration/biopsy of the lower lumbar spine.
  e. Perform a Heaf test.

Answer 87

> d. Plasma exchange with fresh frozen plasma.

The patient is post-partum and presents with an epileptic seizure (*Table A*). She has a fever, thrombocytopenia, microangiopathic haemolytic anaemia and impaired renal function, raising the possibility of either haemolytic uraemic syndrome or thrombotic thrombocytopenic purpura. The two conditions are probably part of the same disorder. Classically TTP is characterized by neurological manifestation and more subtle deterioration in renal function compared with HUS, where neurological dysfunction is relatively infrequent. In TTP neurological manifestations include headache, seizures and coma. Objective localizing signs are rare. Diagnosis of TTP is based on the pentad below (*Table B*).

The differential diagnosis for TTP or HUS includes DIC, anti-phospholipid syndrome, vasculitides and malignant hypertension. TTP or HUS can usually be differentiated from these conditions (*Table C*)

In some patients TTP is secondary to deficiency of the enzyme von Willebrand factor cleaving protease (ADAMTS13). Von Willebrand factor is synthesized in endothelial cells and assembled in larger multimers that are present in normal plasma. The larger multimers, called unusually large von Willebrand factor (ULvWf), are rapidly degraded in the circulation into the normal size range of vWf multimers by a specific von Willebrand factor-cleaving protease (ADAMTS13).

ULvWf multimers (including unique forms arising from proteolytic digestion) accumulate in patients with TTP, being found in the platelet thrombi and serum. These ULvWf multimers can attach to activated platelets, thereby promoting platelet aggregation. ULvWf multimer accumulation in TTP is associated with absent or markedly diminished ADAMTS13 activity due to an inherited or acquired deficiency.

Treatment is with plasma exchange using large volumes of fresh-frozen plasma. The mechanism by which this method is therapeutic is not well understood. One possibility is that plasma exchange allows repletion of the missing enzyme ADAMTS13.

Table A Differential diagnosis in a pregnant woman presenting with epilepsy

- Cerebral neoplasm
- Cerebral haemorrhage
- Eclampsia
- Haemolysis, elevated liver enzymes and low platelets
- Thrombotic thrombocytopenic purpura
- Cerebral vein thrombosis secondary to hyperviscocity

Table B Pentad in TTP*

1. MAHA
2. Thrombocytopenia
3. Fever
4. Renal involvement
5. Neurological involvement

* Not all patients have the classic pentad. Usually 1 and 2 are required to make the diagnosis.

Table C Differentiation of TTP and HUS from other conditions

Medical condition	Differentiation from TTP or HUS
DIC	Abnormal clotting, low fibrinogen, high FDPs, low factors V and VIII
Vasculitides	Usually have history of rash, arthralgia with normal platelets and peripheral nervous system involvement
Antiphospholipid syndrome	Can cause neurological problems but APPT is high
Malignant hypertension	Diastolic blood pressure usually >130 mmHg and evidence of haemorrhages, exudates and papilloedema on retinal examination

Answer 88

> d. Organize CT-guided aspiration/biopsy of the lower lumbar spine.

The presentation of back pain associated with weakness of the lower limbs is consistent with cord compression. The accompanying fever, night sweats and raised inflammatory markers are highly suggestive of infection of the lower spine or a involvement of bone with haematological malignancy. The plain lumbar spine film shows minor destruction of the third lumbar vertebra and reduced joint space between the third and fourth lumbar vertebrae to indicate a discitis. The MRI scan shows destruction of the third and fourth lumbar vertebrae and marked discitis (reduced joint space). There is a collection of pus around the anterior and posterior aspects of the third and fourth lumbar vertebrae. The anterior collection is pressing on the spinal cord. The most probable diagnosis is tuberculous osteomyelitis of the lumbar spine in a female of her ethnicity.

Spinal TB usually occurs in immunocompromised adults and is due to reactivation of TB acquired from a primary infection. The lag period between primary TB and spinal TB may be decades. Spinal TB may occur as an immediate complication of the primary infection and most commonly affects the lower thoracic and lumbar spine. Patients present with back pain, night sweats, weight loss and signs of cord compression from epidural abscess formation. The differential diagnosis is osteomyelitis secondary to *Staphylococcus aureus* infection, in which blood cultures are positive in over 90% of cases.

A chest X-ray is rarely helpful in the diagnosis since it is only abnormal in 50% of cases. Whereas a Heaf test is positive in over 90% of immunocompetent patients with spinal TB, many patients with spinal TB are immunocompromised and may have a negative test. The investigation of choice following MRI of the spine is a CT-guided aspirate/biopsy of the affected area before starting treatment. An attempt to make a tissue diagnosis should be made whenever possible before initiating anti-TB therapy. Treatment is with conventional anti-TB treatment for 12–18 months.

Question 89

A 23-year-old woman with insulin-dependent diabetes mellitus had experienced recurrent episodes of cystitis for which she was taking trimethoprim. She smoked 15–20 cigarettes per day. Her blood pressure measured 120/80 mmHg. Urinalysis did not reveal any evidence of micralbuminuria.

> What is the best method of preserving renal function?
> a. Cessation of smoking.
> b. Strict glycaemic control.
> c. ACE inhibitor therapy.
> d. Lifelong prophylactic antibiotics.
> e. Angiotensin II receptor blocker.

Question 90

A 35-year-old woman presented with vomiting and epigastric discomfort after a weekend of binge drinking. On examination she was alert. She had several spider naevi on the face and chest wall. The heart rate was 100 beats/min and regular. The blood pressure was 160/96 mmHg. The respiratory rate was 20/min. Both heart sounds were normal. The abdomen was soft. Inspection of the fundi was normal.

Initial investigations are shown.

> What is the diagnosis?
> a. Diabetic ketoacidosis.
> b. Methanol poisoning.
> c. Euglycaemic ketoacidosis.
> d. Renal tubular acidosis.
> e. Lactic acidosis.

Hb	12 g/dl
WCC	12×10^9/l
Platelets	100×10^9/l
MCV	102 fl
Sodium	132 mmol/l
Potassium	3.3 mmol/l
Urea	7 mmol/l
Creatinine	80 μmol/l
Bicarbonate	11 mmol/l
Chloride	98 mmol/l
Bilirubin	18 μmol/l
AST	160 iu/l
Gamma GT	100 iu/l
Plasma osmolality	290 mOsm/l
Blood glucose	5 mmol/l
Urinalysis	Ketones ++++
	No crystals

Answer 89

> b. Strict glycaemic control.

The patient does not have hypertension or micro-albuminuria, therefore the best treatment for preventing nephropathy is meticulous glycaemic control. Glycaemic control and blood pressure are the main predictors for the development of microalbuminuria (the earliest marker of diabetic nephropathy) in both type 1 and type 2 diabetes. Data from the DCCT trial in type 1 diabetes and UKPDS trial in type 2 diabetes have shown that meticulous glycaemic control alone delays the onset of diabetic nephropathy in patients who do not have coexistent hypertension. In patients with diabetes and hypertension prevention of diabetic nephropathy requires both meticulous glycaemic control and maintaining a normal blood pressure. Better glycaemic control reduces glomerular basement membrane thickening and microalbuminuria.

Once microalbuminuria has developed there is little evidence that improving glycaemic control alone delays progression of nephropathy. In these circumstances, control of blood pressure and the intraglomerular pressure, particularly using ACE inhibitors or angiotensin II receptor blockers, can greatly retard the progression of nephropathy (see Algorithm).

In young type 1 diabetics with microalbuminuria or proteinuria, an ACE inhibitor should be prescribed regardless of the blood pressure. The target blood pressure (which may require multiple other anti-hypertensive agents in addition to ACE inhibitors) in patients with microalbuminuria is <120/70 mmHg and in patients with proteinuria it is <130/75 mmHg.

In patients with type 2 diabetes there is more compelling evidence from large trials that angiotensin II receptor blockers prevent development of proteinuria in patients with microalbuminuria. Target blood pressure is <130/75 mmHg.

Smoking has also been identified as a risk factor for the development of microalbuminuria. However, there are no prospective studies showing the benefit of cessation of smoking on renal function in type 1 diabetics at least.

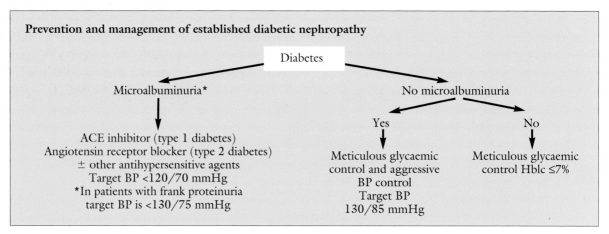

Prevention and management of established diabetic nephropathy

Diabetes

Microalbuminuria* / No microalbuminuria

ACE inhibitor (type 1 diabetes)
Angiotensin receptor blocker (type 2 diabetes)
± other antihypersensitive agents
Target BP <120/70 mmHg
*In patients with frank proteinuria
target BP is <130/75 mmHg

Yes — Meticulous glycaemic control and aggressive BP control Target BP 130/85 mmHg

No — Meticulous glycaemic control Hblc ≤7%

Answer 90

> c. Euglycaemic ketoacidosis.

The patient is admitted after an episode of alcohol bingeing. Apart from the history, her investigations raise the suspicion of alcohol abuse (macrocytosis, low platelets and abnormal liver function tests). Patients who abuse alcohol may present with ketoacidosis in the absence of insulin deficiency. There are several factors that contribute to ketoacidosis. Firstly, alcohol inhibits gluconeogenesis, which offsets glucagon-mediated lipolysis and ketone generation. Secondly, alcohol itself may be metabolized to ketones. Thirdly, patients who abuse alcohol generally have a low calorie intake and are effectively starving on a chronic basis. Patients usually have normal or low blood glucose, but a high glucose is also recognized. There is no clear explanation for high glucose levels except that some patients may have concomitant diabetes mellitus.

The plasma osmolality may also be increased owing to alcohol itself, and the generation of endogenous acids but also raises the differential diagnosis of methanol or ethylene glycol poisoning. Therefore it is important to take a detailed alcohol history and to check the urine for ethylene glycol crystals. Salicylate toxicity may also present in a similar fashion and should be excluded by measuring plasma salicylate levels. The treatment is IV dextrose and saline solutions as well as thiamine replacement. The dextrose replaces the glucose required to inhibit glucagon production and the saline replenishes fluid loss.

Question 91

A 27-year-old female artist was seen in the chest clinic with a three-day history of worsening dyspnoea requiring the use of an inhaled short-acting β_2-agonist every 3–4 hours. Over the past few months she had been using the bronchodilator with increasing frequency. She had also experienced a non-productive cough particularly at night and after exercise. She was diagnosed with asthma since the age of 14 years and was hospitalized on two occasions more than 10 years ago for infective exacerbations of asthma. Her only other medication was a low-dose inhaled steroid, which she takes twice daily.

On examination she was afebrile. She was 1.52 m tall. The peak expiratory flow rate was 365 l/min, with her normal best at 470 l/min. She could complete sentences in one breath. Her respiratory rate was 20/min, pulse rate 80 beats/min and blood pressure 110/70 mmHg. Auscultation of the lungs revealed mild generalized polyphonic wheeze.

Blood gases (air):

$PaCO_2$	5 kPa
PaO_2	12 kPa
pH	7.34

Which two of the following would be possible options in stepping up this patient's asthma management?
   a. Continue current treatment and add regular oral prednisolone.
   b. Continue short-acting β_2-agonist as required and substitute high-dose inhaled steroid twice daily.
   c. Start regular short-acting inhaled β_2-agonist and continue on low-dose inhaled steroid twice daily.
   d. Start regular short-acting β_2-agonist and substitute high-dose inhaled steroid twice daily.
   e. Continue short-acting β_2-agonist as required and continue on low-dose inhaled steroid, add long-acting inhaled β_2-agonist twice daily.
   f. Continue short-acting β_2-agonist as required, add sodium cromoglycate and stop low-dose inhaled steroid.
   g. Continue short-acting β_2-agonist as required, add modified release theophylline and stop low-dose inhaled steroid.
   h. Continue current treatment and add inhaled ipratropium bromide twice daily.
   i. Continue current treatment and add regular oral prednisolone and erythromycin 250 mg QDS.
   j. Continue current treatment and add high-dose inhaled steroid twice daily.

Question 92

A 52-year-old male with non-insulin-dependent diabetes mellitus has a blood pressure of 148/94 mmHg. Fundoscopy reveals evidence of background diabetic retinopathy.

Investigations are shown.

Hb	13.1 g/dl
WCC	5×10^9/l
Platelets	290×10^9/l
Sodium	138 mmol/l
Potassium	4.1 mmol/l
Urea	9 mmol/l
Creatinine	138 µmol/l
Glucose	8 mmol/l
Cholesterol	5.8 mmol/l
Triglycerides	3.2 mmol/l
12-lead ECG	Normal
24-hour urine protein	1g

What is the best treatment for reducing the rate of nephropathy?
   a. Losartan.
   b. Ramipril.
   c. Insulin.
   d. Metformin.
   e. Atenolol.

Answer 91

> b. Continue short-acting β_2-agonist as required and substitute high-dose inhaled steroid twice daily.
>
> e. Continue short-acting β_2-agonist as required and continue on low-dose inhaled steroid, add long-acting inhaled β_2-agonist twice daily.

The British Thoracic Society (BTS) published guidelines for the management of asthma in 1990, which have since been updated (1997), in response to concerns over the increasing prevalence, morbidity, admissions and deaths from asthma. Supported by randomized controlled trials, steroids have since been established as the mainstay of preventative treatment in all but the mildest cases of asthma. This question tests the candidate's knowledge of the BTS guidelines of the stepwise approach to the management of chronic asthma with the introduction of inhaled steroids early in the treatment (*Table A*).

The patient described had none of the features of acute severe or life-threatening asthma and had a PEFR >75% of predicted. She was on step 2 of the management ladder of chronic asthma. She had symptoms indicating loss of control of asthma and the need to step up management (*Table B*).

Patients should start treatment at the step most appropriate to the initial severity. A rescue course of prednisolone may be needed at any time and at any step. Until growth is complete any child requiring inhaled high-dose steroids or oral steroids should be referred to a paediatrician with an interest in asthma. The aim is to achieve control and then to reduce treatment.

A peak-flow meter should be prescribed and the response to treatment should be reviewed every 3–6 months. In patients with chronic asthma a 3–6 month period of stability should be shown before slow stepwise reduction in the treatment is undertaken.

Table A Stepwise management of asthma

Step 1 Occasional use of inhaled short-acting β_2-agonist as required for symptom relief. If needed more than once daily move to step 2

Step 2 Occasional use of inhaled short-acting β_2-agonist as required plus low-dose inhaled steroid twice daily
Alternatively use cromoglycate but start inhaled steroids if control not achieved.

Step 3 Occasional use of inhaled short-acting β_2-agonist as required plus high-dose inhaled steroid daily or low-dose inhaled steroid twice daily plus long-acting β_2-agonist twice daily (especially if experiencing side-effects with high-dose inhaled steroids)
Alternatively use MR theophylline or cromoglycate but start inhaled steroids if control not achieved

Step 4 Occasional use of inhaled short-acting β_2-agonist as required plus high-dose inhaled steroid daily plus sequential therapeutic trial of one or more of the following:
• Long-acting β_2-agonist twice daily
• MR theophylline
• Inhaled ipratropium bromide or oxitropium
• Long-acting β_2-agonist tablets
• Cromoglycate

Step 5 Occasional use of inhaled short-acting β_2-agonist as required plus high-dose inhaled steroid daily plus one or more of the long-acting bronchodilators plus regular prednisolone tablets in a single daily dose

---

Table B Symptoms indicating inadequate control of asthma

• The need for frequent relieving bronchodilator therapy
• Chronic cough and nocturnal symptoms
• Limitations on activity including exercise
• PEFR <80%
• Frequent exacerbations
• Circadian variation in PEFR >20%
• Adverse effects from medications

Answer 92

a. Losartan.

The patient has moderate proteinuria and abnormal renal function. The question specifically relates to the treatment of diabetic nephropathy in a patient with type 2 diabetes mellitus. While ACE inhibitors have been clearly shown to attenuate micro-albuminuria in patients without overt nephropathy and retard progression of nephropathy in those patients with established diabetic nephropathy in type 1 diabetes, the management of nephropathy in type 2 diabetes is still evolving.

It is clear that tight glycaemic control is effective in retarding nephropathy in both type 1 and type 2 diabetes mellitus and that control of hypertension is also necessary in both conditions. In contrast with type 1 diabetes mellitus, there is much less information on the effects of ACE inhibitors in treating diabetic nephropathy in type 2 diabetes mellitus. However, two important studies have shown that in patients with type 2 diabetes, angiotensin receptor blockers are as effective in retarding nephropathy as ACE inhibitors are in type 1 diabetes mellitus.

For example, in the RENAAL trial, 1513 patients with type 2 diabetes and nephropathy were randomly assigned to losartan (50 titrating up to 100 mg once daily) or placebo, both in addition to conventional antihypertensive therapy (but not ACE inhibitors). Compared to placebo, losartan reduced the incidence of a doubling of the plasma creatinine by 25% and end-stage renal disease by 28%; the mean follow-up was 3.4 years. These benefits were not associated with differences in blood pressure levels between the groups. Subsequent analysis found that the most significant risk factor for progressive kidney disease was the initial degree of proteinuria.

Question 93

A 45-year-old man with HIV syndrome presented with weakness affecting the left upper and lower limbs. On examination he was confused and had a temperature of 38°C (100.4°F). He had recently been treated for a *Pneumocystis carinii* infection. The CD4 count was 150. CT scan of the brain with contrast revealed subcortical atrophy and multiple contrast-enhancing ring lesions in the cortex and subcortical areas.

What is the most probable diagnosis?
a. Primary CNS lymphoma.
b. Tuberculous meningitis.
c. CMV encephalitis.
d. Cerebral toxoplasmosis.
e. Progressive multifocal leucoencephalopathy.

Question 94

A 60-year-old male was noted to have an irregular pulse. A subsequent 12-lead ECG showed atrial fibrillation with a ventricular rate of 80 beats/min. The patient was asymptomatic. There was no past medical history of note. The patient consumed 10 units of alcohol per week. His blood pressure was 110/80 mmHg and both heart sounds were normal.

Investigations are shown.

Hb	12 g/dl
Blood glucose	4.2 mmol/l
Total cholesterol	5.4 mmol/l
TSH	1.3 mu/l
Total thyroxine	170 nmol/l
Chest X-ray	Normal
12-lead ECG	Atrial fibrillation
	Normal QRS complexes
Echocardiography	Left atrial diameter 40 mm
	Normal left ventricle
	Normal systolic function
	Normal valves

Which additional treatment is required to reduce the risk of stroke?
a. Warfarin.
b. Clopidogrel.
c. Ramipril.
d. Aspirin.
e. Pravastatin.

Answer 93

> d. Cerebral toxoplasmosis.

The most probable diagnosis is cerebral toxoplasmosis. The CT scan is consistent with the diagnosis; the sub-cortical atrophy probably represents HIV encephalopathy.

The exact cause of CNS involvement in HIV infection is largely influenced by the CD4 count. Patients with CD4 counts >500 have benign and malignant brain tumours similar to those seen in immunocompetent patients. Patients with a CD4 count of between 200 and 500 often have cognitive disorders associated with HIV such as HIV dementia and progressive leucoence-phalopathy, which are not mass lesions. Patients with a CD4 count <200 have either opportunistic CNS infections or HIV-related cerebral tumours.

Opportunistic infections include toxoplasmosis, TB, CMV and cryptococcal meningitis (see Question 277). Toxoplasmosis is by far the commonest cerebral mass lesion seen in HIV patients and is usually associated with multiple ring-enhancing lesions either in the cortico-medullary junction or around the basal ganglia. Patients often have headache, confusion and fever. Focal neurological signs or seizure are common. The other opportunistic infections rarely result in mass lesions in the absence of disseminated infection.

Primary CNS lymphoma does display some degree of contrast enhancement but it is usually nodular or patchy; however, lesions may be multiple and difficult to differentiate from toxoplasmosis. Thallium single photon emission computed tomography has been shown to be useful in differentiating cerebral toxoplasmosis from cerebral lymphoma. Primary CNS lymphoma is rarer than cerebral toxoplasmosis in HIV infection. Generally patients with multiple ring-enhancing lesions on the CT scan with mass effect are treated empirically for toxoplasma infection for two weeks with a combination of pyrimethamine and sulphadiazine. Failure of a radiological response (on CT scan) is an indication for brain biopsy to enable an alternative diagnosis such as lymphoma.

Answer 94

> d. Aspirin.

The patient has atrial fibrillation which is associated with a five-fold increase in stroke secondary to systemic thromboembolism. The two main pharmacological treatments available for preventing systemic thrombo-embolism in AF are antithrombotic agents and oral anticoagulant drugs. Aspirin is the only antithrombotic agent recommended for preventing systemic thrombo-embolism in AF. Warfarin is the most commonly used oral anticoagulant drug used in this particular situation.

Studies have shown that in high-risk patients (see below) warfarin is superior to aspirin in preventing systemic thromboembolism. However, there is no conclusive evidence that warfarin is superior to aspirin in this regard in low-risk patients. In patients at moderate risk both aspirin and warfarin appear to be equally effective in reducing systemic thromboembolism. Patients' age above 75 years of age, rheumatic mitral valve disease and prior embolic events are the greatest risk factors for systemic thromboembolism in AF (*Table*).

The patient in question is at low risk of systemic thromboembolism, therefore he should be treated with aspirin instead of warfarin.

Treatment to prevent systemic thromboembolism in atrial fibrillation

Factor	Risk	Treatment
Any of Age ≥75 years Previous stroke or TIA Uncontrolled hypertension Impaired left ventricular systolic function Rheumatic mitral valve disease	High	Warfarin
Any of Age 65–74 years Controlled hypertension Diabetes mellitus Ischaemic heart disease Thyrotoxicosis	Moderate	Warfarin or aspirin
All of Age <65 years Normal left ventricular function No evidence of rheumatic heart disease Normal hypertension	Low	Aspirin

Question 95

An 84-year-old fully independent male was admitted with very transient episodes of dizziness. The 12-lead ECG showed first degree AV block and left bundle branch block. A subsequent 24-hour ECG revealed episodic third degree AV block.

Which of the following treatments is most suitable for the patient?
a. AAIR pacemaker.
b. VVI pacemaker.
c. DDDR pacemaker.
d. VVIR pacemaker.
e. None of the above.

Question 96

Hb	10 g/dl
WCC	3.1 × 10⁹/l
	(neutrophils, 1.5;
	lymphocytes, 0.7;
	eosinophils, 0.9)
Platelets	108 × 10⁹/l
MCV	80 fl
Bone marrow:	Erythroid hyperplasia,
	myeloid hyperplasia but lack of
	mature forms
	Multiple megakaryocytes

A patient with long-standing rheumatoid arthritis is noted to have splenomegaly. Results of haematological investigations are shown.

What is the cause of the low white cell count?
a. Folate deficiency.
b. Drug-induced marrow aplasia.
c. Myelodysplastic syndrome.
d. Felty's syndrome.
e. Hodgkin's lymphoma.

Question 97

A 50-year-old woman presented with pain in her left shoulder and weight loss of 4 kg over the past four weeks. She had been taking non-steroidal anti-inflammatory drugs with only mild relief of her pain. She smoked 15–20 cigarettes per day.

Investigations are shown.

Hb	11.2 g/dl
WCC	8.2 × 109/l
Platelets	500 × 109/l
ESR	72 mm/h
Chest X-ray (**97**)	

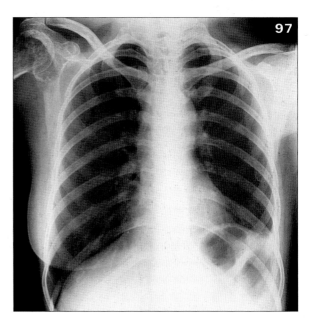

What is the diagnosis?
a. Pancoast's tumour.
b. Multiple myeloma.
c. Osteomyelitis affecting the right shoulder joint.
d. Metastatic bone disease.
e. Avascular necrosis of the head of femur.

Answer 95

> c. DDDR Pacemaker.

The patient has third degree AV block. The condition is associated with an annual mortality exceeding 15% in the absence of permanent cardiac pacing. The aim would be to maintain physiological rhythm and to pace both the atrium and the ventricle, i.e. he should have a dual chamber pacemaker (*Table*). He is fully independent and should have a rate response facility (R).

Choice of pacemaker

Condition	Pacemaker of choice
Pure sustained AF	VVI or VVIR
Pure sinus node dysfunction without AF or evidence of AV block at rapid heart rates (>150/min)	AAIR (or DDDR)*
Second or third degree AVB or other bradyarrhythmias with visible P waves	DDD or DDDR

*Most cardiologists in the UK implant DDD (DDDR) pacemakers in patients with sick sinus syndrome as many patients go on to develop atrioventricular block. First letter, chamber(s) paced; second letter, chamber(s) paced; third letter, mode of sensing (I = inhibition and D = triggering and inhibition); fourth letter (R), rate response facility.

Answer 96

> d. Felty's syndrome.

In a patient with chronic rheumatoid arthritis, neutropaenia and splenomegaly, the most probable diagnosis is Felty's syndrome. However, other conditions associated with a low white cell count in rheumatoid arthritis include drugs such as penicillamine, gold and methotrexate, which are associated with bone marrow aplasia. Folate deficiency may also cause pancytopenia. The bone marrow does not reveal hypoplasia, therefore drug-induced marrow aplasia is unlikely here. The absence of megaloblasts is against the diagnosis of folate deficiency.

While Hodgkin's lymphoma may explain the splenomegaly and eosinophilia (NB: eosinophila is well recognized in rheumatoid arthritis, particularly in patients with skin vasculitis, pulmonary fibrosis and subcutaneous nodules), it is less likely than Felty's syndrome, particularly as the disease would have to be fairly advanced to produce pancytopenia as in this case. Furthermore, at such an advanced state one would expect the bone marrow to have a better yield for the diagnosis than it normally has in the very early stages of Hodgkin's lymphoma. Myelodysplasia may cause a hypercellular marrow and a peripheral eosinophilia but splenomegaly is very uncommon.

Answer 97

> d. Metastatic bone disease.

There are small lucencies in the head of the humerus and a large lucency in the lateral border of the scapula. There is only one breast shadow present (on the left). The right breast shadow is absent, indicating that the patient has had a mastectomy, presumably for treatment of carcinoma. In this case the lucencies have to be assumed to be secondary to disseminated breast carcinoma until proven otherwise. In the exam always ensure both breast shadows are present on chest radiographs in female patients. Evidence of a mastectomy may be a major clue to the answer in a question – as in this case.

Question 98

A 22-year-old medical student developed sudden dysphasia and right-sided weakness while on holiday in Australia. She was afebrile. Apart from the neurological abnormality described, there were no other abnormal physical signs.

Investigations are shown.

Hb	15 g/dl
WCC	$10 \times 10^9/l$
Platelets	$200 \times 10^9/l$
ESR	8 mm/h
Autoantibody screen	Normal
12-lead ECG	Normal
2-D echocardiogram	Normal
Carotid Doppler study	Normal

What is the most probable diagnosis?
  a. Carotid dissection.
  b. Encephalitis.
  c. Small intracerebral haemorrhage.
  d. Paradoxical cerebral embolus via patent foramen ovale.
  e. Cardiac embolus from paroxysmal atrial fibrillation.

Question 99

A 50-year-old Jamaican male was admitted with discomfort in the left shoulder. On examination he had weakness of abduction of the right upper limb.

Investigations are shown.

Hb	11 g/dl
WCC	$11.5 \times 10^9/l$
Platelets	$200 \times 10^9/l$
Sodium	133 mmol/l
Potassium	4.6 mmol/l
Urea	7.4 mmol/l
Calcium	2.76 mmol/l
Albumin	36 g/l
Chest X-ray (**99a**)	

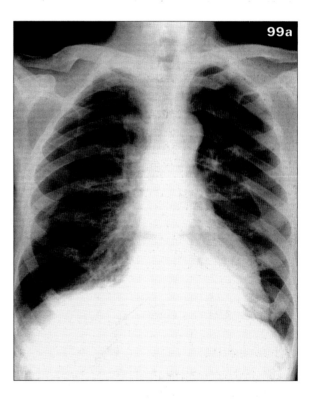

What is the diagnosis?
  a. Sarcoidosis.
  b. Multiple myeloma.
  c. Paget's disease.
  d. Bronchial carcinoma.
  e. Retrosternal goitre.

Answer 98

> d. Paradoxical embolus via patent foramen ovale.

A young patient presenting with stroke with a normal cardiac examination, 2-D echocardiogram, carotid Doppler study, autoantibody screen and inflammatory markers is highly consistent with the diagnosis of paradoxical embolism via a patent foramen ovale.

A PFO occurs when the primum and secundum septa fail to fuse completely leaving a small flap-like communication allowing the possibility of a shunt. She has been on a long flight from Australia and therefore it is possible that she had deep-vein thrombi, which have traversed the PFO and passed into the systemic circulation. PFOs are relatively common and may be present in up to 30% of the general population. PFOs more than 4 mm in diameter and associated with intermittent right-to-left intracardiac shunting are more likely to be associated with systemic emboli. PFOs may not be identified on a 2-D echocardiogram. A transoesophageal echocardiogram with contrast studies is the diagnostic investigation of choice. Patients with systemic embolism in association with a PFO with a demonstrable right-to-left shunt with following Valsalva manoeuvre (provided there is no other obvious cause such as atrial fibrillation or intramural thrombus) may be treated by closure using a mechanical devise (Amplatzer closure device) via the right superficial femoral vein.

While cerebrovascular accidents are uncommon in young individuals, there are several potential causes due to disorders affecting the heart and vasculature supplying the brain and primary central nervous system (*Table*).

Causes of stroke in young (≤35 years of age) individuals

Cause	*Notes*
Cerebral haemorrhage	Sudden onset severe headache and vomiting
Meningoencephalitis	Fever, confusion, meningism, seizures
Neoplasm	Headache, focal neurology, seizures
Carotid or vertebral dissection	Trauma/pain/unilateral lower cranial nerve palsies
Migraine	Usually female; may be precipitated by typical aura
Inflammatory conditions (vasculitides, antiphospholipid syndrome, isolated cranial angitis, Takayasu's disease)	Systemic features, raised inflammatory markers, positive autoantibody screen
Structural arterial disease (Fibromuscular dysplasia)	Involves carotid artery; associated intracranial aneurysms; renal artery commonly affected
Cerebral vein thrombosis	Hyperviscocity, pregnancy, contraceptive pill, ear, sinus or facial skin infection; headache, focal neurology, seizures
Thrombophilic states	Previous arterial or venous thrombosis
Cardiac causes (severe hypertension, AF, rheumatic heart disease, mechanical valves, cardiomyopathy, septal defects, PFOs)	Irregular pulse; murmur
Haematological (polycythaemia, thrombocythaemia, paroxysmal nocturnal haemaglobinuria, sickle cell anaemia)	
Mitochondrial disease, e.g. MELAS	(see Question 315)

Answer 99

> d. Bronchial carcinoma.

There is opacification of the right upper lobe consistent with a mass lesion. The first rib is eroded on the right side indicating involvement of bone. The findings are typical of a Pancoast tumour. The raised calcium may be secondary to bone metastases or secretion of PTH-related peptide by the carcinoma. Patients with Pancoast tumour present with symptoms and signs of pressure on the brachial plexus, the sympathetic trunk (Horner's syndrome) and bone metastases (**99b**, arrows).

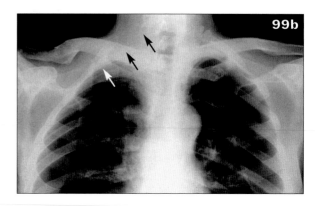

Question 100

A 67-year-old male with dilated cardiomyopathy is admitted for the third time in four months with increasing breathlessness and swollen ankles. He consumed 2 units of alcohol per week. His medications consisted of furosemide 80 mg daily, ramipril 10 mg daily, candesartan 6 mg daily, spironolactone 25 mg daily, bisoprolol 7.5 mg daily and isosorbide mononitrate SR 60 mg daily.

On examination his heart rate was 70 beats/min and regular. The blood pressure measured 80/40 mmHg. The JVP was raised. Examination of the precordium revealed a displaced apex in the sixth intercostal space and a forceful right ventricular impulse. Auscultation of the heart revealed a systolic murmur in the mitral area and a third heart sound. On auscultation of the lungs there was evidence of bilateral pleural effusions. Investigations are shown.

Hb	11 g/dl
WCC	7 × 10⁹/l
Platelets	200 × 10⁹/l
MCV	90 fl
Sodium	129 mmol/l
Potassium	5.9 mmol/l
Urea	17 mmol/l
ECG	Sinus rhythm; LBBB
Chest X-ray	Enlarged heart; bilateral pleural effusions

Echocardiography:
  Dilated left and right ventricles.
  Ejection fraction 20%.
  Severe functional mitral regurgitation

What is the most effective management step to improve his symptoms?
  a. Add digoxin.
  b. Consider mitral valve repair.
  c. Increase dose of bisoprolol to 10 mg.
  d. Implant biventricular pacemaker.
  e. Increase dose of diuretics.

Question 101

A 21-year-old woman presented with a painless swelling in her neck. There was no history of a recent viral illness. The patient did not have symptoms of hyper- or hypothyroidism. She was not taking any medications. On examination she had a 2 cm painless mass thyroid lump associated with cervical lymphadenopathy.

Investigations are shown.

Hb	14 g/dl
ESR	5 mm/h
TSH	2 iu/l
Chest X-ray	Normal

What is the most useful investigation in elucidating the diagnosis?
  a. Thyroid ultrasound.
  b. Radio-iodine thyroid scan.
  c. Fine-needle aspiration of the thyroid gland.
  d. Thyroid myoperoxidase antibodies.
  e. Total plasma thyroxine concentration.

Question 102

Hb	6.1 g/dl
WCC	3.0 × 10⁹/l
Platelets	115 × 10⁹/l
MCV	116 fl
MCHC	37 pg
Ferritin	710 μmol/l
Bilirubin	35 μmol/l
AST	40 iu/l
LDH	1500 iu/l
Alkaline phosphatase	100 iu/l
Albumin	37 g/l

A 70-year-old woman was investigated for lethargy. On examination she appeared slightly pale but all other aspects of physical examination were normal.

Investigations are shown.

What is the diagnosis?
  a. Hodgkin's lymphoma and haemolytic anaemia.
  b. Pernicious anaemia.
  c. Aplastic anaemia.
  d. Paroxysmal nocturnal haemoglobinuria.
  e. Autoimmune haemolytic anaemia.

Answer 100

> d. Implant biventricular pacemaker.

The patient has severe symptoms despite adequate doses of an ACE inhibitor, beta-blocker and spironolactone. His low systolic blood pressure does not allow additional pharmacological therapy such as an angiotensin II receptor blocker. He has poor left ventricular function and an interventricular conduction defect suggesting that he may benefit symptomatically from biventricular pacing (*Table A*). The mitral regurgitation is a consequence of the left ventricular dilatation rather than the cause of it. An internal cardiac defibrillator prevents sudden death in patients at risk of malignant ventricular arrhythmias but does not improve functional capacity.

Patients with cardiomyopathy and interventricular conduction defects are generally more symptomatic than those with normal conduction, owing to the resulting desynchronization of ventricular contraction. Pacing both ventricles (RV is paced conventionally; LV is paced via the coronary sinus) helps resynchronize ventricular contraction and improve functional capacity. Indications for biventricular pacing are listed in *Table A*. Biventricular pacing is associated with significant improvement in quality of life, functional capacity and reduction in hospitalization owing to heart failure (*Table B*). There are preliminary reports that suggest that overall mortality from heart failure is also improved with biventricular pacing.

Table A Indications for biventricular pacing

- Severe NYHA class III–IV failure despite optimal drug therapy
- QRS >130 msec
- Left ventricular end diastolic diameter >55 mm
- Left ventricular ejection fraction <35%

Table B Clinical effects of biventricular pacing

Improves	*Reduces*
Quality of life	Total and heart failure related hospitalizations
Exercise capacity	Heart rate
NYHA functional class	
LV ejection fraction	
LV dimensions	

Answer 101

> c. Fine-needle aspiration of the thyroid gland.

Thyroid lumps may represent simple or multinodular goitres, toxic nodules, neoplastic lesions, inflammatory masses or thyroid cysts. Thyroid carcinomas account for 5–6% of all lumps in the thyroid. Thyroid cancer is most common in patients aged under 30 years or over 60 years. Prior radiation to the head and neck is a recognized risk factor for thyroid carcinoma. Patients with a family history of thyroid carcinoma are at a higher risk of thyroid malignancy than the general population.

A painless swelling in the neck associated with cervical lymphadenopathy is highly suggestive of papillary carcinoma of the thyroid gland. Papillary carcinoma of the thyroid invades local structures quickly and usually presents early as a result. The diagnosis of thyroid carcinoma is usually made by histological sampling of a fine-needle thyroid aspirate. Prior thyroid ultrasound is not necessary. Indeed in patients with a normal TSH, fine-needle aspiration is the investigation of choice to investigate thyroid lumps. In patients with a low TSH a radio-iodine uptake scan is performed to confirm the presence of a hot nodule. Since these are never malignant a fine-needle aspiration is not warranted.

Unfortunately, fine-needle aspiration cannot distinguish between follicular and Hürthle cell adenomas and carcinomas. In these cases the biopsy is termed intermediate rather than obviously benign or malignant. In such cases a radio-iodine uptake scan is performed and if a cold nodule is identified then it is surgically excised.

In patients suspected to have Hashimoto's thyroiditis clinically, or on the basis of high thyroid peroxidase antibodies, a thyroid uptake scan should be performed before fine-needle aspiration as this may reveal functioning thyroid tissue in the entire lobe and obviate the need for biopsy. This is particularly important as patients with Hashimoto's thyroiditis have Hürthle's cells on histology, which may be mistaken for a Hürthle cell carcinoma.

While ultrasonography would provide more detail about the morphology of the gland, it is not diagnostic. Thyroid scintigraphy is sometimes used by some centres to ascertain the functional status of the gland, but in this particular situation it would not provide a diagnosis.

Answer 102

> b. Pernicious anaemia.

This patient with lethargy has a markedly raised MCV and pancytopenia. The best answer is pernicious anaemia. Although paroxysmal nocturnal haemoglobinuria can also be associated with pancytopenia and raised MCV, the actual MCV in PNH is less than in pernicious anaemia. The raised MCV in PNH is due to reticulocytes (newly formed red cell) arising from rapid red cell turnover secondary to haemolysis, whereas in pernicious anaemia the raised MCV is due to large immature red cells (erythroid precursors) secondary to immature nuclear development. Remember hydroxycobalamin is required for thymidine synthesis, an important DNA nucleoside. Erythroid precursors are larger than reticulocytes. Indeed a MCV >115 fl should always raise the possibility of abnormal DNA maturation in red cells, e.g. B_{12} deficiency, folate deficiency, drugs interfering with DNA synthesis.

The raised ferritin is due to iron overload resulting from reduced red cell synthesis. The raised LDH and AST are due to haemolysis. Immature red cell precursors undergo extravascular haemolysis. Aplastic anaemia would explain the pancytopenia and raised ferritin but not the raised MCV or haemolysis. Hodgkin's lymphoma with haemolysis could explain all of the data given in the question but the MCV favours pernicious anaemia. (See Answer 394.)

Question 103

A 64-year-old man presented immediately after recovering from a 20-minute episode of dysphasia and weakness of the right side of the face and arm. He had experienced two episodes of transient loss of vision in the left eye in the past three weeks. There was a past medical history of a myocardial infarction two years ago. His medication comprised 75 mg of aspirin daily. He did not smoke.

On examination there was no evidence of residual neurological deficit. Fundoscopy was normal. The pulse rate was 80 beats/min and regular in nature. His blood pressure measured 138/86 mmHg in both arms. Both heart sounds were normal. Auscultation over the carotid arteries revealed a bruit over the left carotid artery.

Investigations are shown.

Hb	15 g/dl
WCC	8×10^9/l
Platelets	300×10^9/l
ESR	20 mm/h
Sodium	138 mmol/l
Potassium	4.1 mmol/l
Urea	6 mmol/l
Creatinine	100 mmol/l
Glucose	4.7 mmol/l
Total cholesterol	6 mmol/l
CT scan brain	Normal
Carotid Doppler	Stenosis (40%) in left internal carotid artery. Stenosis (80%) in right external carotid artery

Which three treatments have been shown to reduce the risk of recurrent stroke in this type of patient?
a. Add clopidogrel to current therapy.
b. Add dipyridamole to current therapy.
c. Substitute dipyridamole for current therapy.
d. Increase dose of aspirin to at least 150 mg.
e. Perform left carotid endarterectomy.
f. Perform right carotid endarterectomy.
g. Start ACE inhibitor after three days.
h. Anticoagulate with warfarin.
i. Start therapy with a statin drug.

Answer 103

b. Add dipyridamole to current therapy.
g. Start ACE inhibitor after three days.
i. Start therapy with a statin drug.

The patient presents with a transient ischaemic attack which is defined as a neurological deficit lasting <24 hours that is attributed to focal cerebral or retinal ischaemia. The causes of TIAs are the same as those of stroke and include cardiac intramural thrombi, carotid artery disease and disease of the intracranial arteries. Therefore strategies for the prevention of recurrent TIAs are similar to those for stroke.

Aspirin is the drug of choice in patients presenting with TIA or stroke unless there are obvious contraindications. Aspirin reduces the long-term risk of stroke and cardiovascular events after a TIA or stroke, with an overall relative risk reduction of 22%. The dose of aspirin used ranges from 75 mg to 1300 mg, but small doses are as effective as large doses and are associated with a lower rate of gastrointestinal effects. The dose most commonly prescribed in the UK is 75 mg daily. The thienopyridines clopidogrel and ticlopidine are not superior to aspirin in secondary prevention. There are no data on these drugs in primary prevention.

Before commencing therapy, all patients should have imaging of the brain (usually CT scan) to rule out unsuspected cerebral pathology as a cause for a TIA, such as a brain tumour or a subdural haematoma, where therapy with aspirin is contraindicated (algorithm).

Imaging of the carotid arteries using carotid Doppler studies is performed after imaging of the brain to exclude a significant internal carotid artery stenosis. Carotid endarterectomy is of proven benefit in patients with an internal carotid artery stenosis of ≥70% who have had a non-disabling stroke or a TIA attributable to the stenosis. The optimal timing of surgery is currently unknown but greatest benefit appears to be derived if surgery is performed within the first two weeks of a non-disabling stroke, provided there are no contraindications to surgery.

Anticoagulation has not been evaluated specifically in patients with TIA but has been extensively tested after ischaemic stroke. In patients with atrial fibrillation, long-term oral anticoagulation reduces the risk of recurrent stroke. In the absence of AF, oral anticoagulation with warfarin is not superior to aspirin in reducing the risk of recurrent ischaemic stroke.

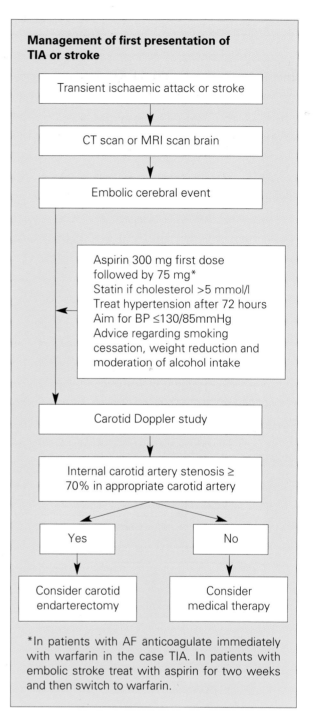

Management of first presentation of TIA or stroke

Transient ischaemic attack or stroke
↓
CT scan or MRI scan brain
↓
Embolic cerebral event
↓
Aspirin 300 mg first dose followed by 75 mg*
Statin if cholesterol >5 mmol/l
Treat hypertension after 72 hours
Aim for BP ≤130/85mmHg
Advice regarding smoking cessation, weight reduction and moderation of alcohol intake
↓
Carotid Doppler study
↓
Internal carotid artery stenosis ≥ 70% in appropriate carotid artery
↓ Yes → Consider carotid endarterectomy
↓ No → Consider medical therapy

*In patients with AF anticoagulate immediately with warfarin in the case TIA. In patients with embolic stroke treat with aspirin for two weeks and then switch to warfarin.

All patients presenting with TIA or stroke require meticulous control of blood pressure. Sudden lowering of the blood pressure may precipitate stroke in patients with TIAs due to carotid artery stenoses or potentiate neurological disability in patients with stroke. It is generally recommended that blood pressure should be reduced cautiously 72 hours after the neurological event. The aim is to keep blood pressure below 130/80 mmHg. All antihypertensive agents protect against stroke; however, the current literature suggests that ACE inhibitors may reduce the risk of further cerebrovascular events even in patients who were normotensive at presentation.

Lipid-lowering therapy with the statin class of drugs has been effective in primary and secondary prevention of stroke. The aim is to treat cholesterol levels above 5 mmol/l in patients with TIA or stroke. In asymptomatic patients treatment of hyper-cholesterolaemia is dependent upon age, and other risk factors for stroke.

It is important not to underestimate the importance of lifestyle modification, and advice regarding smoking cessation, exercise, moderation of alcohol consumption, and weight control is mandatory.

Some patients continue to have TIAs or further strokes despite the use of aspirin. In such patients the addition of extended-release dipyridamole has been shown to reduce the risk of further cerebrovascular embolic events. (European Stroke Prevention Study 2.) A transoesophageal echocardiogram should also be performed to exclude a patent foramen ovale as a cause of paradoxical emboli.

Question 104

A 36-year-old woman presented with a four-week history of intermittent upper abdominal pain and vomiting. Her bowel movements were unaffected and were normal. There was no blood or mucus in the stool. Her appetite was reduced. She had lost 2 kg in weight. She had a past medical history of ulcerative colitis which was diagnosed at the age of 14 years, and was stable on sulphasalazine. In the past she had received several courses of steroids for acute exacerbation of her colitis. Her only other drug history was that she was currently on the contraceptive pill. She had been married for 10 years and had two children, aged 7 and 3 years. She smoked 15 cigarettes per day and consumed 1–2 units of alcohol per week.

On examination, she appeared unwell. Her tongue was dry and there was loss of skin turgor. She had mild lower limb pitting oedema. The heart rate was 98 beats/min and blood pressure was 100/65 mmHg. The temperature was 36.8°C (98.2°F). The abdomen was slightly distended, and there was generalized tenderness. The liver was palpable 4 cm below the costal margin, and was tender. There was no evidence of a palpable spleen or any other palpable masses in the abdomen. Percussion of the abdomen revealed shifting dullness. Rectal examination was normal. Examination of the respiratory and cardiovascular system was normal.

Investigations are shown.

Hb	13 g/dl
WCC	8×10^9/l
Platelets	190×10^9/l
Sodium	131 mmol/l
Potassium	3.1 mmol/l
Urea	7.2 mmol/l
Creatinine	100 μmol/l
Bilirubin	20 μmol/l
AST	24 iu/l
ALT	21 iu/l
Alkaline phosphatase	150 iu/l
Albumin	29 g/l
Chest X-ray	Normal heart size
	Clear lung fields

1. What two investigations would you request to ascertain the cause of the presentation?

2. What is the diagnosis?
   a. Primary sclerosing cholangitis.
   b. Carcinoma of the colon complicated by hepatic metastases.
   c. Hepatic vein thrombosis.
   d. Cirrhosis of the liver.
   e. Chronic active hepatitis.

Answer 104

> 1. i. Liver ultrasound and Doppler studies.
>   ii. Liver biopsy via internal jugular vein.
> 2. c. Hepatic vein thrombosis.

The patient has a long history of relatively quiescent ulcerative colitis and presents with a short history of intermittent upper abdominal pain, vomiting, tender hepatomegaly and ascites. There is no history of weight loss preceding the illness. However, she is a smoker and on the oral contraceptive pill, both of which are recognized risk factors for venous thrombosis. Ulcerative colitis itself is associated with an increased risk of venous thrombosis owing to increased fibrinogen levels and the elevated plasma viscosity. The most likely diagnosis in this patient is hepatic vein thrombosis. Although portal vein thrombosis may also occur in ulcerative colitis, the abnormal LFT and hepatomegaly would be against the diagnosis. The differential diagnosis comprises carcinoma of the colon with hepatic metastases, CAH, cirrhosis of the liver and sclerosing cholangitis. Carcinoma of the colon is ten times more common in a patient with long-standing ulcerative colitis than in the general population; however, it is unusual for a patient with relatively well-controlled colitis to present with extensive metastatic liver disease without a prodrome of ill health or bleeding per rectum. Primary sclerosing cholangitis is strongly associated with ulcerative colitis. Some 75% of all cases with primary sclerosing cholangitis occur in patients with ulcerative colitis. The activity of the colitis is inversely related to the severity of sclerosing cholangitis. It is usually asymptomatic in the early stages, the only indicator being a raised alkaline phosphatase. Pruritis, jaundice, abdominal pain and weight loss are features of advanced cholangitis. Rapid deterioration may occur when sclerosing cholangitis is complicated by a cholangiocarcinoma. If this patient's presentation were due to primary sclerosing cholangitis or cholangio-carcinoma complicating sclerosing cholangitis, one would expect a higher bilirubin level and alkaline phosphatase level, particularly if the associated cirrhosis was severe enough to cause hepatocellular failure, as is suggested by the low albumin and ascites. Chronic active hepatitis is also recognized in ulcerative colitis, but the normal transaminase level is against the diagnosis.

The investigation of choice is liver US with Doppler studies on hepatic venous flow. Liver biopsy and hepatic venography are also useful in making the diagnosis. A liver isotope scan may demonstrate preservation of the Riedel's lobe.

All of the complications mentioned above may also complicate Crohn's disease; however, primary sclerosing cholangitis, cholangiocarcinoma and the predisposition to venous thromboses is much more common in ulcerative colitis. Perianal ulcers are much more common in Crohn's disease and, in addition, patients with Crohn's disease have a higher incidence of gallstones than those with ulcerative colitis. The complications of ulcerative colitis are shown (*Table*). With the exception of ankylosing spondylitis and hepatobiliary disease, all the complications of ulcerative colitis are relieved by proctocolectomy.

Complications of ulcerative colitis

Gastrointestinal
- Haemorrhage
- Toxic dilatation
- Perforation
- Carcinoma of the colon
- Oral and anal ulcers

Hepatobiliary
- Fatty infiltration of the liver
- CAH
- Cirrhosis of the liver
- Sclerosing cholangitis

Dermatological
- Erythema nodosum
- Pyoderma gangrenosum

Ophthalmic
- Episcleritis
- Scleritis
- Anterior uveitis

Rheumatological
- Seronegative arthritis of the small joints
- Ankylosing spondylitis

Haematological
- Predisposition to venous thromboses

Question 105

A 40-year-old woman presented with a five-day history of recurrent falls and an unsteady gait. She had a past history of a stroke causing a right-sided hemiparesis, which resolved spontaneously after a few days. The patient underwent intensive investigation following presentation with the stroke including carotid Doppler studies, transoesophageal echocardiography and CT scan of the brain, which were normal.

On examination she had a broad-based gait. There was evidence of dysdiadochokinesia in both upper limbs and abnormal heel–shin testing. The lower limb reflexes were brisk and the plantar response was extensor. The heart rate was 80 beats/min and regular. The blood pressure was 130/90 mmHg. Both heart sounds were normal.

What is the most probable diagnosis?
- a. Systemic lupus erythematosus with cerebral involvement.
- b. Multiple sclerosis.
- c. Multiple paradoxical emboli.
- d. Friedreich's ataxia.
- e. Multiple cerebral metastases.

Questions 106 and 107

A 30-year-old male presented with weight loss and palpitation for six months. He had lost approximately 4 kg. The patient had been well previously. He was not taking any medication. There was no family history of note. Apart from an orchidopexy affecting the right testicle ten years ago, there was no past history of note. On examination he had a resting tachycardia and evidence of bilateral gynaecomastia. There were no other abnormalities.

Investigations are shown.

Hb	14 g/dl
WCC	6×10^9/l
Platelets	180×10^9/l
Sodium	135 mmol/l
Potassium	4.3 mmol/l
Urea	5 mmol/l
Albumin	38 g/l
Alkaline phosphatase	190 iu/l (NR 25–115 iu/l)
Alpha-fetoprotein	8 ku/l (NR <10 ku/l)
Human chorionic gonadotrophin	1250 iu/l
TSH	<0.01 mu/l
Thyroxine	300 nmol/l (NR 60–160 nmol/l)
Testosterone	60 nmol/l (NR 10–35 nmol/l)
Oestradiol	1300 pmol/l (NR 500–1100 pmol/l)

Question 106

What is the diagnosis?
- a. Leydig cell tumour.
- b. Choriocarcinoma.
- c. Teratoma.
- d. Seminoma.
- e. Thyroid carcinoma.

Question 107

What investigation is required to help make the diagnosis?
- a. Ultrasound testes.
- b. CXR.
- c. CT thorax.
- d. FSH level.
- e. FNA thyroid.

Question 108

A 42-year-old man required ventilation for a prolonged period during an episode of septicaemia. Following this he developed difficulty with walking and required the aid of an assistant to mobilize. On neurological examination there was weakness on dorsiflexion of the toes, as well as ankle eversion. The patient also had reduced sensation, affecting the anterior lateral aspects below the knee and the dorsum of the foot.

What is the neurological diagnosis?
- a. L5 radiculopathy.
- b. L4 radiculopathy.
- c. Common peroneal nerve palsy.
- d. Femoral nerve palsy.
- e. Guillain–Barré syndrome.

Answer 105

| b. Multiple sclerosis. |

The patient has had a previous right hemiparesis and now presents with ataxia. Neurological examination reveals findings consistent with a cerebellar syndrome and bilateral pyramidal tract involvement. The differential diagnosis of cerebellar and pyramidal tract involvement includes multiple sclerosis, subacute combined degeneration of the spinal cord, Friedreich's ataxia, multiple cerebral metastases and multiple cerebral infarcts.

The most probable diagnosis is multiple sclerosis, a demyelinating disorder characterized by involvement of the optic tracts, pyramidal tracts, cerebellar peduncle and the posterior columns of the spinal cord.

The normal CT scan of the brain and carotid Doppler studies are against the diagnosis of multiple cerebral metastases and infarctions. A normal transoesophageal echocardiogram is against the diagnosis of paradoxical emboli. Whereas SLE may manifest with multiple neurological manifestations, the patient does not have any other manifestations of a multi-system disorder. With specific reference to SLE there is no history of arthralgia, myalgia or a rash. Whilst Friedreich's ataxia may be associated with pyramidal tract and cerebellar involvement, the condition usually presents at a much younger age and is associated with progressive neurological deterioration. The condition also affects the dorsal root ganglia, which causes absent peripheral reflexes.

Answers 106 and 107

| **Answer 106**
b. Choriocarcinoma.

Answer 107
a. Ultrasound testes. |

The patient had weight loss, palpitation and suppressed TSH, suggesting hyperthyroidism. Furthermore he has gynaecomastia, raised testosterone and oestrogen levels as well as a high human chorionic gonadotrophin level. This combination is highly suggestive of a chorionic carcinoma; chorionic carcinomas are characterized by high HCG levels. The alpha subunit in HCG is similar to that found in TSH, FSH and LH, therefore patients with choriocarcinoma may be hyperthyroid and have raised testosterone and oestrogen.

Testicular tumours can be divided into germ-cell tumours and sex-cord stromal cell tumours. Germ-cell tumours include seminomas, choriocarcinomas, teratomas, embryonal cell cancer, and yolk sac tumours. Sex-cord tumours comprise Leydig cell tumours and tumours affecting the cells of Sertoli. 95% of all testicular tumours are germ-cell tumours. 50% of all germ-cell tumours are seminomas. Seminomas are most common in the fourth decade. Tumour markers are usually normal. Testicular teratomas are relatively rare. They may be found in prepubertal males and in adults. Tumour markers are usually negative. Choriocarcinomas are associated with high HCG levels.

Leydig cells are the commonest sex-cord stromal tumours that have the ability to produce both oestrogen and testosterone.

Answer 108

| c. Common peroneal nerve palsy. |

Weakness of dorsiflexion and eversion of the foot and reduced sensation over the antero-lateral aspects of the lower leg and dorsum of the foot are typical features of common peroneal nerve palsy. The common peroneal nerve crosses over the fibula, where it may become damaged owing to acute or chronic compression. Common peroneal nerve palsy occurs following compression due to plaster casts below the knee, excessive crossing of the legs, or prolonged pressure on the fibula during general anaesthesia or unconsciousness. The nerve may be also be damaged during trauma or affected by diabetic neuropathy.

Question 109

A 53-year-old male was investigated for recurrent episodes of sinusitis and earache that did not respond to conventional antibiotics. He had experienced several attacks in the past 18 months. Just three months previously he experienced two episodes of epistaxis that were managed at home. He was generally unwell and tired easily. He had taken six weeks of sick leave from work for malaise and fever in the past six months. According to his wife he seemed to be losing weight. On further questioning the patient complained of a dry non-productive cough usually at the same time that he had either sinusitis or earache. He denied haemoptysis or night sweats. He worked as a postman. He did not smoke and consumed alcohol on an infrequent basis. Apart from a holiday in Kenya three years ago, he had not left the country for ten years. There was a family history of adult onset asthma. His father had died from bronchial carcinoma.

On examination, he was thin. There was no clubbing or lymphadenopathy. His heart rate was 98 beats/min. The blood pressure measured 148/96 mmHg. The JVP was not raised. Cardiovascular examination was normal. Examination of the upper respiratory tract revealed crusting of the inner aspect to the nostrils. The throat was normal. Auscultation of the lung fields was normal, as was examination of the abdomen. On neurological examination, Rinne's test was positive in the right ear. There was no skin rash.

Investigations are shown.

Hb	11 g/dl
WCC	15×10^9/l
	(neutrophils 12×10^9/l,
	lymphocytes 2×10^9/l,
	eosinophils 0.35×10^9/l)
Platelets	490×10^9/l
MCV	80 fl
ESR	60 mm/h
CRP	90 g/l
Sodium	138 mmol/l
Potassium	4.1 mmol/l
Urea	7 mmol/l
Creatinine	110 μmol/l
Bilirubin	11 μmol/l
AST	23 iu/l
ALT	25 iu/l
Alkaline phosphatase	156 iu/l (NR <115 iu/l)
Albumin	31 g/l
Immunology:	
pANCA	Positive
(myeloperoxidase)	
cANCA	Negative
ANF	Negative
C3	0.9 g/l (NR 0.55–1.2 g/l)
C4	0.3 g/l (NR 0.2–0.5 g/l)
Chest X-ray	Right middle lobe consolidation
Urinalysis	24-hour protein 0.8g
	Blood ++
	Casts absent

What is the most likely diagnosis?
a. Classic polyarteritis nodosa.
b. Churg–Strauss syndrome.
c. Microscopic polyangiitis.
d. Mixed essential cryoglobulinaemic vasculitis.
e. Wegener's granulomatosis.

Question 110

A 40-year-old homosexual male presented to the Accident and Emergency Department with a four-day history of sore throat and fever. On examination he had cervical and axillary lymphadenopathy and widespread maculopapular rash. An HIV antibody test was negative.

Which one of the following investigations would you perform next to help identify the cause of his illness?
a. Blood film.
b. Monospot test.
c. HIV viral RNA load.
d. CD4 count.
e. CT scan of the thorax and abdomen.

Answer 109

c. Microscopic polyangiitis.

The patient presents with specific symptoms of upper and lower respiratory tract involvement. Additionally, he has malaise, arthralgia, weight loss and raised inflammatory markers suggestive of a systemic illness. The presence of blood and protein in the urine indicates renal involvement. A normal creatinine concentration does not preclude renal involvement. The differential diagnosis is that of a multi-system disease capable of involving the upper and lower respiratory tract as well as the kidneys. The presence of a positive ANCA test is suggestive of a small-vessel vasculitis. Possibilities include Wegener's granulomatosis, microscopic polyangiitis and Churg–Strauss syndrome.

Wegener's granulomatosis and microscopic polyangiitis are both small-vessel vasculitides associated with ANCA. Both are characterized by upper and lower tract involvement (sinusitis, epistaxis, otitis media, haemoptysis) and renal involvement. Other features common to both include episcleritis, peripheral/central nervous system involvement and effects on the gastrointestinal tract. While manifestations of the upper and lower respiratory tract involvement may be identical in both of these small-vessel vasculitides, the presence of granulomata in small vessels in biopsy specimens is specific for Wegener's granulomatosis. The ANCA subtype may also aid differentiation between Wegener's granulomatosis and microscopic polyangiitis. Wegener's granulomatosis is characterized by the presence of

cANCA (antigen is proteinase 3) whereas microscopic polyangiitis is characterized by presence of pANCA (antigen is myeloperoxidase). The presence of pANCA in this case favours the diagnosis of microscopic polyangiitis.

Churg–Strauss syndrome is a small-vessel vasculitis affecting the upper and lower respiratory tract as well as the skin and the peripheral nervous system. Nasal polyps, allergic rhinitis and adult-onset asthma usually predate the vasculitis by many years. Renal involvement is usually mild but can be severe. A mild eosinophilia (usually $<2 \times 10^9/l$) is a recognized feature. Patients have a positive pANCA directed specifically against myeloperoxidase. (See Questions 4, 396.)

Classic PAN is vasculitis that can affect medium and small vessels. It is characterized by micro-aneurysms, tissue infarction, haemorrhage and organ dysfunction. Fever, malaise, gastrointestinal, cardiac, CNS and soft tissue involvement is usual. The diagnosis is best made by arteriography. Renal biopsy is usually not diagnostic unless a medium-sized vessel is included in the biopsy specimen. The glomeruli are normal. ANCA is characteristically absent. (See Question 174.)

Mixed essential cryoglobulinaemia hepatitis C virus is implicated in 80% of cases. Clinical features include pupura, arthralgia, membranoproliferative glomerulonephritis, hepatosplenomegaly and neurological manifestations. Rheumatoid factor levels are often high. Complement levels are low. ANCA is usually absent. (See Question 15.)

Answer 110

c. HIV viral RNA load.

The presentation is consistent with HIV seroconversion. Most patients can be diagnosed by conventional ELISA tests, which identify the presence of HIV antibodies by the time the patient has features of HIV seroconversion. However, if HIV antibody testing proves negative, then the diagnosis can be confirmed by measuring HIV viral RNA load. HIV viral load is not routinely used to diagnose HIV infection because it is labour intensive, but it is useful in diagnosing acute HIV infection, helping to resolve indeterminate HIV antibody results and in newborn babies where there is passive transfer of antibody from the mother to the baby. A low CD4 count alone is not specific for HIV infection.

Question 111

A 68-year-old male complained of dyspnoea on minimal exertion. Respiratory function tests are shown.

FEV1	2.1 l	(predicted 2–3 l)
FVC	2.5 l	(predicted 2.8–4.4 l)
TLC	4.2 l	(predicted 5–7 l)
TLCO	90% predicted value	

With what are the lung function tests most consistent?
    a. Extrinsic allergic alveolitis.
    b. Pulmonary fibrosis.
    c. Asthma.
    d. Ankylosing spondylitis.
    e. Pulmonary hypertension.

Question 112

A 66-year-old female patient presented with transient bilateral loss of vision lasting a few seconds. A few days later she developed a right-sided hemiparesis. There was no history of head injury or headaches. She had a four-year history of hypertension. The patient had smoked for 40 years. Physical examination revealed a right-sided hemiparesis but no other abnormality. The heart rate was 80 beats/min and regular. The blood pressure measured 160/100 mmHg.

The following test results were obtained:

12-lead ECG	Normal
2-D echocardiogram with colour flow	Normal
CT scan brain	Left middle cerebral artery infarction

What is the investigation of choice to ascertain the cause of her presentation?
    a. Carotid Doppler studies.
    b. Transoesophageal echocardiograph.
    c. Carotid angiography.
    d. MRI scan brain.
    e. Thrombophilia screen.

Question 113

A 79-year-old man was admitted with sudden onset of chest pain and breathlessness. On examination he was cyanosed. He had had a total hip replacement ten days previously. The patient smoked ten cigarettes per day and had hypertension for which he took nifedipine. On examination the heart sounds were normal and auscultation of the lungs revealed a clear chest.

Investigations are shown.

Hb	13 g/dl
WCC	13 × 10^9/l
Platelets	250 × 10^9/l
CRP	28 g/l
ECG	Sinus tachycardia and LBBB
Arterial blood gases (air):	
pH	7.49
PaCO$_2$	3.1 kPa
PaO$_2$	8.8 kPa
HCO$_3$	28 mmol/l

What is the most probable diagnosis?
    a. Pulmonary embolism.
    b. Acute myocardial infarction.
    c. Fat embolism syndrome.
    d. Pneumonia.
    e. Pulmonary oedema secondary to hypertensive heart disease.

Answer 111

d. Ankylosing spondylitis.

The patient has a restrictive lung defect (FEV1/FVC ratio approx. 80%), a low total lung capacity and a relatively normal transfer factor. These findings are consistent with either a thoracic cage deformity, a neuromuscular defect affecting the respiratory muscles or massive pleural fibrosis. From the options given, ankylosing spondylitis is the best answer.

Extrinsic allergic alveolitis and pulmonary fibrosis are associated with a low transfer factor. Asthma causes an obstructive respiratory defect and pure pulmonary hypertension does not usually affect the lung volumes.

Answer 112

a. Carotid Doppler studies.

The patient has evidence of multiple transient ischaemic episodes followed by a right-sided hemiparesis. CT scan of the brain reveals a left middle cerebral artery infarction, which is consistent with the final presentation. There is no evidence of any other abnormality in the brain. Possible causes of multiple cerebral emboli in this particular case include thrombi from the carotid arteries, calcific plaques from a degenerative aortic valve, and paradoxical emboli from a patent foramen ovale. In the absence of atrial fibrillation, the commonest cause of thromboembolism to the brain is atheromatous carotid artery disease, particularly in patients with hypertension.

The normal transthoracic echocardiogram certainly excludes calcific thromboemboli from degenerative aortic valve disease, but a patent foramen ovale cannot be excluded with certainty. However, in patients aged over 40, carotid artery disease is a much commoner cause of stroke than a patent foramen ovale.

The initial investigation of choice is a carotid Doppler study (see Answer 166). In the absence of significant carotid artery disease, a transoesophageal echocardiogram should be performed to exclude a patent foramen ovale. A thrombophilia screen is indicated in young patients with stroke and in those with a previous history of arterial and venous thrombosis or a family history of arterial or venous thrombosis.

Answer 113

a. Pulmonary embolism.

The presentation with sudden chest pain, dyspnoea, hypoxia and hypocarbia ten days after a hip replacement is highly suggestive of pulmonary embolism. The ECG reveals LBBB, which may be due to silent coronary disease or long-standing hypertension. The ECG in massive pulmonary embolism classically reveals right ventricular strain pattern or RBBB. Although it is possible that the presentation may represent acute myocardial infarction, the blood gases cannot be explained by the absence of pulmonary oedema, yet his chest is clear on auscultation.

Fat embolism syndrome is a condition that may occur after bony fractures (more common with closed than open fractures). It is characterized by hypoxaemia, peticheal rash and neurological abnormalities usually within 72 hours (but rarely before 12 hours) after the procedure. The patient above does not fulfil the diagnosis of fat embolism syndrome.

Questions 114 and 115

A 56-year-old woman was admitted for a left hip replacement. She had mechanical mitral valve prosthesis. Two days before surgery the patient was commenced on intravenous heparin and was continued on a daily infusion of 28,000 units per day for the next 7 days. On the fifth post-operative day she complained of a painful lower left limb. On examination the lower limb was swollen and tense. Doppler venography confirmed an ileo-femoral deep-vein thrombosis. The patient was commenced on warfarin but developed gangrene of the skin affecting the toes after 12 hours.

Investigations are shown.

Hb	10 g/dl
WCC	$12 \times 10^9/l$
Platelets	$30 \times 10^9/l$
APTT	94 s (control 45 s)
INR	3.8
Factor V Leiden mutation	Absent

Question 114

What is the diagnosis?
  a. Protein S deficiency.
  b. Protein C deficiency.
  c. Heparin-induced thrombocytopenia type I.
  d. Heparin-induced thrombocytopenia type II.
  e. Anti-thrombin III deficiency.

Question 115

What is the next management step?
  a. Stop warfarin and switch to danaparoid.
  b. Switch to therapeutic dose of low-molecular-weight heparin.
  c. Give intravenous protein C concentrate.
  d. Give intravenous protein S concentrate.
  e. Stop all anticoagulation until platelet count is $>100 \times 10^9/l$.

Question 116

A patient with psoriasis was referred to the psychiatrist and found to have manic depression. He was started on medication that resulted in severe exacerbation of the rash shown (**116**).

Which one of the following medications is the most likely cause for the deterioration?
  a. Amitryptilline.
  b. Paroxitene.
  c. Risperidone.
  d. Lithium.
  e. Haloperidol.

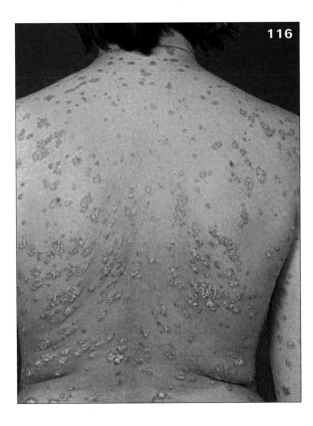
116

Answers 114 and 115

> **Answer 114**
> d. Heparin-induced thrombocytopenia type II.
>
> **Answer 115**
> a. Stop warfarin and switch to danaparoid.

The diagnosis is heparin-induced thrombocytopenia type II, also known as heparin-induced thrombocytopenic thrombosis. In contrast with HIT type I, which is a transient isolated thrombocytopenia usually occurring after 48 hours of therapy with unfractionated heparin, HIT type II is an immune-mediated disorder resulting in the formation of antibodies against the heparin-platelet factor 4 complex. HIT type II has a prevalence of between 0.3 and 3% of patients who have been on heparin for between 4 and 10 days. The condition rarely occurs after 10 days of treatment.

HIT II is characterized by an increased level of IgG and IgM antibodies to heparin, which results in both platelet activation causing venous and arterial thromboses and thrombocytopenia due to immune-mediated destruction of platelets. Venous thromboses are more common than arterial ones. Manifestations include deep-vein thrombosis, pulmonary embolism, sinus vein thrombosis, myocardial infarction, cerebrovascular thrombosis and infarction of any other organ. Another different manifestation is skin necrosis. The condition should be suspected in anyone who develops an abnormally low platelet count or a >50% drop from the original platelet count in association with a thrombotic episode a few days after starting heparin. The platelet count rarely drops below 20,000 (the usual nadir is approximately 60,000), therefore bleeding is rare.

It is important to note that there are reports of delayed onset HIT type II that may occur nine days after heparin has been stopped.

The diagnosis is clinical, being based upon a thrombocytopenia in association with heparin therapy and an associated arterial or venous thrombus. It is confirmed by demonstrating heparin-induced platelet antibodies (serotonin reactive assay, heparin-induced platelet aggregation or solid phase immunoassay).

Type II HIT can be prevented by using low-molecular-weight heparin or limiting the use of heparin to less than five days (i.e switching to warfarin early if long-term anticoagulation is required).

> **Management of HIT (type II)**
> 1. Stop heparin.
> 2. Don't switch from unfractionated heparin to LMWT heparin once the diagnosis is made (10% cross reactivity).
> 3. Danaparoid (heparinoids) or lepirudin (recombinant hirudin) should be started even if the platelet count is very low unless there is active bleeding. These drugs are the mainstay of therapy for HIT type II.
> 4. Don't use warfarin alone if deep-vein thrombosis (can get skin necrosis due to transient acquired protein C deficiency).
> 5. Don't give warfarin until platelet count is >100 $\times$ 10^9/l.

Answer 116

> d. Lithium.

The patient has developed severe psoriasis. Psoriasis may be exacerbated by drugs and infections. With respect to drugs, the commonest culprits are beta-blockers, lithium and antimalarial drugs. Other drugs include ACE inhibitors and NSAIDs.

Viral (including HIV) and bacterial infections are recognized exacerbating factors for psoriasis. Streptococcal infections have been particularly implicated in guttate psoriasis.

Question 117

A 69-year-old woman presented with pain in her shoulders and upper back, polydipsia and polyuria.
Investigations are shown.

Hb	9 g/dl
WCC	14 × 10⁹/l
Platelets	140 × 10⁹/l
MCV	89 fl
Sodium	129 mmol/l
Potassium	3.4 mmol/l
Urea	26 mmol/l
Creatinine	290 µmol/l
Calcium	2.8 mmol/l
Phosphate	1.9 mmol/l
Total protein	98 g/l
Albumin	34 g/l

1. What is the diagnosis?
   a. Multiple myeloma.
   b. Aplastic anaemia.
   c. Hyperparathyroidism.
   d. Chronic renal failure.
   e. Vitamin D toxicity.

2. What is the commonest cause of renal failure in this condition?
   a. Hypercalcaemia.
   b. Amyloid deposition.
   c. Tubular obstruction by light chain.
   d. Analgesic nephropathy.
   e. Hyperuricaemia.

3. Give one possible cause for the low potassium.
   a. Vomiting.
   b. Diarrhoea.
   c. Diuretic therapy.
   d. Proximal renal tubular acidosis.
   e. Distal renal tubular acidosis.

Questions 118 and 119

A 14-year-old Asian boy diagnosed with pulmonary tuberculosis was commenced on antituberculous drugs consisting of isoniazid, rifampicin, pyrizinamide and ethambutol. Four days after commencing treatment he presented with malaise, myalgia, nausea and anorexia. On examination he was febrile with a diffuse erythematous rash. The blood pressure was 90/55 mmHg and there were crackles and bronchial breathing audible over the right upper lobe.
Investigations are shown.

Hb	14 g/dl	
WCC	12 × 10⁹/l	
Neutrophils	7 × 10⁹/l	
Lymphocytes	2.5 × 10⁹/l	
Eosinophils	4 × 10⁹/l	
Basophils	0.1 × 10⁹/l	
Monocytes	0.4 × 10⁹/l	
Platelets	300 × 10⁹/l	
ESR	120 mm/h	
Sodium	130 mmol/l	
Potassium	6.5 mmol/l	
Chloride	87 mmol/l	
Urea	26 mmol/l	
Creatinine	300 µmol/l	
Glucose	9 mmol/l	
Urinary microscopy	White blood cells, red blood cells and white cell casts	
24-hour urinalysis	Sodium	60 mmol/l
	Protein	0.8 g

Question 118

What is the cause of this patient's renal dysfunction?
   a. Renal tuberculosis.
   b. Acute tubular necrosis.
   c. Acute interstitial nephritis.
   d. Acute post-infectious glomerulonephritis.
   e. Rhabdomyolysis.

Question 119

What is the most important initial step in his management?
   a. Renal biopsy.
   b. Haemodialysis.
   c. Corticosteroids.
   d. Discontinuation of isoniazid.
   e. Discontinuation of rifampicin.

Answer 117

> 1. a. Multiple myeloma.
> 2. c. Tubular obstruction by light chain.
> 3. d. Proximal renal tubular acidosis.

The diagnosis of myeloma is based on the very high globulin count (albumin subtracted from total protein content), anaemia, renal failure and hypercalcaemia.

The question tests understanding of the renal and biochemical complications of myeloma.

The causes of anaemia, renal failure and other biochemical abnormalities in myeloma are covered in the answers above. (See also Answer 38.)

Answers 118 and 119

> **Answer 118**
> c. Acute interstitial nephritis.
>
> **Answer 119**
> e. Discontinuation of rifampicin.

The patient presents with fever, rash, eosinophilia and renal impairment shortly after commencing anti-tuberculous therapy. The findings are consistent with acute interstitial nephritis secondary to rifampicin. AIN is most commonly due to drug therapy (*Table*).

The onset of AIN after drug therapy ranges from three to five days following a second exposure, to as long as several weeks with a first exposure. However, the latent period may be as short as one day with rifampicin or as long as 18 months with an NSAID.

Patients typically present with an acute rise in the plasma creatinine concentration temporally related to an offending drug or infection. Fever occurs in most cases and may be accompanied by a rash. The urine sediment usually reveals white cells, red cells, and white cell casts. Eosinophilia and eosinophiluria are present in over 75% of cases with the exception of disease induced by NSAIDs where fever, rash, and eosinophilia are typically absent. Most patients have normal or only mildly increased protein excretion (<1 g/day) although some older individuals have significant proteinuria (approximately 3 g/day). Concurrent nephrotic syndrome due to minimal change disease is often seen with NSAIDs. Signs of tubulo-interstitial damage, such as the Fanconi syndrome and renal tubular acidosis, may also be present.

The diagnosis should be suspected from the temporal relation to an offending drug and the characteristic laboratory findings. The urinary findings usually distinguish AIN from other causes of acute renal failure such as glomerulonephritis and acute tubular necrosis. Acute glomerulonephritis is usually associated with the presence of red cell casts in the urine. In acute tubular necrosis urinalysis typically shows granular and epithelial cell casts and free epithelial cells. Even when none of these other conditions appears to be present, examination of the urine is still important because some of the drugs listed below can produce other forms of acute renal failure.

Genitourinary tuberculosis usually has an insidious presentation, with dysuria and gross haematuria being the most common symptoms, and thus not the most likely diagnosis in this case. Patients with rhabdomyolysis typically present with the triad of pigmented granular casts in the urine, pigmenturia due to myoglobinuria and a marked elevation in the plasma level of creatine kinase.

Although the clinical picture is often highly suggestive of AIN, the diagnosis can be confirmed only by renal biopsy. In the absence of severe disease, it is acceptable to begin by observing the response to discontinuation of the suspected offending drug. No further evaluation or therapy is required if renal function begins to improve within several days.

Indications for biopsy generally include uncertainty as to the diagnosis, advanced renal failure or lack of spontaneous recovery following cessation of drug therapy. An alternative – particularly in those who are poor candidates for renal biopsy – is to initiate a trial of corticosteroids (such as 1 mg/kg of prednisone per day). Patients with AIN typically begin to improve within one to two weeks and rapidly return to their baseline plasma creatinine concentration.

> **Causes of acute tubulo-interstitial nephritis**
>
> *Drug-induced*
> - Non-steroidal anti-inflammatory drugs
> - Penicillins
> - Cephalosporins
> - Sulphonamides
> - Loop and thiazide-type diuretics
>
> *Non drug-induced*
> - Sarcoidosis
> - Legionella infection
> - Leptospirosis
> - Streptococcal infection

Question 120

A 56-year-old male was admitted with weight loss and fatigue. He consumed 40 units of alcohol per week. On examination he was pale and had a palpable spleen 10 cm below the costal margin.

Investigations are shown.

Hb	8 g/dl
WCC	23 × 109/l
Platelets	500 × 109/l
MCV	90 fl
Neutrophils	58%
Lymphocytes	2%
Monocytes	1%
Eosinophils	1%
Basophils	2%
Neutrophil alkaline phosphatase	25 iu/l (NR 35–100 iu/l)

What is the diagnosis?
a. Myelofibrosis.
b. Polycythaemia rubra vera.
c. Myelodysplasia.
d. Chronic myeloid leukaemia.
e. Hypersplenism secondary to cirrhotic portal hypertension.

Question 121

A 67-year-old man presented with central chest pain associated with ST segment depression in the inferior and lateral leads. He had smoked 20–30 cigarettes per day for over 40 years. Troponin T 12 hours after admission was 0.4 ng/l (NR <0.05 ng/l). The patient remained pain free for three days and the ECG changes resolved. He was treated with antiplatelet agents, a statin, ACE inhibitor and a beta-blocker.

What is the next step in his management?
a. Echocardiography prior to discharge.
b. Coronary angiography prior to discharge.
c. Exercise stress test prior to discharge.
d. CRP.
e. Discharge home and arrange outpatient exercise test in six weeks.

Question 122

A 24-year-old woman presented with a swollen left lower limb when she was eight weeks pregnant. Lower limb vein Doppler studies confirmed a femoral vein deep-vein thrombosis. There was no family history of thrombophilia.

What is the management of the patient?
a. Consider termination of pregnancy.
b. Start subcutaneous fractionated heparin and continue for the entire pregnancy, maintaining an antifactor Xa >1.0 (four hours after injection). After pregnancy give warfarin for six weeks.
c. Start fractionated heparin initially and switch to warfarin in the second trimester. Continue warfarin until the middle of the third trimester and then switch patient back to heparin until term.
d. Start warfarin and continue throughout pregnancy.
e. Use high-dose aspirin during pregnancy and switch to warfarin for six weeks post-partum.

Answer 120

> d. Chronic myeloid leukaemia.

The patient has large splenomegaly and a high white cell count consisting predominantly of neutrophils. The differential diagnosis is between CML and myelofibrosis. Both conditions may be associated with much higher white cell counts; however, CML can be differentiated from myelofibrosis by karyotyping for Philadelphia chromosome, measurement of neutrophil leucocyte alkaline phosphatase level and bone marrow analysis. Patients with CML usually have the Philadelphia chromosome abnormality and low neutrophil alkaline phosphatase levels. Further support for the diagnosis of CML in this question is the relatively high basophil count. (See Question 392.)

Answer 121

> b. Coronary angiography prior to discharge.

The patient has chest pain and raised troponin in the absence of ST elevation. By definition this patient has suffered a non-ST elevation myocardial infarction. Such patients have a relatively low risk of in-hospital mortality compared with ST segment elevation myocardial infarction; however, six-month mortality exceeds that of patients with STEMI and is around 20%. Therefore, it is prudent that all appropriate patients with NSTEMI have coronary angiography and revascularization (if required) prior to discharge from hospital. The same applies to patients who present with chest pain and marked ST segment depression even if the serum cardiac troponin is not elevated (*Table A*).

In the interim the management of both groups of patients is essentially the same and consists of anti-thrombotic agents (aspirin and clopidogrel together), fractionated heparin, and IIb/IIIa platelet receptor blocking agents (*Table B*). High-dose statins may play a role in plaque pacification in the peri-infarction period. In addition beta-blockers may reduce myocardial oxygen demand. GTN infusion is useful in reducing symptoms of acute myocardial ischaemia.

The benefits of aspirin in myocardial infarction are well established. Over the past few years the CURE study demonstrated that the addition of clopidogrel to aspirin in patients with non-ST elevation acute coronary syndrome was associated with a lower rate of adverse cardiac events in the ensuing nine months. Both drugs are initiated on admission. Aspirin is continued indefinitely whereas clopidogrel should be continued for up to 12 months. Glycoprotein IIb/IIIa inhibitors are started at the same time as antithrombotic therapy and subcutaneous fractionated heparin in all patients with NSTEMI and in patients with unstable angina who continue to have pain and/or dynamic ECG changes representative of myocardial ischaemia. Eptifibatide and tirofiban are the most commonly used IIb/IIIa glycoprotein receptor inhibitors. IIb/IIIa glycoprotein receptor blockers are continued for up to 72 hours, by which time most patients should have undergone coronary angiography.

Table A Indications for in-patient coronary angiography in patients with non-ST elevation coronary syndromes

- Raised serum troponin T or I
- Chest pain with dynamic ST segment changes of myocardial ischaemia
- Chest pain with clinical evidence of left ventricular dysfunction
- Chest pain associated with malignant ventricular arrhythmias

---

Table B Management of non-ST elevation myocardial infarction

1. Relieve pain as in ST elevation myocardial infarction
2. Aspirin loading dose of 300 mg followed by 75–150 mg daily indefinitely
3. Clopidogrel loading dose 300 mg followed by 75 mg daily for 12 months
4. Fractionated heparin, usually enoxaparin (subcutaneously), until coronary angiography.
5. IIb/IIIa glycoprotein receptor blockers for up to 72 hours. Ideally most patients should have had coronary angiography within 72 hours of presentation
6. Initiate high-dose statin therapy
7. Beta-blocker therapy on admission as with ST elevation myocardial infarction
8. Coronary angiography in all patients where general health and comorbidities allow for the procedure to be performed safely
9. ACE inhibitor prior to discharge

Early use of high-dose statins, such as simvastatin 40 mg or atorvastatin 40–80 mg, has been shown to reduce adverse cardiac events 30 days after the initial insult. There are no trials assessing the effect of beta-blockers in NSTEMI; however, given the magnitude of prognostic benefit of this group of drugs in patients with STEMI, it seems reasonable to deduce that they are probably effective in the management of patients with NSTEMI.

It is unclear whether early initiation of an ACE inhibitor alters the immediate prognosis in patients with NSTEMI unless the patient has left ventricular dysfunction. However, the long-term benefits of ACE inhibitor therapy in patients with coronary artery disease are now well established (EUROPA and HOPE studies) and it is recommended that all patients presenting with NSTEMI are initiated on an ACE inhibitor prior to discharge home, provided there are no contraindications.

Answer 122

> b. Start subcutaneous fractionated heparin and continue for the entire pregnancy, maintaining an antifactor Xa >1.0 four hours after injection of heparin. After pregnancy give warfarin for six weeks.

The patient requires anticoagulation but warfarin is contraindicated in the first 13 weeks of pregnancy as it is teratogenic (skeletal, cartilage and foetal CNS abnormalities). Heparin, on the other hand, does not cross the placenta and has not been associated with teratogenic effects. The recommendation is to use either unfractionated or low-molecular weight heparin, at least in the first 13 weeks.

Following this there are three options, as follows:

1. Continue dose-adjusted unfractionated heparin throughout pregnancy, maintaining an APPT twice that of the normal range. However, treatment with unfractionated heparin requires daily monitoring of the APTT, which is inconvenient and impractical. Long-term unfractionated heparin injections are associated with a high risk of osteoporosis.

2. Continue weight-adjusted low-molecular weight heparin aiming for a 4-hour post injection antifactor Xa of 1.0 u. Antifactor Xa levels need to be measured once or twice a month as the patient is gaining weight. This is currently the anticoagulant strategy of choice.

3. Start with either unfractionated or low-molecular weight heparin during the first trimester and then switch to warfarin until the mid-third trimester (maintenance INR of 2). During the mid-third trimester the patient should be switched back to heparin until term because warfarin is associated with a higher risk of foetal haemorrhage during vaginal delivery and the baby's INR cannot be reversed by giving the mother fresh-frozen plasma during labour.

In all three cases above the patient should be anticoagulated with warfarin for six weeks following delivery, as these women have low antithrombin III levels, increase in factors I, II, VII, VIII and X and have increased venous stasis.

Aspirin is not effective in preventing propagation of a venous thrombus or preventing pulmonary embolism in pregnancy.

Question 123

A 70-year-old obese male saw his GP and was noted to have a blood pressure of 170/98 mmHg. The fundi were normal. Urinalysis was normal. Urea, electrolytes and blood sugar were normal. The total cholesterol measured 6 mmol/l. The patient was advised to lose weight and adhere to a low-salt diet. Blood pressure readings over the next six months were 170/96 mmHg, 168/96 mmHg and 166/96 mmHg.

> What is the treatment for the hypertension?
> a. Continue lifestyle modification for another six months.
> b. Bendroflumethiazide (bendroflumethazide).
> c. Ramipril.
> d. Atenolol.
> e. Doxososin.

Answer 123

> b. Bendroflumethiazide (bendroflumethazide).

The patient has moderate to severe hypertension and requires lifestyle modification advice as well as pharmacological therapy to help control his blood pressure. Hypertension in the elderly is best treated with calcium channel blockers or a thiazide diuretic. The use of thiazide diuretics as first line in most elderly patients with hypertension is supported by the recently published ALLHAT study, which was the largest study ever in the hypertensive population. The study showed that thiazide diuretics were more effective than beta-blockers, calcium channel blockers and angiotensin-converting enzyme inhibitors at reducing cardiovascular mortality in diabetics and non-diabetics.

All patients should receive advice regarding lifestyle modification to help reduce the blood pressure (*Table A*). Lifestyle modification alone without antihypertensive drug therapy for a period of six months to one year is reserved for patients with mild hypertension (BP 140–159/ 90–99 mmHg) who do not have any evidence of end-organ damage such as retinopathy, abnormal renal function, proteinuria, or any history of diabetes, nephropathy, stroke, coronary artery disease or heart failure (*Table A*). Most patients with hypertension require antihypertensive drug therapy.

The British Hypertension Society recommends that any one of the five major classes of antihypertensive drugs (thiazides, beta-blockers, calcium channel blockers, ACE inhibitors and angiotensin II receptor blockers) may be used as first-line monotherapy, although most patients require two or even three antihypertensive drugs to help control blood pressure. All of these groups of drugs have been shown to reduce cardiovascular mortality and stroke. The aim is to bring down the blood pressure to ≤140/90 mmHg. In patients with diabetes, stroke, coronary disease, heart failure or nephropathy the goals are more stringent and the aim is to reduce blood pressure to ≤130/85 mmHg.

During initiation of antihypertensive drugs, the ABCD method of prescription is useful for stepwise management of hypertension. The system is based on the fact that most young patients (aged ≤55 years) and non-black patients have high plasma renin levels and respond best to drugs primarily targeting the renin–angiotensin–aldosterone system when used as monotherapy. These patients respond to **A**CE inhibitors, **A**ngiotensin receptor blockers, or **B**eta-blockers as monotherapy (i.e. the A and B drugs). In contrast older patients and black patients (Afro-Caribbean in origin) respond better to drugs promoting natriuresis and reducing plasma volume such as **C**alcium channel blockers and **D**iuretics (i.e. the C and D drugs) when used as single agents (*Table B*). Addition of an A or B drug to a patient whose blood pressure is still elevated while taking a C or D drug and *vice versa* has an additive effect because in combination, these drugs counteract different mechanisms responsible for high blood pressure.

This particular system should not be applied to every case as there may be compelling indications to use A or B class drugs in patients aged >55 years or black patients if there is a history of diabetes (ACE inhibitor or A II receptor blocker) or heart failure (all of the A or B drugs).

Table A Lifestyle modification

- Lose weight to bring BMI down below 30
- Reduce alcohol consumption
- Regular exercise for 30–45 min three times per week
- Reduce salt intake to 6 g/day
- Increase potassium to 90 mmol/day
- Smoking cessation

Table B The stepwise management of hypertension using the ABCD system

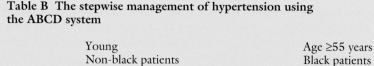

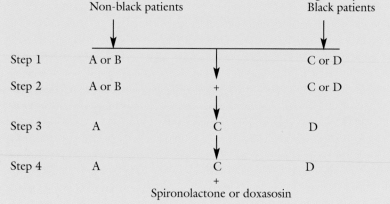

	Young Non-black patients		Age ≥55 years Black patients
Step 1	A or B		C or D
Step 2	A or B	+	C or D
Step 3	A	C	D
Step 4	A	C	D

Spironolactone or doxasosin

Question 124

A 70-year-old male presented with a four-week history of increasing dyspnoea and swollen ankles. There was no evidence of ischaemic heart disease, diabetes or alcohol abuse. On examination he had clinical and radiological evidence of pulmonary oedema. The blood pressure measured 180/100 mmHg. He was treated with intravenous furosemide with good results.

Investigations are shown.

Hb	10 g/dl
WCC	10×10^9/l
Platelets	200×10^9/l
Sodium	139 mmol/l
Potassium	5.1 mmol/l
Urea	14.9 mmol/l
Creatinine	250 µmol/l
Albumin	29 g/l
Chest X-ray after diuretic treatment (**124**)	
ECG	Sinus rhythm; small complexes; Q waves inferior and lateral leads
Urinalysis	Protein ++
Renal ultrasound	Normal kidneys

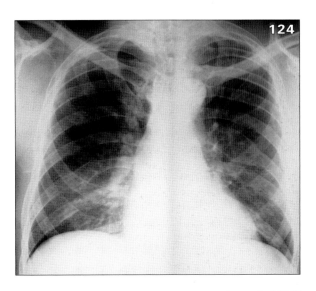

What is the most probable cause for the heart failure?
a. Hypertensive heart disease.
b. Anaemia.
c. Ischaemic heart disease.
d. Cardiac amyloid.
e. Renal artery stenosis.

Question 125

A 54-year-old non-insulin-dependent diabetic patient was referred to the blood pressure clinic for assessment and control of blood pressure. He was a non-smoker. He had a body mass index of 28. The blood pressure in clinic measured 180/98 mmHg on three successive occasions. His medication comprised metformin 1 g twice daily, simvastatin 40 mg od, aspirin 75 mg and amlodipine 10 mg od. Renal function was normal but urinalysis revealed proteinuria +. The HbA1c was 7%. The total cholesterol was 5.2 mmol/l. The 12-lead ECG revealed voltage criteria for left ventricular hypertrophy.

What is the most effective initial pharmacological step in reducing cardiovascular mortality?
a. Weight loss.
b. Increase dose of statin.
c. Start atenolol.
d. Start bendroflumethiazide.
e. Start losartan.

Answer 124

d. Cardiac amyloid.

The commonest causes of heart failure in the UK are ischaemic heart disease and hypertension. However, the clue to the answer in this question is in the interpretation of the chest X-ray, which shows expansile lytic lesions in the ribs consistent with the diagnosis of multiple myeloma. A significant proportion of patients with multiple myeloma develop amyloidosis. Cardiac amyloid is associated with restrictive dilated cardiomyopathy, conduction disturbance and angina due to amyloid deposits in the coronary arteries. The characteristic features of cardiac amyloid on the 12-lead ECG include small complexes, pseudo-infarcts (q-waves) and heart block (see Question 389). Amyloidosis commonly cause renal failure in multiple myeloma as in this case (see Question 38).

Almost 80% of patients have evidence of bone involvement from myeloma at the time of diagnosis.

Bone involvement is characterized by expansile lytic lesions, osteopenia and pathological fractures. Osteolytic lesions are thought to be due to stimulation of osteoclastic activity. The vertebral bodies, skull thoracic cage, pelvis and proximal aspects of the humeri and femora are the commonest sites of bone lesions. The most serious complication of bone involvement is cord compression from vertebral body collapse.

Technetium bone scans, which primarily detect osteoblastic activity, are not as useful as conventional plain radiographs (skeletal survey) at identifying the extent of bone involvement in multiple myeloma.

All patients with multiple myeloma should be treated with bisphosphonates to reduce the risk of skeletal complications. Treatment with bisphosphonates reduces bone pain, and the rate of pathological fractures and cord compression. A small proportion of patients on bisphosphonates for myeloma may develop nephrotic syndrome due to focal segmental glomerulosclerosis.

Answer 125

e. Start losartan.

The most effective method of reducing cardiovascular mortality in this patient with non-insulin-dependent diabetes would be to control the blood pressure effectively. Weight loss alone in a patient with this magnitude of hypertension would not be enough to reduce blood pressure.

While all groups of antihypertensive drugs listed have been shown to be equally efficacious in bringing the blood pressure down in 40–60% of patients when used as monotherapy, there are clinical settings in which certain groups of drugs may have additional benefits on cardiovascular mortality. In patients with non-insulin-dependent diabetes mellitus, both angiotensin II receptor blockers and angiotensin-converting enzyme inhibitors have been particularly effective in reducing cardiovascular mortality, as shown in the HOPE study and LIFE studies, respectively.

The LIFE trial evaluated the specific cardiovascular benefits of losartan in high-risk patients with moderate to severe hypertension (resting BP 160–200/95–115 mmHg) and electrocardiographic evidence of left ventricular hypertrophy.

Patients were randomly assigned to either losartan or atenolol therapy, with dose increases and the addition of hydrochlorthiazide (as well as other agents) to attain the target blood pressure levels (resting BP <140/90 mmHg). The initial and subsequent doses of both losartan and atenolol were 50 and 100 mg/day, respectively. The fall in blood pressure was similar in the two groups (30/17 mmHg).

The study showed that losartan was more effective than atenolol in reducing mortality, primarily owing to a reduction in fatal or non-fatal stroke. The benefit from losartan was more pronounced among diabetics compared to non-diabetics. The benefit was most prominent in diabetic patients who had not previously received antihypertensive therapy.

The recently published ALLHAT study, which was the largest study ever in the hypertensive population, showed that thiazide diuretics were more effective than beta-blockers, calcium channel blockers and angiotensin-converting enzyme inhibitors at reducing cardiovascular mortality in diabetics and non-diabetics. However, patients in the ALLHAT study did not have severe hypertension and not all had ECG criteria for left ventricular hypertrophy. Furthermore, the ALLHAT study did not evaluate angiotensin receptor blockers specifically. In this particular case one would add up to 100 mg losartan initially and introduce a thiazide diuretic if the BP was still >140/90 mmHg.

The patient will also require additional cholesterol lowering therapy in the form of a statin; however, in this case BP reduction is the priority.

Question 126

A 69-year-old male was seen in the renal clinic complaining of fatigue and dyspnoea. He had chronic renal impairment secondary to focal segmental glomerulonephritis and had been on haemodialysis for six months. The patient was noted to have been anaemic three months ago for which he was commenced on oral iron supplements. He had controlled hypertension but no other medical history. Medication comprised amlodipine 10 mg od, ferrous sulphate 200 mg bd and simvastatin 40 mg od.

On examination he appeared pale. There was no evidence of oedema. The heart rate was 90 beats/min and regular. The blood pressure measured 140/80 mmHg. The JVP was not raised. On examination of the precordium the apex was not displaced. Auscultation of the heart was normal and the chest was clear.

Investigations are shown.

Hb	9.9 g/dl
WCC	5×10^9/l
Platelets	200×10^9/l
MCV	88 fl
Sodium	138 mmol/l
Potassium	5.1 mmol/l
Urea	20 mmol/l
Creatinine	340 µmol/l
Calcium	2.0 mmol/l
Phosphate	1.3 mmol/l
Albumin	38 g/l
Glucose	4 mmol/l
Iron	9 mmol/l (NR 14–32 mmol/l)
TIBC	50 mmol/l (NR 40–80 mmol/l)
Ferritin	36 mg/l (NR 15–250 mg/l)
ECG	Left ventricular hypertrophy
Chest X-ray	Slight cardiac enlargement; clear lung fields

How would you treat the anaemia?
  a. Transfuse two units of packed red cells.
  b. Increase dose of oral iron therapy.
  c. Intravenous iron therapy.
  d. SC erythropoietin.
  e. IV iron and SC erythropoietin.

Question 127

A 17-year-old boy was referred to the local paediatrician because he had not grown very much in the past four years. Apart from feeling more lethargic than his school friends, he gave no other history of note. He measured 1.53 m. He had never needed to shave. His younger brother, aged 16, measured 1.73 m and had already started shaving. There were no other siblings. Both parents were well. The father was 1.76 m tall and the mother was 1.63 m tall.

On examination, he was slightly pale. He did not have any facial hair. He was below the third centile for height and was just at the 10th centile for weight. He did not have any evidence of secondary sexual characteristics, and his testes were small. The blood pressure was 115/70 mmHg.

Investigations are shown.

Hb	10 g/dl
WCC	7×10^9/l
Platelets	200×10^9/l
MCV	102 fl
Sodium	138 mmol/l
Potassium	4.3 mmol/l
Urea	4 mmol/l
Calcium	2.1 mmol/l
Phosphate	1.1 mmol/l
Albumin	38 g/l
Glucose	4.3 mmol/l

List two possible diagnoses.
  a. Coeliac disease.
  b. Growth hormone deficiency.
  c. Constitutional delay in puberty.
  d. Hypothyroidism.
  e. Vitamin D resistant hypophosphataemic rickets.

Answer 126

> c. Intravenous iron therapy.

The patient has chronic renal failure and is anaemic. Anaemia is a common complication of chronic renal failure. The cause of anaemia in CRF is multifactorial but deficiency of erythropoietin plays an important role. Anaemia is associated with a reduced quality of life and worse clinical outcomes as well as a higher prevalence of left ventricular hypertrophy and left ventricular cavity size in patients with chronic renal failure.

Anaemia is defined as an Hb <11g/dl in pre-pubertal children and pre-menopausal women and an Hb <12 g/dl in adult males and post-menopausal women. Patients with chronic renal failure should be maintained on an Hb of at least 11–12 g/dl.

Other causes of anaemia, including iron deficiency, should be excluded before attributing the anaemia to chronic renal failure (*Table*). Iron stores should be replenished before considering therapy with erythropoietins. In patient with chronic renal failure, the most useful markers of iron stores are the serum ferritin and the transferrin saturation which = Fe/TIBC × 100. A serum ferritin <100 mg/l and a TSAT ≤20% is indicative of absolute iron deficiency in a patient with chronic renal failure. The patient in question has evidence of absolute iron deficiency and requires iron supplements before considering the need for EPO. Patients with iron deficiency usually require intravenous iron supplements to replenish iron stores, particularly patients receiving haemodialysis. A treatment algorithm for anaemia in chronic renal failure is shown below. Patients who are not iron deficient generally respond to erythropoietin.

Causes of anaemia in renal failure

- Erythropoietin deficiency
- Chronic blood loss (iron deficiency)
- Hypothyroidism
- Vitamin B_{12} or folate deficiency
- Chronic infection or inflammation
- Aluminium toxicity
- Malignancy
- Haemolysis
- Myeloma
- Bone marrow infiltration
- Marrow aplasia

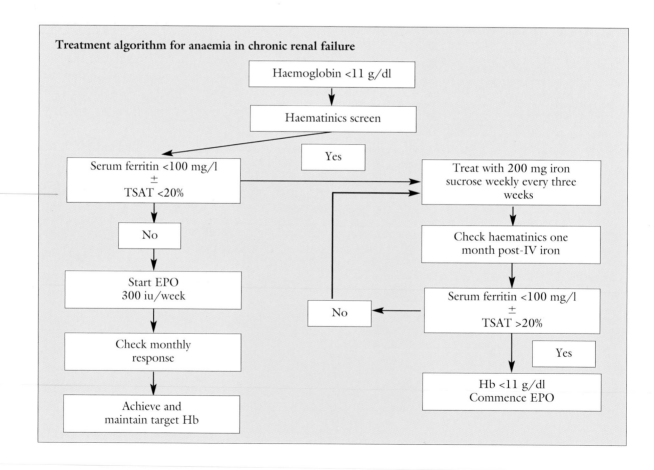

Answer 127

a. Coeliac disease.

This is a difficult question. There is evidence of short stature, delayed puberty and a macrocytosis. These three features can be best explained by malabsorption. The commonest cause of malabsorption in the Western world is coeliac disease. The macrocytosis in this respect is due to folate deficiency. It is unusual, however, not to also have biochemical evidence of osteomalacia. The differential diagnosis here is hypothyroidism, which may explain the short stature, delayed puberty and macrocytosis; however, the problem has been present for approximately four years and one would expect a history of performing poorly at school or the presence of dry skin on examination. In addition, many children with hypothyroidism are relatively overweight in relation to their height.

GH deficiency or gonadotrophin deficiency could explain short stature and delayed puberty, but they do not explain the macrocytosis. As with hypothyroidism, children with GH deficiency are relatively plump.

Question 128

A 15-year-old male presented with a four-day history of severe right-sided headaches affecting the orbit and right maxillary area. On examination he had acneform lesions around the nose and cheeks. Shortly after admission he became drowsy and developed a high temperature. He complained of diplopia. Subsequent physical examination revealed swelling of the right eye, a partial ptosis of the right eye and a lateral gaze palsy affecting the same eye. Fundoscopy revealed papilloedema. There was no evidence of nuchal rigidity.

What is the diagnosis?
  a. Septic cavernous sinus thrombosis.
  b. Viral encephalitis.
  c. Bacterial meningitis.
  d. Cerebral abscess.
  e. Cogan's syndrome.

Question 129

A 60-year-old man presents with general malaise and drowsiness. On examination, the blood pressure was 120/70 mmHg. Investigations are shown.

Sodium	108 mmol/l
Potassium	4 mmol/l
Urea	3 mmol/l
Creatinine	56 μmol/l
Bicarbonate	23 mmol/l
Random blood sugar	4.2 mmol/l
Urine glucose	Not detected
Urine ketones	Not detected

What is the diagnosis?
  a. Addison's disease.
  b. Hypothyroidism.
  c. SIADH secretion.
  d. Ectopic ACTH-secreting tumour.
  e. Gastric outlet obstruction.

Answer 128

> a. Septic cavernous sinus thrombosis.

The patient has septic dural sinus thrombosis syndrome. Three main types of dural sinus thrombosis are recognized, notably cavernous sinus thrombosis, lateral sinus thrombosis and superior saggital sinus thrombosis.

The commonest variety is the cavernous sinus thrombosis syndrome, possibly because the facial veins drain into the sinus and the most common source of infection is due to squeezing of nasal furuncles without antibiotic cover. Other sources of infection include otitis media, sinusitis and dental infections (*Table*). The commonest organism implicated is *Staphylococcus aureus*. Patients with cavernous sinus thrombosis present with severe peri-orbital headache, which also affects areas innervated by the ophthalmic and maxillary branches of the trigeminal nerve. Fever and peri-orbital oedema usually develop afterwards. Ocular swelling, chemosis, ophthalmoplegia and drowsiness are recognized complications. Ophthalmoplegia is due to compression of the third, fourth and sixth cranial nerves. Headache and associated ophthalmoplegia should always alert the clinician to the possible diagnosis of cavernous sinus thrombosis.

The diagnosis of cavernous sinus thrombosis is either with high resolution CT scan of the orbit with contrast or a gadolinium-enhanced MRI scan of the orbit. Management comprises intravenous flucloxacillin and intravenous heparin. Corticosteroids may be used (after the infection has been cleared with antibiotics) to improve inflammation around the cranial nerves. Corticosteroids are mandatory if pituitary infarction, a recognized complication of cavernous sinus thrombosis, occurs.

Lateral sinus thrombosis is rare and almost always complicates otitis media. It is characterized by fifth and sixth nerve palsy and papilloedema. It may be complicated by hydrocephalus. Treatment is as above but a radical mastoidectomy is also necessary.

Superior saggital venous thrombosis may complicate sinusitis. Thrombosis of the anterior segment of the sinus causes headaches, which resolve on the development of collaterals. Complete thrombotic occlusion of the superior saggital sinus is invariably fatal, resulting in large venous cortical infarction.

Cogan's syndrome is a chronic inflammatory disorder characterized by interstitial keratitis and vestibulo-auditory dysfunction, which may be associated with a systemic vasculitis.

> **Causes of dural sinus thrombosis**
>
> - Infections of the face, ear and sinuses
> - Hereditary thrombophilic states
> - Hyperviscocity states
> - Oral contraceptive pill/pregnancy
> - Behçet's disease

Answer 129

> c. SIADH secretion.

Syndrome of inappropriate ADH secretion (see *Table* for causes) is the most likely diagnosis when the serum sodium is <115 mmol/l. Hypothyroidism can cause failure to excrete water, and produce a similar biochemical picture to SIADH. The diagnosis is confirmed by demonstrating a low plasma osmolality and an inappropriately high urine osmolality.

> **Causes of SIADH**
>
> *Central nervous system*
> - Head injury
> - Encephalitis/meningitis
> - Cerebral abscess
> - Cerebral neoplasm
> - Cerebral haemorrhage
>
> *Respiratory system*
> - Bronchial carcinoma (particularly oat cell)
> - TB
> - Pneumonia (Legionnaire's is the college favourite)
> - Empyema
>
> *Drugs*
> - Chlorpropamide
> - Chlorpromazine
> - Carbamazepine
> - Opiates
> - Vincristine
>
> *Miscellaneous*
> - Guillain–Barré syndrome
> - Acute intermittent porphyria
> - Carcinoma pancreas/thymoma

Questions 130–132

A 32-year-old woman who was 12 weeks into her first pregnancy presented with headache and malaise. Her blood pressure in the antenatal clinic four weeks previously was 120/70 mmHg. The current blood pressure reading was 220/112 mmHg.

Investigations are shown.

Hb	13 g/dl
WCC	7×10^9/l
Platelets	180×10^9
ESR	12 mm/h
Sodium	140 mmol/l
Potassium	4 mmol/l
Urea	6 mmol/l
Creatinine	110 μmol/l
Autoantibody screen	Normal
ECG	Normal
Urinalysis	Normal
Renal ultrasound	12 cm kidney on the right and a 7 cm kidney on the left

Question 130

What is the most probable cause for the hypertension?
  a. Atheromatous left-sided renal artery stenosis.
  b. Fibromuscular dysplasia of the left renal artery.
  c. Unilateral reflux nephropathy affecting left kidney.
  d. Congenital atrophic kidney.
  e. Pre-eclampsia.

Question 131

If the patient has papilloedema what is the drug treatment of choice?
  a. IV labetolol.
  b. Oral methyldopa.
  c. Oral bendroflumethiazide.
  d. Oral nifedipine.
  e. IV nitroprusside.

Question 132

Which one of the following drugs should not be used to treat hypertension in pregnancy?
  a. Labetolol.
  b. Methyldopa.
  c. Lisinopril.
  d. Nifedipine.
  e. Hydralazine.

Question 133

A 22-year-old male was admitted to hospital after an episode of haematemesis preceded by profuse vomiting. The patient had been on an alcoholic binge drinking session 12 hours previously. On examination his heart rate was 90 beats/min. The blood pressure was 100/60 mmHg. The Hb was 15 g/dl. An upper gastrointestinal endoscopy performed 24 hours after admission was normal.

What is the next management step?
  a. Start ferrous sulphate.
  b. Start lansoprazole.
  c. Allow home.
  d. Coeliac axis angiogram prior to discharge.
  e. Technetium scan for Meckel's diverticulum.

Answers 130–132

> **Answer 130**
> b. Fibromuscular dysplasia of the left renal artery.
>
> **Answer 131**
> a. IV labetolol.
>
> **Answer 132**
> c. Lisinopril.

The onset of severe hypertension within a few weeks of pregnancy in the setting of unilateral kidney disease is highly suggestive of renal artery stenosis. Two distinct forms of renal artery stenosis are recognized, notably atheromatous renal artery disease, which is more common in middle-aged males with risk factors for atherosclerosis, and fibromuscular dysplasia, which usually occurs in younger females and is characterized by narrowing of the distal main renal artery or the intrarenal arteries.

The most probable diagnosis in this particular case is fibromuscular dysplasia affecting the left renal artery. Affected patients may present with severe exacerbations of an otherwise relatively stable (normal or slightly elevated) blood pressure. In pregnancy, for example, the increase in blood volume results in increased vascular oxidative stress in the kidney in patients with renal artery stenosis, which is a stimulus for increased production of angiotensin II, a potent vasoconstrictor. Increased angiotensin II levels have the effect of large increases in blood pressure and precipitation of left ventricular failure or encephalopathy.

While unilateral pyelonephritis is a recognized cause of unilateral small kidney, it does not usually result in disturbed renal function unless there is an intrinsic abnormality affecting the contralateral kidney.

Pre-eclampsia usually occurs after 20 weeks' gestation, complicates 5–6% of all pregnancies and is much more common in women with pre-existing hypertension. It is defined as hypertension and proteinuria (>0.3 g/24 hours). Up to 2% of patients with pre-eclampsia develop seizures and the condition is then termed eclampsia. Pre-eclampsia may not be associated with any symptoms, but in severe cases women may present with headache, papilloedema and abdominal pain due to liver oedema or hepatic haemorrhage. The management of hypertension in pre-eclampsia does not halt the progression of the disease but does reduce the risk of complications such has cerebral haemorrhage. Delivery is the definitive method of treating the progression of pre-eclampsia but the usual practice is to allow the pregnancy to proceed as long as possible with control of hypertension without unduly risking the mother or the foetus. The management of hypertension in pre-eclampsia and all other causes of hypertension in pregnancy is outlined below.

In the presence of severe symptoms or evidence of end-organ damage such as heart failure, renal failure or raised intracranial pressure, the management of severe hypertension (BP >170/110 mmHg) includes either IV hydralazine or labetolol. Even in the absence of end-organ damage or symptoms there is evidence that failure to treat severe hypertension increases the risk of cerebral haemorrhage and should be treated. IV nitroprusside is contraindicated in pregnancy.

In patients who do not have severe hypertension, the drug of choice is methyldopa. Second-line agents are hydralazine and nifedipine, which should be added if the blood pressure is not adequately controlled with methyldopa. Third-line agents include alpha- and beta-blockers (labetolol and oxprenolol). Beta-blockers are generally avoided in the first half of pregnancy as they are associated with foetal growth retardation. Thiazide diuretics may be used to treat hypertension in women with pre-existing hypertension but should be avoided in patients with pre-eclampsia, as many such patients are volume depleted.

ACE inhibitors and possibly also angiotensin II receptor blockers are contraindicated in pregnancy. Although there is no evidence that they are teratogenic, their use has been associated with foetotoxic effects such as growth retardation.

Answer 133

> c. Allow home.

Patients with a bleeding Mallory–Weiss tear, but without risk factors for re-bleeding, clinical features indicating severe bleeding, or active bleeding at endoscopy will almost always heal spontaneously. They can be managed medically with a brief hospitalization of 24 hours.

Patients with an actively bleeding Mallory–Weiss tear at endoscopy should be treated with endoscopic haemostasis (either adrenaline injection or thermocoagulation). They should be hospitalized for at least 48 hours because re-bleeding generally occurs within 24 hours of the initial therapeutic endoscopy.

Question 134

A 48-year-old post-menopausal woman with asthma was taking hormone replacement therapy to prevent progression of osteoporosis, which was thought to be due to steroid therapy. While on hormone replacement therapy she developed a deep-vein thrombosis.

Which alternative treatment would you use to treat the osteoporosis?
  a. 1,25-Dihydrocholecalciferol.
  b. Calcitonin.
  c. Alendronate.
  d. Raloxifene.
  e. Vitamin D and calcium supplements.

Question 135

A 38-year-old man was recently diagnosed with polycystic kidney disease after being investigated for hypertension. His father and brother also had hypertension but had never been screened for polycystic kidney disease. His paternal uncle had died from heart failure. There was no family history of sudden death or cerebral haemorrhage. His blood pressure measured 150/94 mmHg.

Which of the following statements is correct?
  a. Aggressive management of hypertension will reduce the rate decline of renal function.
  b. There is a high chance that the patient will be dialysis-dependent by the age of 60 years.
  c. The patient should undergo magnetic resonance angiography of the brain to exclude berry aneurysms.
  d. Angiotensin-converting enzyme inhibitor therapy is beneficial in retarding the rate of decline of renal function.
  e. Renal failure is the commonest cause of death in this condition.

Question 136

A 20-year-old male was admitted with hypertension and malaise. His blood pressure on admission was 210/124 mmHg. The mini-mental test score was 10/10. Both heart sounds were normal and the chest was clear. There was mild ankle swelling. Inspection of the fundi revealed grade I hypertensive retinopathy.
  Investigations are shown.

Hb	11 g/dl
WCC	$12 \times 10^9/l$
Platelets	$120 \times 10^9/l$
ESR	60 mm/h
Sodium	138 mmol/l
Potassium	7.4 mmol/l
Urea	28 mmol/l
Creatinine	500 μmol/l
Glucose	4 mmol/l
24-hour urinalysis	Volume 400 ml
	Protein 1.4 g
	Blood ++

What is the immediate management step?
  a. Haemodialysis.
  b. IV actrapid and dextrose 50%.
  c. IV labetolol.
  d. IV calcium gluconate.
  e. High-dose IV furosemide.

Answer 134

> c. Alendronate.

All patients with or at risk of osteoporosis should have a diet containing 800 iu of vitamin D and take supplemental calcium 1.2 g per day. Regular exercise (30 minutes three times per week) and cessation of smoking are also recommended.

Drug treatment of choice in established osteoporosis is a bisphosphonate, of which alendronate has been used most successfully. Other drugs include selective oestrogen receptor modulators such as raloxifene, oestrogen itself, calcitonin and vitamin D. The selective receptor modulator raloxifene has been shown to be effective in the treatment of osteoporosis, and – unlike oestrogen – does not promote endometrial hyperplasia or vaginal bleeding. It may reduce the risk for breast cancer but the risk of venous thromboembolism is similar to that of oestrogens; therefore, the drug should not be used in this particular case.

Since the Women's Health Initiative study, which demonstrated that HRT did not reduce the risk of cardiovascular disease and increase the risk of stroke, breast cancer and venous thromboembolism, oestrogen therapy is no longer first line and is only reserved for patients who do not tolerate other treatments. Calcitonin is effective but less practical to take because it is administered nasally and furthermore, calcitonin therapy exhibits tachyphylaxis.

Answer 135

> b. There is a high chance that the patient will be dialysis-dependent by the age of 60 years.

The features of polycystic kidney disease are covered in Question 382. Hypertension is common in patients with PKD, and patients with hypertension have a faster decline in renal function than patients who are normotensive. However, there is no conclusive trial demonstrating that treatment of hypertension reduces the rate of decline of renal function. ACE inhibitors and AIIRBs do not have an effect on renal function but may improve prognosis by preventing left ventricular hypertrophy.

Cardiovascular disease is the commonest cause of death in PKD. Renal failure is the most serious renal complication of PKD. The median age of end-stage renal failure is 54 years; 74 years in patients with PKD1 and PKD2. There is a high probability that this patient has PKD1 since PKD1 accounts for the vast majority of cases of PKD and has an earlier presentation. The most serious extra-renal manifestation of PKD is subarachnoid haemorrhage due to intracerebral aneurysms. Patients with PKD should be screened for intracranial aneurysms with magnetic resonance angiography if there is a family history of subarachnoid haemorrhage.

Answer 136

> d. IV calcium gluconate.

The patient has life-threatening hyperkalaemia, which is defined as a serum potassium level ≥7 mmol/l or hyperkalaemia <7 mmol/l that is associated with typical electrocardiographic changes or muscle weakness, the latter occur owing to antagonistic effects of potassium on the membrane potential. In these circumstances the immediate treatment is to stabilize the membrane potential with intravenous calcium gluconate. Intravenous calcium acts within minutes. Its effects last for up to 60 minutes, which allows definitive treatment with intravenous dextrose and insulin to take effect (*Table*).

Management of hyperkalaemia

Method	Agent
Antagonism of membrane actions of potassium	Calcium gluconate
Drive extra-cellular potassium into cells	Dextrose and insulin Sodium bicarbonate if acidotic Beta-agonists
Removal of potassium from cells	Diuretics Cation exchange resins Haemodialysis if severe or in patients with renal failure

Question 137

A 5-year-old male was admitted for investigation of ankle swelling and abdominal distension that had occurred over three months. His appetite was satisfactory, and there was no history of diarrhoea, breathlessness, arthralgia or syncope. He was born by a normal vaginal delivery and weighed 3.6 kg at birth. He was well as a neonate and had achieved his milestones normally thus far. Apart from having mild eczema there was no past medical history of note. His father was a solicitor, and his mother had just returned to full-time teaching after giving birth to his 16-month-old brother, who was the only other sibling. There was no history of travel abroad or any drug history.

On examination, he had facial swelling. There was no pallor or cyanosis. The most striking feature was pitting oedema of the lower limbs from the ankles to the thighs. The heart rate was 100 beats/min and regular. The blood pressure was 95/55 mmHg. The JVP was not raised. Palpation of the precordium was normal. On auscultation, heart sounds I and II were normal, but there was an additional third heart sound. Examination of the respiratory system revealed dullness to percussion at the right lung base and reduced air entry on auscultation. Abdominal examination demonstrated a non-tender, distended abdomen with shifting dullness. There was no palpable organomegaly.

Investigations are shown.

The patient was treated with 60 mg prednisolone and 40 mg furosemide. The oedema started improving after one week, and renal function remained normal. After two weeks he was discharged and seen at weekly intervals. In the sixth week the oedema had completely subsided, and his abdomen was soft and non-distended. A 24-hour urinary protein estimation was 0.7 g. The furosemide was stopped and plans were made to review the patient again in two weeks, but three days later he was admitted with right upper quadrant pain and abdominal distension. On examination, the JVP was not raised. There was palpable tender hepatomegaly and shifting dullness. There was no lower-limb oedema.

Further investigations are shown.

Hb	10 g/dl
WCC	$5 \times 10^9/l$
Platelets	$166 \times 10^9/l$
MCV	80 fl
Urinalysis	Microscopy revealed occasional transitional cells
	24-hour urinary protein 5.2 g
	Selective protein clearance ratio was low
Ascitic fluid	Protein 8 g/l
Chest X-ray	Normal
Sodium	135 mmol/l
Potassium	3.7 mmol/l
Urea	2.1 mmol/l
Creatinine	65 μmol/l
Bilirubin	10 μmol/l
AST	19 iu/l
Alkaline phosphatase	80 iu/l
Total protein	36 g/l
Albumin	13 g/l
Glucose	4 mmol/l

Bilirubin	15 μmol/l
AST	90 iu/l
Alkaline phosphatase	89 iu/l
Albumin	35 g/l

1. What was the original cause of oedema?
2. What was the subsequent cause of abdominal pain and distension?
3. List two tests which will help confirm the cause of abdominal pain.
4. In one step, what is the management?

Question 138

What is the rhythm disturbance in this rhythm strip (**138**)?

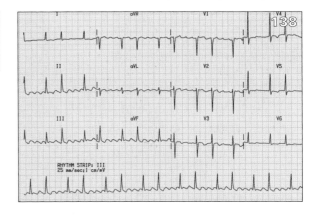

Answer 137

1. Nephrotic syndrome.
2. Hepatic vein thrombosis.
3. i. Ultrasound or CT scan of the liver looking particularly at the hepatic and portal veins.
   ii. Liver biopsy.
4. Thrombolysis to prevent severe hepatic congestion.

The combination of hypoalbuminaemia, heavy proteinuria and oedema is strongly suggestive of the diagnosis of nephrotic syndrome, which in young children is most often due to minimal change glomerulonephritis. Minimal change glomerulonephritis is thought to be an auto-immune disorder, and usually responds extremely well to steroids and other immunosuppressants such as cyclophosphamide and chlorambucil. There is a well-recognized association of the disorder with Hodgkin's lymphoma, bee stings, cow's milk allergy and ingestion of NSAIDs. Minimal change nephropathy is found in 80% of children with nephrotic syndrome. Treatment is with high-dose steroids, and diuretics are often necessary to treat the oedema. Relapses are common and are treated with steroids until the urine is completely free of protein for three days. Steroids are prescribed for a maximum of four weeks. Recurrent relapses are managed with cyclophosphamide or chlorambucil. Complications of nephrotic syndrome include susceptibility to infection due to loss of immunoglobulins in the urine, protein malnutrition, hyperlipidaemia, arterial and venous thromboses and acute renal failure.

Thrombosis is a frequent and serious complication; corticosteroids and diuretic therapy contribute to thrombosis. Whole blood viscosity is increased, and there is alteration in the concentration of clotting factors in the blood. The levels of antithrombin III and plasminogen are reduced, increasing the tendency to thrombosis. In this case the onset of abdominal pain, tender right upper quadrant, ascites and abnormal LFT reflect hepatic vein or portal vein thrombosis. Patients may present rapidly with fulminant hepatic failure or with gradual-onset ascites and jaundice. Early revascularization with a thrombolytic agent is important to prevent hepatic infarction and fibrosis leading to chronic portal hypertension. In patients where thrombolysis is contraindicated, a shunt procedure is necessary.

The diagnosis can be confirmed by ultrasonography and Doppler. The hepatic veins, portal vein and inferior vena cava should be examined by venography. Liver biopsy helps make the diagnosis, and is also important to assess hepatic necrosis and fibrosis.

Answer 138

Atrial flutter with 2:1/3:1 atrioventricular block.

There is an irregular narrow complex tachycardia, and the differential diagnosis is between atrial fibrillation, atrial flutter with varying atrioventricular block, and an atrial tachycardia with varying atrioventricular block. The clue is in the rhythm strip which reveals a 'saw-tooth' pattern to the ECG complexes, indicating flutter. The RR-interval is not constant, therefore there is flutter with varying block. In this case there are between two and three flutter waves between each RR-interval, and hence the diagnosis is atrial flutter with 2:1/3:1 atrioventricular block. The causes of atrial flutter are the same as those for AF. The most effective treatment for atrial flutter is DC cardioversion, delivering small energy shocks of between 50 and 100 J. Chemical cardioversion is difficult, but the most effective drugs for this purpose are flecainide and amiodarone. Like AF, patients with atrial flutter should be anticoagulated to prevent the risk of thromboembolism.

Causes of atrial flutter/fibrillation

- Ischaemic heart disease
- Hypertension
- Mitral stenosis
- Thyrotoxicosis
- Myocarditis
- Cardiomyopathy
- Pericarditis
- Bronchial carcinoma
- Severe pneumonia
- Chronic lung disease
- Pulmonary emboli
- Wolff–Parkinson–White syndrome
- Alcohol abuse
- Cocaine abuse

Question 139

A 66-year-old retired school teacher presented with a six-month history of progressive weakness, fatigue and breathlessness which was accompanied by weight loss of 5 kg. He had difficulty climbing stairs because his 'legs would not carry him', and had noticed that he had difficulty holding light objects with his left hand without dropping them. Over the past week his wife had noticed that his speech appeared slurred and nasal, and he was having difficulty swallowing his meals. He had a past history of pernicious anaemia for which he was taking regular intramuscular B_{12} injections. On examination, he was thin. There was no evidence of pallor or clubbing. The patient had dysarthria. Examination of the cranial nerves revealed normal eye movements, but tongue movement was sluggish and there was reduced palatal movement. The jaw jerk was brisk. On examination of his limbs there was wasting and fasciculation of the small muscles of the left hand. The tone and power in the left upper limb was generally reduced. The upper-limb reflexes were brisk. There was wasting and fasciculation in both thigh muscles. The tone was increased and the power was reduced. The ankle and knee jerks were brisk, and there was obvious clonus at the ankle joint. Sensation was normal and Romberg's test was negative. Examination of the fundi revealed bitemporal pallor.

Investigations are shown.

Hb	12 g/dl
WCC	5×10^9/l
Platelets	180×10^9/l
MCV	86 fl
Sodium	137 mmol/l
Potassium	4.1 mmol/l
Urea	6 mmol/l
Creatinine	110 µmol/l
Chest X-ray	Normal

1. What is the diagnosis?
   a. Cervical myelopathy.
   b. Subacute combined degeneration of the spinal cord.
   c. Multiple sclerosis.
   d. Motor neurone disease.
   e. Polymyositis.

2. What two investigations could be performed to confirm your suspicion?
   a. Anti-Hu antibodies.
   b. MRI scan brain.
   c. CSF analysis for oligoclonal bands.
   d. Visual evoked potentials.
   e. Nerve conduction studies.
   f. MRI scan of cervical spine.
   g. Serum creatinine kinase.
   h. Serum B_{12} concentration.
   i. Muscle biopsy.
   j. Electromyography.

Question 140

An 86-year-old male was found collapsed in his home by his neighbour after his son raised concern about not being able to contact him by telephone. There was no significant past medical history. He was independent. He was last seen two days earlier when he joined his neighbour for Christmas dinner.

On examination, he was unconscious and had a Glasgow coma scale of 5 out of 15. There was no nuchal rigidity. Pupillary reflexes were sluggish, but examination of the fundi was normal. Tone was slightly increased in all the limbs. The peripheral reflexes were present and both plantar reflexes were flexor. The heart rate was 40 beats/min, and blood pressure was 80/40 mmHg. Heart sounds were normal, and the chest was clear.

An ECG was performed in the Accident and Emergency Department (**140**).

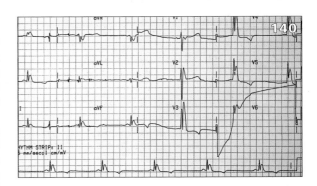

1. List four abnormalities on the ECG.
2. Which single investigation should the medical officer have performed?
3. In one sentence, what is the management of this case?

Answer 139

> 1. d. Motor neurone disease.
> 2. e. Nerve conduction studies.
>   j. Electromyography.

There is evidence of combined lower motor neurone and upper motor neurone lesions and a pseudobulbar palsy. There is no sensory abnormality, and ocular movements are normal. These findings are characteristic of motor neurone disease, which is characterized by a progressive degeneration of the motor neurones in the cortex, spinal cord and motor nuclei of the cranial nerves. The breathlessness is probably due to involvement of the respiratory muscles. The bitemporal pallor is a 'red herring', and although it may have led some readers to diagnose multiple sclerosis, it is important to note that bitemporal pallor is a normal finding in some individuals. Moreover, wasting and fasciculation are not features of multiple sclerosis because it does not affect lower motor neurones. Although the patient has a history of pernicious anaemia, his blood count does not suggest B_{12} deficiency and therefore subacute degeneration of the spinal cord is unlikely. The absence of a sensory neuropathy is also against the diagnosis.

The cause of motor neurone disease is unknown. In approximately 15% of cases the disease is familial and is due to mutations in the copper/zinc superoxide dismutase gene on chromosome 21. The incidence is 1/50,000, and the male-to-female ratio is 1.5:1. There are three distinct patterns known as progressive muscular atrophy, amyotrophic lateral sclerosis and progressive bulbar palsy which are characterized by predominantly lower motor lesions, predominantly upper motor neurone lesions, and bulbar and pseudobulbar palsy, respectively. Usually, a combination of all three is present. Female sex, bulbar onset and old age are poor prognostic markers. The disease usually progresses inexorably and death is usually from bronchopneumonia within five years of onset of symptoms.

The diagnosis is clinical, but electromyography characteristically reveals a reduced number of action potentials in the muscles which have an increased amplitude and duration. Nerve conduction studies reveal normal motor conduction and exclude an underlying neuropathy, particularly in patients with the progressive muscular atrophy variety of the disorder.

There are no curative therapies, but glutamate antagonists such as riluzole appear promising, as does ciliary neurotrophic factor, which has been shown to promote survival of cultured rat and human motor neurones. Both agents are currently being tested on affected humans.

Answer 140

> 1. i. Bradycardia.
>   ii. Tremor artefact.
>   iii. J-waves.
>   iv. Prolonged QT-interval.
> 2. Rectal (core) temperature with a low-reading thermometer.
> 3. Gradual rewarming using space blankets and possibly warmed intravenous fluids, depending on the severity of hypothermia.

Hypothermia is common among the elderly. It is usually attributable to cold environment (no heating at home), inadequate clothing, poor nutrition, neuroleptic drugs, alcohol and hypothyroidism. Hypothermia is defined as a fall in the core temperature to below 35°C (95°F). Severe hypothermia causes impaired consciousness and cardiac embarrassment. Bradycardia, hypotension, hypopnoea, sluggish pupillary and peripheral reflexes, muscle rigidity and coma are recognized features of severe hypothermia. Ventricular fibrillation and asystole are the usual causes of death.

ECG abnormalities include bradycardia, atrial fibrillation with a slow ventricular rate, prolonged PR- and QT-intervals and J-waves. A baseline artefact due to muscle tremor may also be seen, and should help make the diagnosis in the examination situation.

Gentle rewarming is indicated. If the temperature is above 32°C (89.6°F), space blankets and warm oral fluids are usually sufficient. If the temperature is lower than this, and the patient is unconscious, then warmed intravenous fluids should be given. In this situation there is a danger of severe metabolic acidosis due to sluggish circulation, which should be corrected promptly. The aim is to increase the temperature by 1°C (1.8°F) per hour.

Question 141

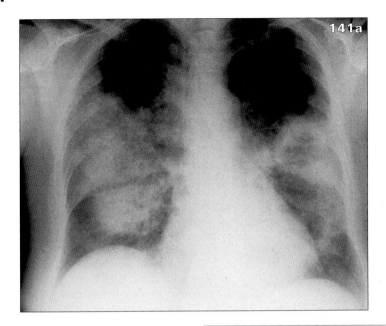

141a

A 21-year-old chef presented with a two-week history of general malaise, cough and headaches. He had just returned from a ten-day holiday in a hotel resort in Spain. He consulted his GP on arrival, who diagnosed a respiratory tract infection and prescribed erythromycin. Despite this, the patient's symptoms continued to persist. He had now developed a foul-smelling, blood-stained nasal discharge and was deaf in his left ear. His cough was worse, but was non-productive. He felt 'hot and cold' and had a reduced appetite due to nausea. He was a non-smoker and consumed 20 units of alcohol per week.

On examination, he appeared relatively well. There was no skin rash, pallor, cyanosis, clubbing, lymphadenopathy or ankle oedema. He was tender over his frontal sinuses, and had crusting around the nasal septum on the right side. Inspection of the outer ears and tympanic membranes was normal. The Rinne's test revealed reduced air and bone conduction on the left side. Weber's test lateralized to the right side. Apart from the abnormal hearing tests, all other neurological examination was normal. The heart rate was 96 beats/min and blood pressure 140/90 mmHg. The patient was tachypnoeic on mild exertion, and had a respiratory rate of 20/min. Chest expansion was moderate. The trachea was central. On auscultation of the lung fields there was evidence of bronchial breathing at the left lung base and a few inspiratory crackles at the right lung base. Examination of the heart and abdomen was normal.

Investigations are shown.

Hb	11 g/dl
WCC	$14 \times 10^9/l$ (neutrophil leucocytosis)
Platelets	$480 \times 10^9/l$
ESR	110 mm/h
CRP	209 g/l
Sodium	134 mmol/l
Potassium	4.1 mmol/l
Urea	6 mmol/l
Creatinine	89 μmol/l
Urinalysis	Protein +1
	Blood not detected
Chest X-ray (**141a**)	

1. Describe the abnormalities on the chest X-ray.
2. How would you interpret the findings from the Rinne's and Weber's tests?
3. What two tests could you perform to help achieve the diagnosis?
4. What is the underlying diagnosis?

Answer 141

1. The chest X-ray demonstrates alveolar shadowing affecting the right middle and lower lobes and in the left lower lobe. In addition, there is a round cavitating lesion in the left lower lobe. The findings are consistent with either a purulent pneumonia with left lower lobe abscess formation, or pulmonary haemorrhage and a cavitating granuloma due to Wegener's granulomatosis.
2. The Rinne's test reveals reduced bone and air hearing conduction, suggesting sensorineuronal deafness on the left side. The Weber's test does not normally lateralize to either ear, but in this case it lateralized to the right. This is in keeping with sensorineuronal hearing loss in the left ear. Because both air and bone conduction are impaired in sensorineuronal deafness, the sound from the tuning fork (which is conducted via bone in the Weber's test) is heard loudest in the ear which is not affected. In the case of pure conduction deafness, the Weber's test lateralizes to the affected ear. Wegener's granulomatosis can produce conduction and sensorineuronal deafness by blockage of the Eustachian tube when it involves the upper respiratory tract and 8th cranial nerve, respectively.
3. i. Nasal or transbronchial lung biopsy.
   ii. c-ANCA (antiproteinase 3).
4. Wegener's granulomatosis.

Wegener's granulomatosis is a necrotizing granulomatous vasculitis affecting the upper and lower respiratory tracts and the kidneys, although several other organs can be affected. Granulomas occur in small arterioles. The diagnosis should be suspected when two of these systems are involved in the presence of systemic features such as malaise, night sweats, fever and weight loss. This patient has features of upper and lower respiratory tract involvement which include frontal sinusitis, purulent nasal discharge and nasal septal crusting, dry cough and evidence of gross respiratory involvement on the chest X-ray. The deafness in the left ear is indicative of 8th nerve

involvement. The kidneys do not appear to be significantly affected. The trace of protein may be a response to a febrile illness. Upper respiratory involvement can also lead to hoarseness and stridor due to vocal cord and tracheal involvement, respectively, and lower respiratory involvement may present with pleurisy and haemoptysis. Renal involvement can vary from asymptomatic proteinuria and haematuria to fulminant renal failure due to crescentic glomerulonephritis. Other organs affected include the eye, cardiovascular system, central nervous system and the skin. In the eye, the disease can present with scleritis, uveitis and pseudotumour due to retro-orbital granuloma formation. Cardiovascular involvement is rare. The most common manifestation is pericarditis, but conduction tissue involvement produces tachy- and bradyarrhythmias. Involvement of the central nervous system is also rare and comprises a mononeuritis multiplex, isolated cranial nerve palsies and meningeal involvement.

The diagnosis is based on demonstrating a necrotizing granulomatous vasculitis biopsy of the affected tissue. The best yield of a positive biopsy comes from the kidney or the lungs when they are involved. ANCA are present in over 80% of untreated cases. Immunofluorescence studies have revealed two main types of ANCA which are determined by the pattern of cytoplasmic staining. c-ANCA stains the outer cytoplasm, whereas p-ANCA stains the perinuclear cytoplasm. It is now clear that c-ANCA binds the enzyme proteinase 3 (PF3) and is specific for Wegener's granulomatosis. p-ANCA is heterogeneous. One subset binds the cytoplasmic enzyme MPO, which is positive in microscopic polyangiitis and idiopathic crescentic glomerulonephritis. Other subsets of p-ANCA bind elastase, lactoferrin, lysozyme and cathepsin G and are present in a variety of auto-immune conditions including CAH, sclerosing cholangitis, ulcerative colitis and SLE (**141b**).

The management of Wegener's granulomatosis is with steroids and other immunosuppressants such as cyclophosphamide. Disease progress is monitored by estimating ANCA titres. There is good correlation between ANCA titres and underlying inflammatory activity in most patients.

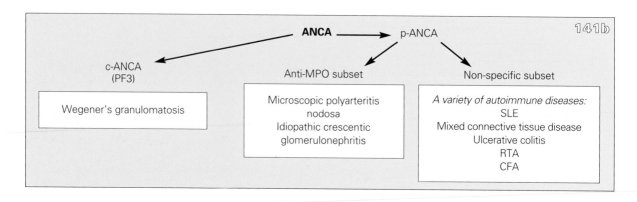

Question 142

A 28-year-old male presented with a three-day history of rigors and pleuritic pain affecting the left lung, where there were signs of consolidation. There was no evidence of lymphadenopathy or hepatosplenomegaly.
  Investigations are shown.

Hb	12 g/dl
WCC	$24 \times 10^9/l$
Platelets	$149 \times 10^9/l$
Neutrophils	85%
Normoblasts	7%
Myeloblasts	3%
Myelocytes	2%
Lymphocytes	3%

1. What is the characteristic term given to this blood picture?
2. Which two features on the blood film would confirm your suspicions?

Question 143

The following are serial LFT on a 51-year-old married schoolteacher who had a partial gastrectomy for a perforated peptic ulcer ten years previously. He was asymptomatic. He was currently taking ranitidine. He consumed approximately 4 units of alcohol per week. Apart from very slight jaundice, the physical examination was normal.

	1987	1988	1990	1992	1993
Alanine aminotransferase (normal 5–30 iu/l)	30	36	40	44	49
Aspartate aminotransferase (normal 10–40 iu/l)	42	65	69	73	78
Alkaline phosphatase (normal 25–115 iu/l)	100	112	118	125	135
Bilirubin (normal <17 µmol/l)	17	20	24	29	36

1. What is the most likely cause for the abnormality of the LFT?
2. Which two investigations would you perform?
3. What treatment should be considered?

Question 144

The following are cardiac catheter data on a 4-year-old male with cyanosis and failure to thrive:

Chamber	Pressure (mmHg)	Oxygen saturation (%) (on air)	Oxygen saturation (%) (on 28% oxygen)
Right atrium	8	52	52
Right ventricle	90/30	53	54
Pulmonary artery	22/12	53	54
PCWP	4		
Left ventricle	80/20	82	81
Aorta	77/50	66	66

1. List four abnormalities.
2. What is the underlying diagnosis?
3. Explain the lack of rise in oxygen tension after inspiring 28% oxygen.

Answer 142

1. 'Leukaemoid reaction'.
2. i. The presence of toxic granulations or Dohle bodies in the white cells.
   ii. Neutrophils exhibiting a toxic shift to the left, i.e. three or fewer segments of the nucleus.

A leukaemoid reaction is a descriptive term given to a leucoerythroblastic blood picture which follows sepsis. In some cases of overwhelming infection, the 'sick' marrow releases immature cells into the blood stream; thus, there is an abundance of myelocytes and normoblasts. In contrast to a true leucoerythroblastic anaemia where the marrow is characteristically replaced by neoplastic cells, there is no lymphadenopathy or hepatosplenomegaly.

Answer 143

1. Chronic active hepatitis due to hepatitis B or hepatitis C.
2. i. Hepatitis B and C serology.
   ii. Liver biopsy.
3. Interferon therapy.

The patient has had major surgery in the past that almost certainly required blood transfusion. Both hepatitis B and C are readily contracted from blood transfusions. Since screening donated blood for hepatitis B was initiated in the 1980s, hepatitis C has become the most common cause of post-transfusion hepatitis in the Western world.

Almost 20% of patients with hepatitis B infection will develop CAH. The cause is unknown, but is thought to be a defective T-cell immune response. Most patients affected are male. The condition is usually asymptomatic, or may present as very slowly progressive hepatitis. About 50% of those affected present with established chronic liver disease.

CAH may also occur following hepatitis C infection. The acute hepatitic event is usually very mild, and often goes unnoticed. The sequelae are similar to those of hepatitis B infection; however the incidence of CAH is almost 50%. Other causes of CAH are given (Table). There is nothing in the patient's history to suggest any of these other causes.

The aminotransferases and bilirubin are usually modestly raised and the alkaline phosphatase is very slightly raised. The blood transaminase level bears no correlation with the severity of the hepatic damage. In hepatitis B-related CAH, the hepatitis B surface antigen and the e antigen is present. In hepatitis C-related CAH, antihepatitis C antibodies are present. The histological landmark of CAH is piecemeal necrosis. There is destruction of the liver cells between the interface of the hepatic parenchyma and the connective tissue. In hepatitis B-related CAH, the presence of hepatitis B surface antigen in the hepatocytes produces a ground-glass appearance on haematoxylin and eosin staining.

Patients with evidence of CAH should be treated with intravenous interferon for several months to prevent viral replication and allow seroconversion. The success rate is below 30%, and relapse often occurs soon after cessation of therapy.

Other causes of CAH

Autoimmune
- Lupoid hepatitis
- Anti-LKM antibody-associated CAH

Drugs
- Methyl dopa
- Isoniazid
- α-1 antitrypsin deficiency
- Wilson's disease
- Inflammatory bowel disease (usually ulcerative colitis)

Answer 144

(See Interpretation of Cardiac Catheter Data, page 418.)

1. i. Elevated right ventricular pressure.
   ii. Pressure drop across the pulmonary valve, suggesting pulmonary stenosis.
   iii. Low oxygen saturation in the left ventricle, suggestive of a VSD with a right-to-left shunt.
   iv. Saturation in the ascending aorta much lower than the left ventricle, indicating an overriding aorta.
2. Fallot's tetralogy.
3. The right-to-left shunt means that the majority of the blood does not pass through the lungs to be oxygenated.

Question 145

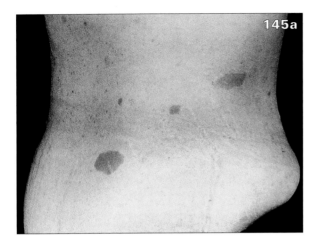

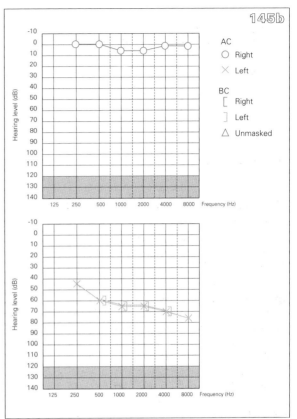

A 30-year-old male presented with vertigo and deafness in the left ear. His trunk was examined (**145a**), and he had an audiogram as part of the investigation for his symptoms (**145b**). There was no air–bone gap.

1. What is the audiographic abnormality?
2. What is the unifying diagnosis?

3. What other abnormalities would you expect to find on neurological examination?

Question 146

A 17-year-old male was referred with poorly developed secondary sexual characteristics. He was a slow developer, and had been to a special school for his entire education. He had a brother who was severely handicapped and wheelchair-bound who had died at the age of 17 years.

On examination, there was absence of axillary and pubic hair. His penis and testicles were small. There was bilateral gynaecomastia. Neurological examination was normal.

Investigations are shown.

Hb	12 g/dl
WCC	5 × 10⁹/l
Platelets	190 × 10⁹/l
Sodium	137 mmol/l
Potassium	3.7 mmol/l
Urea	5 mmol/l
Creatinine kinase	350 iu/l
Testosterone	4 nmol/l
LH	35 iu/l (normal range 1–10 iu/l)
FSH	30 iu/l (normal range 1–7 iu/l)

1. What is the endocrine abnormality?
2. What is the most probable diagnosis?
3. How would you confirm the diagnosis?
4. How would you explain the abnormal creatinine kinase level?

Answer 145

1. There is severe hearing loss at progressively higher frequencies in the left ear.
2. The trunk demonstrates café au lait spots, a feature of neurofibromatosis. An important association of neurofibromatosis is acoustic neuroma, which is a recognized cause of sensorineuronal deafness (*Table A*).
3. On neurological examination, the patient may also have an absent ipsilateral corneal reflex and ipsilateral cerebellar signs. In a minority of cases acoustic neuromas may be bilateral.

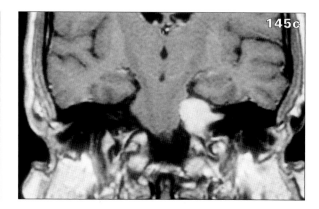

Neurofibromatosis is inherited as an autosomal dominant condition. Abnormalities on two chromosomes may cause disease with either a predominantly peripheral or central manifestation (*Table B*). Regular audiometry is mandatory to detect acoustic neuroma early. MRI of the brain revealed an acoustic neuroma (**145c**).

(See Audiograms, page 416.)

Table A Causes of sensorineuronal deafness

Unilateral (lesion in the cerebellopontine angle)
- Meningioma
- Acoustic neuroma
- Granuloma
- Metastasis

Bilateral
- Degenerative (presbycusis)
- Aminoglycosides
- Amphotericin
- High-dose loop diuretics
- Mumps
- Rubella

Table B Other associations of neurofibromatosis

Chromosome 17 (peripheral abnormalities)
- Renal artery stenosis
- Pulmonary fibrosis
- Cardiomyopathy (hypertrophic, restrictive and dilated)
- Fibrous dysplasia of bone
- Phaeochromocytoma

Chromosome 22 (central abnormalities)
- Acoustic neuroma
- Meningioma
- Optic glioma
- Ependymoma

Answer 146

1. Primary hypogonadism (hypergonadotrophic hypogonadism).
2. Kleinfelter's syndrome.
3. Demonstration of Barr body on buccal smear or karyotyping.
4. Carrier for Duchenne muscular dystrophy.

The most common cause of primary hypogonadism is Kleinfelter's syndrome, which has an incidence of 1/1,000 births. Patients are tall, lack secondary sexual characteristics, have gynaecomastia, and are often mentally subnormal. The condition is characterized by failure of development of Leydig cells and seminiferous tubules. Other causes of primary hypogonadism include Prader–Willi syndrome, Lawrence–Moon–Biedel syndrome, Leydig cell agenesis (Castelli's syndrome), 5α-reductase deficiency, mumps orchitis, renal failure, sickle cell disease, alcohol excess, chemotherapy and radiotherapy (*Table*, Answer 260).

Patients have XXY karyotype due to non-dysjunction and have the potential of being carriers for X-linked recessive conditions (as with females) such as Duchenne muscular dystrophy, glucose-6-phosphate dehydrogenase deficiency and haemophilia A. Kleinfelter patients are infertile. They are capable of having erections and ejaculation, but the semen does not contain spermatozoa.

Kleinfelter's syndrome is associated with a higher incidence of carcinoma of the breast, hypothyroidism, diabetes mellitus and chronic respiratory disease than the general male population.

Question 147

A 17-year-old female was admitted with a seven-hour history of severe central abdominal pain radiating to her back, which was accompanied by bilious vomiting. She had been constipated for 72 hours. There was no significant past medical history; in particular there was no history of abdominal surgery. She was a non-smoker and had a very occasional glass of wine. She was an only child. Her father died when she was aged two. She was not certain about the cause of death, but mentioned that he had a history of psychosis and epilepsy. Her mother had gallstones, but was otherwise well. She took paracetamol for infrequent 'period pains'. The only other drug history was that of the contraceptive pill, which had been commenced 10 days previously.

On examination she was unwell and distressed with pain. She was sweating profusely. Her heart rate was 130 beats/min and blood pressure 190/110 mmHg. Examination of the precordium revealed normal heart sounds. Peripheral pulses were easily palpable. The chest was clear. The abdomen was generally very tender, with guarding around the umbilical area. The hernial orifice was normal. There was a positive succussion splash and the bowel sounds were present. Rectal examination revealed an empty rectum. Neurological examination was normal.

The patient was prescribed pethidine for her pain and metoclopramide for the vomiting. She received intravenous saline. A few hours later she complained of weakness affecting her left shoulder. She was unable to abduct or adduct the shoulder. Shortly afterwards she developed weakness in both her legs, in addition to urinary retention. She was due to be catheterized when she had a grand mal epileptic seizure.

Investigations are shown.

Hb	13 g/dl
WCC	19×10^9/l
Platelets	400×10^9/l
ESR	12 mm/h
Sodium	121 mmol/l
Potassium	3 mmol/l
Urea	5 mmol/l
Calcium	2.5 mmol/l
Albumin	44 g/l
Bilirubin	15 μmol/l
AST	44 iu/l
Blood glucose	4 mmol/l
Abdominal X-ray	Normal
Chest X-ray	Normal
CT scan brain	Normal
Lumbar puncture	1 lymphocyte/mm³
	No red cells
	Protein 0.3 g/l
	Glucose 3.3 mmol/l

1. What is the diagnosis?
2. Which two investigations would you perform to confirm the diagnosis?
3. What is the precipitating factor?
4. List four management steps which you would take in this patient.
5. How will you manage her epileptic seizures?

Question 148

A 68-year-old male presented with a 48-hour history of right upper quadrant pain, dark urine and pale stools. Shortly after admission he had an investigation (**148**).

1. What investigation has been performed?
2. What does it reveal?
3. What is the diagnosis?

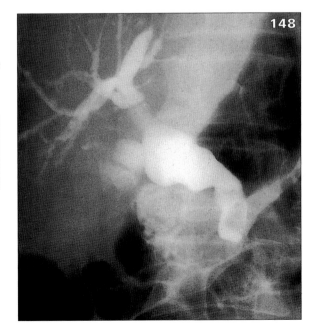

148

Answer 147

1. Acute intermittent porphyria (AIP). The combination of abdominal pain, neurological features, hypertension and tachycardia in a young person should raise the suspicion of AIP.
2. i. Urinary PBG.
   ii. Assay red cells for the enzyme PBG deaminase.
3. The oral contraceptive pill.
4. i. Stop oral contraceptive pill.
   ii. High calorie intake with intravenous infusion 500 ml of 50% dextrose per 24 hours via a large central vein in this case. The normal regime is 2 litres of 20% dextrose per 24 hours; however, in the case of syndrome of inappropriate ADH secretion, fluid restriction demands the use of smaller volumes of high-concentration dextrose.
   iii. Start intravenous haematin.
   iv. Intravenous beta-blocker to control tachycardia and hypertension.
5. Intravenous diazepam or chlormethiazole.

Acute intermittent porphyria is the most common type of acute porphyria. It is a rare condition caused by a genetic mutation in the gene encoding the enzyme PBG deaminase on chromosome 11, and is inherited as an autosomal dominant trait. A family history is usually present, but in up to one-third of cases this may be absent, either because the condition has not been diagnosed in first-degree relatives, or because the condition is running a latent course. It is five times more common in females than males, and usually presents between the ages of 14 and 30 years. The absence of PBG deaminase leads to elevated δ-ALA and PBG in the blood stream (**147**), both of which are responsible for the clinical manifestations of the condition. AIP is characterized mainly by gastrointestinal and neurological symptoms. Unlike the chronic porphyrias, skin photosensitivity is extremely unusual in AIP. Attacks are usually precipitated by drugs, alcohol, fasting and sepsis. Several drugs, particularly barbiturates and other anticonvulsants, have been implicated. The oral contraceptive pill has also been associated with acute attacks of porphyria and is the most likely precipitating factor in this case. The most common symptoms are acute abdominal pain which can simulate a surgical emergency, nausea, vomiting and constipation. Abdominal guarding may be present, but bowel sounds are usually present. There is often evidence of delayed gastric emptying, and it is not unusual to elicit a succussion splash due to a stomach full of gastric contents. The abdominal X-ray is normal. Neurological manifestations of the disease include a peripheral and autonomic neuropathy. Autonomic neuropathy most commonly manifests as tachycardia which is out of proportion to the extent of abdominal pain, hypertension and excess sweating. In approximately 50% of cases there is evidence of a motor neuropathy which often affects the proximal muscles. Both bulbar palsy and quadriplegia are recognized manifestations. Respiratory muscle paralysis is life-threatening, and requires assisted ventilation. In this case there was involvement of the left shoulder girdle and then a paraparesis. Epilepsy occurs when the disease is in its most aggressive phase. It often heralds the onset of hyponatraemia due to SIADH.

The management is by withdrawing the offending drug, if this is applicable. A high calorie intake reduces precursors of haem synthesis in the blood by reducing the activity of the rate-limiting enzyme ALA synthetase. Intravenous haematin is used in the acute situation and also acts by inhibiting the action of ALA synthetase. The control of abdominal pain requires narcotic analgesia. Vomiting can be prevented by insertion of a nasogastric tube to empty the stomach contents.

Metoclopramide is another drug which can precipitate acute porphyria, and should be avoided. Beta-blockers are used to manage the tachycardia and hypertension.

The management of epilepsy is by trying to abate the condition with a high calorie intake and by fluid restriction to prevent further hyponatraemia from SIADH. Epilepsy in the acute situation is managed with chlormethiazole, which is one of the very few anticonvulsant agents not known to cause acute porphyria. Prevention of the condition is mainly based on avoiding precipitating drugs and recognizing warning symptoms early.

The diagnosis is made by demonstrating high levels of δ-ALA and PBG in the urine. The addition of Ehrlich's dye to the urine will cause a red discoloration in the presence of PBG; however, this phenomenon is also observed in the

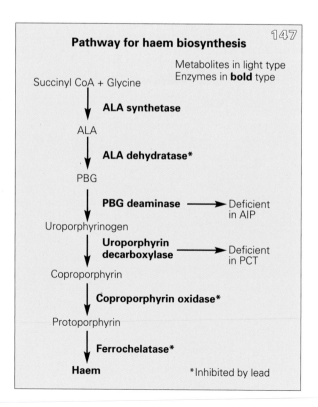

Pathway for haem biosynthesis 147

Metabolites in light type
Enzymes in **bold** type

Succinyl CoA + Glycine

↓ **ALA synthetase**

ALA

↓ **ALA dehydratase***

PBG

↓ **PBG deaminase** ⟶ Deficient in AIP

Uroporphyrinogen

↓ **Uroporphyrin decarboxylase** ⟶ Deficient in PCT

Coproporphyrin

↓ **Coproporphyrin oxidase***

Protoporphyrin

↓ **Ferrochelatase***

Haem   *Inhibited by lead

presence of urobilinogen in the urine. Differentiation of urobilinogen from PBG involves the addition of chloroform, which will cause PBG to separate out in the aqueous layer as a purple sediment, whereas the urobilinogen is soluble and becomes colourless. This is the basis of the Watson–Schwartz test. The urinary levels of ALA and PBG are always elevated during an attack, though they may be normal when the patient is well. The red cells can also be assayed for the enzyme PBG deaminase, which is very low in AIP. The enzyme ALA dehydratase is elevated. (See Answer 400).

Answer 148

1. The investigation is a percutaneous transhepatic cholangiogram.
2. Both the common bile duct and the internal hepatic ducts are dilated. There is a large filling defect at the distal end of the common bile duct.
3. A gall stone in the common bile duct causing obstructive jaundice.

Question 149

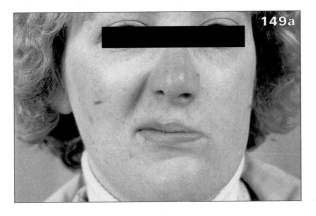

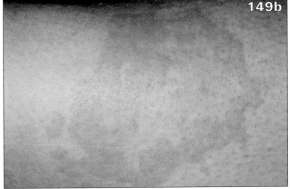

A 25-year-old female presented to her GP after noticing asymmetry of her face (**149a**). For the past two days she had also experienced dizziness and lethargy, particularly on exertion. She had no past medical history. Six weeks previously she had been to visit friends in North America. While on holiday, she developed a painful rash on her left arm which she described as a small red nodule which gradually expanded over the next few days before subsiding. A friend had taken a photograph of the rash (**149b**).

On examination, she had a temperature of 37°C (98.6°F) and a slow pulse. Examination of the ears was normal. The doctor was concerned and performed an ECG (**149c**).

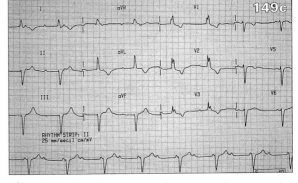

1. What is the cause of the abnormality on her face?
2. What is the characteristic name given to the rash?
3. Give two other dermatological manifestations of this disorder.
4. What is the ECG diagnosis?
5. What is the overall diagnosis?
6. List two therapeutic steps in the management of this patient.

Answer 149

> 1. Left facial nerve palsy.
> 2. Erythema chronicum migrans.
> 3. i. *Borrelia* lymphocytoma.
>   ii. Acrodermatitis chronica atrophicans.
> 4. Complete heart block. (Third-degree atrioventricular block.)
> 5. Lyme disease.
> 6. i. Therapy with doxycycline, benzyl penicillin, azithromycin, or cefotaxime.
>   ii. Temporary cardiac pacing.

The patient presented with a facial palsy and has ECG evidence of third-degree atrioventricular block. In addition, she had a macular rash which appears to be fading in the centre (**149b**) and is characteristic of erythema chronicum migrans. While there are several medical conditions which may involve the cardiovascular and central nervous system simultaneously (*Table*), the rash makes Lyme disease the most likely diagnosis.

Lyme disease is caused by the spirochaete, *Borrelia burgdorferi*. It is transmitted by hard-bodied ticks (*Ixodes* species). The disease has a wide clinical spectrum, ranging from asymptomatic infection to multi-system involvement. The first presentation is a characteristic skin lesion at the site of the tick bite, which begins as a macule between 2–40 days after exposure, and expands with central clearing. This is termed erythema chronicum migrans and may be associated with fever and regional lymphadenopathy. Early localized infection may present as *Borrelia* lymphocytoma, which is a bluish-red nodule on the ear lobe or nose. The second stage of the disease occurs several weeks or months after exposure, and is due to spread of the organism via the blood or the lymphatics. At this stage there may be fever and flu-like symptoms, several skin lesions similar to erythema chronicum migrans and cardiac and neurological involvement. Cardiac disease occurs in 5% of affected individuals and is characterized by varying degrees of heart block and myopericarditis. It is usually brief and seldom lasts more than one week. Temporary pacing is only indicated in patients who are symptomatic from heart block, as in this case. Neurological disease comprises a mild meningoencephalitis, peripheral neuritis, cranial nerve involvement, particularly the facial nerve and Bannworth's syndrome (lymphocytic meningoradiculitis).

Chronic Lyme disease may manifest years later as an erosive oligoarthritis or as acrodermatitis chronica atrophicans, which is characterized by atrophy of the skin on the lower limbs.

The diagnosis is clinical and confirmed by serological testing. Serology may be negative during the early erythema chronicum migrans stage. All stages of the disease are amenable to therapy with antibiotics, and the clinical response is usually good. The antibiotics used with success include doxycycline, benzyl penicillin, cefotaxime, amoxycillin and azithromycin.

Conditions simultaneously affecting the cardiovascular and central nervous system

Infections
- TB
- HIV
- Syphilis
- Lyme disease
- Rheumatic fever
- Infective endocarditis

Multi-system conditions
- Connective tissue diseases
- Vasculitides
- Sarcoidosis

Toxins
- Alcohol

Drugs
- Amphetamines
- Tricyclic antidepressant drugs
- Lithium

Neuroectodermal syndromes
- Neurofibromatosis
- Tuberose sclerosis

Hereditary neuropathies
- Friedreich's ataxia
- Dystrophia myotonica
- Duchenne muscular dystrophy

Miscellaneous
- AIP
- Guillain–Barré syndrome

Question 150

A 69-year-old male was admitted to the Coronary Care Unit after presenting with a three-hour history of chest pain, palpitations and breathlessness. He had a past history of hypertension and three myocardial infarctions. His regular medication comprised aspirin 150 mg once daily, captopril 50 mg three times daily, furosemide 40 mg once daily, and simvastatin 10 mg once daily. An ECG performed on admission is shown in **150a**. (Do not answer 4 until you have finished answering 1–3.)

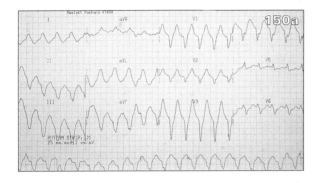

1. What is the ECG diagnosis?
2. Give four reasons in favour of your diagnosis.
3. What is the drug of choice?
4. Shortly after administering the drug, the patient becomes very clammy and cyanosed. His conscious level deteriorates and his blood pressure recording is 70/40 mmHg. What is the next step in his management?

Question 151

A deaf couple both have a hereditary form of deafness. They have recently married, and want advice on the chances of their children being affected. The family tree of both parents is shown (**151**).

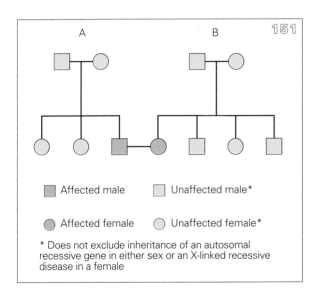

Affected male   Unaffected male*

Affected female   Unaffected female*

* Does not exclude inheritance of an autosomal recessive gene in either sex or an X-linked recessive disease in a female

1. What is the pattern of inheritance for family A?
   a. Autosomal dominant.
   b. Autosomal recessive.
   c. X-linked recessive.
   d. X-linked dominant.
   e. Autosomal dominant with incomplete penetrance.

2. What is the inheritance for family B?
   a. Autosomal dominant.
   b. Autosomal recessive.
   c. X-linked recessive.
   d. X-linked dominant.
   e. Autosomal dominant with incomplete penetrance.

3. Assuming that both families have the same mutation causing deafness, what is the chance of their children being affected?
   a. None.
   b. 1/4.
   c. 1/2.
   d. 100%.
   e. 3/4.

Answer 150

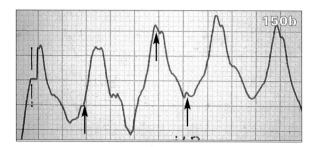

1. Ventricular tachycardia (VT).
2. i. Broad complex tachycardia.
   ii. Extreme axis deviation.
   iii. Concordance in the precordial leads.
   iv. Dissociated P waves (**150b**).
3. Intravenous amiodarone.
4. DC cardioversion.

Factors favouring VT rather than supraventricular tachycardia include all of those in (**150b**) above (see also *Table*). The diagnosis of VT rather than SVT in a patient with a broad complex tachycardia is also more likely when there is a history of ischaemic heart disease or cardiomyopathy.

Most VT has a RBBB morphology because it arises from the left ventricle; however, VT from the right ventricle is also recognized, in which case it has a LBBB morphology. Examples of right ventricular VT include right ventricular outflow tachycardia, congenital heart disease with right-to-left shunts, and arrhythmogenic right VT.

The management of sustained VT is dependent on haemodynamic status. Patients who are haemodynamically stable (not hypotensive or clammy) should be treated with amiodarone. Other effective drugs include sotalol, procainamide and lignocaine. Sotalol and procainamide are more effective than lignocaine. Amiodarone is the least negatively inotropic agent and is the drug of choice when there is suspicion that left ventricular function may be impaired. Patients with haemodynamic collapse should be cardioverted immediately.

Features of ventricular tachycardia

- Broad complex (QRS usually >140 ms)
- Extreme axis deviation
- Positive or negative concordance in the precordial leads
- RSr pattern in V1
- Deep S-wave in V6
- Fusion and capture beats
- Dissociated P-waves

Answer 151

1. b. Autosomal recessive.
2. b. Autosomal recessive.
3. d. 100%.

In both families neither parent is affected, which excludes an autosomal dominant or an X-linked dominant condition in any of the parents and an X-linked recessive condition in both fathers (the presence of a defective X-linked gene in the fathers would manifest as abnormal phenotype). This leaves the possibility of an autosomal recessive condition, or that the mothers are carriers of an X-linked condition. However, an X-linked recessive mode of inheritance is excluded by the fact that there are affected daughters in both families. If a mother is a carrier for an X-linked recessive condition there is a 50% chance that her daughters will be carriers, but none will have the disease, and there is a 50% chance that her sons will be affected. If both parents are carriers of autosomal recessive genes for deafness, then there is a 25% chance that their children will be affected, irrespective of their sex.

Both the couple in question are affected, which implies that both carry two autosomal recessive genes for deafness. The chance of their children being affected is 100%, because they will inherit one autosomal recessive gene for deafness from each parent.

Question 152

A 5-year-old male was admitted with a two-day history of blood-stained diarrhoea. Three days after, he felt nauseous and generally unwell. On examination he had periorbital oedema and a blood pressure of 150/95 mmHg.

Investigations are shown.

Hb	8 g/dl
WCC	13 × 10⁹/l
Platelets	36 × 10⁹/l
PT	13 s (control 13 s)
APTT	34 s (control 36 s)
Blood film (**152**)	
Sodium	138 mmol/l
Potassium	5.9 mmol/l
Creatinine	130 µmol/l
Urea	11 mmol/l

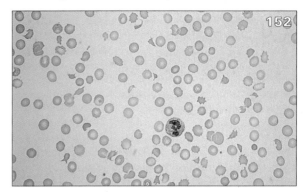

1. What is the diagnosis?
   a. Nephrotic syndrome secondary to minimal change glomerulonephritis.
   b. IgA nephritis.
   c. Haemolytic uraemic syndrome.
   d. Thrombotic thrombocytopenic purpura.
   e. Chronic pyelonephritis.

2. What investigation would you request to confirm your suspicion?
   a. 24 hour urine collection.
   b. Intravenous pyelogram.
   c. Stool culture for *Escherichia coli* 0157:H7.
   d. Renal biopsy.
   e. Auto-antibody screen.

Question 153

Hb	9.8 g/dl
WCC	14 × 10⁹/l
Platelets	350 × 10⁹/l
MCV	84 fl
Clotting	Normal
Sodium	135 mmol/l
Potassium	6.8 mmol/l
Urea	16 mmol/l
Creatinine	670 µmmol/l
Bicarbonate	15 mmol/l
Calcium	2.0 mmol/l
Phosphate	2.8 mmol/l
Bilirubin	14 µmol/l
AST	26 iu/l
Alkaline phosphatase	100 iu/l
Albumin	40 g/l
Glucose	9 mmol/l
Urinalysis	Blood +++
	Protein +
Chest X-ray	Normal
X-ray of left hip	Fracture and dislocation of the neck of femur
ECG	Minor T-wave abnormalities in the lateral leads

A 67-year-old patient with diet-controlled diabetes was found collapsed at the bottom of the stairs in his home by his daughter. The only other medical history available was that he had a history of hypertension, for which he was taking bendroflumethiazide. On examination he was drowsy. His heart rate was 41 beats/min, and blood pressure 140/90 mmHg. The temperature was 36.8°C (98.2°F). The JVP was not raised. The heart sounds were normal, and his chest was clear. Abdominal examination was normal. His left lower limb was externally rotated and painful to move, and there was extensive bruising of the buttock and left thigh.

Investigations are shown.

1. What is the diagnosis?
2. List two investigations you would perform to confirm the cause of the metabolic abnormality.

Answer 152

> 1.c. Haemolytic uraemic syndrome.
> 2.c. Stool culture for *Escherichia coli* 0157:H7.

E. coli 0157:H7 is most commonly transmitted by eating under-cooked beef. The bacterium produces a toxin that is responsible for the gastrointestinal effects, which include colicky pain and diarrhoea, which may be blood-stained. Fever is very mild or completely absent. Symptoms of infection usually subside after about a week; however, the HUS develops in approximately 6% of patients. This is characterized by an MAHA, which is a result of endothelial damage by the toxin, leading to adherence of fibrin strands which trap and fragment red cells and platelets. This produces a characteristic blood picture of anaemia, red cell fragments, thrombocytopenia and increased reticulocytes. Small vessel fibrin deposition and thrombosis resulting from MAHA lead to renal damage and oliguric renal failure. Bleeding and bruising are common. In pure MAHA clotting is usually normal; however, MAHA often coexists with disseminated intravascular coagulation, where clotting is impaired and the serum fibrinogen degradation product level is elevated. Treatment of HUS complicated by MAHA and renal failure is supportive. Blood transfusions are often necessary. Some 50% of patients require dialysis. The mortality rate is 3–5%.

A variant of HUS occurring in the same circumstances and characterized by neurological involvement is known as thrombotic thrombocytopenic purpura. This is caused by a circulating inhibitor for the Von Willebrand Factor protease enzyme. This results in uncontrolled thrombotic tendencies in small vessels.

The combination of MAHA and DIC occurs in sepsis, malignancy and obstetric emergencies such as septic abortion, abruptio placentae and amniotic fluid embolism.

The presence of blood in the urine is against the diagnosis of nephrotic syndrome.

> **Causes of MAHA**
>
> - HUS
> - Thrombotic thrombocytopenic purpura
> - Accelerated hypertension
> - Septicaemia
> - Vasculitides
> - Connective tissue diseases
> - Mucinous adenocarcinoma
> - Burns
> - Prosthetic valve-induced haemolysis
> - Drugs (cyclosporin, mitomycin)

Answer 153

> 1. Rhabdomyolysis.
> 2. i. Measuring creatinine kinase levels, which are elevated due to skeletal muscle damage
>   ii. Detection of myoglobin in the urine.

There are two important clues for diagnosing rhabdomyolysis. Firstly, the patient has had a fall. Secondly, there is renal failure with a disproportionately raised creatinine level. Other causes of rhabdomyolysis are tabulated below (*Table A*). The common pathology is myositis, skeletal muscle trauma or infarction leading to raised myoglobin levels in the blood. Myoglobin is toxic to the renal tubules and precipitates renal failure. In rhabdomyolysis, the serum calcium is low because free calcium becomes bound by myoglobin. The serum potassium and phosphate are high because large amounts of these electrolytes are released from damaged muscle cells (*Table B*)

The management involves adequate hydration and alkalinization of the urine to reduce precipitation of myoglobin in the renal tubules. Loop diuretics should be avoided as they result in an acidic urinary pH.

> **Table A Causes of rhabdomyolysis**
>
> - Muscle trauma/infarction
> - Electrocution
> - Hypothermia
> - Status epilepticus
> - Neuroleptic malignant syndrome
> - Ecstasy/amphetamine abuse
> - Burns
> - Septicaemia
> - Therapy with statins
> - Very strenuous exercise (e.g. marathon running)

> **Table B Causes of low calcium and high phosphate**
>
> - Chronic renal failure
> - Hypoparathyroidism
> - Pseudohypoparathyroidism
> - Magnesium deficiency*
> - Rhabdomyolysis
>
> * Due to end-organ resistance to the effects of PTH

Question 154

A 16-year-old male presented with a four-day history of a dry cough, right-sided pleuritic chest pain and increasing breathlessness. On examination, he had a temperature of 38°C (100.4°F). He had a widespread rash affecting his arms and legs and his face (**154**).

Investigations are shown.

Hb	9 g/dl
WCC	$5 \times 10^9/l$
Platelets	$150 \times 10^9/l$
Blood film	Red cell agglutination
Sodium	131 mmol/l
Potassium	4.0 mmol/l
Urea	4.0 mmol/l
Creatinine	70 µmol/l
Bilirubin	26 µmol/l
AST	60 iu/l
ALT	83 iu/l
Alkaline phosphatase	110 iu/l
Albumin	36 g/l
Chest X-ray	Right middle lobe consolidation

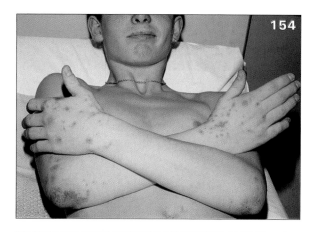

154

1. What is the rash?
2. What is the cause of the low sodium?
3. What is the cause of his anaemia?
4. Which single investigation would you perform to confirm the cause of the anaemia?
5. What is the cause of his chest X-ray findings?
6. Which two tests would you perform to confirm the diagnosis?

Question 155

A 14-year-old female was admitted for investigation of intermittent colicky abdominal pain associated with vomiting. She had experienced several episodes in the past six months requiring hospital admissions. Physical examination during these episodes revealed a distended abdomen which was tympanic to percussion. Bowel sounds were tinkling. Hernial orifice examination was normal. The patient usually developed two painful 4 cm macular lesions on her left hand and forearm respectively which were only present while she was symptomatic. She was never in hospital for more than 48 hours, during which time she was managed with intravenous fluids and resting the bowel. She always made a spontaneous recovery. In between episodes of abdominal pain she was perfectly well. She had a 5-year-old cousin who had also recently been admitted to hospital on three occasions with the same symptoms.

These investigations were performed while the patient was symptomatic.

The patient had a small bowel meal when her symptoms had recovered, which was also normal.

Hb	12 g/dl
WCC	$6 \times 10^9/l$
Platelets	$390 \times 10^9/l$
U&E	Normal
LFT	Normal
Thyroid function tests	Normal
Bone biochemistry	Normal
Blood glucose	5 mmol/l
Serum amylase	Normal
Serum lead	Undetectable
Urinary δ-ALA	Undetectable
Urinary PBG	Undetectable
Serum immunoglobulins	Normal

1. What is the cause of the abdominal pain?
2. How would you manage her symptoms if she remained symptomatic for several days, or if her symptoms deteriorated?

Answer 154

1. Erythema multiforme.
2. Syndrome of inappropriate ADH secretion.
3. Autoimmune haemolytic anaemia.
4. Direct Coomb's test at 4°C (39.2°F).
5. *Mycoplasma* pneumonia.
6. i. *Mycoplasma* serology.
   ii. Cold agglutinin estimation.

The patient has a right middle lobe pneumonia and a rash which is characterized by blistering target lesions (erythema multiforme). The patient has an anaemia, and the agglutination on the blood film points to an immune haemolytic anaemia. *Mycoplasma* pneumonia is associated with both erythema multiforme and a cold autoimmune haemolytic anaemia. Other causes of erythema multiforme and complications of *Mycoplasma* pneumonia are listed in *Tables A* and *B*. The low sodium is a consequence of SIADH complicating pneumonia. The causes of SIADH are discussed in Answer 129.

Table A Causes of erythema multiforme

Infections
- *Mycoplasma* pneumonias
- Herpes simplex virus
- Orf
- TB

Drugs
- Penicillins
- Sulphonamides
- Barbiturates
- NSAID

Miscellaneous
- Connective tissue diseases
- Vasculitides
- Internal malignancy

Table B Complications of *Mycoplasma* pneumonia

Neurological	Aseptic meningitis
	Encephalitis
	Transverse myelitis
	Guillain–Barré syndrome
	Peripheral neuropathy
Cardiac	Myocarditis
	Pericarditis
Haematological	Thrombocytopenia
	Cold autoimmune haemolytic anaemia
Locomotor	Myositis
	Arthritis
Skin	Erythema multiforme
Gastrointestinal	Diarrhoea/vomiting
Endocrine	SIADH
Miscellaneous	Bullous myringitis

Answer 155

1. Hereditary angio-oedema.
2. Use fresh-frozen plasma or C1 esterase inhibitor concentrates.

Hereditary angio-oedema is inherited as an autosomal dominant trait. It is associated with C1 esterase inhibitor deficiency, resulting in high C1 esterase levels. Deficiency of C1 esterase inhibitor (which modulates complement) can lead to angio-oedema. A positive family history is very common, although there is a similar condition associated with an acquired lymphoproliferative disorder in which C1 esterase inhibitor levels are also low. Clinical features can occur late in adult life. Attacks are preceded with a painful macular rash, or even a rash simulating erythema marginatum. Triggering factors include trauma to the skin. Laryngeal oedema can be life-threatening. Abdominal pain occurs due to visceral oedema. Attacks can exceed 72 hours. Treatment is supportive, although fresh-frozen plasma can be given to abort severe or prolonged attacks. Inhibitors of plasmin, such as danazol, are used for long-term treatment. Hydrocortisone and chlorpheniramine are not as effective in the management of this condition as they are in acute anaphylaxis. The diagnosis is made by quantifying the C1 esterase level (high) and C1 esterase inhibitor level (low). C2 and C4 levels are also low.

Question 156

A 30-year-old male presented with a four-day history of passing dark urine. He had passed dark urine intermittently for six months, though such passage had never exceeded 24 hours, except on this occasion. More recently, he complained of malaise, lethargy and weakness. His GP thought he appeared pale, and prescribed iron tablets. Two days before coming to the hospital, the patient developed sharp right lower chest pain which was worsened on inspiration, and a cough productive of bright red sputum. On further questioning, he volunteered a six-month history of intermittent abdominal pain and episodes of abdominal distension.

He had never taken any regular medication and had not travelled abroad for a year. He consumed 5–7 litres of lager on weekends, and occasionally had a glass of wine with a meal.

On examination, he was pale and slightly jaundiced. He had a temperature of 37.5°C (99.5°F). There was no lymphadenopathy. The JVP was not raised. Examination of the respiratory system revealed dullness of the right base associated with reduction of air entry. Abdominal examination demonstrated firm, palpable hepatomegaly 4 cm below the costal margin. There were no other palpable masses. There was no clinical evidence of peripheral oedema.

Investigations are shown.

Hb	7.3 g/dl
WCC	2.8 × 10⁹/l
Platelets	200 × 10⁹/l
MCV	93 fl
Reticulocyte count	15%
Direct Coomb's test	Negative
Chest radiograph	Atelectasis at the right lung base
Urinalysis	Urobilinogen +++
	Haemosiderin ++
	Cell 0
Sodium	136 mmol/l
Potassium	4.8 mmol/l
Urea	5.3 mmol/l
Bilirubin	33 μmol/l
AST	40 iu/l
Alkaline phosphatase	94 iu/l
Albumin	36 g/l

1. What is the cause of the dark urine?
   a. Bilirubinuria.
   b. Urobilinogenuria.
   c. Myoglobinuria.
   d. Haemoglobinuria.
   e. Haemosiderinuria.

2. What is the cause of jaundice?
   a. Haemolysis.
   b. Hepatitis.
   c. Gall stones.
   d. Hepatic metastases.
   e. Pancreatitis.

Question 157

An 18-year-old male developed sharp left-sided chest pain on running up a flight of stairs, followed by slight breathlessness on exertion. On examination, he appeared relatively well. His heart rate was 90 beats/min, and the respiratory rate was 18/min. On auscultation of the heart there was a clicking sound synchronous with the heart sounds.

1. What is the most probable cause of his symptoms?
   a. Mitral valve prolapse.
   b. Pericarditis.
   c. Left-sided apical pneumothorax.
   d. Pulmonary embolism.
   e. Aortic dissection.

2. What investigation would you perform to confirm the diagnosis?
   a. Echocardiogram.
   b. ECG.
   c. Serum cardiac troponin measurement.
   d. CT pulmonary angiogram.
   e. Chest X-ray in end expiration.

Answer 156

> 1. d. Haemoglobinuria.
> 2. a. Haemolysis.

Bilirubinuria does not occur in haemolytic anaemia because bilirubin is in the unconjugated form and therefore is not water-soluble and cannot be excreted in the urine. Urobilinogen does stain urine, but not enough to give it the red colour of haemoglobinuria. Myoglobin is produced in large amounts in rhabdomyolysis, and while it may produce red discoloration of urine, there is no evidence for rhabdomyolysis in this case. Haemosiderinuria occurs in intravascular haemolyis, but can only be detected on staining the urine with Prussian blue.

Hepatitis, gallstones and pancreatitis do not account for the severity of the anaemia. Although haemolyis and thrombotic episodes can be present in a patient with malignancy, it does not account for the dark urine that is present in the absence of red cells in the urine.

The diagnosis is PNH. This is an acquired disorder of the haematopoietic cells which usually occurs after an episode of aplastic anaemia, leading to increased susceptibility of red cells to complement lysis. White cells and platelets are also affected. The onset of the disease is often insidious. The disorder is characterized by non-immune haemolytic anaemia, variable pancytopenia and thrombotic episodes. The MCV may be normal, depending on the extent of reticulocytosis. The molecular basis of the membrane defect has recently been unfolded and attributed to abnormalities in the synthesis of the phospholipid GPI, which serves an anchoring function for important cell surface proteins such as CD59 on red cells, which is a complement lysis inhibitor. Lack of GPI does not permit red cells to express the antigen CD59 on their cell surface, leading to complement lysis. The thrombotic tendency results from inappropriate activation of platelets that are abnormally sensitive to complement. Intravascular haemolysis is reflected by an increased reticulocyte count, raised bilirubin levels, reduced serum haptoglobins, methaemoglobinaemia, increased urinary urobilinogen, haemoglobinuria and haemosiderinuria. The latter is only detectable by staining the urine with Prussian blue agent. Haemolysis is increased during sleep, hence the term PNH. It is not clear why haemolysis should increase during sleep. Haemolysis is usually worse after infections, following inoculations, blood transfusions and surgery. Anaemia causes fatigue and dyspnoea. Some patients present with intermittent abdominal pain which is worse during episodes of active haemolysis. There is mild jaundice and intermittent passage of dark urine. On examination the patient may be pale and jaundiced. The spleen is sometimes palpable and the liver may be enlarged.

Complications include venous thrombosis, increased susceptibility to infection due to granulocytopenia, iron deficiency, pigment gallstones and transformation to acute myeloid leukaemia. Thrombosis is the most frequent complication. Small vessel thrombosis may be the cause of abdominal pain, and swelling may be due to intermittent ascites, as in this patient. Portal vein or hepatic vein thrombosis is a serious complication. Pulmonary embolism is a recognized complication. In this case the pleuritic chest pain and haemoptysis may be due to pulmonary embolism or infection, the latter worsening the haemolytic event. Acute myeloid leukaemia complicates a few cases of PNH and is characterized by rapid pancytopenia and blast cells in the peripheral blood film.

The diagnosis of PNH is made by addition of acidified serum to the red cells, which will cause rapid haemolysis (the Ham's test). The reason for acidification of the serum is to activate the alternative complement pathway.

The definitive treatment is marrow transplantation. Leucocyte-depleted blood transfusions are often necessary.

Answer 157

> 1. c. Left-sided apical pneumothorax.
> 2. e. Chest X-ray in end expiration.

A systolic click that is synchronous with heart sounds is a rare but recognized sign of a small left apical pneumothorax. It is often referred to as Hamman's sign. A differential diagnosis of this sign is the systolic click of mitral valve prolapse; however, this is not consistent with chest pain and breathlessness on exertion of sudden onset in a young man.

An inspiratory X-ray alone may fail to detect small apical pneumothoraces. The management is conservative. Patients are advised not to engage in strenuous exertion for at least two weeks.

Question 158

A 33-year-old male returned from Mombasa, East Africa with a high fever, headaches and rigors. On examination, he had a temperature of 40°C (104°F). A blood film performed on admission is shown (**158a**).

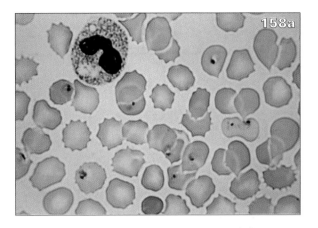

What is the diagnosis?

Question 159

A 15-year-old female was investigated for short stature. She measured 1.22 m tall. Her sister aged 14 was 1.53 m tall. She was born three weeks prematurely, and was noted to have a divergent squint affecting her left eye in childhood. She had achieved her milestones in a normal manner, but school performance had been below average. On examination, the patient weighed 42 kg. She had a left-sided divergent squint. Her neck was short and her hands were small. Breast development had just begun and there was scanty pubic and axillary hair growth. The heart rate was 90 beats/min and regular, and the blood pressure was 110/70 mmHg. The heart sounds were normal and the chest was clear. Abdominal and neurological examination was also normal.

Initial investigations are shown.

Hb	13 g/dl
WCC	4.2 × 10⁹/l
Platelets	410 × 10⁹/l
Sodium	136 mmol/l
Potassium	3.8 mmol/l
Urea	5.1 mmol/l
Creatinine	90 µmol/l
Glucose	5.2 mmol/l
Calcium	1.96 mmol/l
Phosphate	1.3 mmol/l
Alkaline phosphatase	90 iu/l
Albumin	39 g/l
TSH	2 mu/l
Thyroxine	87 nmol/l (normal 60–160 nmol/l)
LH	4 iu/l (normal 1–12 iu/l)
FSH	6 iu/l (normal 1–9 iu/l)
GH	2 mu/l
X-ray	Left wrist, lateral skull – normal bone age

1. List two possible causes for her short stature.
2. Give one test you would perform to confirm the diagnosis.

Answer 158

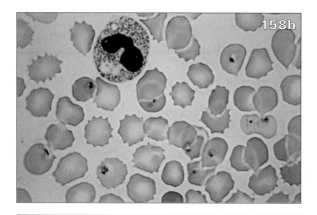

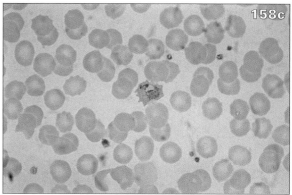

Plasmodium falciparum malaria.

The two malaria parasites commonly shown on blood films in higher examinations are *P. falciparum* and *P. vivax* (for comparison, the blood films of both parasites are shown side-by-side [**158b**, **c**]). *P. falciparum* can be differentiated from *P. vivax* by the following features:

- The parasite count is high, whereas in *P. vivax* it is low.
- The affected cells are small and/or crenated, whereas in *P. vivax* the cells are large.
- The ring form has two chromatin dots, whereas *P. vivax* has just one.
- The actual ring is thin, whereas in *P. vivax* it is thick.

Answer 159

1. i. Pseudohypoparathyroidism.
   ii. Idiopathic hypoparathyroidism.
2. Serum PTH level.

A low serum calcium, raised phosphate and normal alkaline phosphatase are suggestive of either idiopathic hypoparathyroidism or pseudohypoparathyroidism. The short stature, short neck and squint are characteristic of pseudohypoparathyroidism. In addition, the patient has small hands – presumably secondary to short metacarpals – which are also associated with pseudohypoparathyroidism. However, these morphological changes are also infrequently present in idiopathic hypoparathyroidism. Pseudohypoparathyroidism results from resistance of some target tissues to the actions of PTH. The disorder may be asymptomatic, present with lethargy, neuromuscular irritability or psychosis. Neuromuscular irritability is only present in profound hypocalcaemia, and consists of paraesthesia of the face and extremities, carpopedal spasm, and latent tetany. Convulsions are relatively common.

The serum PTH distinguishes between idiopathic hypoparathyroidism and pseudohypoparathyroidism. In idiopathic hypoparathyroidism, PTH level is extremely low or absent. The diagnosis of pseudohypoparathyroidism is also confirmed by measuring urinary cyclic AMP and phosphate concentration after infusion of PTH (Howard–Ellsworth test). The normal response is an increase in both cyclic AMP and phosphate in the urine after PTH. In patients with end-organ resistance to PTH, i.e. pseudohypoparathyroidism, there is no such response. In a small proportion there is a normal response (type II pseudohypoparathyroidism). In these cases the diagnosis is based on the identification of a relatively high level of PTH in relation to the low serum calcium level.

Question 160

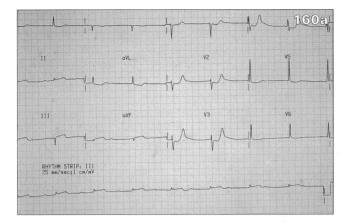

160a

A 55-year-old West Indian male presented with severe anterior chest pain. On arrival, he was hypotensive. An ECG performed in the Accident and Emergency Department is shown (**160a**). Shortly after admission, the patient had an echocardiogram (**160b**).

1. What is the complete diagnosis?
2. What would be the next step in your management?

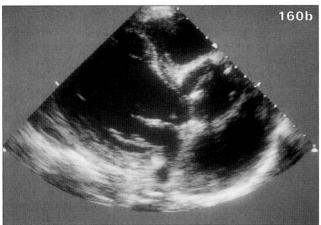

160b

Question 161

A 70-year-old male presents to the Accident and Emergency Department in the morning with a painful swelling on the anterior aspect of his left thigh which he had noticed on the previous evening. The swelling had become bigger and he was having difficulty walking due to the pain. He denied any recent trauma to the leg. Apart from a past history of TB 30 years ago, there was no other history of note. He was widowed three years ago and lived alone. He took paracetamol infrequently for aches and pains in his limbs.

On examination, he appeared unkempt and was thin. There was no pallor or oedema. Vital parameters were normal and he was apyrexial. There was a 6 cm, tender swelling on the anterior aspect of the left thigh. There was also evidence of widespread bruising on his forearms and legs.

Investigations are shown.

Hb	11 g/dl
WCC	5 × 10⁹/l
Platelets	170 × 10⁹/l
MCV	90 fl
PT	14 s (control 14 s)
APTT	45 s (control 45 s)
BT	12 min (control <10 min)

What is the diagnosis?
  a. Vitamin C deficiency (scurvy).
  b. Folate deficiency.
  c. B_{12} deficiency.
  d. Von Willebrand's disease.
  e. Chronic liver disease.

Answer 160

> 1. Acute inferior myocardial infarction with complete heart block complicating an acute proximal aortic dissection. The echocardiogram demonstrates an enlarged aortic root with an obvious dissection flap. (See Echocardiography, page 421.)
> 2. Immediate referral to the cardiothoracic surgeons.

> **Conditions predisposing to aortic dissection**
>
> - Hypertension in patients of Afro-Caribbean origin
> - Marfan's syndrome
> - Ehlers–Danlos syndrome
> - Pregnancy
> - Coarctation of the aorta
> - Relapsing polychondritis

Patients with proximal dissections should undergo urgent surgical repair, but those with distal dissection are treated conservatively. Repair is by resection of the ascending aorta and replacement with dacron. In the interim, it would be important to relieve the severe pain with opiates and insert a temporary pacing wire to treat the complete heart block and help maintain circulation as he is hypotensive. In acute dissection, hypotension is due to rupture of the proximal dissection into the pericardial space, which is not present in this case; therefore, complete heart block is contributing to the hypotension in this case. In contrast with this case, most patients presenting with acute dissection are hypertensive and in these circumstances it is prudent to treat the hypertension aggressively to obtain a systolic blood pressure equal to or less than 100 mmHg. Drugs most commonly used include intravenous beta-blockers, for example, labetolol, or intravenous nitroprusside. It is very important to recognize that the cause of myocardial infarction is a proximal dissection, and not coronary thrombosis. While thrombolytic therapy has revolutionized the management of acute coronary thrombosis, it is an absolute contraindication in a patient who has sustained a myocardial infarction secondary to aortic dissection.

Aortic dissection is catastrophic, with a mortality rate of 1% per hour for the first 48 hours in untreated patients. Some 95% of dissections originate at the site of the intimal tear. Most tears occur in the ascending aorta (65%), followed by the proximal descending aorta (20%), in the transverse arch (10%) and in the distal thoracic aorta (5%). Predisposing factors are tabulated above.

Clinical features of acute dissection include very sudden onset of chest pain, either in the chest or between the shoulder blades. Syncope from tamponade, neurological deficit from involvement of the carotid artery, abdominal pain from mesenteric ischaemia, ischaemic upper limbs from brachiocephalic and left subclavian involvement and acute renal failure from involvement of the renal arteries are other presentations.

The diagnosis may be made by transthoracic echocardiography; however, transoesophageal echocardiography is the 'gold standard' test in the diagnosis of suspected dissection. MRI scanning is superior to transoesophageal echocardiogaphy, but its main disadvantage is that it is not portable.

Answer 161

> a. Vitamin C deficiency (scurvy).

The normocytic anaemia, bruising and abnormal bleeding time in an elderly patient point to the diagnosis of vitamin C (ascorbic acid) deficiency, or scurvy. Vitamin C is abundant in fresh greens, citrus fruits, liver and kidney. Nutritional deficiency is relatively common in the elderly, who eat predominantly tinned foods. Vitamin C is required for the hydroxylation of proline in collagen synthesis. Deficiency results in abnormal connective tissue, resulting in easy bruising, bleeding gums, periosteal haemorrhage and muscle haematomas. The characteristic signs of vitamin C deficiency are perifollicular haemorrhages, widespread bruising and 'corkscrewing' of the body hair. The latter may be normal in the elderly. Patients may have coexistent iron and folate deficiency. The marrow is megaloblastic when there is folate deficiency. The bleeding time is prolonged, although platelet function is normal. The diagnosis is made by the demonstration of a low platelet or leucocyte ascorbate concentration. Treatment is with high doses of ascorbic acid.

The normal MCV is not consistent with the diagnosis of B_{12} deficiency or chronic liver disease. There is no previous history of haemorrhage to indicate Von Willebrand's disease.

Question 162

A 48-year-old female had an 11-month history of abdominal cramps and diarrhoea. She moved her bowels twice daily; the stool was loose and foul-smelling. There was no history of bleeding per rectum or tenesmus. Her appetite was unchanged, but she had lost 8 kg in weight. Two years ago she had a total abdominal hysterectomy and salpingo-oophorectomy for carcinoma of the cervix, followed by a course of external radiotherapy. She had been followed up regularly by her gynaecologist, and was free from recurrence of the malignancy. She was married with two sons, aged 10 and 12. She worked as a secretary. She consumed 1 unit of alcohol daily and was a non-smoker. There was no history of travel abroad. She had a long history of Raynaud's phenomenon. She took paracetamol for very infrequent headaches.

On examination she was thin. There was no pallor, clubbing, lymphadenopathy or oedema. The temperature was normal. Inspection of the oral cavity revealed two small, non-tender, shallow ulcers. The abdomen was thin. There was a lower, midline scar. Mild tenderness was elicited on palpation of the right iliac fossa. Rectal examination was normal. Investigations are shown.

Hb	10g/dl
WCC	8×10^9/l
Platelets	199×10^9/l
MCV	106 fl
ESR	16 mm/h
Serum B_{12}	98 pmol/l
Serum folate	18 µg/l
Calcium	2.12 mmol/l
Phosphate	0.9 mmol/l
Alkaline phosphatase	112 u/l
Albumin	38 g/l
U&E	Normal
Total thyroxine	110 nmol/l
TSH	1.9 mu/l
Abdominal X-ray	Normal
Chest X-ray	Normal

1. What is the diagnosis?
   a. Crohn's disease.
   b. Coeliac disease.
   c. Small bowel lymphoma.
   d. Radiation enteritis.
   e. Tuberculous ileitis.

2. Which investigation would you perform to reach a diagnosis?
   a. Schilling test.
   b. Duodenal biopsy.
   c. Small bowel meal.
   d. $^{14}CO_2$ breath test.
   e. Duodenal aspiration for culture.

Question 163

An 18-year-old female had blood tests as part of a routine medical (below).

Hb	10.5 g/dl
WCC	6×10^9/l
Platelets	300×10^9/l
MCV	61 fl
MCHC	28 g/l
MCH	19 pg
Red cell count	6.8×10^{12}/l
Blood film	Hypochromia, anisocytosis, poikilocytosis, target cells
Sodium	136 mmol/l
Potassium	4.1 mmol/l
Urea	4 mmol/l
Creatinine	72 µmol/l

1. What is the most probable diagnosis?
   a. β-thalassaemia major.
   b. Anaemia of chronic disease.
   c. β-thalassaemia minor.
   d. Iron deficiency anaemia.
   e. Paroxysmal nocturnal haemoglobinuria.

2. What two investigations should be performed?
   a. Blood film.
   b. Ham's test.
   c. Serum ferritin.
   d. Serum B_{12}.
   e. Serum folate.
   f. Thyroid function.
   g. Haemoglobin electrophoresis.
   h. Coomb's test.
   i. Liver function tests.
   j. Red cell sequestration study.

Answer 162

> 1. d. Radiation enteritis.
> 2. c. Small bowel meal.

The patient has a malabsorption syndrome. The B_{12} level is low in the presence of a normal folate level. This suggests either selective B_{12} malabsorption due to terminal ileal disease (Crohn's disease, terminal ileal resection, ileal TB), pernicious anaemia or excess utilization of B_{12} within the gut itself (bacterial overgrowth which occurs in the presence of a structural abnormality of the small bowel, e.g. after Billroth II gastric surgery, jejunal diverticula, Crohn's disease, intestinal fistulae, radiation enteritis and small bowel involvement in systemic sclerosis, amyloidosis and diabetic autonomic neuropathy).

Symptoms of malabsorption are absent in pernicious anaemia. The differential diagnosis is, therefore, between terminal ileal disease or bacterial overgrowth. There is no mention of small bowel surgery in the question. Ileal TB is unlikely in the absence of a febrile illness, night sweats, only slightly elevated ESR, absent past history or contact with TB, and a normal chest X-ray. Although Crohn's disease is a possibility, the most likely answer is radiation enteritis. Radiation enteritis can complicate radiotherapy to the abdominal region. In the acute phase this may remain silent or present as diarrhoea. The sequel is fibrotic strictures or adhesions causing cramp-like abdominal pain. Strictures predispose to bacterial overgrowth, which in turn leads to steatorrhoea due to deconjugation of bile salts. Vitamin B_{12} is metabolized by the bacteria, whereas folate absorption is left unhindered. Moreover, some bacteria actually produce folate, often leading to elevated levels in the blood. Investigation involves small bowel meal, which will demonstrate the structural abnormality. Hydrogen or carbon dioxide breath tests will confirm the diagnosis.

Small bowel meal is regarded as the investigation of choice in this question because it will detect Crohn's disease, ileal TB, radiation enteritis and small bowel lymphoma. The latter occasionally complicates radiotherapy, but it does not lead to a selective B_{12} deficiency.

Answer 163

> 1. c. β-thalassaemia minor.
>   d. Iron-deficiency anaemia.
> 2. c. Serum ferritin.
>   g. Haemoglobin electrophoresis.

The best answer is β-thalassaemia minor. The clue lies in the fact that the MCV is disproportionately low compared with the Hb. In β-thalassaemia trait (minor), the cells are small due to defective globin synthesis and are removed relatively rapidly from the circulation by the spleen. As a consequence, the marrow produces large amounts of red cells and, provided that iron and folate stores remain replenished, the Hb is only modestly reduced but the cells are relatively small. The red cell count itself, however, may be high. In iron deficiency, the marrow is unable to produce red cells to maintain a normal Hb because haem synthesis is incomplete without iron. Therefore, the number of cells produced (and hence the red cell count) is small compared with β-thalassaemia trait; however, the size is similar. By the time the iron deficiency has become severe enough to cause a reduction in the MCV as low as 61 fl, the Hb is much lower than in β-thalassaemia trait.

In β-thalassaemia major the Hb, red cell count and MCV are all very low, and such patients require life-long blood transfusions to maintain a Hb around 10 g/dl. α-thalassaemia trait may present with a similar picture as β-thalassaemia trait if two of the four genes which code for α-globin chains are defective. When only one gene is defective the Hb and MCV are usually normal.

The investigation of choice is Hb electrophoresis. This is normal in a patient with iron deficiency, revealing approximately 98% HbA (i.e. normal Hb comprising two α- and two β-globin chains) and 2% HbA2 (two α- and two δ-globin chains). In β-thalassaemia trait the HbA is reduced to approximately 90%, the HbA2 is slightly increased to 6%, and in addition may be the presence of some HbF (fetal Hb; two α- and two γ-globin chains). The reason for this is that in β-thalassaemia trait the deficiency of normal β-globin means that α-globin chains combine with either γ-globin or δ-globin. In β-thalassaemia major, where there is no normal β-globin production, almost all the Hb is HbF.

The serum ferritin is also useful because it is low in iron deficiency but normal or increased in β-thalassaemia trait, unless there is coexisting iron deficiency. The slightly elevated ferritin in some patients with β-thalassaemia trait may be explained by the fact that defective β-globin synthesis prevents the marrow utilizing all the iron which is absorbed from the gastrointestinal tract, resulting in some iron accumulation.

Patients with megaloblastic marrow as seen in B_{12} or folate deficiency and those with hypothyroidism and chronic liver disease have a raised MCV. Patients with anaemia of chronic disease generally have a normal MCV. There is nothing in this patient's history to indicate paroxysmal nocturnal haemoglobinuria, therefore a Ham's test is not necessary.

Question 164

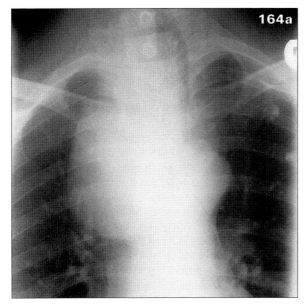

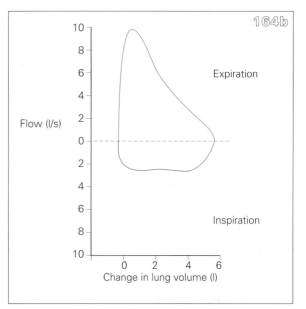

A 76-year-old female developed gradual onset of breathlessness over the past three weeks. On admission, she had stridor. Her respiratory rate was 30/min, and she was not cyanosed. Her trachea was slightly deviated to the right, and there was a mass just palpable in front of it, which moved slightly with swallowing. The lower margins of the mass could not be defined. Auscultation of the lungs revealed stridor-type sounds transmitted from the upper airways. She was managed with oxygen and saline nebulizers in the Accident and Emergency Department, and felt considerably better. She mentioned having a problem with her thyroid gland, and over 20 years ago was told she did not need any treatment. She had lost 5 kg in weight over the past two months.

She had a chest radiograph (**164a**) in the Accident and Emergency Department.

Lung function tests and a thyroid scan were performed the following day. Results of the flow loop curve (**164b**) and thyroid scan (**164c**) are shown.

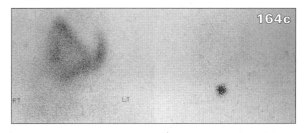

1. What is the abnormality on the chest radiograph? List four possible causes for this appearance.
2. What is the abnormality on the flow loop curve and what does this suggest?
3. Give three possible causes for the abnormality in the flow loop curve in our patient.
4. What is the abnormality on the thyroid scan?
5. List two tests which would help confirm the cause of her breathlessness.

Question 165

The blood results shown were performed two months apart in a patient with HIV infection.

	October	December
Hb (g/dl)	11.8	7.6
WCC ($\times 10^9$/l)	3.0	3.1
Platelets ($\times 10^9$/l)	160	90
MCV (fl)	86	110
Reticulocyte count (%)	1.5	4
CD4	24	120

What is the most likely cause for the discrepancy between the results?
   a. Development of B_{12} deficiency.
   b. Development of folate deficiency.
   c. Development of systemic lupus erythematosus.
   d. The patient has become pregnant.
   e. Zidovudine toxicity.

Answer 164

1. The lateral chest X-ray reveals a mass in the superior mediastinum. Possible causes of a superior mediastinal mass include (i) retrosternal goitre, (ii) thymoma, (iii) lymphoma, (iv) malignant lymphadenopathy, (v) teratoma, and (vi) aneurysm of the aortic arch. The most likely cause of the mass in this situation is a retrosternal goitre.
2. There is evidence of reduced airflow rate which is more pronounced in the inspiratory phase of respiration. This is suggestive of extrathoracic large airways obstruction. Typical examples include retrosternal goitre and its complications, compression by malignant lymph nodes and bilateral vocal cord paralysis.
3. i. Compression from a retrosternal multinodular goitre which has undergone malignant change.
   ii. Compression from a retrosternal multinodular goitre due to spontaneous haemorrhage within the gland.
   iii. Compression from locally metastasized lymphatic deposits from carcinoma of the thyroid.
4. A large 'cold nodule' in the left lobe of the thyroid gland.
5. i. CT scan of the neck and upper thorax.
   ii. Fine-needle aspirate of the thyroid gland for histology.

There is a history of a chronic thyroid disorder in this elderly woman. She is clinically and biochemically euthyroid, and has a palpable mass in the suprasternal area which moves with swallowing. The most probable cause for the mass in the superior mediastinum is a retrosternal extension of a goitre. The reason for sudden deterioration is tracheal compression due to rapid enlargement of the goitre. This may occur as a result of haemorrhage or malignant change within the goitre. An additional cause of tracheal compression in this situation is compression from malignant lymph nodes. Tracheal compression causes stridor when it is severe. It is potentially a medical emergency requiring rapid relief of the compression, the speed of which is determined by the extent of respiratory embarrassment.

Carcinoma of the thyroid complicates approximately 4% of multi-nodular goitres. Most patients are asymptomatic, but some experience symptoms as a result of local compression of structures which include dysphagia, dysphonia, stridor and haemoptysis. Technetium scanning is the most widely used imaging agent of a goitre. Lack of uptake of technetium in parts of the thyroid gland is suggestive of hypofunction. Such 'cold' nodules are associated with carcinoma of the thyroid in 20% of cases. Cold areas can also occur with cysts, colloid adenomas, degenerative nodules and thyroiditis. The differentiation from a cyst is possible with US scanning. This patient has a very large area in the left lobe where there is no uptake (cold area). An US will confirm whether this is a cystic or a solid lesion; however, in this case the symptom of stridor raises the suspicion of sinister pathology and therefore a CT scan of the neck and thorax is more likely to provide extra information about the gland, its pathology and the extent of direct invasion from a probable malignant process. Fine-needle aspiration of the lesion is an invaluable means of making a histological diagnosis, provided an experienced cytopathologist is available to interpret the histology. The main limitation of this procedure is that it does not necessarily allow differentiation between a follicular adenoma and follicular carcinoma, and in a few cases false-negative results are generated due to sampling error. The results of the aspirate should be interpreted in the context of the patient's presentation and results from other imaging techniques.

Answer 165

e. Zidovudine toxicity.

The patient has become more anaemic, has developed a macrocytosis, thrombocytopenia and an increase in the CD4 count. The most likely cause of these abnormalities is treatment with AZT. AZT is a nucleoside analogue that inhibits the viral enzyme reverse transcriptase and is a DNA chain terminator. It is widely used in symptomatic HIV infection. In such patients it has been shown to reduce mortality by reducing the incidence of opportunistic infections owing to a significant but transient improvement in the CD4 count. The drug has important haematological side-effects, which include a reduction in all cell lines and a megaloblastic change in the marrow. The general side-effects of the drug include nausea, vomiting, myalgia, headaches, neuropathy and myopathy.

Other drugs which cause pancytopenia and macrocytosis in HIV patients are co-trimoxazole (used in the treatment of *Pneumocystis carinii* infection) and 2',3'-deoxynucleoside analogues other than AZT, such as dideoxyadenosine and dideoxyinosine. The latter drugs have less marrow toxicity.

Marrow suppression may occur in HIV as a direct result of the virus.

Another important haematological manifestation of HIV in relation to the MRCP and similar examinations is the presence of a circulating anticoagulant in some cases. All the other options except pregnancy may result in a pancytopenia and raised MCV. While pregnancy may cause anaemia it would usually have no bearing on the white cells or platelets in the early stages.

Question 166

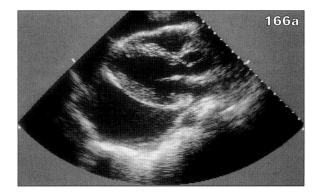

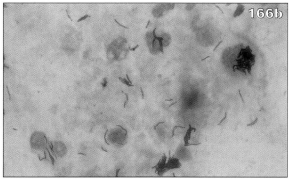

A 30-year-old Bangladeshi female was admitted to hospital with a two-month history of increasing lethargy and ankle swelling. One week before admission she developed right upper quadrant pain, nausea and anorexia. She had immigrated from Bangladesh two years ago, and ever since coming to this country she had noticed a troublesome cough which was productive of yellow sputum and for which she had been prescribed several courses of oral antibiotics. She lived with her husband in a rented flat.

On examination she was thin and slightly pale. Her temperature was 37.5°C (99.5°F). The heart rate was 110 beats/min and regular; the blood pressure was 95/55 mmHg. The JVP was grossly elevated. On examination of the precordium the apex was not palpable, and on auscultation both heart sounds were soft. On examination of the respiratory system there were harsh breath sounds on auscultation of the left upper zone. Abdominal examination demonstrated smooth and tender hepatomegaly palpable 6 cm below the costal margin. In addition, there was clinical evidence of moderate ascites. The lower limbs had pitting oedema to the shins.

Investigations are shown.

Hb	11 g/dl
WCC	$10 \times 10^9/l$
Platelets	$180 \times 10^9/l$
MCV	85 fl
ESR	80 mm/h
Sodium	129 mmol/l
Potassium	4.3 mmol/l
Urea	8 mmol/l
Creatinine	90 µmol/l
Glucose	5 mmol/l
Echocardiogram (**166a**)	
Sputum microscopy (**166b**)	

1. What is demonstrated on the echocardiogram?
2. What is the most probable cause for the abnormality on the echocardiogram?
3. List two therapeutic steps in your management of this patient.
4. What other step would you take after initiating therapy for the patient?

Question 167

The data are from cardiac catheter traces of a 14-year-old male, taken five years apart.

	5 years ago		Present	
	Pressure (mmHg)	Satn (%)	Pressure (mmHg)	Satn (%)
Superior vena cava		68		49
Right atrium	8	68	12	50
Right ventricle	40/5	94	120/20	50
Pulmonary artery	40/18	94	115/55	50
Pulmonary capillary wedge pressure	6		8	
Left ventricle	110/4	95	115/15	57
Aorta	115/60	95	100/50	50

1. List three abnormalities in the catheter performed five years ago.
2. List three abnormalities in the catheter performed most recently.
3. What is the unifying diagnosis?

Answer 166

1. The echocardiogram demonstrates a large pericardial effusion. (See *Table* for causes.) (See Echocardiography, page 421.)
2. Tuberculous pericardial effusion.
3. i. Pericardiocentesis.
   ii. Empirical antituberculous therapy with rifampicin, isoniazid and ethambutol. In patients of ethnic origin, or where multi-resistant bacilli are suspected, there is a case for adding pyrazinamide.
4. Contact tracing.

Causes of pericardial effusion

- Any infective pericarditis
- Uraemia
- Post myocardial infarction
- Post cardiotomy
- Dressler's syndrome
- SLE
- Rheumatoid arthritis
- Malignancy
- Hypothyroidism
- Trauma
- Aortic dissection
- Drugs, e.g. practolol, phenylbutazone, procainamide, hydralazine

The most likely underlying cause is TB, considering that the woman has a productive cough and the sputum, which is stained with the Ziehl–Neelsen stain, reveals acid-fast bacilli. In the UK, the incidence of TB in immigrants from the Asian subcontinent is 40 times higher than in the native white population. Primary TB is usually without symptoms in the majority of individuals, although in a few cases there may be a cough, wheeze and fever. The primary complex heals with calcification; however, there may be reactivation of infection several years later due to malnourishment or conditions predisposing to immunosuppression resulting in pulmonary TB and possible dissemination to other organs via the lymphatics and the bloodstream.

The diagnosis is based on identifying the organism from pericardial fluid. In the simplest form this may be done by staining the fluid with Ziehl–Neelsen to reveal acid-fast bacilli; however, the yield is only 25% with this method. The organism may be cultured on Lowenstein-Jensen medium but this can take over eight weeks. The quickest method of making the diagnosis in the event of a negative acid-fast stain is by PCR to tuberculous protein or by demonstrating evidence of the disease elsewhere, for example in the patient's sputum.

Treatment is with empirical antituberculous therapy. Because TB is spread from person to person, and effective tracing of close contacts helps limit spread of the disease, it is important to identify all individuals who may have come into close contact with the patient or those who share the same bathroom facilities. Individuals who are traced should have a chest X-ray and a tuberculin test. In adults, a normal chest X-ray positive test is a sign of immunity and nothing more needs to be done. In children who have not had a BCG vaccine, a positive tuberculin test is taken as evidence of infection, and treatment is instituted. If the test is negative, it is repeated again in six weeks and if remains negative the patient is given the BCG vaccine. In children under the age of one year who have a family member with TB, isoniazid is given as chemoprophylaxis for six months, together with immunization with a strain of BCG which is resistant to isoniazid.

Answer 167

1. i. Elevated right ventricular pressure.
   ii. Elevated pulmonary artery pressure.
   iii. Increase in oxygen saturation in the right ventricle, suggesting a left-to-right shunt at the level of the ventricle.
2. i. Huge increase in right ventricular pressure in the following five years.
   ii. Huge increase in pulmonary artery pressure in the following five years.
   iii. Reduction in oxygen saturation in the left ventricle, suggesting a right-to-left shunt at the level of the ventricles.

3. There has been a large increase in right ventricular pressure, leading to shunt reversal. The patient has developed Eisenmenger's phenomenon.

(See Interpretation of Cardiac Catheter Data, page 418.)

Question 168

A 45-year-old male was referred to the local psychiatrist by his GP with a three-month history of lethargy, loss of appetite, nausea, early morning wakening and loss of libido. He had recently lost his job as a clerk for making three serious errors in the space of a fortnight. There was no history of headaches or weight loss. He had experienced intermittent abdominal pain after meals which was investigated with upper gastrointestinal endoscopy four weeks earlier and attributed to a small gastric ulcer. Biopsy from the ulcer demonstrated an inflammatory infiltrate but there was no evidence of malignancy or *Helicobacter pyloris*. He had a long history of constipation which had not caused him any concern, and more recently complained of pains in his hands and feet. He was not sleeping well and awoke between two and three times a night to pass urine, which was extremely unusual for him. His wife was concerned that he was worried about loss of earnings and had become very depressed. He had no other significant past medical history. He was a non-smoker and consumed half a bottle of wine daily.

On examination, he had a reduced affect. There was no pallor, clubbing or lymphadenopathy. He was apyrexial. The heart rate was 96 beats/min and blood pressure 160/95 mmHg. Examination of his eye is shown (**168a**). On abdominal examination, a mass was identified in the right iliac fossa which was indentible. There was no tenderness and the bowel sounds were audible. A rectal examination was not performed. The examination of the cardiovascular and respiratory system was normal. He had painful hands, but there was no evidence of joint swelling or restriction of movements. Examination of his central nervous system, including his higher mental function was entirely normal.

Investigations are shown.

1. List two tests you would perform to come to a rapid diagnosis.
2. What is the definitive treatment?
3. How would you manage the patient after he has had the definitive treatment?

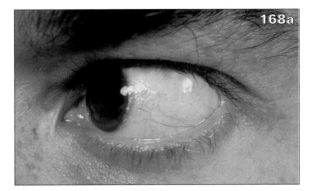

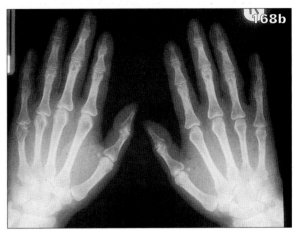

Hb	15 g/dl
WCC	5×10^9/l
Platelets	306×10^9/l
ESR	18 mm/h
Sodium	136 mmol/l
Potassium	4.2 mmol/l
Bicarbonate	19 mmol/l
Chloride	115 mmol/l
Urea	7 mmol/l
Creatinine	89 µmol/l
Bilirubin	12 µmol/l
AST	24 iu/l
Alkaline phosphatase	300 iu/l
Total protein	78 g/l
Albumin	44 g/l
X-ray of hands (**168b**)	

Answer 168

1. i. Serum calcium.
   ii. PTH level.
2. Parathyroidectomy.
3. Vitamin D supplements.

The symptoms of hypercalcaemia are rather non-specific, and include nausea, anorexia, weight loss, abdominal pain, bone pain, polyuria, polydipsia, lack of concentration, depression and occasionally acute psychosis. The abdominal pain may be non-specific or due to constipation, peptic ulcer disease, pancreatitis and renal colic, all of which are recognized complications of hyperparathyroidism. It is worth remembering that while nephrocalcinosis is also a complication of hyperparathyroidism, it is not associated with abdominal pain. This man has several of these symptoms, as well as recent peptic ulcer disease. The eye in **168a** reveals corneal calcification which occurs in hypercalcaemic states. The calcification is usually seen at the 3 and 9 o'clock positions. The hand X-ray (**168b**) demonstrates periosteal bone resorption which is characteristic of hyperparathyroidism. Hyperparathyroid-related bone disease is further supported by the raised alkaline phosphatase level. Bone changes are seen in 2% of cases of hyperparathyroidism. Cystic lesions may be present, and can result in pathological fractures. Extensive bone resorption affecting the skull gives it a characteristic 'salt-and-pepper' appearance on the skull X-ray.

Hyperparathyroidism is diagnosed by demonstrating elevated or normal levels of PTH in the presence of a high serum calcium. Primary hyperparathyroidism is usually secondary to a single, benign parathyroid adenoma. Hyperparathyroidism due to carcinoma of the parathyroid glands is extremely rare. Hyperparathyroidism can be part of MEN syndromes. Secondary hyperparathyroidism results from chronic calcium deficiency, and is a compensating mechanism whereby all four parathyroid glands undergo hyperplasia. In this situation, the calcium may be low or normal, but the PTH level is elevated. The condition is treated with vitamin D and calcium supplements. Tertiary hyperparathyroidism complicates some cases of secondary hyperparathyroidism where autonomous production of PTH occurs, leading to hypercalcaemia which is not controlled with vitamin D or calcium supplements. In this case, there is no underlying disorder to predispose to secondary or tertiary hyperparathyroidism, and so the most likely answer is primary hyperparathyroidism.

Other causes of hypercalcaemia are given below (*Table*). Myeloma is unlikely in the presence of a normal full blood count, ESR and globulin level. Sarcoidosis is associated with hypercalcaemia and band keratopathy, but is less likely in the presence of a normal chest X-ray. Moreover, it would not explain the X-ray changes in the hands. This patient is not taking regular antacids, which excludes the milk-alkali syndrome, a condition caused by chronic ingestion of calcium-based antacids and milk for the relief of dyspepsia or peptic ulcer disease. Metastatic bone disease is a possibility, but the majority of patients with bony metastases have overt metastatic deposits, particularly in areas where pain is experienced. In such cases, the albumin level is also low due to cachexia and the plasma bicarbonate is normal or high because bony destruction often releases bicarbonate from the bone. In hyperparathyroidism in the absence of renal disease, a mild metabolic acidosis is common. It is due to RTA and is reflected by a slightly low bicarbonate and a high chloride level.

In the past, other causes of hypercalcaemia – particularly malignancy – could be differentiated from hyperparathyroidism by the hydrocortisone suppression test, where high doses of hydrocortisone given daily for a week would fail to reduce the serum calcium level in hyperparathyroidism but not in other cases; however, the more sensitive PTH assays used nowadays have made this test obsolete.

Treatment of primary hyperparathyroidism is with total parathyroidectomy following transplantation of a small amount of parathyroid tissue into the forearm muscles. Following surgery, calcium levels have to be monitored because they fall rapidly and tetany can be precipitated. Hypocalcaemia can persist for several months during which time it is important to continue vitamin D supplements.

(See Calcium Biochemistry, page 415.)

Causes of hypercalcaemia	
1° hyperparathyroidism	Paget's disease (immobility)
3° hyperparathyroidism	Familial hypocalcuric hypercalcaemia
Sarcoidosis	
Multiple myeloma	
Thiazide diuretics	
Milk-alkali syndrome	
Addison's disease	
Acromegaly	
Phaeochromocytoma	
Thyrotoxicosis	
Vitamin D intoxication	

Question 169

A 44-year-old female was persuaded to come into hospital after she was seen in the out-patient clinic with jaundice. She was diagnosed as having auto-immune CAH five months ago and was successfully treated with high-dose steroids, which had gradually been withdrawn. She had not been taking any medication before admission and denied alcohol consumption. On examination, she was thin and deeply jaundiced. She was alert and orientated, and did not demonstrate any signs of cognitive impairment. Abdominal examination was essentially normal. Investigations on admission are shown. Two days following admission, the patient became suddenly very aggressive, and soon after collapsed and was comatosed.

Hb	12.3 g/dl
WCC	8×10^9/l
Platelets	45×10^9/l
MCV	109 fl
PT	59 s (control 13 s)
APTT	90 s (control 45 s)
Bilirubin	300 µmol/l
AST	350 iu/l
Alkaline phosphatase	340 iu/l
Albumin	26 g/l

Which urgent investigation would be most useful in determining the cause of collapse?
a. CT scan of the head.
b. EEG.
c. Drug screen for sedatives.
d. Blood cultures.
e. Blood glucose.

Question 170

This pedigree chart (**170**) is from a family with a very rare condition.

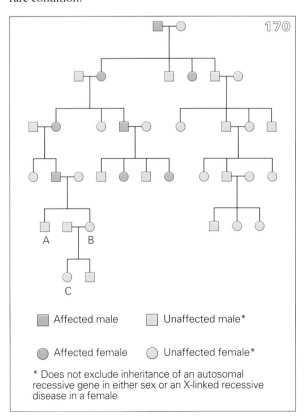

Affected male ☐ Unaffected male*

Affected female ◯ Unaffected female*

* Does not exclude inheritance of an autosomal recessive gene in either sex or an X-linked recessive disease in a female

1. What is the mode of inheritance?
a. Autosomal dominant.
b. Autosomal recessive.
c. X-linked dominant.
d. X-linked recessive.
e. Autosomal dominant with incomplete penetrance.

2. What are the chances of A being affected?
a. None.   d. 50%.
b. 100%.   e. 75%.
c. 25%.

3. What are the chances of B being affected?
a. None.   d. 50%.
b. 100%.   e. 75%.
c. 25%.

4. What are the chances of C being affected?
a. None.   d. 50%.
b. 100%.   e. 75%.
c. 25%.

Answer 169

> e. Blood glucose.

The patient was admitted with gross hepatic dysfunction. She had previously been successfully treated with corticosteroids, and had a relapse after they were gradually withdrawn. She became aggressive and then comatosed. The most probable diagnosis is hepatic encephalopathy. Precipitating factors include gastrointestinal haemorrhage, sepsis, hypokalaemia, drugs promoting catabolism, sedatives and hypoglycaemia. In hepatic encephalopathy it is possible for both hypoglycaemia and hyperglycaemia to occur because glucose homeostasis is disturbed. Glycogen is neither efficiently stored nor mobilized and gluconeogenesis is impaired. Early features of encephalopathy include confusion, irritation, aggressiveness or psychosis. Coma can ensue rapidly. The test which would be most useful in determining the cause of collapse is the serum blood glucose, because its correction and therapeutic effect are almost immediate. There is nothing in the history or examination to suggest sepsis, although it must be noted that patients with chronic liver disease do not always have a pyrexia. There is no history of sedative drug ingestion, and in practice screening for sedative drugs is unhelpful because it seldom influences the management. A cerebral haemorrhage is possible in the presence of a raised PT and low platelets. If the blood glucose is normal, a cerebral haemorrhage should be excluded by CT scanning of the head. If this is normal, the diagnosis is encephalopathy. An EEG is not necessary to diagnose encephalopathy, but at the onset of encephalopathy the EEG shows an alpha rhythm and as drowsiness worsens this is replaced by lower frequency theta activity. In deep coma, high-amplitude delta waves are present.

Answer 170

> 1. c. X-linked dominant.
> 2. a. None.
> 3. b. 100%.
> 4. d. 50%.

In X-linked conditions there is no male-to-male transmission. In X-linked dominant conditions, the female offspring of affected males have an abnormal phenotype, and in X-linked recessive conditions all female offspring are carriers but do not have the disease. In X-linked dominant conditions, an affected female will transmit the disorder to 50% of her daughters and 50% of her sons. In X-linked recessive conditions, an affected female will transmit the disease to 50% of her sons, and 50% of the daughters will be carriers, i.e. none will have the disease phenotype.

Examples of X-linked dominant conditions include vitamin D-resistant rickets, Rett's syndrome and incontinentia pigmentii.

Question 171

A 65-year-old male was admitted with a six-week history of progressive dyspnoea. One week before admission he had developed dyspnoea at rest, orthopnoea and paroxysmal nocturnal dyspnoea. He had lost his appetite, and had lost over 3 kg in weight in six weeks. He had a cough productive of yellow sputum initially which was treated with antibiotics; however, the cough persisted and three days before admission he had an episode of frank haemoptysis. The patient had enjoyed a very active and independent life and, apart from a truncal vagotomy and drainage procedure for a perforated duodenal ulcer 20 years ago, he had been very well. He was a non-smoker.

On examination, he appeared pale and was dyspnoeic. The heart rate was 144 beats/min and irregular; the blood pressure was 160/100 mmHg. The JVP was not raised. The respiratory rate was 30/min and temperature was 38°C (100.4°F). The heart sounds appeared normal; there were no audible murmurs. Auscultation of the lung fields revealed fine inspiratory crackles both anteriorly and posteriorly. Examination of the abdomen and central nervous system was normal.

A subclavian line was inserted which revealed a CVP of 3 cmH$_2$O. A urinary catheter drained a residual urine volume of 300 ml.

Investigations were as follows:

Hb	5.3 g/dl	Arterial blood gases (on 40% oxygen):	
WCC	17×10^9/l	pH	7.32
Platelets	249×10^9/l	PaCO$_2$	5.6 kPa
MCV	89 fl	PaO$_2$	14 kPa
MCHC	34 g/dl	Bicarbonate	14 mmol/l
ESR	102 mm/h	O$_2$ saturation	99%
Sodium	131 mmol/l	Blood cultures	No growth
Potassium	5.7 mmol/l	Urinalysis	Blood +++
Urea	29 mmol/l		Protein +++
Creatinine	560 μmol/l		Pus cells +++
Calcium	2.1 mmol/l		Granular casts +++
Phosphate	1.5 mmol/l		
Albumin	33 g/l	Urine culture	No growth
Bilirubin	14 μmol/l	ECG	Atrial fibrillation;
AST	19 iu/l		ventricular rate of 154/min
Alkaline phosphatase	113 iu/l		Non-specific T-wave
LDH	1320 iu/l		changes
Thyroid function tests	Normal	Chest X-ray (**171**)	
CRP	316 g/l	Echocardiogram	Biatrial enlargement
PT	12 s (control 12 s)		Mild left ventricular
APTT	43 s (control 41 s)		hypertrophy with good
Renal US	Normal-sized kidneys with		systolic function
	echogenic renal parenchyma		The mitral valve appeared
	No evidence of obstruction		normal

The patient was treated with intravenous cefuroxime and erythromycin, and gently transfused with 3 units of packed cells. The temperature came down, CVP increased to 9 cmH$_2$O, and urine output averaged 420 ml/24 h. The Hb following transfusion was 6.4 g/dl. While on the ward, the patient had three episodes of frank haemoptysis.

Serial chest X-rays over four days remained unchanged. He reverted to sinus rhythm three days after commencing digoxin.

Serum biochemistry on day four is shown.

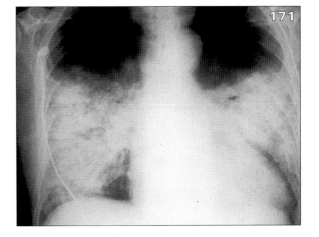

171

Sodium	131 mmol/l
Potassium	6.0 mmol/l
Urea	35 mmol/l
Creatinine	780 μmol/l

1. Describe the chest X-ray and give two possible pathological causes for this appearance.
2. List three possible diagnoses.
3. List at least four further tests which would be useful in confirming the diagnosis.
4. The patient was given 120 mg of intravenous furosemide, with no increase in urine output. What would be the next step in your management?

Answer 171

1. The chest X-ray reveals bilateral, widespread alveolar shadowing with sparing of the apices. Possible causes of alveolar shadowing on the chest X-ray include:
   i. Pulmonary oedema.
   ii. Pulmonary haemorrhage.
   iii. Pulmonary consolidation.
   In this case, pulmonary oedema is unlikely if the apices are spared, and this could only be explained if there was pre-existing, severe bilateral apical emphysema.

2. The patient has a relatively acute illness involving the respiratory and renal system. Possible cause of a systemic illness causing respiratory and renal impairment include:
   The vasculitides (in order of decreasing frequency):
   • Anti-GBM disease or Goodpasture's syndrome.
   • Polyarteritis nodosa.
   • Wegener's granulomatosis.
   • Systemic lupus erythematosus.

Infection:
   • Legionnaire's disease and secondary interstitial nephritis.
   • Pneumococcal pneumonia with mycotic emboli to the kidneys.

3. i. Anti-GBM antibodies.
   ii. ANCA.
   iii. Renal biopsy with immunofluoresence studies.
   iv. Transbronchial lung biopsy if the patient's respiratory status permits.
   v. Antinuclear factor.
   vi. *Legionella* antigen in the urine or *Legionella* RMAT on the serum.
   vii. TLCO.
4. Haemodialysis.

The history of continuing haemoptysis and failure of the haemoglobin to rise sufficiently after blood transfusion strongly suggest that the chest X-ray appearances are secondary to pulmonary haemorrhage rather than any other cause. The presence of normal-sized kidneys is suggestive of an acute renal process. In chronic renal disease, the kidney size is usually small, although there are a few exceptions (*Table A*). Pulmonary haemorrhage and acute renal failure are best explained by a systemic vasculitis. The best answers are, therefore, anti-GBM, polyarteritis nodosa or Wegener's granulomatosis in decreasing frequency. Anti-GBM disease is a rare condition where antibodies to the basement membrane of the glomeruli and alveoli lead to acute nephritis and pulmonary haemorrhage, respectively. The disease presents with cough, fatigue, dyspnoea or haemoptysis followed days, weeks or months later, by glomerulonephritis.

Wegener's granulomatosis would be the best answer if there was additional upper respiratory tract involvement. Although it is also possible, involvement of the upper respiratory tract is much more common in Wegener's than in any of the other vasculitides. SLE is rare in males and in this age group. Pulmonary haemorrhage is much less common in SLE than in the other vasculitides mentioned above. Although Legionnaire's disease is possible, there is no history of travel abroad or being in an environment with air conditioning, and it does not easily explain the pulmonary haemorrhage. Fever is a recognized feature of both infection and the vasculitides. The initial cough productive of yellow-brown sputum may have been secondary to a respiratory tract infection which is of interest because pulmonary haemorrhage is more common in anti-GBM disease if there has been a recent respiratory infection. Other factors predisposing to

Table A Causes of chronic renal impairment with normal-sized kidneys

• Myeloma
• Diabetes mellitus
• Amyloidosis
• Polycystic kidney disease (kidneys are usually huge by the time renal impairment becomes apparent)

pulmonary haemorrhage in anti-GBM disease are smoking, coexisting pulmonary oedema and exposure to organic solvents.

Other conditions which affect the respiratory and renal system include IgA nephritis, which occurs following upper respiratory tract infections. Respiratory involvement can occur as an indirect consequence of glomerulonephritis if the ensuing renal failure is complicated by fluid overload, producing pulmonary oedema. A rare situation where a primarily renal disorder affects the respiratory system to produce haemoptysis is renal vein thrombosis complicated by pulmonary embolism.

The tests should be based around making the most probable diagnosis where two or three diagnoses are possible. The presence of anti-GBM antibodies will make the diagnosis of anti-GBM disease, which can be confirmed on renal biopsy, and immunofluorescence studies which will demonstrate IgG deposits around the GBM. A lung biopsy would be dangerous in the presence of frank pulmonary haemorrhage. High titres of serum ANCA may support a vasculitic process, particularly if the anti-GBM antibody is absent. Again, a renal or lung biopsy with immunofluoresence should help make the final diagnosis. The TLCO is raised in pulmonary haemorrhage. It is useful in the assessment of haemorrhage in the acute situation because the chest X-ray appearance takes several days to improve, even if the haemorrhage has ceased. The causes of raised TLCO are listed (*Table B*).

If Legionnaire's disease is suspected, and a rapid diagnosis is required, the best tests are estimation of the *Legionella* antigen and the RMAT. *Legionella* antigen is present in the urine of 90% of patients within 48 hours. The RMAT can be performed on the serum and respiratory secretions, and a result is available on the same day. Testing for raised levels of *Legionella* antibodies is possible in this case because the disease has been present for a little while, but if the illness had started in the previous week then this test would not be useful in making a rapid diagnosis as it can take up to 10 days for the *Legionella* antibodies to rise appreciably.

The patient is oliguric, acidotic, has a rapidly rising creatinine, and has developed hyperkalaemia. Haemodialysis is indicated in all of these situations and when the patient shows evidence of fluid overload. It allows the opportunity for plasmapheresis, which is successful in some patients with anti-GBM disease, particularly with respect to pulmonary haemorrhage. However, results on the renal system are not very satisfactory if plasmapheresis is initiated after significant renal impairment has occurred. Subsequent management will be with high-dose steroids and cyclophosphamide.

Table B Causes of raised TLCO

- Pulmonary haemorrhage
- Polycythaemia
- Left-to-right shunts
- Asthma

Question 172

An 18-year-old male was admitted following a collapse at a local night club. On examination he was drowsy. His temperature was 40°C (104°F), and he was sweating profusely. His heart rate was 120 beats/min, and regular. The blood pressure was 160/110 mmHg. His pupils were dilated and reacted poorly to light.

Investigations are shown.

Hb	11 g/dl
WCC	11×10^9/l
Platelets	100×10^9/l
PT	20 s
APTT	70 s
TT	16 s
Sodium	125 mmol/l
Potassium	7.4 mmol/l
Urea	10 mmol/l
Creatinine	123 µmol/l
Phosphate	1.7 mmol/l
Urine	Blood +++

1. What is the underlying cause of his presentation?
2. Explain his serum potassium and phosphate levels.
3. What is the cause of his abnormal clotting?
4. List two therapeutic steps in the management of his temperature.
5. Give two explanations for the hyponatraemia.

Answer 172

1. 'Ecstasy' (3, 4-methylenedioxymetamphetamine; MDMA) abuse.
2. Rhabdomyolysis.
3. DIC.
4. i. Cooling/tepid sponging.
   ii. Intravenous dantrolene.
5. i. Syndrome of inappropriate antidiuretic hormone.
   ii. Excess sodium loss from skin during profuse perspiration.

The history is of collapse at a local night club, and on examination the patient has a very high temperature, is sweating profusely, has dilated pupils, and is hypertensive. The blood tests reveal evidence of renal failure with a disproportionately high potassium and phosphate, hinting that the patient may have rhabdomyolysis; the haematological tests suggest underlying DIC. In this case, the most probable diagnosis is Ecstasy abuse. The case would have been more difficult if he was hypotensive because then the differential diagnosis would have included septicaemia, encephalitis or meningitis, all of which must also be borne in mind when attending to a young patient with any of these features.

Ecstasy abuse has become an increasingly common problem over the past few years, and therefore knowledge of its recognition and management have become almost mandatory. The clinical features are basically those of a large concentration of circulating catecholamines in the blood. In the acute situation it may present as collapse, convulsions and hyperpyrexia, i.e. a core temperature of 39–42°C (102.2–107.6°F) (see *Table* for causes of hyperpyrexia). Other features comprise profuse sweating, tachycardia, hypertension and dilated pupils.

The blood pressure may also be low due to shock from excessive fluid loss secondary to perspiration. Complications of Ecstasy abuse include rhabdomyolysis, acute renal failure (either from reduced renal perfusion or myoglobin-induced tubular damage), DIC, acute hepatitis, myocardial infarction and cerebrovascular accident.

Hyponatraemia is a common problem and may be due to excess sodium loss from the skin during perspiration. The problem is compounded because most Ecstasy abusers are advised to drink large amounts of water which may replenish fluid, but not the actual salt loss. Furthermore, Ecstasy is thought to cause SIADH which may exacerbate the hyponatraemia. In some cases the sodium concentration may be low enough to precipitate cerebral oedema and intractable seizures.

The management of the patient involves cooling with tepid sponging, and rectal paracetamol. Intravenous dantrolene is useful in controlling the hyperpyrexia. Diazepam is effective in controlling seizures. Fluid replacement will depend on the sodium concentration and the CVP. The general rule is to administer 1 litre of saline to all patients with a high temperature and low blood pressure before inserting a central venous catheter, irrespective of the sodium concentration. If the blood pressure goes up and the heart rate comes down, this is followed by another litre. After this, any further fluid replacement is determined by the CVP and the sodium concentration. If the sodium is low and the CVP is low, the patient is infused with normal saline until the CVP is normal. Following this, the sodium and fluid intake and output is observed carefully and fluid restriction is instituted to help combat possible SIADH. In the patient where the sodium is low and the venous pressure is high/normal, fluid restriction is instituted for the same reasons; however, if the sodium is low enough to cause coma and seizures, then therapy is with mannitol or hypertonic saline and furosemide. In patients who are hypertensive on admission, fluid replacement should be guided by the CVP from the beginning, and all other rules are the same as those for patients who are hypotensive at presentation.

Causes of hyperpyrexia

- Septicaemia
- Viral infections
- Malaria
- Neuroleptic malignant syndrome
- Malignant hyperpyrexia
- Ecstasy or other amphetamine abuse
- Cocaine abuse
- Malignancy
- Aspirin toxicity
- Prostaglandins

Question 173

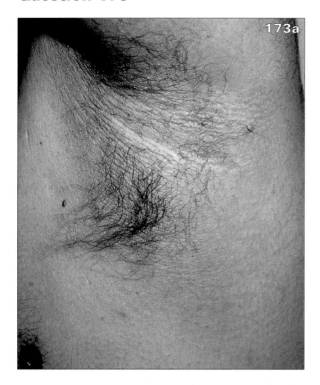

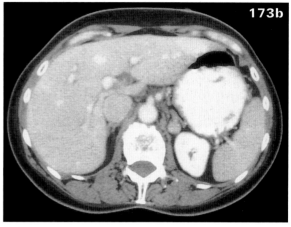

A 52-year-old male was investigated for obesity of recent onset, polydipsia and polyuria. On examination, he had a blood pressure of 180/105 mmHg, and was obese. Examination of the arm pit is shown (**173a**). He underwent routine investigations which are shown.

Hb	14 g/dl	
WCC	12×10^9/l	
Platelets	230×10^9/l	
Sodium	139 mmol/l	
Potassium	3.2 mmol/l	
Urea	7 mmol/l	
Bicarbonate	30 mmol/l	
Glucose	16 mmol/l	
Serum cortisol (nmol/l)	*9.00 a.m.*	*Midnight*
	940	1,000
After dexamethasone 2 mg q.i.d. for 48 h	900	800
Chest X-ray	Normal	
CT scan abdomen (**173b**)		

1. What is shown on inspection of this patient's arm pit?
2. Comment on the dexamethasone suppression test.
3. What is the differential diagnosis for the patient's presentation?
4. Which single biochemical test would you perform to confirm the diagnosis?
5. What is demonstrated on the CT scan of the abdomen?
6. Which other condition does the patient have?
7. What is the management of this patient?

Answer 173

1. The arm pit demonstrates acanthosis nigricans.
2. The high dose of dexamethasone fails to suppress the elevated cortisol down to normal.
3. The differential diagnosis is between ectopic ACTH and an autonomous glucocorticoid-secreting adrenal tumour (**173d**).
4. Plasma ACTH level, which will be elevated in ectopic ACTH secretion and suppressed in a cortisol-secreting tumour.
5. The CT scan demonstrates an adrenal tumour on the left side (see also detail, **173c**, arrowed).
6. Diabetes mellitus.
7. Surgical excision of the affected adrenal gland.

Acanthosis nigricans is characterized by velvety hyperpigmentation and overgrowth of skin affecting the neck, axilla, groin or the face. The condition may be a normal variant in the Asian race. It is associated with internal malignancy, particularly carcinoma of the stomach and the lung and lymphoma. It is also associated with a variety of endocrine disorders causing insulin resistance and hyperandrogenic states (*Table A*). In this case, it is due to Cushing's syndrome (*Table B*). Complications are shown in *Table C*.

The high-dose dexamethasone test suppresses the serum cortisol in over 60% of patients with Cushing's

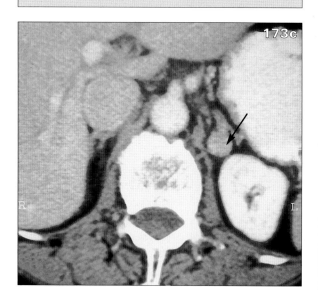

Table A Causes of acanthosis nigricans

- Normal variant (Asian race)
- Obesity
- Carcinoma stomach, lung
- Lymphoma
- Cushing's syndrome
- Acromegaly
- Insulin-resistant diabetes
- Polycystic ovary syndrome
- Androgen-secreting tumours

Table B Causes of Cushing's syndrome

- Pituitary basophil adenoma
- Ectopic ACTH secretion
- Adrenal adenoma
- Adrenal carcinoma
- Iatrogenic

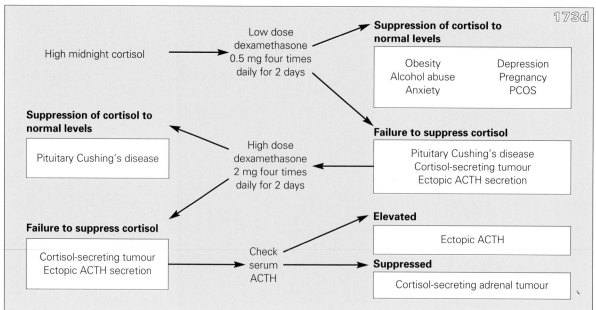

Table C Complications of Cushing's syndrome

- Obesity
- Diabetes mellitus
- Hypertension
- Premature coronary artery disease
- Osteoporosis

- Myopathy
- Psychosis
- Immunosuppression
- Poor wound healing
- Hypokalaemia

suppress. The serum cortisol in patients with autonomous glucocorticoid-secreting adenomas and those with ectopic ACTH production does not suppress to high-dose dexamethasone. In the normal clinical situation, the differential diagnosis between the three conditions, based on the dexamethasone suppression test, is not necessarily resolved; however, in the examination situation it is almost always assumed that suppression with high-dose dexamethasone excludes Cushing's syndrome.

Most tumours are benign; however, in rare instances adrenal carcinoma may result in Cushing's syndrome. Malignant tumours are highly aggressive and the prognosis is poor.

syndrome (bilateral hyperplasia of the adrenal glands due to autonomous production of ACTH by a pituitary basophil adenoma); however, nearly 40% of cases fail to

---

Question 174

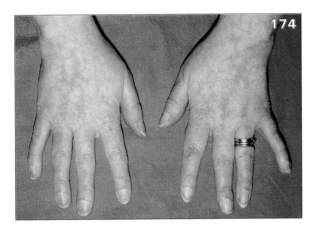

174

Hb	9.5 g/dl
WCC	15.1×10^9/l
Platelets	591×10^9/l
MCV	90 fl
ESR	104 mm/h
CRP	82 g/l
Sodium	136 mmol/l
Potassium	5.3 mmol/l
Urea	6.5 mmol/l
Creatinine	99 µmol/l
Calcium	2.31 mmol/l
Phosphate	0.9 mmol/l
Albumin	35 g/l
Bilirubin	7 µmol/l
AST	22 iu/l
Gamma GT	43 iu/l
Alkaline phosphatase	162 iu/l
Total protein	77 g/l
Glucose	5.4 mmol/l
ANF	Negative
Rheumatoid factor	Not detected
Immunoelectrophoresis	Polyclonal increase in gamma-globulin region. No paraprotein
Blood cultures × 6	No growth
Urinalysis	Blood ++. 24 hour urine protein 2.4g
Urine culture	Negative. AAFB not detected on early morning urine specimens
Chest X-ray	Normal

A 69-year-old male was referred with a five-month history of pains in his shoulders and thighs, night sweats and weight loss of approximately 3 kg. The pain was worse in the mornings and during episodes of the night sweats. Two months previously the patient was seen in the Accident and Emergency Department for ongoing testicular pain, but no obvious cause was found.

On examination, he appeared unwell and pale. He was apyrexial. There was no lymphadenopathy. His hands were examined (174). The heart rate was 104 beats/min and regular, and the blood pressure was 170/100 mmHg. The heart sounds were normal and the chest was clear. Abdominal examination was normal. On examination of the genitalia, there was testicular tenderness, but no swelling or erythema. There was no inguinal lymphadenopathy. Neurological examination demonstrated normal power, although hip extension was difficult due to painful quadriceps muscles. There was no fasciculation. Both ankle jerks, the left knee jerk and right supinator reflex were absent. There was loss of light touch sensation in both toes, extending to the medial border of the dorsal aspect of the left foot.

Investigations are shown.

1. Give at least two possible diagnoses.
2. List at least three useful investigations.

Answer 174

1. i. Polyarteritis nodosa.
   ii. Polymyalgia rheumatica.
   iii. Lymphoma.
   iv. Testicular seminoma.
   v. Post-primary TB.
2. i. Renal biopsy.
   ii. Skin biopsy.
   iii. Muscle biopsy may help in the differentiation of vasculitis from polymyalgia rheumatica.
   iv. Renal or hepatic angiography to demonstrate micro-aneurysms.
   v. Serum ANCA lends support to a vasculitic process.
   vi. CT scan thorax/abdomen to check for intra-abdominal malignancy, splenomegaly and para-aortic lymphadenopathy.
   vii. Ultrasound of the testes.
   viii. Bone marrow examination/culture for AAFB.
   ix. Mantoux test.

This is a case where several diagnoses are possible. The patient is in his seventh decade and has evidence of general malaise, night sweats, weight loss and myalgia, associated with a very high ESR (Table C). There is clinical evidence of peripheral neuropathy. The inflammatory markers are elevated and the possible differential diagnoses in an elderly patient includes PAN, malignancy (including lymphoma), PMR and sepsis. TB is a possibility; however, a completely normal chest X-ray makes post-primary infection less probable. The main differentials are PAN and PMR. Factors differentiating between PAN and PMR have been tabulated below (Table A). Neuropathy can only be explained by PAN. The slide reveals livedo reticularis, which is a skin manifestation associated with connective tissue disease and the vasculitides. It is due to random spasm of cutaneous arterioles and secondary dilatation of capillaries and venules. The presence of livedo reticularis favours the diagnosis of PAN, which is a non-granulomatous vasculitis affecting medium-sized arteries. It is more common in males, and is most prevalent in the sixth and seventh decades. It may manifest with myalgia, night sweats and weight loss, and is a recognized cause of pyrexia of unknown origin. The disorder can affect the kidneys, cardiovascular system, gastrointestinal tract and nervous system. Arteritis leads to aneurysm formation, with subsequent thrombosis and infarction of the supplied organs. Clinical features include progressive glomerulonephritis, myocardial infarction, mesenteric ischaemia, peripheral neuropathy, CVA and vasculitic areas affecting the skin. Testicular pain is a recognized manifestation of PAN (Table B).

Inflammatory markers are elevated. ANCA may be detected and lend support for a vasculitic process, but it is not specific for PAN. The diagnosis is made by biopsying the affected organ or demonstrating micro-aneurysms on angiography. Treatment is with steroids.

Table A Differentiation between PMR and PAN in this case

	PMR	PAN
Age	7th decade onwards	Middle age onwards
Sex	Male	Male
Symptoms	As above	As above
Neuropathy	Absent	Present
Testicular pain	Absent	Recognized
Livedo reticularis	Absent	Present
Raised ESR, CRP	Common	Common
Raised WCC, alkaline phosphatase	Common	Common
Raised ANF/Rh factor	Absent	Uncommon

Table B American College of Rheumatology criteria for PAN

- Weight loss of more than 4 kg
- Livedo reticularis
- Testicular pain
- Myalgia, leg tenderness
- Mono/polyneuropathy
- Hepatitis B sAg positive
- Arterographic abnormality
- Positive biopsy

Table C Causes of a very high (>100 mm/h) ESR

- Multiple myeloma
- Giant cell arteritis/polymyalgia rheumatica
- Sepsis
- Occult malignancy
- SLE

Question 175

A 45-year-old female on treatment for ulcerative colitis complained of increasing tiredness, while her bowel problems seemed well controlled.

Some of her results are shown.

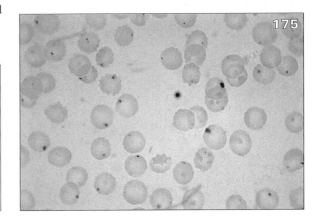

Hb	7.5 g/dl
MCV	95 fl
MCHC	34%
WCC	$10.5 \times 10^9/l$
Neutrophils	$8.4 \times 10^9/l$
Platelets	$290 \times 10^9/l$
Reticulocytes	9.8%
Blood film (**175**)	

1. What type of anaemia do these results suggest?
   a. Iron deficiency anaemia.
   b. Anaemia of chronic disease.
   c. Oxidative haemolytic anaemia.
   d. Immune haemolytic anaemia.
   e. Anaemia secondary to folic acid deficiency.

2. What is the likely cause?
   a. Azathioprine-induced folic acid deficiency.
   b. Chronic blood loss secondary to ulcerative colitis.
   c. Splenic atrophy.
   d. Septicaemia secondary to steroid-induced immunosuppression.
   e. Sulphasalazine-induced anaemia.

Question 176

A 26-year-old male presented to the Accident and Emergency Department with a stiff jaw and being unable to open his mouth. Three days previously he was immunized with tetanus toxin after lacerating his finger at work. On examination, he had evidence of 'lock jaw'. His injured finger was swollen, painful and exuding pus.

What is the immediate management?
   a. Debridement and cleansing of the wound.
   b. Injection of tetanus antitoxin into the wound.
   c. Oral penicillin V.
   d. Intramuscular human tetanus immunoglobulin.
   e. Intravenous pancuronium.

Answer 175

> 1. c. Oxidative haemolytic anaemia.
> 2. e. Sulphasalazine-induced anaemia.

The patient has a low Hb and a high reticulocyte count, suggesting either haemolysis or recent blood loss. The blood film is diagnostic. It is stained with methyl violet to reveal small inclusions within red cells termed Heinz bodies, which are essentially precipitated Hb. These inclusion bodies are visualized with methyl violet stain. They occur in patients with genetic Hb abnormalities (unstable Hb), or when the iron within the haem molecule is oxidized from the ferrous state (Fe^{2+}) to the ferric state (Fe^{3+}) to produce methaemoglobin. Causes of methaemoglobinaemia are discussed in Answer 316. In this case, therapy for ulcerative colitis with sulphasalazine (sulphonamide) is the culprit. Patients taking sulphonamides may develop a chronic haemolytic anaemia owing to the oxidative action of the drugs on the Hb. Haemolysis is particularly severe in patients with glucose-6-phosphate dehydrogenase deficiency. Management involves drug withdrawal; however, if this is not possible then a lower dosage should be prescribed, together with iron and folate supplements. Azathioprine is not associated with oxidative haemolytic anaemia. Splenic atrophy is also associated with inclusions within red cells termed Howell–Jolly bodies, which represent particles of denatured DNA. They are visible when the blood film is stained with Wright's stain. In contrast, Heinz bodies cannot be seen when stained with Wright's stain because they are the same colour as the red cell.

Answer 176

> 1. d. Intramuscular human tetanus immunoglobulin.

Tetanus is caused by the anaerobic, Gram-positive bacillus *Clostridium tetani*. The organism produces spores that are commonly found in soil and faeces of domestic animals. Soil is the natural habitat for *C. tetani*. The organism gains entry into the body through traumatic wounds, where it multiplies under anaerobic conditions and produces tetanospasmin, a potent neurotoxin. The toxin reaches the spinal cord via the blood or by retrograde axon transport and increases excitability in motor neurones by interfering with the function of inhibitory neurones. The toxin may also produce overactivity of the sympathetic nervous system. The incubation period after injury is less than 14 days and can be as early as 2 days.

The dominant features of tetanus are rigidity and reflex spasms. Rigidity may affect any muscle, including the jaw muscles, so the mouth cannot be fully opened, as in this case. This is known as 'trismus' or 'lock jaw'. Stiffness may affect the facial muscles, altering facial appearance. Risus sardonicus (pursing of the lips with retraction of the angles of the mouth) is a characteristic feature of this phenomenon. Pharyngeal involvement may produce dysphagia early in the disease. Rigidity of the muscles of the back causes the body to curve back excessively with the head fully retracted (ophisthotonus). Reflex spasms are a sudden exacerbation of underlying rigidity which last 1–2 seconds. The time of onset of spasms from the first symptoms of rigidity is known as the 'period time'. This is usually within 72 hours. The shorter the period time, the worse the prognosis. Large groups of muscles are affected at any one time. Relaxation may take a few seconds, which is particularly hazardous when thoracic muscles are involved because respiration is impeded until relaxation of the muscles occurs. Laryngeal spasm is probably the most dangerous event in tetanus.

Autonomic overactivity has effects on the cardiovascular system. Tachycardia, massive swings in blood pressure and cardiac arrhythmias are recognized complications. Haemodynamic instability may produce hypoperfusion of vital organs leading to multi-system failure and death. Most deaths are from respiratory failure, either due to laryngeal spasms, respiratory muscle fatigue and paralysis or pulmonary aspiration.

The mainstay of treatment in an affected individual is to give intramuscular human immunoglobulin immediately. Human immunoglobulin will remove circulating tetanospasmin from the blood. Fixed neurotoxin has to be removed from the wound by aggressive cleansing and, if necessary, by surgical debridement of the wound. Despite such measures the organism may not be entirely removed from the wound and added protection with intravenous penicillin is mandatory. Diazepam is useful in controlling spasms. In severe cases total paralysis with curarization (using intravenous pancuronium) and artificial ventilatory support are necessary to reduce mortality from respiratory failure.

Prevention is by active immunization and meticulous wound cleansing as soon as possible after trauma.

Question 177

A 33-year-old Indian male presented with a four-week history of a painful swollen knee, which he attributed to a fall during a game of tennis. The knee was painful after the fall, but over the next two weeks he developed swelling and increasing pain which was only partially relieved by paracetamol. He had never had a similar problem in the past. Apart from feeling slightly more breathless than usual while playing tennis over the past three months, he had no other complaints. There was no significant family history except that his grandparents had both had TB. He could not ever recall having had a BCG vaccine, but did have several chest X-rays in his early teenage years. On examination, he appeared well. He had a temperature of 37.5°C (99.5°F). Examination of his upper arms did not reveal a BCG scar. Examination of the left knee demonstrated a painful erythematous joint with a large synovial effusion. On examination of the respiratory system there were some harsh breath sounds in anterior aspect of the chest. The attending rheumatologist requested some investigations, which are shown.

On the basis of these investigations, the patient was commenced on empirical antituberculous therapy. He was reviewed four months later and had an ESR check, which measured 57 mm/h. The swelling in the left knee had subsided, but the changes on the chest X-ray persisted. Six months later he presented to the Accident and Emergency Department with swelling in his right knee and both ankles. In addition, he complained of pain in the cervical area and lower back pain that radiated into the buttocks and was worse in the mornings.

1. What is the diagnosis?
2. How would you explain the changes on the chest X-ray?
3. Give two diagnostic tests.
4. Apart from diagnostic tests, which other investigation would you perform to help his further management?
5. What is the management of his condition?

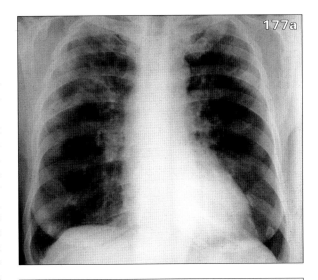

177a

Hb	12 g/dl
WCC	7×10^9/l
Platelets	308×10^9/l
ESR	107 mm/h
Chest X-ray (**177a**)	
Rheumatoid factor	Negative
X-ray of left knee	Soft-tissue swelling
	No bony involvement
Aspirate of knee joint	Yellow fluid; low viscosity; WCC 50/mm³; culture sterile
Synovial biopsy	Thickened synovium macroscopically with histological evidence ofincreased inflammatory infiltrate

Answer 177

1. Ankylosing spondylitis.
2. Bilateral apical fibrosis.
3. i. X-ray of the sacroiliac joints, which will demonstrate sacroiliitis and may demonstrate squaring of the lumbar vertebrae with thickening and calcification of the interspinous ligaments.
   ii. HLA typing for B27; however, one must remember that this is found in 5% of the general population.
4. Respiratory function tests given the history of breathlessness on exertion and the lung fibrosis.
5. NSAID and physiotherapy.

While the inflamed knee joint in association with the abnormal chest X-ray may be highly suggestive of TB in an Asian patient, the failure to improve with anti-tuberculous therapy is against this diagnosis. In a young male with a synovitis of the knee joint followed by pain in the ankle joints and in the lumbar and cervical area, the differential diagnosis is between rheumatoid arthritis, adult Still's disease and a seronegative arthropathy, particularly ankylosing spondylitis. The absence of the rheumatoid factor is against the diagnosis of rheumatoid arthritis. Still's disease is not sufficient to explain the chest X-ray abnormalities, which in this case are due to apical fibrosis (**177a**) (*Table A* lists other causes), a well-recognized complication of ankylosing spondylitis. Other complications of ankylosing spondylitis are listed below (*Table B*). In addition, there is an increased incidence of scleritis and scleromalacia.

Ankylosing spondylitis is a chronic inflammatory disorder that predominantly affects the spinal joints. It is strongly associated with the presence of HLA B27, which is present in 95% of all cases, and the disease is more prevalent in males in their second and third decades. The exact aetiology of the disorder is unknown. Most patients present with a sacroiliitis causing back pain and stiffness, which is worse in the mornings (*Table C*). There is a characteristic loss of lumbar lordosis and a reduced ability to flex the spine. An asymmetric peripheral large joint arthropathy may be the presenting feature in some patients – as in this case. Enthesopathy causes pain in the tendons, particularly the Achilles tendon. Weight loss, low-grade fever and high inflammatory markers in the blood are recognized. Extra-articular complications occur in approximately 15% of patients. The diagnosis is a clinical one, but is helped by the demonstration of sacroiliitis on the X-ray of the pelvis and the demonstration of thickening and calcification of the interspinous ligament, which may give the appearance of a bamboo spine (**177b**).

Table A Causes of apical lung fibrosis

- TB
- Extrinsic allergic alveolitis
- Ankylosing spondylitis
- Allergic bronchopulmonary aspergillosis
- Radiation
- Sarcoidosis
- Histiocytosis X

Table C Causes of sacroiliitis

- Ankylosing spondylitis
- Reiter's syndrome
- Psoriatic arthropathy
- Enteropathic arthritis (inflammatory bowel disease)
- Whipple's disease
- Osteoarthritis

Table B Ankylosing spondylitis is easily remembered as the 'A' disease

- Arthritis
- Atlano axial subluxation
- Arachnoiditis (spinal)
- Apical fibrosis
- Anterior uveitis
- Aortitis
- Aortic regurgitation
- Atrioventricular block
- Amyloidosis
- IgA nephropathy
- Achilles tendinitis
- Plantar fAsciitis

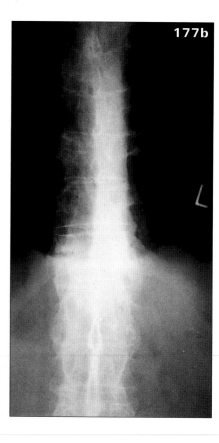

177b

Question 178

A 21-year-old female developed a sudden left hemiparesis followed by loss of vision in her left eye 24 hours afterwards. For three months she had felt generally listless, experienced frequent night sweats and had lost 4 kg in weight. Over the past two weeks she had become breathless on exertion and could not sleep unless she was propped up on three pillows. She lost consciousness on two occasions and was seen in the local Accident and Emergency Department with a suspected epileptic seizure three days earlier, but was not admitted. The medical officer had arranged an out-patient appointment with a cardiologist because he had heard an interesting murmur. The patient had enjoyed a healthy life before this illness and had never travelled abroad.

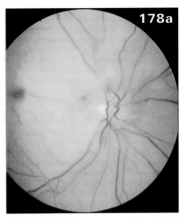

On examination, she was unwell. The temperature was 37.6°C (99.7°F). She had a heart rate of 110 beats/min, which was regular, and the blood pressure was 90/60 mmHg. The JVP was elevated 4 cm above the sternal angle. The cardiac apex was not displaced. On auscultation, the heart sounds were normal but there was a soft mid-diastolic murmur in the mitral area, as well as a mitral regurgitant murmur. Auscultation of the lung fields revealed fine inspiratory crackles at both lung bases. Neurological examination demonstrated a left hemiparesis. The speech was intact. Examination of the left fundus is shown (**178a**). Investigations are shown.

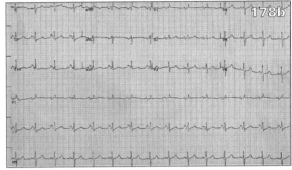

Hb	10 g/dl
WCC	8×10^9/l
Platelets	360×10^9/l
ESR	90 mm/h
Sodium	135 mmol/l
Potassium	4.1 mmol/l
Urea	8 mmol/l
Glucose	5 mmol/l
ECG (**178b**)	
Chest X-ray	Cardiac silhouette slightly enlarged Upper lobe vein distension and bibasal interstitial lung shadowing

1. What is the diagnosis?
   a. Mitral valve endocarditis.
   b. Left atrial myxoma.
   c. Systemic lupus erythematosus.
   d. Polyarteritis nodosa.
   e. Sarcoidosis.

2. What investigation is required to confirm the diagnosis?
   a. Serial blood cultures.
   b. Serum ANCA.
   c. Double stranded DNA antibodies.
   d. Coronary angiography.
   e. Echocardiography.

Question 179

A 15-year-old male is admitted for parathyroidectomy. His father had a parathyroidectomy 20 years previously.

Pre-operative blood and post-operative blood (two months later) results are shown.

Pre-operative:	Calcium	2.8 mmol/l
	Phosphate	0.8 mmol/l
	Albumin	44 g/l
	PTH	40 ng/l
Post-operative:	Calcium	2.9 mmol/l
	Phosphate	0.9 mmol/l
	Albumin	43 g/l
	PTH	Undetectable

1. What is the diagnosis?
2. How would you confirm the diagnosis?

Answer 178

> 1. b. Left atrial myxoma.
> 2. e. Echocardiography.

The patient presents with a fever, systemic illness, a murmur and retinal artery occlusion. The differential diagnosis is between atrial myxoma and endocarditis affecting a stenosed mitral valve. Both may present in identical fashion and may be associated with left atrial enlargement and right ventricular hypertrophy, as seen on the 12-lead ECG. In this particular case mitral stenosis is less likely for three main reasons: (i) there is no past history of rheumatic fever to account for mitral stenosis (congenital mitral stenosis is rare and would have presented at a much younger age); (ii) endocarditis is rare in mitral stenosis owing to the low pressure proximal to the valve surface; and (iii) it is unusual for a patient with mitral stenosis to be in sinus rhythm in the presence of symptomatic mitral stenosis. Left atrial myxoma (**178c**) would explain the dyspnoea, constitutional upset, fever, cardiac signs and the cerebral emboli.

Atrial myxomata are the most common tumours of the heart, with 75% being found in the left atrium. The tumours are benign and characteristically attached to the fossa ovalis by a pedicle. They are highly mobile and prolapse to and fro through the mitral valve orifice. The movement through the valve produces an added sound in diastole known as a 'tumour plop', which sounds like a third heart sound, and a mid-diastolic murmur, which

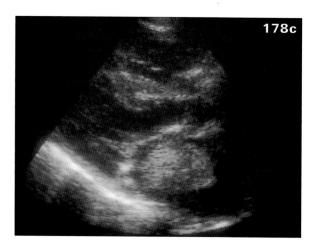

178c

may be confused with mitral stenosis. However, third heart sounds do not occur in mitral stenosis. Breathlessness owing to increased left atrial pressure is common. Mechanical obstruction of the mitral valve orifice may cause syncope or even sudden death. Constitutional upset and pyrexia are common, as are raised inflammatory markers and hypergamma-globulinaemia. Haemolysis is also recognized. Systemic emboli from the gelatinous tumour may complicate atrial myxoma. Arrhythmias, including atrial fibrillation, are uncommon. The diagnosis is made by echocardiography and the management is surgical excision.

Answer 179

> 1. Familial benign hypocalcuric hypercalcaemia.
> 2. 24-hour urinary calcium estimation or a urinary calcium clearance to creatinine clearance (CaCl/CrCl) ratio.

Familial benign hypocalcuric hypercalcaemia is an autosomal dominant disorder which is characterized by life-long, asymptomatic hypercalcaemia. However, some patients develop acute pancreatitis, gallstones and chondrocalcinosis. The abnormality is in the calcium-sensing receptor, a G-protein-coupled receptor. It may be difficult to distinguish from primary hyperparathyroidism, and in 20% of cases the PTH is mildly elevated. The serum phosphate values are usually normal or slightly reduced. In contrast to other causes of hypercalcaemia, the 24-hour urinary calcium is reduced; 75% of patients have values <2.5 mmol/l, and 95% have values <5 mmol/l. The serum calcium level may vary from mild elevation to marked hypercalcaemia with values exceeding 3.5 mmol/l. The CaCl/CrCl ratio can be used to improve differentiation between hyperparathyroidism and familial benign hypocalcuric hypercalcaemia:

$$CaCl/CrCl = Ur_{Ca} \times P\,Cr/P\,Ca \times Ur_{Cr}$$

Some 80% of patients with familial benign hypocalcuric hypercalcaemia have a ratio of <0.01, whereas more than 70% of those with primary hyperparathyroidism have values above this cut-off.

The management is conservative.

Question 180

A 43-year-old male was admitted with a 2-hour history of malaise and nausea. A 12-lead ECG revealed an acute inferior myocardial infarction and third degree AV block. He had type 1 diabetes mellitus. The heart rate at rest was 34 beats/min. The blood pressure was 80/50 mmHg. Both heart sounds were normal. A temporary pacing wire was inserted via the right superficial femoral vein and the patient was successfully paced. The BP improved to 90/60 mmHg.

Blood results were as follows:

Hb	13 g/dl
WCC	17×10^9/l
Platelets	380×10^9/l
Sodium	140 mmol/l
Potassium	4.2 mmol/l
Urea	8 mmol/l
Creatinine	126 μmol/l
Glucose	17 mmol/l

What is the next management step?
   a. IV heparin.
   b. IV recombinant tissue plasminogen activator.
   c. IV metoprolol.
   d. IV streptokinase.
   e. IV glyceryl trinitrate.

Question 181

A 16-year-old female was investigated for lethargy and polyuria. Her blood pressure measured 116/70 mmHg. Investigations are shown.

What is the diagnosis?
   a. Laxative abuse.
   b. Addison's disease.
   c. Thiazide diuretic abuse.
   d. Self-induced vomiting.
   e. Bartter's syndrome.

Hb	13 g/dl
WCC	7×10^9/l
Platelets	300×10^9/l
Sodium	129 mmol/l
Potassium	3.0 mmol/l
Urea	7 mmol/l
Creatinine	80 μmol/l
Bicarbonate	33 mol/l
Calcium	2.0 mmol/l
Phosphate	1.3 mmol/l
Albumin	40 g/l
Glucose	4 mmol/l
24-hour urinalysis:	
Sodium	30 mmol/l (<20 mmol/l in hyponatraemia)
Potassium	40 mmol/l (<10 mmo/l in presence of hypokalaemia)
Calcium	10.6 mmol (NR <7.5 mmol/24h)
Chloride	42 mmol/l (NR <25 mmol/l)
Serum renin	960 pmol/l (NR 100–500 pmol/l)

Answer 180

> b. IV recombinant tissue plasminogen activator.

There is good evidence that the patient should either undergo primary coronary angioplasty or receive thrombolysis to reduce his immediate risk of sudden death. The angioplasty option is not provided, therefore the candidate is left to decide between streptokinase and recombinant TPA. Streptokinase carries the risk of an allergic/anaphylactic reaction, which may compromise the blood pressure further. Streptokinase should be used with caution in a patient with hypotension. Recombinant TPA is not usually associated with such reactions and is marginally superior to streptokinase in achieving vessel patency.

Answer 181

> E. Bartter's syndrome.

The patient has hypokalaemia and metabolic alkalosis associated with a normal blood pressure. The differential diagnosis is between self-induced vomiting, chronic thiazide diuretic use (or abuse) and Bartter's syndrome. Although laxative abuse can also be associated with hyponatraemia and hypokalaemia, most patients who abuse laxatives have a metabolic acidosis rather than alkalosis (loss of bicarbonate via the gastrointestinal tract). Addison's disease is usually associated with hypotension, hyperkalaemia, reduced potassium excretion in the urine and metabolic acidosis.

The differentiation between thiazide drug abuse, self-induced vomiting and Bartter's syndrome is dependent upon the history and the urinary electrolytes. Patients who lose sodium or potassium via the gastrointestinal tract usually have low urinary sodium (<10 mmol/l) and potassium (<20 mmol/l) levels. The patient in question has inappropriately high urinary sodium and potassium, indicating primary renal tubular dysfunction or lack of mineralocorticoid. Mineralocorticoid deficiency is characterized by low serum sodium, high serum potassium and metabolic acidosis.

The remaining differential diagnosis is between thiazide diuretic abuse and Bartter's syndrome. Thiazides may cause all of the biochemical abnormalities in the blood shown in the question. Raised plasma renin is due to hypovolaemia or hyponatraemia. Furthermore thiazides are also associated with high urine sodium, potassium and chloride levels. However, urinary calcium is low in patients taking thiazide diuretics since thiazides increase absorption of calcium in the distal convoluted tubule. Chronic frusemide abuse can cause a metabolic syndrome identical to Bartter's syndrome. Unlike thiazide diuretics, loop diuretics promote calcium excretion by the kidneys by inhibiting sodium re-absorption in the loop of Henle.

Bartter's syndrome is a rare syndrome with a characteristic set of metabolic abnormalities that include hypokalaemia, metabolic acidosis, hyponatraemia, hyperaldosteronism, and hyperplasia of the juxta-glomerular apparatus (source of renin in the kidney). Most cases present early in life and may be associated with short stature and mental retardation. The condition is due to abnormal sodium concentration ability in the loop of Henle. This results in increased sodium and chloride excretion via the kidney. The resulting hyponatraemia that is associated with hyperreninaemia and hyperaldosteronism causes hypokalaemia and metabolic alkalosis. Because urinary calcium reabsorption in the loop of Henle is dependent on sodium absorption, urinary calcium excretion is also increased. Similarly magnesium reabsorption is impaired and may result in hypomagnesaemia. Urinary calcium is typically >40 mmol/l. In relation to the differential diagnosis above, self-induced vomiting is associated with low urinary calcium levels (<25 mmol/l).

Prostaglandin levels are raised in Bartter's syndrome, which may explain why these patients are normotensive. Treatment is aimed at minimizing the effects of prostaglandins and aldosterone. Non-steroidal anti-inflammatory drugs and high dose spironolactone or amiloride are the drugs of choice. Magnesium supplements may also be required in those patients with hypomagnesaemia.

Question 182

A 60-year-old obese male was referred to a gastroenterologist with a 4-month history of right upper quadrant pain and abnormal liver function tests. He did not have nausea, vomiting or steatorrhoea. He consumed 24 units of alcohol per week. He had an 8-year history of non-insulin-dependent diabetes mellitus and had been diagnosed as having hypertension 1 year previously. He had chronic pain in both knees that was attributed to osteoarthritis.

On examination he was obese. He measured 1.8 m and weighed 105 kg. He was not jaundiced and there were no peripheral stigmata of chronic liver disease. The heart rate was 70 beats/min and regular. The blood pressure measured 150/90 mmHg. Both heart sounds were normal and the chest was clear. Abdominal examination revealed a palpable liver edge 4 cm below the costal margin. The spleen was not palpable.

Investigations are shown.

Hb	14 g/dl
WCC	6×10^9/l
Platelets	200×10^9/l
Sodium	36 mmol/l
Potassium	4.1 mmol/l
Urea	6 mmol/l
Creatinine	100 μmol/l
AST	60 iu/l
ALT	78 iu/l
Alkaline phosphatase	180 iu/l
Bilirubin	12 μmol/l
Albumin	38 g/l
Total cholesterol	7.2 mmol/l
Triglyceride	6.1 mmol/l
Blood glucose	13 mmol/l
Serum ferritin	400 μg/l
Serum iron	20 μmol/l
TIBC	60 μmol/l
IgG	22 g/l
IgA	4.8 g/l
IgM	3.1 g/l
Hep B sAg	Not detected
HCV antibodies	Not detected

What is the most probable diagnosis?
  a. Autoimmune hepatitis.
  b. Non-alcoholic steatohepatitis.
  c. Primary biliary cirrhosis.
  d. Haemochromatosis.
  e. Wilson's disease.

Question 183

This is a chest X-ray (**183**) of a 70-year-old Indian female who presented with dyspnoea and a low-grade fever.

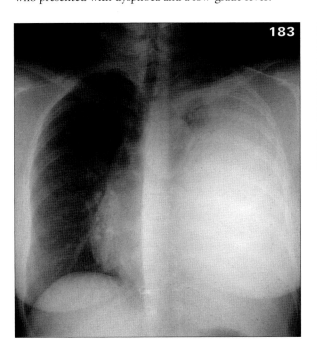

What is the next most important management step?
  a. Commence IV cefuroxime and oral clarithromycin.
  b. Arrange urgent bronchoscopy.
  c. Commence antituberculous treatment.
  d. Aspirate left-sided pleural effusion and send fluid for microscopy and culture.
  e. Start intravenous diuretics.

Answer 182

> b. Non-alcoholic steatohepatitis.

The patient is obese. He has non-insulin-dependent diabetes mellitus, hypertension and mixed hyperlipidaemia. The findings are compatible with insulin resistance or metabolic syndrome. Additionally, the patient has right upper quadrant pain, hepatomegaly and a transaminitis in the absence of alcohol abuse, specific drug therapy or hepatitis B or C infection. The most probable diagnosis is non-alcoholic steatohepatitis.

NASH is associated with obesity and the metabolic syndrome. It is characterized by fatty infiltration of the liver associated with hepatitis or even cirrhosis in the absence of alcohol abuse, specific drug therapy (amiodarone, tamoxifen, oestrogens) or chronic viral hepatitis. Liver biopsy is identical to alcoholic hepatitis. Both AST and ALT are raised. The AST/ALT ratio is usually <1, unlike in alcohol abuse where the ratio is usually >2. Alkaline phosphatase is only modestly raised but hyperbilirubinaemia is rare. Serum ferritin is raised as in certain other chronic liver disorders such as alcohol abuse and chronic viral hepatitis. The diagnosis of NASH is confirmed by liver biopsy (*Table*). Patients with alcohol abuse or chronic hepatitis B/C infection should not be diagnosed as having NASH. Other differential diagnoses are tabulated below.

The condition is more common in females. Most patients present with abnormal liver function tests although malaise and right upper quadrant pain are recognized presenting features. Hepatomegaly is common. Insulin resistance is thought to play a primary role in NASH.

The prognosis is relatively benign although some patients, particularly elderly diabetic females, may develop cirrhosis. There is no specific treatment but gradual weight loss has been shown to improve liver function. The role of insulin sensitizing drugs such as metformin is not well established. Treatment with $\beta 1$ cannabanoid receptor blockers appears promising.

Differential diagnosis of NASH

Condition	Differentiating features*
Alcohol-related liver disease	History of alcohol abuse/AST:ALT >2
Chronic viral hepatitis (B or C)	Virology
Auto-immune hepatitis	Autoantibody screen shows raised SMA or ANA
	Hypergammaglobulinaemia is also a feature
Primary biliary cirrhosis	Predominant cholestasis on blood tests and positive antimitochondrial antibodies
Haemochromatosis	Serum TIBC >90%; ferritin >300
Primary sclerosing cholangitis	History of inflammatory bowel disease
	Predominantly cholestatic picture
	Hypergammaglobulinaemia
Drugs	History

*In the absence of liver biopsy

Answer 183

> d. Aspirate left-sided pleural effusion and send fluid for microscopy and culture.

There is a large area of opacification affecting the left lung without any visible lung markings, and marked mediastinal shift to the right. The diagnosis is consistent with a large pleural effusion. Given her ethnicity it is possible that this may represent a tuberculous pleural effusion, although a malignant pleural effusion cannot be excluded by the history. The next management step would be to perform a diagnostic/therapeutic pleural aspirate before starting any antibiotic treatment.

Question 184

A 24-year-old man presented with sudden onset of palpitations while walking to work. He had no past medical history of note. He consumed two units of alcohol per day. He did not smoke or abuse illicit drugs.

Hb	15 g/dl
WCC	5 × 10⁹/l
Sodium	138 mmol/l
Potassium	3.8 mmol/l
Blood glucose	4.2 mmol/l
Serum TSH	2 mu/l
ECG	Atrial fibrillation with a ventricular rate of 132 beats/min but no other abnormality
Chest X-ray	Normal
Echocardiogram	Normal study

On examination his heart rate was 132 beats/min and irregular. The blood pressure measured 105/70 mmHg. Both heart sounds were normal and his chest was clear.

Investigations are shown.

What is the most effective drug in restoring sinus rhythm quickly in this patient?
  a. IV digoxin.
  b. IV flecanide infusion.
  c. IV esmolol.
  d. Oral sotalol.
  e. IV amiodarone.

Question 185

An 18-year-old male navy cadet presented with a 2-day history of headache, fever and sore throat. On examination he was noted to have cervical lymphadenopathy. His heart rate was 80 beats/min and BP was 170/100 mmHg. There was a soft systolic murmur at the left lower sternal edge, which did not radiate. All other examination was normal.

Investigations are shown.

Hb	13.6 g/dl
WCC	12.0 × 10⁹/l
Platelets	180 × 10⁹/l
ESR	36 mm/h
Sodium	136 mmol/l
Potassium	4.8 mmol/l
Urea	7.3mmol/l
Creatinine	143 μmol/l
Blood cultures	No growth
Throat swab culture	No growth
Urinalysis	10–20 rbc ++, granular casts, no growth

He was treated with antibiotics for one week and he made an unremarkable recovery. Review in the outpatients clinic following this revealed the following results:

Hb	14.1 g/dl
WCC	8.2 × 10⁹/l
Platelets	191 × 10⁹/l
Sodium	136 mmol/l
Potassium	4.1 mmol/l
Urea	5.1 mmol/l
Creatinine	92 μmol/l
ANA and ds DNA binding	Negative
Urinalysis	Blood ++ Protein ++

What diagnosis would you consider most likely?
  a. Post-streptococcal glomerulonephritis.
  b. Berger's nephritis.
  c. Infective endocarditis.
  d. Henoch–Schönlein purpura.
  e. Focal segmental glomerulonephritis.

Answer 184

> b. IV flecanide infusion.

The patient has atrial fibrillation (AF) that is definitely less than 48 hours in duration. In such patients sinus rhythm can be safely restored immediately without prior anticoagulation if the patient does not have left ventricular dysfunction or rheumatic mitral valve disease (see below).

In patients with haemodynamic embarrassment due to atrial fibrillation with a rapid ventricular rate the treatment of choice is urgent electrical cardioversion, as it is more effective than pharmacological therapy at restoring sinus rhythm.

In patients who are haemodynamically stable and do not have dilated cardiomyopathy or suspicion of rheumatic mitral valve disease, either electrical cardioversion or anti-arrhythmic drugs may be used to restore sinus rhythm. The drugs commonly used are class I and class III anti-arrhythmic agents. The class III anti-arrhythmic agents commonly used are sotalol and amiodarone. Recent evidence suggests that sotalol is not superior to conventional beta-blockers at restoring sinus rhythm. Amiodarone is not as effective as some of the class I anti-arrhythmic drugs and should be reserved for use in patients with underlying cardiomyopathy.

Commonly used class I anti-arrhythmic agents used to restore sinus rhythm in atrial fibrillation include flecanide, propafenone and dofetilide. Of these, flecanide is the most effective agent at restoring sinus rhythm early and is effective in 72–95% of cases. Flecanide is avoided in patients who have any form of cardiomyopathy or have atrial fibrillation in the context of a myocardial infarction.

Digoxin is not effective at restoring sinus rhythm, but plays an important role in controlling ventricular rate when given with beta-blockers or calcium antagonists with AV nodal blocking properties such as verapamil or diltiazem. Beta-blockers are less effective than flecanide at restoring sinus rhythm.

Anticoagulation in atrial fibrillation

Patients with AF associated with haemodynamic collapse should have electrical cardioversion irrespective of prior anticoagulation. Patients with stable AF of <48 hours duration may undergo electrical or pharmacological cardioversion without prior anticoagulation if they do not have any evidence of left ventricular dysfunction or rheumatic mitral valve disease on echocardiography. Patients with left ventricular dysfunction or rheumatic mitral valve disease should have TOE prior to restoring sinus rhythm.

Patients who have been in stable atrial fibrillation for >48 hours should undergo transoesophageal echocardiography to exclude thrombus in the left atrial appendage before restoring sinus rhythm. If a thrombus is identified, the patient should be anticoagulated for at least three weeks, following which a TOE should be repeated to ensure resolution of thrombus before attempting restoration of sinus rhythm. In the absence of transoesophageal echocardiography the patient should be anticoagulated for at least three weeks before safely attempting to restore sinus rhythm.

After successful restoration of sinus rhythm the patients should continue anticoagulation for four weeks. Anticoagulation may be stopped after four weeks if the patient remains in sinus rhythm and does not have risk factors for further episodes of atrial fibrillation (such as left ventricular dysfunction or rheumatic mitral valve disease). Patients who have suffered prior systemic thrombo-embolism secondary to AF should continue anticoagulation despite restoration of sinus rhythm, as one cannot predict if the patient will revert to atrial fibrillation.

Answer 185

> b. Berger's nephritis.

There is a short history of upper respiratory tract infection with transient deterioration in renal function and persistent proteinuria and microscopic haematuria. The most probable diagnosis is Berger's nephritis (IgA nephritis). The history is not long enough for classic post-streptococcal glomerulonephritis, which usually occurs 10–14 days after the initial respiratory infection. Apart from the nephritis there is nothing to suggest Henoch–Schönlein vasculitis such as a rash, arthralgia or abdominal symptoms. Although there is a soft murmur at the lower sternal edge, the preceding symptoms of an upper respiratory tract infection favour IgA nephritis rather than nephritis complicating infective endocarditis. Treatment is not usually required.

Proteinuria exceeding 1g per 24 hours or the persistence of haematuria would be an indication for renal biopsy to exclude another cause of nephritis.

Patients with chronic proteinuria following IgA nephropathy should receive ACE inhibitors or AIIRBs. There is some evidence currently that the addition of an AIIRB to ACE inhibitor provides additional antiproteinuric effects. The blood pressure should be managed aggressively. Steroids and other immuno-suppressive therapy are reserved for patients with nephritic syndrome or an active and persistent nephritis.

Apart from being secondary to viral illness, IgA nephritis has also been associated with cirrhosis of the liver, coeliac disease, HIV infection, certain bacterial infections (*Staphylococcus aureus*) and Wegener's granulomatosis. A familial form of IgA nephritis is also recognized.

Question 186

A 45-year-old man was involved in a motorbike accident resulting in a fractured femur. He underwent internal fixation of the hip. While in theatre the temperature rose to 39°C (102.2°F). The heart rate was 140 beats/min. There was evidence of hypertonia. Blood results were as follows:

Arterial blood gases:	
pH	7.3
PCO$_2$	6.2 kPa
PO$_2$	12 kPa
Bicarbonate	18 mmo/l
Sodium	136 mmol/l
Potassium	7.1 mmol/l
Urea	7 mmol/l
Creatinine	130 μmol/l

What is the immediate management step?
a. Stop anaesthesia.
b. IV dantrolene.
c. Haemodialysis.
d. IV bromocryptine.
e. IV calcium gluconate.

Question 187

A 70-year-old male who presented with anterior chest wall pain had a chest X-ray (**187**).

What is the diagnosis?
a. Cannon ball metastases.
b. Multiple myeloma.
c. Bony metastases.
d. Left lower lobe collapse.
e. Fractured ribs on the right side.

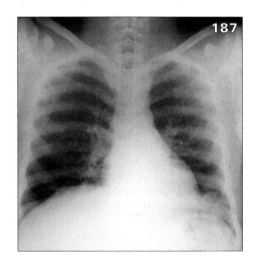

Question 188

A 69-year-old woman attended her GP complaining of lethargy and pruritis. She also complained of difficulty on climbing stairs because she felt her thighs could not carry her. She had always led a very healthy lifestyle and was not taking any medications. On examination she appeared slightly icteric and had xanthelasma. There were several scratch marks on the skin. The heart rate, temperature and blood pressure were normal. The liver was palpable 3 cm below the costal margin and the spleen could just be felt. There was no evidence of lymphadenopathy.

Investigations are shown.

Hb	11 g/dl
WCC	6 × 10^9/l
Platelets	120 × 10^9/l
Sodium	133 mmol/l
Potassium	4.1 mmol/l
Urea	3 mmol/l
Creatinine	110 μmol/l
Bilirubin	56 mmol/l
AST	58 iu/l
Alkaline phosphatase	230 iu/l
Total protein	70 g/l
Albumin	32 g/l

Give two explanations for the raised alkaline phosphatase.
a. Cholestasis.
b. Haemolysis.
c. Bony metastases.
d. Hypothyroidism.
e. Osteomalacia.
f. Osteoporosis.
g. Hepatic metastases.
h. Choriocarcinoma.
i. Paget's disease.
j. Hepatitis.

Answer 186

a. Stop anaesthesia.

Hyperpyrexia, hypertonia and hyperkalaemia during anaesthesia raise the possibility of malignant hyperpyrexia.

Malignant hyperthermia is a rare genetic disorder, which manifests following treatment with anaesthetic agents, most commonly succinylcholine and halothane. The onset of malignant hyperthermia is usually within one hour of the administration of general anaesthesia but rarely may be delayed as long as 11 hours. 50% of cases are inherited in an autosomal dominant fashion. Susceptible patients with autosomal dominant disease have any one of eight distinct mutations in the ryanodine receptor calcium channel receptor found in the sarcoplasmic reticulum of skeletal muscle.

In the presence of anaesthetic agents, alterations in the hydrophilic, amino-terminal portion of the ryanodine receptor result in uncontrolled efflux of calcium from the sarcoplasmic reticulum with subsequent tetany, increased skeletal muscle metabolism, and heat production.

Early clinical findings in malignant hyperthermia include muscle rigidity (especially masseter stiffness), sinus tachycardia, increased CO_2 production, and skin cyanosis with mottling. Marked hyperthermia (up to 45°C [113°F]) occurs minutes to hours later; core body temperature tends to rise 1°C every 5 to 60 minutes. Hypotension, complex dysrhythmias, rhabdomyolysis, electrolyte abnormalities, disseminated intravascular coagulation, and mixed acidosis commonly accompany the elevated temperature. Rectal temperature should be determined in all patients. Abnormalities of vital signs in severe hyperthermia include sinus tachycardia, tachypnoea, a widened pulse pressure, and hypotension.

The diagnosis of malignant hyperthermia can be confirmed by an *in vitro* muscle contracture test following recovery from the acute hyperthermic episode. Abnormal augmentation of *in vitro* muscle contraction following treatment with halothane or caffeine is diagnostic of the disorder.

Management of malignant hyperthermia requires immediate cessation of any triggering anaesthetic agent, ensuring adequate airway, breathing, and circulation; initiation of rapid cooling; and treatment of complications such as DIC and rhabdomyolysis. Alpha-adrenergic agonists should be avoided, since the resultant vasoconstriction decreases heat dissipation. Continuous core temperature monitoring with a rectal or oesophageal probe is mandatory, and cooling measures should be stopped once a temperature of 39.5°C (103°F) has been achieved.

Dantrolene administration is the mainstay of treatment of malignant hyperthermia, and should be initiated as soon as the diagnosis is suspected. Since the introduction of dantrolene, the mortality of the fulminant syndrome has fallen from close to 70% to less than 10%. Dantrolene is a non-specific skeletal muscle relaxant that acts by blocking the release of calcium from the sarcoplasmic reticulum. This, in turn, decreases the myoplasmic concentration of free calcium and diminishes the myocyte hypermetabolism that causes clinical symptoms. The drug is most effective when given early in the illness (i.e. before hyperthermia occurs), when maximal calcium can be retained within the sarcoplasmic reticulum.

Although the patient also has dangerous hyperkalaemia and would normally also receive intravenous calcium gluconate to reduce the risk of cardiac arrest, the priority is to stop the causal anaesthetic agent first.

Answer 187

c. Bony metastases.

The chest X-ray shows multiple sclerotic areas affecting the ribs. These areas are characterized by loss of distinction between the cortex and the medulla. The commonest cause of sclerotic metastases in a male patient is carcinoma of the prostate.

Answer 188

a. Cholestasis.
e. Osteomalacia.

The patient has primary biliary cirrhosis. Vitamin D deficiency is a well recognised complication.

Question 189

A 66-year-old white female slipped and fell on an icy walkway. When seen in the Accident and Emergency Department she complained of pain in the left hip. Her left leg was shortened and externally rotated. X-rays confirmed a diagnosis of fractured neck of the femur, for which she underwent arthroplasty. Two days after surgery, she complained of difficulty breathing. On examination her heart rate was 110 beats/min, respiratory rate was 20/min, and BP was 90/50 mmHg. The JVP was elevated and there was a right parasternal heave. Auscultation revealed a gallop rhythm and loud P2. She had a fever of 38.5°C (101.3°F). Inspection of the trunk revealed reddish-brown non-palpable petechiae. There were also subconjunctival and oral haemorrhages and petechiae. ECG showed sinus tachycardia. CXR showed diffuse bilateral pulmonary infiltrates. Investigations are shown.

Arterial blood gases:

PaO_2	8 kPa
$PaCO_2$	4 kPa
pH	7.55
Haemoglobin	8.0 g/dl
MCV	80 fl
WCC	11×10^9/l
Platelets	100×10^9/l
Fibrinogen	0.95 g/l (NR 2–4 g/l)

What is the most likely diagnosis?
 a. Meningitis.
 b. Pulmonary embolism.
 c. Fat embolism.
 d. Subacute bacterial endocarditis.
 e. Endotoxic shock.

Question 190

A 30-year-old woman with a history of epilepsy since childhood was 12 weeks pregnant. Her epilepsy had been very well controlled on carbamazepine 200 mg tds and she had been completely free from epileptic seizures for eight years.

What is the best management of her seizures during pregnancy?
 a. Continue with the current dose of carbamazepine.
 b. Stop the carbamazepine.
 c. Halve the dose of carbamazepine.
 d. Switch to sodium valproate.
 e. Switch to phenytoin.

Question 191

A 26-year-old female patient developed severe abdominal pain and vomiting. The haemoglobin on admission was 9.6 g/dl. A blood film is shown (**191**).

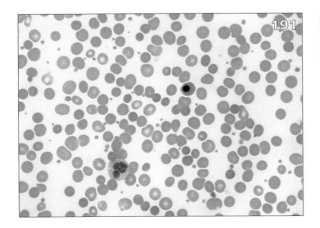

What is the cause of her abdominal pain?
 a. Biliary colic.
 b. Small bowel obstruction.
 c. Lead poisoning.
 d. Haemolytic uraemic syndrome.
 e. Mesenteric ischaemia.

Answer 189

> c. Fat embolism.

Fat embolism is a clinical diagnosis. In many patients the diagnosis is missed owing to subclinical illness or confounding injury or illness. Mortality rate is 10–20%. It is usually caused by trauma to a long bone or the pelvis, including orthopaedic procedures, as well as parenteral lipid infusion or recent corticosteroid administration (*Table*).

Early persistent tachycardia may herald the onset of the syndrome. Patients become tachypnoeic, dyspnoeic and hypoxic owing to ventilation–perfusion abnormalities 12–72 hours after the initial injury. A high fever is common. Between 20 and 50% of patients develop reddish-brown non-palpable petechiae over the upper body, particularly in the maxillae, within 24–36 hours of insult or injury; these resolve quickly. The presence of petechiae in this setting is virtually diagnostic of fat embolism. Subconjunctival and oral haemorrhages are also recognized.

Central nervous system dysfunction initially manifests as agitated delirium but may progress to stupor, seizures, or coma and frequently is unresponsive to correction of hypoxia. Retinal haemorrhages with intra-arterial fat globules are visible upon fundoscopic examination.

Arterial blood gas shows an otherwise unexplained increase in pulmonary shunt fraction alveolar-to-arterial oxygen tension difference.

Thrombocytopenia, anaemia, and hypofibrino-genaemia are indicative of fat embolism syndrome; however, they are non-specific.

Serial chest X-rays reveal increasing diffuse bilateral pulmonary infiltrates within 24–48 hours of the onset of clinical findings. Nuclear medicine ventilation–perfusion imaging of the lungs may be normal or may demonstrate subsegmental perfusion defects.

Medical care is supportive in nature and includes maintenance of adequate oxygenation and ventilation, stable haemodynamics, blood products as clinically indicated, hydration, prophylaxis of deep venous thrombosis and stress-related gastrointestinal bleeding, and adequate nutrition.

Causes of fat embolism

- Blunt trauma (associated with 90% of FES cases)
- Acute pancreatitis
- Diabetes mellitus
- Burns
- Joint reconstruction
- Liposuction
- Cardiopulmonary bypass
- Decompression sickness
- Parenteral lipid infusion
- Sickle cell crisis

Answer 190

> a. Continue with the current dose of carbamazepine.

Most anticonvulsant drugs have teratogenic properties. However, in patients with epilepsy the benefits of treatment with anticonvulsant drugs outweigh the risks of teratogenicity, and anticonvulsant therapy is continued. The risk of teratogenicity is reduced if the treatment of epilepsy is limited to a single drug in pregnancy.

Neural tube defects are probably the most serious teratogenic effect of anticonvulsants and are particularly important in patients taking carbamazepine, oxycarbamazepine, phenytoin and valproate. The risk of neural tube defects may be reduced by folic acid supplements. Pregnant females taking anticonvulsant medications should be advised to take folic acid supplements before and during pregnancy.

Women with epilepsy wishing to become pregnant should be informed of the potential consequences of anticonvulsant medications on the foetus. Women who are already pregnant should be counselled and offered antenatal screening with alpha-fetoprotein measurements and second-trimester foetal ultrasound scan.

Answer 191

> a. Biliary colic.

The blood film shows numerous spherocytes (red cells without the central punched out doughnut ring). The presence of more than 50% spherocytes on the blood film is highly suggestive of hereditary spherocytosis. Patients with hereditary spherocytosis have chronic haemolysis and are prone to pigment gallstones at a young age. The commonest complications of gallstones are biliary colic, cholecystitis and pancreatitis.

Question 192

A 20-year-old woman gave birth to a full term baby who was floppy at birth and required resuscitation followed by assisted ventilation. The mother had ptosis, muscle weakness and bilateral cataracts. Her father also had premature cataracts.

What is the baby's diagnosis?
a. Galactosaemia.
b. Hypoparathyroidism.
c. Hypothyroidism.
d. Myasthenia gravis.
e. Myotonic dystrophy.

Question 193

A 29-year-old Tanzanian woman presented with a one-week history of increasing dyspnoea, orthopnoea and paroxysmal nocturnal dyspnoea. She had undergone a Caesarean section for an uncomplicated twin pregnancy two weeks previously. This was her first pregnancy. The blood pressure throughout the pregnancy was normal. The first trimester was complicated by hyperemesis, which resolved spontaneously. The patient had noticed increasing dyspnoea and swollen ankles just prior to delivery but attributed this to her advanced pregnant state.

A murmur was heard on routine examination in the second trimester, which was investigated with a 12-lead ECG and echocardiogram that were both reported as normal. There was no family history of cardiac disease.

On examination the pulse was 120/min and regular. The temperature was 37.2°C (99.0°F). The blood pressure measured 100/60 mmHg. The JVP was raised. Palpation of the precordium revealed a displaced and prominent apex. On auscultation both heart sounds were normal. In addition there was a systolic murmur of mitral regurgitation and a third heart sound. Auscultation of the lungs revealed inspiratory crackles at both bases.

Investigations are shown.

Hb	10.8 g/dl
WCC	13 × 10⁹/l
Platelets	368 × 10⁹/l
ESR	38 mm/h
CRP	13 g/l
CXR	Pulmonary oedema
12-lead ECG (**193a**)	
Echocardiogram	Dilated left ventricle with globally impaired systolic function
	Ejection fraction 35%
	Mitral regurgitation
	No obvious vegetations on the valves
Blood cultures	Awaited
Arterial blood gases:	
pH	7.38
PaCO₂	4.3 kPa
PaO₂	7.3 kPa
Bicarbonate	25 mmol/l

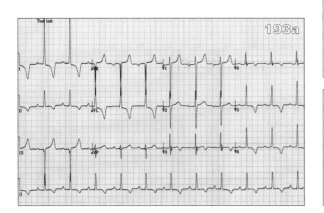

What is the most probable diagnosis?
a. Idiopathic dilated cardiomyopathy.
b. Infective endocarditis.
c. Forward output heart failure due to anaemia.
d. Viral myocarditis.
e. Peri-partum cardiomyopathy.

Answer 192

> e. Myotonic dystrophy.

The mother has ptosis, muscle weakness and bilateral cataracts indicating that she has myotonic dystrophy. Her baby is also affected. Whereas the classical form of dystrophia myotonica presents in adolescence or young adulthood, babies born to mothers with dystrophia myotonica may have the manifesting features of myotonic dystrophy at birth, i.e. hypotonia and respiratory muscle weakness.

Dystrophia myotonica is inherited as an autosomal dominant trait. The condition is due to mutation comprising a triple nucleotide repeat (CTG) expansion in the gene encoding a serine threonine protein kinase on chromosome 19. Another locus on chromosome 3 comprising a CCGT repeat has also been identified.

Affected individuals usually present with myotonia with subsequent progressive muscle weakness and wasting affecting the face, neck and distal limb muscles. Cataracts, frontal balding, diabetes due to insulin resistance, cardiac conduction tissue disease, cardiomyopathy, hypogonadism and low intelligence are also recognized features.

The severity of the condition appears to be related to the number of triple nucleotide repeats. The higher the number or repeats the more severe the manifestations. There can be further amplification of the triple nucleotide repeats in successive generations, resulting in increased disease severity in future generations (genetic amplification). Myotonia is treated primarily with mexiletine, although phenytoin, procainamide and carbamazepine and quinine have also been used. Weakness is treated with mechanical devices.

Answer 193

> e. Peri-partum cardiomyopathy.

The patient presents with pulmonary oedema in the puerperium associated with systolic heart failure. She had previously documented normal LV function and there is no obvious cause for her heart failure other than pregnancy. Although she has a low-grade fever and a murmur of mitral regurgitation, the CRP is not high enough to indicate overwhelming sepsis, and the echocardiogram does not show any vegetations or valve dysfunction as would be expected in this situation.

Peri-partum cardiomyopathy affects 1 in 3,000 live-birth pregnancies. The aetiology is unknown but the condition is much more common in African women. Other predisposing factors include advanced age, multiple pregnancy, multi-parity and a history of hypertension in pregnancy. The condition presents in the last month of pregnancy or within five months post delivery, whereas females with idiopathic dilated cardiomyopathy present in the second trimester when the burden of volume overload is greatest (**193b**).

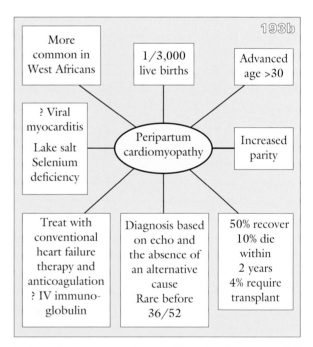

Diagnosis requires the following four criteria:
1. Presentation in the last month or within five months of delivery.
2. Absence of an obvious cause for heart failure.
3. Previously normal cardiac status.
4. Echocardiographic evidence of systolic left ventricular dysfunction.

The patient fulfils all four criteria. The ECG may show multiple abnormalities that include voltage criteria for left ventricular hypertrophy and ST/T wave abnormalities, as in this case. There are no symptoms of myocardial ischaemia as expected in a thrombotic myocardial infarction that may rarely complicate pregnancy.

The management is with conventional heart failure therapy. ACE inhibitors should be avoided during pregnancy. Patients with very dilated or poorly contracting left ventricles should be anticoagulated, as the risk of intramural thrombus is high in peripartum cardio-myopathy. The prognosis is guarded with up to 25% of females dying in the first three months. Approximately 50% recover full cardiac function within six months. Around 5% of females require cardiac transplantation. Future pregnancies should be avoided in females who have not recovered normal cardiac size and function.

Questions 194 and 195

Symbol definitions

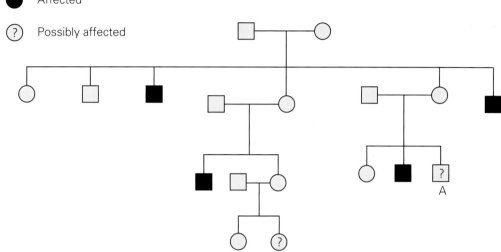

□	○	Clear
■	●	Affected
?	?	Possibly affected

Question 194

What are the chances of A being affected?
- a. None.
- b. 100%.
- c. 50%.
- d. 25%.
- e. 12.5%.

Question 195

What are the chances of B being a carrier?
- a. None.
- b. 100%.
- c. 50%.
- d. 25%.
- e. 12.5%.

Question 196

A 60-year-old female, who was diagnosed as having rheumatoid arthritis eight years previously, presented with a two-month history of progressive dyspnoea. She was on a non-steroidal agent and methotrexate for control of her rheumatoid arthritis. There was no history of cough productive of sputum.

On examination her heart rate was 80 beats/min and regular. Her blood pressure measured 106/68 mmHg. The JVP was not raised. Both heart sounds were normal and the chest was clear. The oxygen saturation on air was 96% but desaturated to 85% after walking for two minutes. The chest X-ray was normal.

What investigation would you perform first to investigate the cause of her breathlessness?
- a. Pulmonary function tests.
- b. Ventilation/perfusion scan.
- c. Bronchial washings for *Pneumocystis jerovecii*.
- d. High-resolution CT scan.
- e. Echocardiogram.

Answers 194 and 195

Answer 194
c. 50%.

Answer 195
d. 25%.

This is a family pedigree with an X-linked recessive condition. The mother of A in generation 2 is a definite carrier as his brother is affected. Since females pass the

abnormal X-chromosome to 50% of all their children there is a 50% chance that A will have the disease. (A cannot be a carrier as this is an X-linked condition.) The grandmother of B (see generation 2) is a definite carrier as her son is affected (generation 3). Therefore there is a 50% (or a 1/2) chance of B's mother being a carrier. The chances of B being a carrier are 1/2 × 1/2 since a carrier female will only pass the abnormal gene to half of all her offspring. B will not be affected, as this is an X-linked recessive condition.

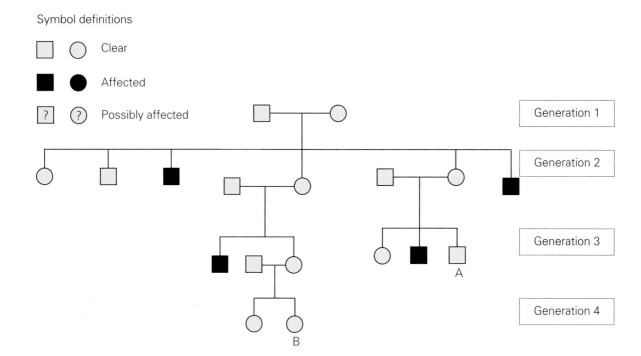

Answer 196

b. Ventilation/perfusion scan.

This is a difficult question. Progressive dyspnoea and oxygen desaturation during exercise in patients with rheumatoid arthritis are suggestive of pulmonary fibrosis. However multiple pulmonary emboli may also present in a similar fashion. The presence of sharp chest pains does not differentiate small pulmonary emboli from pulmonary fibrosis due to rheumatoid arthritis because sharp chest pain is common to both. The absence of inspiratory crackles and a normal chest X-ray are not characteristic of

rheumatoid lung disease such as pulmonary fibrosis and obliterative bronchiolitis, respectively. While it is still possible that the patient's symptoms are related directly to rheumatoid arthritis or the treatment of rheumatoid arthritis, the diagnosis of pulmonary embolism should be considered. Therefore the first investigation in a patient presenting in this fashion is a ventilation/perfusion scan or a CT pulmonary angiography. The identification and treatment of pulmonary embolism should prevent further pulmonary emboli. The absence of fever is against the diagnosis of *Pneumocystis jerovecii* pneumonia.

Question 197

A 57-year-old woman presented with a six-hour history of severe central chest pain. The 12-lead ECG revealed ST elevation in the antero-lateral leads. Apart from a history of a perforated duodenal ulcer requiring surgery five weeks previously, there was no other past medical history of significance.

What would be the most effective treatment in the management of this patient?
  a. Aspirin and IV heparin.
  b. IV tenectoplase.
  c. Aspirin and beta-blocker.
  d. Aspirin, clopidogrel and heparin.
  e. Primary coronary angioplasty.

Question 198

A 50-year-old West African woman was admitted to hospital with a 48-hour history of generalized headache and dyspnoea at rest. The patient had a cough productive of white frothy sputum. There was no history of fever, haemoptysis or drowsiness. The patient had been treated for hypertension for five years; blood pressure control over the past two years had been satisfactory. She was known to have mild asthma that was usually precipitated by cold weather. She had Raynaud's disease that was controlled with nifedipine and had recently been referred to a gastroenterologist for investigation of difficulty in swallowing. Current medications included nifedipine SR 20 mg bd and ranitidine 150 mg bd.

On examination she appeared unwell. Her temperature was 36.8°C (98.2°F) and her heart rate was 110 beats/min and regular. The blood pressure was 220/130 mmHg. The JVP was not raised. On examination of the precordium, the apex was not displaced. Auscultation revealed normal heart sounds and an added fourth heart sound at the apex. The respiratory rate was 28/min. Auscultation of the lungs revealed bibasal inspiratory crackles. The ankles were mildly swollen. Neurological examination was normal with the exception of the fundi, which revealed grade hard exudates, cotton wool spots and flame-shaped haemorrhages.

Investigations are shown.

Hb	11 g/dl
WCC	11 × 109/l
Platelets	100 × 109/l
Blood film	Shistocytes
	Microspherocytes
Sodium	138 mmol/l
Potassium	4.8 mmol/l
Urea	28 mmol/l
Creatinine	490 µmol/l
ECG	Left ventricular hypertrophy
Chest X-ray	Bilateral basal alveolar shadows
	and small pleural effusions
Urinalysis	Protein ++
	Blood 0

What is the best treatment for her hypertension?
  a. Prednisolone.
  b. IV nitroprusside.
  c. Plasma exchange.
  d. ACE inhibitor.
  e. Labetolol.

Answer 197

e. Primary coronary angioplasty.

The patient's chest pain and ST elevation in the anterior leads are consistent with the diagnosis of acute anterior myocardial infarction. The usual treatment would be to thrombolyse the patient. However, the patient does have a major contraindication as she had major surgery only five weeks previously (*Table*). The safest and most effective therapy in this situation would be to perform coronary angiography with a view to primary angioplasty. Patients who undergo primary angioplasty are usually given intravenous abciximab (which itself may promote haemorrhage) to reduce the risk of acute stent occlusion; however, the drug would be used with great caution in a patient who had recently had major surgery.

While aspirin and heparin have been shown to reduce mortality in acute myocardial infarction, they are not as effective as thrombolysis or angioplasty.

Contraindications for thrombolysis

Absolute contraindications for thrombolysis
- Aortic dissection
- Cerebral haemorrhage (ever)
- Intracranial neoplasm
- Active severe bleeding at time of presentation

Major contraindications
- CVA (embolic) within three months
- Major surgery within three months
- INR more than 4 in patient taking warfarin or equivalent

Relative contraindications
- Pregnancy
- Uncontrolled hypertension
- Concomitant use of anticoagulant drugs
- Active peptic ulcer disease

Answer 198

d. ACE inhibitor.

The patient has a history of well-controlled hypertension and then presents with headache and breathlessness. The presence of grade III hypertensive retinopathy and pulmonary oedema in association with severe hypertension is consistent with the development of accelerated or malignant hypertension.

While there are potentially several conditions associated with malignant hypertension – such as renal artery stenosis, hypertensive nephrosclerosis, haemolytic uraemic syndrome, anti-phospholipid syndrome – the presence of Raynaud's syndrome and possible oesophageal problems is highly suggestive of systemic sclerosis. In the context of this history the micro-angiopathic haemolytic blood picture reflects malignant hypertension rather than haemolytic uraemic syndrome or a vasculitis.

Renal disease is frequently present in patients with scleroderma. Up to 80% of patients have renal disease and 50% actually have signs of renal problems, e.g. abnormal electrolytes, hypertension and proteinuria. Around 10% of patients develop scleroderma renal crisis owing to fibrinoid necrosis within the interlobular arteries and the glomeruli. It is characterized by acute renal failure, abrupt onset of hypertension or sudden acceleration of otherwise mild hypertension. Proteinuria is common but haematuria is not a feature.

Risk factors for the development of sclerodrema renal crisis include diffuse skin involvement in association with the scleroderma, use of corticosteroids, cool weather and black race.

Blood pressure control is the mainstay of treatment. ACE inhibitors are the drugs of choice and lead to BP improvement in up to 90% of patients by inhibiting angiotensin II mediated vasoconstriction. ACE inhibitors have significantly improved the prognosis in this condition. Best benefit is achieved by gradual BP reduction (10–15 mmHg per day) until diastolic BP reaches 85–90 mmHg. Rapid reduction in BP may worsen renal function, therefore IV nitroprusside and labetolol are relatively contraindicated. Despite treatment with ACE inhibitors up to 50% of patients develop end-stage renal failure.

Question 199

A 70-year-old man was awoken with retrosternal chest pain radiating into his left arm in the early hours of the morning. The pain was persistent for 5 hours, and unrelieved by taking antacids before finally subsiding. The following day he consulted his daughter over the telephone, who persuaded him to make an urgent appointment with his GP. There was a past history of mild hypertension and hypothyroidism. The latter was diagnosed over a year ago after the patient presented with lethargy and was treated with 25 mg of thyroxine; however, the drug was stopped by the patient within three months because he felt well again. He was a non-smoker and consumed alcohol on a very infrequent basis. Over the past two months he had felt lethargic and saw another doctor, who diagnosed depression. He lived alone. He had been widowed three years previously. He took antacids for infrequent indigestion.

On visiting his GP, an ECG was performed (**199**). The patient was referred to the local hospital immediately for further evaluation. On arrival at hospital he appeared pale, but was well perfused. His heart rate was 50 beats/min, and blood pressure was 150/95 mmHg. The heart sounds were normal and the chest was clear. There was no clinical evidence of cardiac failure. Neurological examination was normal.

Further investigations are shown.

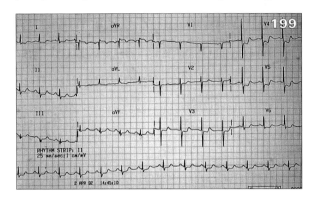

Hb	9.6 g/dl
WCC	4×10^9/l
Platelets	150×10^9/l
MCV	108 fl
Sodium	132 mmol/l
Potassium	3.8 mmol/l
Urea	3 mmol/l
Creatinine kinase	300 iu/l
Troponin T	5.3 ng /l (NR < 0.1 ng/l)
TSH	21 mu/l
Thyroxine	30 nmol/l
Thyroid microsomal antibodies	Positive 1/3,000
Morning cortisol	800 ng/l
LH	8 iu/l (normal, 1–10 iu/l)
FSH	5 iu/l (normal, 1–7 iu/l)
Prolactin	550 mu/l

1. Give one reason for the elevated troponin.
   a. Anterior ST elevation MI.
   b. Non-ST elevation anterolateral infarction.
   c. Inferior ST elevation MI.
   d. Hypothyroidism.
   e. Intramuscular injection.

2. What is the most likely cause of the abnormal thyroid function tests?
   a. Secondary hypothyroidism.
   b. Tertiary hypothyroidism.
   c. Auto-immune hypothyroidism.
   d. de Quervain's thyroiditis.
   e. Sick euthyroid syndrome.

3. What single investigation would you perform to investigate the cause of this patient's anaemia?
   a. Serum B_{12} level.
   b. Serum folate.
   c. Gastric parietal antibodies.
   d. Serum ferritin.
   e. Hb electrophoresis.

Question 200

A 50-year-old woman presented with a two-day history of increasing difficulty with swallowing and regurgitation of food. Over the preceding two to three months she had also experienced difficulty climbing stairs, raising her arms above her head, and arising from a sitting or lying position, with some associated lower back pain. On examination she was found to have symmetrical proximal muscle weakness with normal tone, sensation and deep tendon reflexes. Cranial nerve examination revealed weakness of the bulbar muscles.

What is the most likely cause of her muscle weakness?
   a. Motor neurone disease.
   b. Myasthenia gravis.
   c. Hypothyroidism.
   d. Polymyositis.
   e. Polymyalgia rheumatica.

Answer 199

> 1. b. Non-ST elevation anterolateral infarction.
> 2. c. Auto-immune hypothyroidism.
> 3. a. Serum B_{12} level.

The patient presents with a non-ST elevation anterolateral myocardial infarction as evidenced by the ST depression and elevated troponin level. The blood results suggest that he has primary hypothyroidism. The very high titre of anti-microsomal antibodies indicates atrophic auto-immune hypothyroidism or Hashimoto's hypothyroidism. Hypothyroidism is a well-recognized cause of secondary hypercholesterolaemia (*Table A* for other causes) and ischaemic heart disease. Other cardiac manifestations of the condition include pericarditis, dilated cardiomyopathy and pericardial effusion. In this case, the raised creatinine kinase level could be explained by myocardial infarction and by hypothyroid induced myositis. Other causes of raised creatinine kinase are listed (*Table B*). Kleinfelter's syndrome is associated with hypothyroidism, but the normal LH level (usually high in Kleinfelter's syndrome) is against the diagnosis.

Hypothyroidism may cause normochromic normocytic anaemia, macrocytic anaemia or microcytic anaemia. The latter is usually seen in menstruating women who develop menorrhagia as a consequence of hypothyroidism. Macrocytosis in hypothyroidism may be directly due to hypothyroidism or associated pernicious anaemia, which is common in patients with auto-immune hypothyroidism. Pernicious anaemia is best diagnosed by the demonstration of low serum B_{12} and the presence of gastric, parietal and intrinsic factor antibodies. Coincidental folate deficiency may also cause macrocytosis.

Table A Causes of secondary hypercholesterolaemia

• Alcohol abuse	• Obesity
• Diabetes mellitus	• Chronic liver disease
• Hypothyroidism	• Myeloma
• Primary biliary cirrhosis	• Nephrotic syndrome

Table B Causes of a raised creatinine kinase

- Normal variant in the black population (up to 300 iu/l)
- Muscle injury or trauma
- Septicaemia
- Leptospirosis
- Polymyositis
- Muscular dystrophy
- Hypothyroidism
- Cholesterol-lowering statin and fibrate drugs

See Answer 323.

Answer 200

> d. Polymyositis.

The patient has symmetrical distribution of proximal muscle weakness as well as weakness of the bulbar muscles. The most probable diagnosis is polymyositis. Muscle weakness is the most common presenting feature of polymyositis. The onset is usually insidious, with gradual worsening over a period of several months before medical attention is sought. Occasionally, however, it shows acute onset of symptoms.

Diagnostic criteria:
- Symmetric proximal muscle weakness.
- Elevated plasma muscle enzymes.
- Myopathic changes on electromyography.
- Characteristic muscle biopsy abnormalities and the absence of histopathologic signs of other myopathies.

There is a female to male predominance of about 2:1 and, in adults, the peak incidence occurs in the fifth decade, although all age groups may be affected.

Muscle atrophy may occur in severe, long-standing disease. 30% develop weakness of the oropharyngeal muscles or the striated muscle of the upper one-third of the oesophagus, leading to dysphagia, nasal regurgitation or aspiration.

Arthralgias and joint pain can occur. Myalgias and muscle tenderness occur in 25–50% of cases. These symptoms tend to be mild, unlike those which occur in viral or bacterial myositis, the inherited metabolic myopathies, fibromyalgia or polymyalgia rheumatica. The latter predominantly affects the hip and shoulder girdles with accompanying morning stiffness (see Question 340).

Motor neurone disease can present with elevated plasma muscle enzymes, dysphagia, and proximal muscle weakness. However, distal motor weakness is more common, there are associated pyramidal tract signs and the EMG does not show myopathic changes.

Myasthenia gravis presents in women in their 20s and 30s and men over the age of 60. Weakness often begins in the eyes, causing ptosis and/or diplopia, but may begin in the bulbar and neck muscles or the muscles of the limbs and trunk. One important feature of myasthenia is the marked association with fatiguability. Occasionally it can cause diffuse weakness without prominent fatiguability symptoms. The respiratory muscles can be affected in advanced disease. Myasthenia gravis is distinguished from myositis by the frequent presence of facial muscle weakness, normal muscle enzymes, characteristic EMG changes, and the presence of antiacetylcholine receptor antibodies.

Question 201

A 29-year-old male presented with a three-hour history of severe epigastric pain and profuse vomiting. The pain radiated into his back, and was not relieved by any of the antacid therapies which he had tried at home. There was no previous history of abdominal pain. He was a non-smoker and consumed 1–2 units of alcohol on an infrequent basis.

On examination, he was distressed with pain. On inspection of the trunk there were several raised lesions (**201**). There was no pallor. His heart rate was 100 beats/min and blood pressure 140/80 mmHg. On examination of the abdomen, he was very tender in the epigastrum but there was no abdominal rigidity. Bowel sounds were reduced.

Investigations are shown.

Hb	15 g/dl
WCC	16×10^9/l
Platelets	200×10^9/l
Sodium	128 mmol/l
Chloride	98 mmol/l
Potassium	3.6 mmol/l
Urea	6 mmol/l
Creatinine	100 µmol/l
Calcium	2.1 mmol/l
Albumin	42 g/l
Glucose	6 mmol/l
Chest X-ray	Normal
Abdominal X-ray	Normal

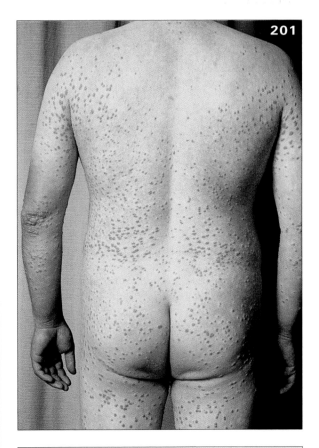

1. Which urgent test would you request to confirm the diagnosis?
2. Which two other investigations would you request to aid your management?
3. What is the full diagnosis?
4. Give two possible explanations for the low sodium.

Question 202

A patient collapsed during an ECG (**202a**).

1. What is the cause of collapse?
2. What is the immediate management?

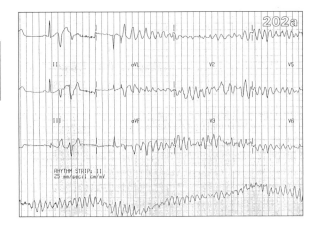

Answer 201

1. Serum amylase.
2. i. Arterial blood gases.
ii. Clotting studies.
3. Acute pancreatitis secondary to hypertrigly-ceridaemia.
4. i. Vomiting.
ii. Pseudohyponatraemia secondary to hyper-lipidaemia.

Causes of acute pancreatitis

- Alcohol abuse
- Cholelithiasis
- Coxsackie and mumps virus
- Hypercalcaemia
- Hypertriglyceridaemia
- Drugs: thiazides, steroids, azathioprine
- ERCP
- Trauma

The history of acute abdominal pain radiating to the back and associated with profuse vomiting is consistent with acute pancreatitis, although a perforated duodenal ulcer and cholecystitis may present similarly. The slightly low serum calcium supports the diagnosis of acute pancreatitis because the associated rise in serum lipase resulting from pancreatic damage leads to an increase in the free fatty acid concentration in the blood, which has the effect of binding calcium and thus reducing the 'free calcium' in the serum.

A very high serum amylase is usually diagnostic of acute pancreatitis, but acute parotitis may cause similarly high levels. However, in the latter case the history is of painful parotid glands. A modestly elevated level is seen in perforated duodenal ulcer, cholecystitis and aortic aneurysm.

A neutrophil leucocytosis is common. The serum calcium may be low for reasons explained above. It is mandatory to check urea, electrolytes, glucose, arterial blood gases, chest X-ray and clotting. The most common cause of mortality is renal failure and respiratory failure due to hypovolaemia and ARDS, respectively. The latter is thought to be due to the effects of high levels of trypsin that has leaked from the pancreas on lung surfactant. DIC is another important cause of mortality.

In this case, the cause of pancreatitis is hypertriglyceridaemia, as evident by the multiple eruptive xanthomata on the trunk of this young male patient. Causes of acute pancreatitis are tabulated above. In the UK, the most common cause of acute pancreatitis is alcohol abuse, followed by cholelithiasis ('gallstones').

The low sodium is either due to vomiting or is a result of pseudohyponatraemia resulting from hyperlipidaemia. In hyperlipidaemia and paraproteinaemias, the serum sodium is falsely low because only the sodium in free water space is measured. True hyponatraemia can be differentiated from pseudohyponatraemia by measuring the plasma osmolality, which is low in the former and normal in the latter.

Answer 202

1. Ventricular fibrillation precipitated by the 'R on T' phenomenon.
2. DC cardioversion using 200 J.

The rhythm is broad complex, and the QRS-complexes are very irregular and are of varying amplitude and duration. This is typical of ventricular fibrillation.

There is only one effective method of reverting ventricular fibrillation to sinus rhythm, and that is DC cardioversion using a high-energy shock. The quicker this is given, the higher the chance of reverting to sinus rhythm. The window for success is around 2 minutes, following which reversion becomes increasingly difficult. The most common cause of ventricular fibrillation is myocardial infarction; however, the cardiomyopathies, ventricular aneurysms, electrolyte imbalances (particularly hypokalaemia) and certain drug overdoses (e.g. cocaine or tricyclic antidepressant drugs) are also recognized causes. Following myocardial infarction, multiple ventricular

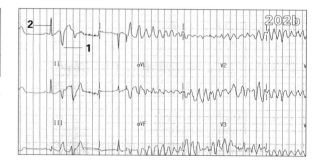

ectopics occurring on the preceding T-wave may cause monomorphic ventricular tachycardia which can degenerate into ventricular fibrillation. Post-myocardial infarction patients with 'R on T' ventricular ectopics are treated prophylactically with a lignocaine infusion to reduce the frequency of the ectopics.

In this case (202b), there is clear evidence of the R-wave of an ectopic beat (1) on the T-wave of the preceding sinus beat (2).

Question 203

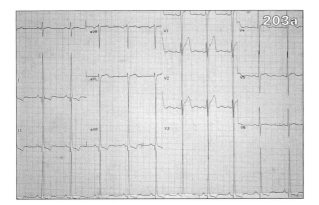

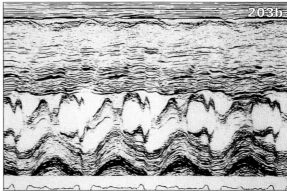

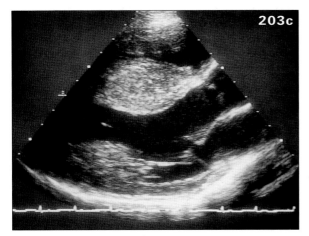

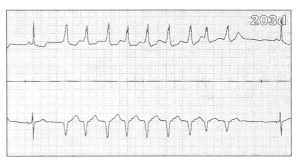

A 24-year-old basketball player was referred to the local cardiologist after experiencing two episodes of dizziness while playing basketball in one week. During the last episode he almost lost consciousness. There were no other associated symptoms. He had similar dizzy episodes one month previously, but attributed these to a coryzal illness. There was no history of headaches. He had no past medical history of significance. His father died in Mexico at the age of only 27 years but the patient was not sure about the cause of death. He had a step brother and sister who were well.

On examination, he appeared well. He weighed 90 kg and was 1.85 m tall. His heart rate was 68 beats/min and his blood pressure was 130/60 mmHg. The JVP was not raised. On examination of the precordium, he had a double apical impulse. On auscultation, there was a loud pansystolic murmur in the mitral area, and an ejection systolic murmur at the left lower sternal edge. His chest was clear. Examination of his peripheral pulses was normal, as was examination of the central nervous system.

The patient had a 12-lead ECG, echocardiogram and 24-hour ECG (**203a–d**).

1. What is the significance of the double apical impulse?
2. With respect to auscultation, what other manoeuvres could you have performed to try and ascertain the cause of the murmurs?
3. What are the abnormalities on the ECG and how would you interpret them?
4. What are the abnormalities on the two-dimensional and M-mode echocardiograms?
5. What is the significance of the abnormality on the 24-hour ECG?
6. What is the diagnosis?
7. What implications (if any) does this have on the patient's career?

Answer 203

1. A double apical impulse is the result of a palpable fourth heart sound which occurs when there is forceful left atrial contraction against a non-compliant left ventricle. This sign is often present in conditions which produce significant left ventricular hypertrophy. Examples include aortic stenosis, hypertrophic cardiomyopathy and occasionally severe left ventricular hypertrophy due to hypertension.

2. In the absence of hypertension, the differential diagnosis is between aortic stenosis and hypertrophic cardiomyopathy. In hypertrophic cardiomyopathy, an obstructive element is present in approximately 30% of patients. The obstruction is variable and thought to be due to anterior motion of the mitral valve towards the hypertrophied interventricular septum in systole, thus narrowing the left ventricular outflow tract. The exact mechanism for this is not clearly understood. The obstruction is worsened by manoeuvres which reduce LVEDP, and in these circumstances the murmur is louder. The Valsalva manoeuvre (blowing against a closed glottis) increases intrathoracic pressure and therefore reduces venous return to the heart, reducing LVEDP. Standing from a squatting position has similar consequences. In aortic stenosis these manoeuvres reduce the intensity of the systolic murmur.

3. The ECG reveals sinus rhythm with voltage criteria for left ventricular hypertrophy and deep S-waves in the septal (V2–V3) leads. In addition, there is T-wave inversion in the inferior leads. Regular physical training can also produce left ventricular hypertrophy; however, the extent of hypertrophy seldom exceeds the upper limit of normal. While it is common to have voltage criteria of left ventricular hypertrophy in athletes, accompanying T-wave inversion in any lead other than V1–V2 should raise the suspicion of organic heart disease and the need for further investigation.

4. The two-dimensional echocardiogram reveals asymmetrical left ventricular hypertrophy. The septum is grossly hypertrophied. The left ventricular cavity size is small. Both these features suggest the diagnosis of hypertrophic cardiomyopathy. The M-mode study demonstrates systolic anterior motion of the mitral valve, which is also suggestive of hypertrophic cardiomyopathy. Other echocardiographic features of hypertrophic cardiomyopathy include an enlarged left atrium and evidence of diastolic dysfunction on Doppler studies. The systolic function is usually excellent.

5. The 24-hour ECG demonstrated a run of non-sustained ventricular tachycardia. This occurs in approximately 25% of patients with hypertrophic cardiomyopathy, and is a high-risk marker of sudden death. Other markers of high risk include syncopal episodes and a family history of sudden death. The patient is experiencing syncopal episodes. The patient's father died aged 27, and in this context we have to assume that he may have had hypertrophic cardiomyopathy. This combination classifies the patient into the high-risk category for sudden death. These patients are treated with an implantable automatic cardiovertor defibrillator.

6. Hypertrophic cardiomyopathy.

7. The diagnosis of hypertrophic cardiomyopathy in an athlete leads to disqualification from competitive sport, in order to minimize the risk of sudden death.

Hypertrophic cardiomyopathy has a prevalence of 0.1–0.2%. It is inherited as an autosomal dominant trait in over 70% of cases, but sporadic cases are recognized. It is a genetically heterogeneous condition which is caused by mutations within genes encoding the sarcomeric proteins. The disease has been assigned to eight separate chromosomal loci (*Table*). Mutations within genes encoding β-myosin heavy chain and troponin T account for over half of all patients with HCM. Some 50% of patients have chest pain and breathlessness; 20% present with dizziness or syncope. Sudden death is frequently the first presentation, particularly in adolescents, young adults and athletes. The overall mortality rate is 3%. Sudden death commonly occurs during or immediately after strenuous exertion. The diagnosis is made using echocardiography to demonstrate left ventricular hypertrophy, which is usually asymmetric, but can be concentric in up to 40% of cases.

Molecular genetics of hypertrophic cardiomyopathy

Chromosome	Gene affected	Chromosome	Gene affected
14	β-myosin heavy chain	11	Myosin-binding protein C
1	Troponin T	7	?
19	Troponin I	3	Myosin essential light chain
15	α-tropomyosin	12	Myosin regulatory light chain

Question 204

A 68-year-old male was admitted for investigation of increasing weakness and recent onset of jaundice. There was no other relevant past medical history. In particular, there was no travel abroad and he was not taking any medication.

On examination, he had non-tender lymphadenopathy in the cervical, axillary and inguinal areas. Abdominal examination revealed an enlarged spleen 6 cm below the costal margin.

Investigations are shown.

Hb	10.1 g/dl
WCC	60×10^9/l
Platelets	190×10^9/l
Reticulocyte count	12%
MCV	101 fl
Blood film (**204**)	
Bilirubin	39 µmol/l
AST	20 iu/l
Alkaline phosphatase	70 iu/l
Albumin	36 g/l
Total protein	56 g/l
Chest X-ray	Normal
Urinalysis	Urobilinogen ++
	Bilirubin 0

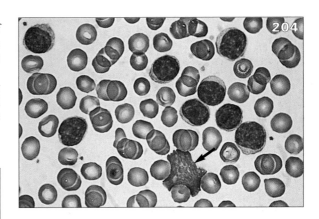

1. List three abnormalities on the blood film.
2. Explain the cause of the phenomenon indicated by the arrow.
3. What is the cause for the jaundice?
4. Give two possible explanations for the raised MCV.
5. Which single investigation would you perform to ascertain the cause of this patient's anaemia?

Question 205

A 19-year-old medical student was admitted to the Accident and Emergency Department with headache and drowsiness on a cold winter's morning. He shared a house with three fellow students, who found him in bed after he failed to answer several wake-up calls to attend an anatomy viva. On examination, he was flushed and drowsy. He was apyrexial. There was no evidence of a skin rash. His heart rate was 100 beats/min and regular, and the blood pressure was 120/80 mmHg. Neurological examination revealed a Glasgow coma score of 11/15. There was no nuchal rigidity. The cranial nerves, motor and sensory systems were normal. Examination of all other systems was normal.

Investigations are shown.

Hb	14 g/dl
WCC	9×10^9/l
Platelets	370×10^9/l
Sodium	135 mmol/l
Potassium	4.4 mmol/l
Urea	4 mmol/l
Creatinine	80 µmol/l
Arterial blood gases:	
pH	7.37
PaO_2	7.2 kPa
$PaCO_2$	3.8 kPa
Bicarbonate	23 mmol/l
O_2 saturation	98%
Chest X-ray	Normal
ECG	Sinus tachycardia

What is the diagnosis?
  a. Herpes simplex encephalitis.
  b. Tricyclic antidepressant overdose.
  c. Subarachnoid haemorrhage.
  d. Carbon monoxide poisoning.
  e. Hypothermia.

Answer 204

1. i. Numerous mature lymphocytes.
   ii. Smudge or smear cell.
   iii. Red cell agglutination.
2. Smudge or smear cells are an artefact phenomenon which arises during blood film preparation due to the fragility of lymphocytes in chronic lymphatic leukaemia.
3. Warm auto-immune haemolytic anaemia (see *Table* for other causes).
4. i. Reticulocytosis secondary to haemolysis.
   ii. Megaloblastic anaemia due to folate deficiency from increased cell turnover.
5. Direct Coomb's test.

Causes of autoimmune haemolytic anaemia for higher examinations

Warm
(IgG antibody attaches to red cells at 37°C (98.6°F))
- SLE
- Lymphoma
- Carcinoma
- Chronic lymphatic leukaemia
- Methyl dopa

Cold
(IgM antibody attaches to red cells below 37°C (98.6°F))
- Mycoplasma pneumonia
- Infectious mononucleosis
- Paroxysmal cold haemoglobinuria (IgG)
- Lymphoma

Chronic lymphatic leukaemia usually affects the middle-aged and the elderly. It is a malignancy of B-cell lymphocytes. The clinical features are insidious, and the diagnosis may be made incidentally on a blood film. The main features are lethargy, night sweats, weight loss and recurrent infections due to hypogammaglobulinaemia. Physical examination reveals generalized lymphadenopathy and hepatosplenomegaly. The characteristic blood picture is of a lymphocytosis and a mild normochromic normocytic anaemia. Smudge or smear cells are common. As disease progresses, the anaemia becomes more severe, partly owing to marrow suppression and partly owing to an auto-immune haemolytic anaemia, and a thrombocytopenia becomes evident. Patients presenting with low platelets have advanced disease and a poor prognosis. Folate deficiency may occur secondary to increased cell turnover and haemolysis. Therapy is commenced in symptomatic patients. The drug of choice is chlorambucil. Severely immunosuppressed individuals may be treated with intravenous gammaglobulin preparations.

Answer 205

d. Carbon monoxide poisoning.

The clue for the diagnosis of carbon monoxide poisoning comes from the arterial blood gases, which reveal hypoxia but a normal oxygen saturation. Carbon monoxide displaces oxygen from Hb and displaces the oxygen dissociation curve to the left. It also inhibits cellular respiration by inhibiting the cytochrome oxidase system. This results in tissue hypoxia, which may manifest as headaches, dizziness, convulsions, nausea and vomiting. On examination, patients may have tachycardia, tachypnoea, ataxia and cherry red discoloration of the lips; however, the latter is a relatively rare and late manifestation of the condition. Retinal haemorrhages are a recognized complication of carbon monoxide poisoning. Late complications include basal ganglia infarction and parkinsonism, and sometimes neuropsychiatric symptoms. Oxygen saturation is normal because automated biochemical and pulse oximeter analysers cannot differentiate between oxyhaemoglobin and carboxyhaemoglobin; however, PaO_2 is low when there is significant carbon monoxide poisoning. It is worth noting that arterial PaO_2 is often normal in patients with carbon monoxide poisoning; therefore, a high index of suspicion is needed to diagnose the condition. Carbon monoxide poisoning is caused by combustion engines, faulty stoves or paraffin heaters when facilities for ventilation are poor.

The diagnosis is made by direct measurement of arterial carboxyhaemoglobin level. Levels of 40–60% are associated with neurological symptoms and signs (described above), as well as cardiac brady- and tachyarrhythmias. Levels above 60% are associated with coma and death.

The management of carbon monoxide poisoning involves administration of 100% oxygen via a tight-fitting mask. This reduces the half-life of carboxyhaemoglobin from 4 hours to approximately 90 minutes. During this period, carboxyhaemoglobin levels should be measured 2-hourly, and the oxygen continued until the carboxyhaemoglobin level is below 10%. Patients with neurological signs and symptoms, ECG abnormalities, myocardial ischaemia, pulmonary oedema and shock require hyperbaric oxygen (3 atm) at a specialized centre. Some would agree that any individual with a carboxyhaemoglobin level exceeding 25% should also be considered for hyperbaric oxygen, even if symptoms are absent.

Question 206

A 38-year-old businessman was admitted to hospital with nausea, vomiting and drowsiness. He had been in Thailand for 10 days and returned back to England two days previously. He was well in Thailand, but on arrival to England developed general malaise and a headache. He attributed his symptoms to excess alcohol ingestion while abroad, and attempted to relieve his symptoms with two paracetamol tablets. He continued to have a headache the following morning, and took another two tablets of paracetamol, without much relief of his symptoms. Following this, he took two paracetamol tablets every four hours. He gradually became more unwell, nauseous and started vomiting. There was no neck stiffness, photophobia or diarrhoea. He normally consumed two bottles of wine and occasional spirits per day and smoked 30 cigarettes a day. While abroad, he had drunk more alcohol than usual. There was no significant past medical history.

On examination, he was tanned and had a flushed face. He was mildly icteric. He had a fever of 39°C (102.2°F). He was slightly drowsy, but could hold a normal, coherent conversation. There was no evidence of asterixis. Examination of the fundi was normal. The heart rate was 110 beats/min and blood pressure 105/70 mmHg. Examination of the precordium revealed a very soft third heart sound. His chest was clear. Abdominal examination revealed a slightly tender palpable liver edge 4 cm below the costal margin. The spleen was not palpable.

Investigations are shown.

Hb	15.8 g/dl
WCC	$9 \times 10^9/l$
Platelets	$105 \times 10^9/l$
MCV	102 fl
PT	20 s (control 14 s)
Malaria parasite	Not detected
Sodium	133 mmol/l
Potassium	3.5 mmol/l
Urea	5 mmol/l
Creatinine	98 µmol/l
Bilirubin	30 µmol/l
AST	1500 iu/l
Alkaline phosphatase	110 iu/l
Serum ferritin	500 µg/l
Chest X-ray	Normal

1. Which test would you perform immediately?
   a. Blood cultures.
   b. Hepatitis serology.
   c. Blood ethanol level.
   d. Serum paracetamol level.
   e. Liver biopsy.

2. What is the cause of the deterioration of his symptoms?
   a. Paracetamol poisoning/viral hepatitis.
   b. Paracetamol poisoning/alcohol abuse.
   c. Haemochromatosis/hepatoma.
   d. Viral hepatitis/paracetamol intoxication.
   e. Haemochromatosis/paracetamol poisoning.

Question 207

A 42-year-old female presented with increasing dyspnoea on exertion. She had a past history of rheumatic fever. Left and right cardiac catheter data were as follows:

Chamber	Pressure (mmHg)	Oxygen saturation (%)
Right atrium	10	68
Right ventricle	40/10	68
Pulmonary artery	40/22	68
PCWP	16	
Left ventricle	160/10	96
Aorta	110/70	96

What statement fits best with the data provided?
   a. Mitral stenosis, aortic stenosis and pulmonary hypertension.
   b. Mitral regurgitation and pulmonary hypertension.
   c. Aortic stenosis and pulmonary hypertension.
   d. Atrial septal defect, aortic stenosis and pulmonary hypertension.
   e. Mixed aortic valve disease.

Answer 206

> 1. d. Serum paracetamol level.
> 2. b. Paracetamol poisoning/alcohol abuse.

There is a history of alcohol abuse and consumption of 6–7 g of paracetamol in 24 hours. Ingestion of 15 g of paracetamol is regarded as a significant overdose in normal healthy individuals; however, the dose of paracetamol required to cause hepatotoxicity in individuals with chronic, heavy alcohol ingestion is much lower. This is explained by the ability of alcohol to induce hepatic microsomal enzymes and to deplete hepatic intracellular levels of glutathione. Paracetamol itself is not hepatotoxic, but it is usually metabolized to NAPQI, a potent oxidative agent with potential to cause massive hepatic necrosis. The metabolite is normally rapidly conjugated with glutathione, which renders it inactive and it is excreted. In patients with heavy alcohol ingestion the detoxifying microsomal enzyme concentration is increased to metabolize alcohol. Although this is a beneficial effect when dealing with alcohol, it can have serious consequences when large amounts of paracetamol are ingested because it leads to rapid metabolism of the drug to NAPQI. The hepatocytes are relatively depleted of glutathione owing to hepatic damage from alcohol and soon become completely depleted in an attempt to conjugate NAPQI. The result is an excess of NAPQI, causing hepatic necrosis, which can have profound effects if hepatic reserve has already been severely affected by alcohol abuse. Alcohol abusers are more likely to develop massive hepatic necrosis and have a worse prognosis from paracetamol overdose.

Hepatitis A infection is possible and in the early stages does produce general malaise, fever, nausea and elevated hepatic transaminases. Hepatitis A has an incubation period of two weeks and has a hepatitic and a cholestatic phase. It is feasible that the patient contracted the virus abroad and is now in the hepatitic phase; however, given the history of alcohol abuse and self-administration of a significant amount of paracetamol, this is less likely than the answer given above.

The diagnosis of haemochromatosis is raised owing to the high serum ferritin level of 500 μg /l; however, high ferritin levels and deposition of iron in the liver also occur in alcohol-related disease and patients with regular blood transfusions (secondary haemochromatosis). Liver biopsy is the main way of distinguishing between primary and secondary haemochromatosis. In secondary haemochromatosis the biopsy will reveal changes of alcoholic hepatitis (Mallory bodies) as well as iron deposition. Moreover, primary haemochromatosis is not usually associated with significant derangement of LFT unless the disease is very advanced or there is development of hepatocellular carcinoma, which is a recognized complication of cirrhosis of the liver due to any cause, but particularly haemochromatosis. In this case there would be a history of poor health before travelling abroad, as well as other features of haemochromatosis such as diabetes mellitus and hypogonadism, which are absent. The LFT usually demonstrate a high alkaline phosphatase and a raised bilirubin in the presence of hepatocellular carcinoma.

Answer 207

> a. Mitral stenosis, aortic stenosis and pulmonary hypertension.

The right ventricular pressure and pulmonary artery pressures exceed 35mmHg, indicating pulmonary hypertension. The PCWP exceeds the LVEDP by 6 mmHg, indicating significant mitral stenosis. There is a pressure drop of 50 mmHg across the aortic valve, indicating moderate to severe aortic stenosis.

There is no evidence of step-up in oxygen saturation in the right heart to indicate a left-to-right intracardiac shunt. (See Interpretation of Cardiac Catheter Data, page 418.)

Question 208

A 15-year-old male was admitted with sudden onset of rapid palpitations which were not associated with chest pain or dizziness. On examination, he was well-perfused and his blood pressure was 110/65 mmHg. An ECG performed in the Accident and Emergency Department is shown (**208a**). He was treated by the medical officer, and his ECG afterwards is shown (**208b**).

1. What is shown in the 12-lead ECG while the patient is having palpitations?
2. List two forms of treatment with which the medical officer may have attempted to treat the palpitation.
3. Which cardiac condition does this patient have?
4. List four forms of drug therapy which could be safely used to prevent the patient's symptoms.
5. What is the definitive treatment in a young patient with this disorder?

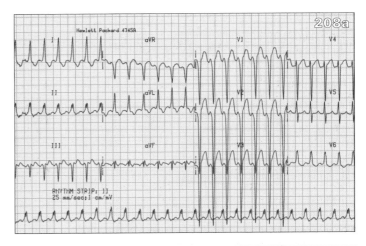

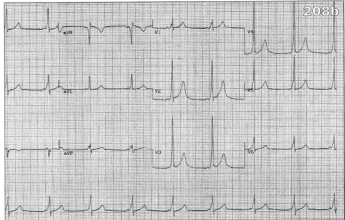

Question 209

A 33-year-old male with recently diagnosed acute schizophrenia was referred to the Accident and Emergency Department after he was found collapsed on the psychiatric ward. On examination, the patient was very drowsy and appeared rigid. The heart rate was 120 beats/min, and regular; blood pressure was 110/60 mmHg.

The temperature was 40°C (104°F). Examination of the cardiovascular, respiratory and abdominal system was normal. Neurological examination demonstrated generalized rigidity of all muscle groups.

Investigations are shown.

Hb	15 g/dl
WCC	10×10^9/l
Platelets	300×10^9/l
Urinalysis	Protein +
Sodium	138 mmol/l
Potassium	4 mmol/l
Urea	10 mmol/l
Creatinine	160 µmol/l

1. What is the diagnosis?
2. Which investigation would you perform to confirm the diagnosis?
3. Briefly, list three management steps.

Answer 208

1. An atrioventricular tachycardia with LBBB.
2. i. Vagotonic manoeuvres such as carotid sinus massage, Valsalva manoeuvre, compression of the eyeball.
   ii. Intravenous adenosine.
3. Wolff–Parkinson–White syndrome (type A).
4. i. Sotalol.
   ii. Flecanide.
   iii. Disopyramide.
   iv. Amiodarone.
5. Radiofrequency ablation of the accessory pathway.

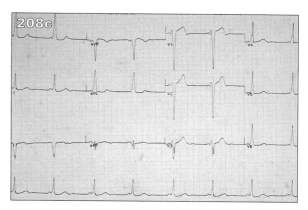

Wolff–Parkinson–White syndrome (WPW), a congenital illness with a prevalence of 1 in 1,500, is characterized by an accessory conduction pathway between atria and ventricles (bundle of Kent) which predisposes to an electrical re-entrant circuit and tachycardia. During sinus rhythm the electrical impulse conducts rapidly over the accessory conduction pathway and depolarizes the ventricles prematurely, resulting in a short PR-interval and a wide QRS-complex with slurred upstroke, often called a delta wave. Anterograde conduction through the accessory pathway and retrograde conduction via the atrioventricular node may predispose to two types of tachyarrhythmias which are atrioventricular re-entrant tachycardia or atrial fibrillation. Two variants of WPW are recognized: type A (left-sided pathway), with an upright (positive) delta wave in V1, as in this case; and type B (right-sided pathway), with negative delta wave in V1 (**208c**). The former is more common.

In atrioventricular tachycardia the ventricular rate is between 140–280 beats/min and the P-wave is seen just after the QRS-complex, usually in the ST-segment In atrial fibrillation, there is a rapid irregular rhythm with some QRS-complexes exhibiting delta waves.

Management of atrioventricular re-entrant tachycardia involves vagotonic manoeuvres such as carotid sinus massage, Valsalva manoeuvre, eyeball compression or intravenous adenosine. AF does not usually respond to vagotonic manoeuvres, but may be abolished by adenosine. DC cardioversion is reserved for patients who are haemodynamically unstable and unresponsive to adenosine. Drugs to prevent arrhythmias include class I and class III antiarrhythmic agents (e.g. sotalol). Both digoxin and verapamil are contraindicated in WPW as they increase conduction through the accessory pathway and increase the risk of malignant ventricular arrhythmias. Radiofrequency ablation of the accessory pathway is the definitive treatment for AF or frequent atrioventricular re-entrant tachycardia.

Answer 209

1. Neuroleptic malignant syndrome secondary to the use of phenothiazines.
2. Serum creatinine kinase.
3. i. Stop drug.
   ii. Intravenous diazepam.
   iii. Adequate hydration to prevent renal failure.

The neuroleptic malignant syndrome is a rare but life-threatening condition that can occur with any anti-psychotic drug, irrespective of dose. It is most common when starting treatment or increasing the dose. Symptoms include fever, muscle rigidity, confusion and impaired consciousness. Autonomic instability is well recognized and is associated with excessive sweating, labile blood pressure and tachycardia. The diagnosis is made by demonstrating a grossly elevated creatinine kinase. Rhabdomyolysis may precipitate renal failure, which can be avoided by adequate hydration. Other complications include aspiration pneumonia and respiratory failure. The management of this condition involves stopping the neuroleptic drug immediately, antipyretics and rehydration. The drug dantrolene may be useful in some cases. Collapse in a psychiatric patient is a common scenario in the exam. While many general medical conditions may cause collapse in patients with psychiatric disease, specific things to consider are tabulated below.

Specific things to consider in a collapsed patient on a psychiatric ward
- Neuroleptic malignant syndrome
- Drug overdose
- Torsades de pointes (polymorphic VT) secondary to neuroleptic agents, lithium or tricyclic antidepressant overdose
- Epilepsy secondary to neuroleptic agents
- Epilepsy secondary to hyponatraemia of psychogenic polydipsia
- Diabetic emergencies secondary to olanzepine

Question 210

A 59-year-old male presented with a three-week history of cough and progressive breathlessness and three episodes of haemoptysis in 24 hours. At the onset of the initial symptoms he visited his GP, who diagnosed a respiratory tract infection and prescribed a course of broad-spectrum antibiotics. The cough persisted and the patient remained breathless. His effort tolerance had become significantly reduced from walking two miles daily to being breathless at rest. He had felt increasingly lethargic and nauseous for a week before being seen in the Accident and Emergency Department. Twenty-four hours previously he had coughed an egg-cup-full of fresh clots of blood on three separate occasions. There was no history of sore throat or night sweats. Prior to a week previously, his appetite was good. There was no history of weight loss. He had a past history of haemorrhoids which were surgically ligated two years ago.

The patient was married with one son and worked as a mechanic. He smoked 10 cigarettes per day and consumed 2–3 units of alcohol per week. There was no history of travel abroad. There was no family history of note, with the exception that his mother had been treated for pulmonary TB 16 years ago.

On examination, he appeared pale and centrally cyanosed. There was no evidence of clubbing or lymphadenopathy. There was bilateral pitting ankle oedema. The heart rate was 110 beats/min, and regular, and blood pressure was 176/105 mmHg. The JVP was raised 4 cm above the sternal angle. On examination of the respiratory system chest expansion was symmetrically reduced. The trachea was central. Percussion note was dull at both bases, and on auscultation there was widespread bronchial breathing at both mid-zones and bases. Precordial and abdominal examination was normal.

Investigations are shown.

Hb	7.2 g/dl
WCC	12×10^9/l
Platelets	500×10^9/l
Sodium	137 mmol/l
Potassium	5.2 mmol/l
Urea	19 mmol/l
Creatinine	400 µmol/l
Calcium	2.1 mmol/l
Phosphate	2 mmol/l
Albumin	40 g/l
ECG	Sinus tachycardia. Partial RBBB
Chest X-ray	Alveolar shadowing affecting both lower zones
Urinalysis	Blood +++
	Protein ++
	Numerous blood cells and red cell casts

Lung function:

FEV_1	65% predicted
FVC	60% predicted
TLC	68% predicted
RV	66% predicted
TLCO	110% predicted

1. Comment on the respiratory function tests.
2. What is the most likely diagnosis?
3. List two tests you would request to confirm the diagnosis.
4. What are the four predisposing factors for producing the changes seen in the chest?

Question 211

Red cell count	8×10^{12}/l
Hb	14.2 g/dl
PCV	0.55
MCV	69 fl
MCH	18.2 pg
WCC	15×10^9/l
Neutrophils	88%
Lymphocytes	8%
Monocytes	4%
Platelets	475×10^9/l
Blood film	Hypochromia ++

A 60-year-old male presents with an episode of amaurosis fugax. On examination, apart from splenomegaly, there are no abnormal neurological or other clinical findings.

Investigations are shown.

What is the diagnosis?
   a. Pseudopolycythaemia.
   b. Secondary polycythaemia.
   c. Primary polycythaemia (polycythaemia rubra vera).
   d. Chronic myeloid leukaemia.
   e. Essential thrombocythaemia.

Answer 210

1. Restrictive lung defect with a raised TLCO. (See Respiratory Function Tests, page 419.)
2. Goodpasture's syndrome. Other possible diagnoses include microscopic polyarteritis nodosa and Wegener's granulomatosis.
3. i. Renal biopsy.
   ii. Anti-GBM disease.
4. i. Smoking.
   ii. Lower respiratory tract infection.
   iii. Pulmonary oedema.
   iv. Inhalation of organic solvents.

The patient has evidence of acute glomerulonephritis. The breathlessness, haemoptysis, raised TLCO and bilateral alveolar shadows on the chest X-ray are highly suggestive of pulmonary haemorrhage. The combination of acute nephritis and pulmonary haemorrhage may occur in anti-GBM disease, Wegener's granulomatosis, microscopic polyarteritis nodosa and SLE. In anti-GBM disease, patients who are smokers are more predisposed to lung haemorrhage, as are patients who are exposed to hydrocarbons. The patient is both a smoker and has been exposed to hydrocarbons from his occupation as a garage mechanic. The most probable diagnosis is anti-GBM disease.

Anti-GBM disease is rare, with prevalence 1 case per million. The male to female ratio is 2:1. The age of onset has two peaks which are the third and the seventh decades. There is a strong association between HLA DR2 and anti-GBM disease, the antigen being present in approximately 80% of affected patients. Other HLA associations include HLA DR4 and HLA DR2. Circulating anti-GBM antibodies are responsible for both the nephritis and pulmonary haemorrhage.

Clinical features are those of rapidly progressive nephritis and/or pulmonary haemorrhage. Fatigue and breathlessness may pre-date the onset of nephritis or frank haemoptysis. Glomerulonephritis is of the rapidly progressive type, and renal function may be completely lost within a week. Some 60% of patients have pulmonary haemorrhage. Smokers, patients with coexisting lower respiratory tract infections and pulmonary oedema, and patients exposed to hydrocarbons are more prone to haemorrhage.

The chest X-ray may reveal alveolar shadowing in the presence of pulmonary haemorrhage. The differentiation from pulmonary oedema (which looks the same) requires determination of the TLCO, which is raised in haemorrhage and reduced in oedema.

Investigations include renal biopsy with immunofluorescent agent which demonstrate rapidly progressive glomerulonephritis and linear IgG deposits along the basement membrane. Transbronchial lung biopsy may be useful, but has a lower histological yield.

Management is with early plasmapharesis, methylprednisolone and cyclophosphamide.

Answer 211

c. Primary polycythaemia (polycythaemia rubra vera).

The patient has a normal Hb but the PCV and the red cell count are elevated. Furthermore, he has associated leucocytosis, thrombocytosis and splenomegaly, which should raise the suspicion of PRV. The normal (as opposed to high Hb) is due to coexisting iron deficiency. The diagnosis of iron deficiency is supported by the low MCV.

PRV has an insidious onset. It rarely occurs before the fifth decade. Symptoms include lethargy, depression, vertigo, tinnitus and amaurosis fugax. On examination, the patient may have a plethoric facial complexion, hypertension, and a palpable spleen in approximately 70% of cases. Complications include bleeding due to thrombocythaemia, stroke from hyperviscosity, and gout from increased cell turnover. Bleeding is most commonly from the upper gastrointestinal tract. PRV may progress to myelofibrosis or acute myeloid leukaemia.

Management is by venesection, although this may result in iron deficiency. Busulphan or hydroxyurea are effective in controlling the thrombocytosis.

Question 212

A 54-year-old Turkish male was admitted to hospital with a three-week history of malaise, headaches, pain in his arms, legs and lower back and night sweats. His appetite was poor, and he had lost almost 3 kilograms in three weeks. He worked as a butcher. He had returned from a holiday in Turkey six weeks ago where he lived on his brother's farm for two weeks.

On examination, he was unwell. He had generalized cervical lymphadenopathy. His temperature was 38.5°C (101.3°F). The blood pressure was 120/60 mmHg. Cardiovascular examination revealed a soft systolic murmur at the apex. Examination of the respiratory system was normal. On examination of his abdomen he had a palpable spleen 4 cm below the costal margin. The liver edge was also palpable 3 cm below the costal margin. Genital examination demonstrated an erythematous scrotum with a swollen, tender left testicle. Examination of the central nervous system, including the fundi, was normal. His lower back was tender, but movements were not restricted. Similarly, his limbs were tender but there was no fasciculation and power was preserved. He had tender, red, macular lesions on his shins which varied between 2–5 cm in diameter.

Investigations are shown.

Hb	11.8 g/dl
WCC	2 × 10⁹/l (neutropenia)
Platelets	440 × 10⁹/l
ESR	66 mm/h
CRP	210 mg/l
U&E	Normal
LFT	Normal
Chest X-ray	Few calcified paratracheal lymph nodes

1. What is the diagnosis?
2. List three tests you would perform to help confirm the diagnosis.
3. What is the management?

Question 213

A 24-year-old Jamaican painter and decorator was admitted with acute colicky central abdominal pain associated with vomiting. The only past history was that of a viral illness associated with a rash two weeks previously. On examination, he appeared pale. The heart rate was 110 beats/min and the blood pressure was 140/90 mmHg. The abdomen was generally tender, but there was no guarding, and bowel sounds were infrequent. Examination of the central nervous system revealed reduced power and tone in the lower limbs, and absent ankle and knee reflexes.

Investigations are shown.

Hb	10 g/dl
WCC	7 × 10⁹/l
Platelets	170 × 10⁹/l
MCV	63 fl
MCHC	28 g/dl
Blood film (**213**)	
Urinary d-ALA	100 mmol/day (normal range 11–57 mmol/day)
Sodium	134 mmol/l
Potassium	3.2 mmol/l
Bicarbonate	15 mmol/l
Chloride	115 mmol/l
Urea	7 mmol/l
Creatinine	80 μmol/l
Calcium	2.32 mmol/l
Albumin	40g/l
Glucose	4 mmol/l
CT of brain	Normal

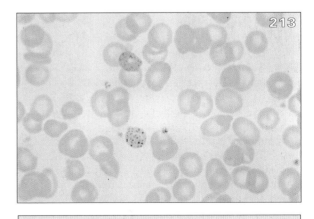

What is the diagnosis?
  a. Sarcoidosis.
  b. Acute intermittent porphyria.
  c. Lead poisoning.
  d. Arsenic poisoning.
  e. Polyarteritis nodosa.

Answer 212

> 1. Brucellosis.
> 2. i. Blood culture.
>   ii. Marrow culture.
>   iii. *Brucella* agglutination test or *Brucella* immunoglobulins (ELISA).
> 3. Tetracycline and rifampicin; co-trimoxazole.

The history of malaise, myalgia, headaches and weight loss in association with neutropenia, hepatosplenomegaly and erythema nodosum is highly suggestive of brucellosis.

Brucellosis is caused by *Brucella*, a Gram-negative bacillus, which may be contracted from cows, goats, pigs or sheep. It has a wide animal reservoir. Three main species cause infection in man: *B. abortus* (cattle), *B. melitensis* (goats/sheep), and *B. suis* (pigs). The organism usually gains access into the human body through the gastrointestinal tract as a result of consuming unpasteurized milk; however, contact with animal carcasses may also increase risk of oral ingestion of the bacterium. Brucellosis is virtually eliminated in the UK due to the strict policy of pasteurization of milk. Once in the gastrointestinal tract, the bacilli travel to the lymphatics and infect lymph nodes, and eventually there is haematogenous spread to many other organs.

The onset is usually insidious. General malaise, headaches, myalgia, weakness and night sweats are common. There is an undulant high fever. Lymphadenopathy is common. Hepatosplenomegaly may be present, but an acute hepatitis is rare. Splenomegaly usually indicates severe infection. Spinal tenderness is relatively common. Haematogenous spread may be complicated by arthritis, orchitis, endocarditis, osteomyelitis, and meningoencephalitis.

Brucellosis may become chronic when it is undiagnosed and is associated with fatigue, myalgia, depression, and occasionally fever. Palpable splenomegaly is characteristic. In a few cases the infection may be localized to specific organs such as the bones, heart or central nervous system. In these circumstances, systemic features are absent in over 60% of cases and antibody titres are low.

The diagnosis is based on positive blood cultures and rising anti-*Brucella* immunoglobulin titres. Blood cultures are positive in only half the cases. The *Brucella* agglutination test is positive within four weeks of the onset of illness. Treatment is with tetracycline and rifampicin for six weeks, although co-trimoxazole is also effective.

Answer 213

> c. Lead poisoning.

In a young man with abdominal pain, vomiting, neuropathy and anaemia, the most likely diagnosis is lead poisoning, although several other conditions may also cause the same symptoms (*Table*). The diagnosis is confirmed by measuring the serum lead concentration. A lead concentration above 4 mmol/l is toxic. Treatment is with D-penicillamine therapy.

Acute lead poisoning is rare, but chronic poisoning may occur in scrap-metal workers or plumbers, in individuals ingesting water from lead pipes, in children ingesting old lead-based paint in the house, and painters and decorators. Lead interferes with haem and globin synthesis (see Answer 147). The effects are a microcytic anaemia and raised precursors of haem synthesis. The latter cause abdominal symptoms, autonomic and motor neuropathy which are identical to those seen in AIP. In both lead poisoning and AIP the δ-ALA is elevated; however, lead poisoning is differentiated from AIP by the relatively severe anaemia, basophilic stippling affecting the red cells and the elevated proto- and coproporphyrins. Basophilic stippling is caused by aggregates of RNA resulting from inhibition of the enzyme pyrimidine-5-nucleotidase. Other features include haemolytic anaemia, lead encephalopathy (which is characterized by a high CSF protein), a blue line on the gums, and dense metaphyseal bands at the end of long bones in children (known as lead lines). Proximal RTA is recognized and comprises a hypokalaemic, hyperchloraemic acidosis, as well as loss of amino acids in the urine.

Although sarcoidosis may be associated with abdominal pain and polyneuropathy and is more common in patients of Afro-Caribbean origin, there is no evidence of pulmonary symptoms, bone pain, iritis or hypercalcaemia. The raised δ-ALA cannot be explained by sarcoidosis.

Arsenic poisoning may affect patients working in some metal and glass production industries and patients who have deliberately or accidentally ingested certain rodenticides. It presents acutely with severe abdominal cramps and profuse diarrhoea. Chronic exposure usually presents with a painful peripheral neuropathy, hyperkeratosis, microcytic anaemia and white horizontal lines on the nails (Mee's lines). Arsenic does not interfere with haem biosynthesis. (See Question 257.)

> **Causes of abdominal pain and neuropathy**
> - AIP
> - Lead poisoning
> - Arsenic poisoning
> - Guillain–Barré syndrome
> - Polyarteritis nodosa
> - Diabetic ketoacidosis
> - Intra-abdominal malignancy
> - Sarcoidosis
> - Alcohol abuse

Question 214

A 52-year-old obese hypertensive female was seen in the Emergency Department with sudden onset of palpitations and breathlessness. She had a history of hypertension, congestive cardiac failure and non-insulin-dependent diabetes mellitus. She was taking captopril 50 mg twice daily, nifedipine slow release 20 mg twice daily, metformin 500 mg three times daily, and furosemide 80 mg daily. The furosemide dose had recently been doubled by her GP to control her persistently elevated blood pressure and help her breathlessness. She had previously undergone several investigations to exclude a secondary cause for the hypertension.

On examination, the patient appeared breathless, but was not cyanosed. She was well perfused. The heart rate was 100 beats/min, and regular; blood pressure was 150/100 mmHg. The JVP was not elevated. On examination of her precordium, the apex was not palpable, but the heart sounds were normal. There were no murmurs. Respiratory examination revealed good chest expansion. The trachea was central and percussion was normal. Auscultation of the lung fields was normal. There was no evidence of peripheral oedema, but she had an erythematous skin rash on her shins. Blood results are shown.

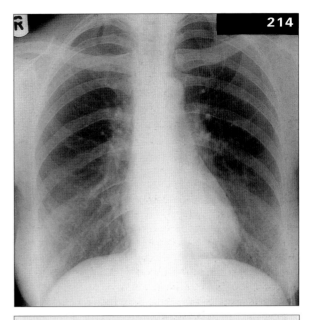

1. Interpret the blood gases.
2. What is the single most likely explanation for the abnormal blood gas results?

Sodium	134 mmol/l	Arterial blood gases:	
Potassium	4.3 mmol/l	pH	7.5
Creatinine	120 µmol/l	PaCO$_2$	1.8 kPa
Urea	8 mmol/l	PaO$_2$	15 kPa
ECG	Sinus tachycardia	Bicarbonate	19.3 mmol/l
Chest X-ray (**214**)		Base excess	+7

Question 215

A 25-year-old Malaysian male was admitted to hospital as an emergency when he noticed that he was completely paralysed for two hours after waking from his sleep in the early hours of the morning. He had experienced this type of severe weakness on four occasions over the past few months, and remarked how they always occurred during sleep and on waking he could not move. He drank four units of alcohol every night. He had recently seen his GP for anxiety attacks and was being counselled. He emigrated to England in 1994 and worked as a chef. He was single. All his family members were in Malaysia and were well.

On examination, he was thin; otherwise, physical examination was normal. Investigations are shown.

FBC	Normal
Sodium	136 mmol/l
Potassium	2 mmol/l
Urea	5 mmol/l
Bicarbonate	23 mmol/l
TSH	<0.1 mu/l
Thyroxine	190 nmol/

1. What is the cause of the intermittent episodes of profound weakness?
   a. Epilepsy.
   b. Periodic paralysis.
   c. Cataplexy.
   d. Narcolepsy.
   e. Brugada's syndrome.

2. List two important steps in the management of this patient.
   a. Implantation of an internal cardiovertor defibrillator.
   b. Perform an EEG.
   c. Treat hypokalaemia.
   d. Perform electrophysiological ventricular stimulation study.
   e. Start carbimazole.
   f. Institute IV dextrose 50% and 16 units of short acting insulin.
   g. Perform MRI scan of the brain.
   h. 24-hour ECG monitoring.
   i. Give a trial of modenifil.
   j. Perform a sleep study.

Answer 214

> 1. The blood gases demonstrate a partially compensated respiratory alkalosis.
> 2. Hyperventilation.

Respiratory alkalosis is characterized by a low $PaCO_2$ and a high pH. Respiratory alkalosis may be seen in hyperventilation and artificial ventilation. In these situations it is associated with a high or normal PaO_2. It is also seen in conditions predisposing to ventilation/perfusion mismatch such as pneumonia, pulmonary oedema, pulmonary embolus and parenchymal lung disease. In this particular case, the patient has a normal PaO_2 and clear lung fields on the chest X-ray, suggesting that she is hyperventilating (see *Table* for causes of respiratory alkalosis).

In all chronic respiratory alkalotic states the kidneys compensate by excreting excess bicarbonate to produce a relative metabolic acidosis in an attempt to normalize the blood pH. Therefore, in compensated respiratory alkalosis the plasma bicarbonate is low.

Acute salicylate poisoning also produces a combined respiratory alkalosis and metabolic acidosis. In toxic doses, salicylates stimulate hyperventilation through effects on the respiratory regulatory system. Renal compensation leads to increased excretion of bicarbonate, resulting in metabolic acidosis. In addition, salicylates interfere with oxidative phosphorylation and lead to lactic acidosis, further exacerbating the metabolic acidosis.

(See Acid–base Disturbance, page 426.)

> **Causes of respiratory alkalosis**
>
> *Due to stimulation of the central nervous system*
> * Anxiety
> * Hypoxia
> * Salicylate poisoning
> * Encephalitis
> * Brainstem injury
>
> *Due to pulmonary disease*
> * Asthma
> * Pneumonia
> * Lung fibrosis
> * Pulmonary oedema
> * Pulmonary embolus

Answer 215

> 1. b. Periodic paralysis.
> 2. c. Treat hypokalaemia.
>   e. Start carbimazole.

Hypokalaemic periodic paralysis is a rare condition that is often inherited as an autosomal dominant trait. It is characterized by episodic paralysis, which classically occurs at night while the patient is asleep. The cause of hypokalaemia is not clear, but shifts in potassium from the extracellular fluid to the intracellular fluid are thought to be responsible. Symptoms can be precipitated by administering intravenous glucose and insulin into such patients, which would lend support to the potassium shift theory. Other precipitating factors include alcohol, large carbohydrate meals, anxiety and tension. Recovery is usually rapid, but can be expedited by intravenous potassium supplements. Long-term treatment is with potassium supplements or potassium-sparing diuretics.

In oriental males, aged between 20 and 50 years, the condition is associated with thyrotoxicosis. The symptoms of thyrotoxicosis may precede the paralysis, or may not be apparent. Paralysis occurs during sleep and periods of prolonged rest. Arrhythmias associated with hypokalaemia are a recognized feature in this condition. Treatment of the thyrotoxicosis prevents further attacks of paralysis. In the meantime, the potassium needs to be corrected. Propranolol is successful in preventing attacks in approximately 60% of cases. Although thyrotoxicosis is more common in females, periodic paralysis only affects males. The mechanism of hypokalaemia is the same as in familial periodic paralysis. *An important differential diagnosis when the patient is in the paralysed state is Guillain–Barré syndrome and acute myasthenia gravis.*

Narcolepsy and cataplexy have been discussed in Question 67 and Brugada's syndrome is discussed in Question 353.

Question 216

A 39-year-old male was admitted with malaise, lethargy and bleeding gums. Investigations on admission were as follows:

Hb	4 g/dl
WCC	70 × 10⁹/l (predominantly blasts)
Platelets	26 × 10⁹/l
Blood film (**216**)	
Sodium	137 mmol/l
Potassium	3.7 mmol/l
Urea	4 mmol/l
Creatinine	74 μmol/l

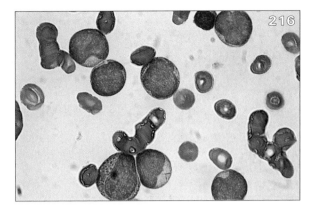

The patient received chemotherapy which he tolerated well, but on the second day post-chemotherapy he complained of severe nausea. Biochemical results were as follows:

Sodium	136 mmol/l
Potassium	7.2 mmol/l
Urea	23 mmol/l
Creatinine	300 μmol/l
Urate	1.2 mmol/l
Phosphate	3 mmol/l

1. What was the haematological diagnosis?
2. How do you account for the abnormal biochemistry?
3. What is the cause of the renal failure?
4. State two steps which should have been taken to prevent this complication.

Question 217

A 59-year-old headmaster was referred to a chest unit with a six-month history of progressive breathlessness. His effort tolerance one year previously was very good, allowing him to jog 10 km, twice a week. Since then he has had to give up running due to fatigue and breathlessness. His condition had continued to deteriorate, despite the use of steroid and salbutamol inhalers prescribed by his GP. He was now breathless after walking just 200 m. He was a non-smoker. He had been a headmaster in a London public school for nearly 25 years. There was no family history of lung disease. He had never worked with asbestos, and did not keep pets.

On examination, the patient was cyanosed and tachypnoeic. His hands and feet were clubbed. The JVP was not raised, and heart sounds were normal. On auscultation of the lung fields there were bilateral fine end-inspiratory crackles at both lung bases.

Investigations are shown.

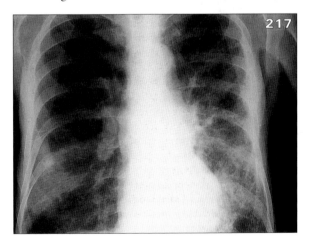

FEV₁ (% predicted)	50	Blood gases on air:
FVC (% predicted)	52	pH 7.45
FEV₁/FVC (%)	89	PaCO₂ 3.5 kPa
TLC (% predicted)	56	PaO₂ 6.4 kPa
KCO (% predicted)	60	Bicarbonate 22 mmol/l

Bronchoalveolar lavage revealed increased number of cells which were predominantly neutrophils
Chest X-ray (**217**)

1. What is the diagnosis?
2. Which two investigations will you perform to confirm the diagnosis?

Answer 216

1. Acute myeloid leukaemia. Myeloblasts are large round cells with a round nucleus and prominent nucleoli. In addition, they may contain cytoplasmic inclusions known as Auer rods, which are almost pathognomonic of the condition.
2. Tumour lysis syndrome. The large numbers of blasts destroyed by chemotherapy liberate large amounts of intracellular contents into the bloodstream, as evidenced by the high potassium and phosphate concentrations. The nucleic acid from the cell nuclei is metabolized to produce urate, which is excreted by the kidney.
3. Hyperuricaemic nephropathy. High concentrations of urate may cause crystallization within renal tubules and acute renal failure.
4. i. Pre-hydration with intravenous fluids.
    ii. Allopurinol, a xanthine oxidase inhibitor that inhibits the synthesis of urate.
    iii. Rasburicase, a recombinant urate oxidase inhibitor.

Answer 217

1. i. Restrictive lung defect with reduced KCO.
   ii. Cryptogenic fibrosing alveolitis.
2. i. High-resolution CT scan.
   ii. Transbronchial lung biopsy.

In the absence of an obvious underlying cause (occupational, drugs, connective tissue disorder) for the symptoms and signs, the most likely diagnosis is CFA, which is a disorder of unknown aetiology which usually occurs in middle age. It is characterized by progressively worsening dyspnoea, eventually leading to respiratory failure and cor pulmonale from pulmonary hypertension. The cardinal signs include cyanosis, clubbing and fine inspiratory crackles at both lung bases. The chest X-ray demonstrates a ground-glass appearance in the mid-zones and bases of the lung which progresses to nodular shadows and streaky fibrosis. The end result is a 'honeycomb appearance of the lung on the chest X-ray'.

Lung function tests demonstrate a restrictive lung defect and a low KCO.

Blood gases demonstrate a low arterial oxygen content and a normal CO_2 content unless the patient develops end-stage respiratory failure. The quality of high-resolution CT scans obviate the need for lung biopsy to diagnose the condition in the majority of patients, but in younger patients biopsy may be useful in differentiating the condition from other causes of a similar chest X-ray appearance. Bronchoalveolar lavage reveals large numbers of neutrophils, and transbronchial biopsy will demonstrate cellular infiltration and thickening and fibrosis of the alveolar walls.

Some 50% of patients are positive for rheumatoid factor, and 33% are positive for ANF.

CFA is associated with other auto-immune conditions such as coeliac disease, primary biliary cirrhosis, ulcerative colitis and RTA.

The management is with prednisolone. Azathioprine or cyclophosphamide may be used as steroid-sparing drugs. Most patients also require oxygen therapy. The median survival is five years.

Causes of lung fibrosis

- CFA
- Extrinsic allergic alveolitis (farmer's lung; bird-fancier's disease)
- Sarcoidosis
- Connective tissue disease (SLE, rheumatoid arthritis, systemic sclerosis)
- Vasculitides
- Drugs (busulphan, bleomycin, cyclophosphamide)
- Pneumoconiosis
- Asbestosis
- Neurofibromatosis
- Tuberous sclerosis
- Histiocytosis
- Ankylosing spondylitis
- TB
- Radiation

Question 218

A 76-year-old female was admitted after being found on the floor by the home help. She complained of frequent dizzy spells, particularly after standing from a recumbent position. She had experienced several falls at home, but never required hospital admission. She had become housebound due to the dizzy spells and falls and was increasingly dependent on the social services. She also complained of lethargy, hoarse voice, intermittent confusion, and weight gain of almost 7 kg over the past seven months. She had a history of arthritis for which she took paracetamol when in pain. She was not taking any other regular medications.

On examination, she was pale and frail. The heart rate was 60 beats/min and regular. The blood pressure was 200/60 mmHg when lying, and 90/50 mmHg when standing. The JVP was not raised. The apex was displaced slightly. Auscultation of the heart revealed soft first and second heart sounds. There were no added sounds or murmurs. Auscultation of the lungs was normal, as was examination of the abdomen. Central nervous system examination was essentially normal, with the exception of bilateral absence of the ankle jerks.

Investigations are shown.

1. What is the most likely explanation for the dizzy spells and falls?
2. What is the explanation for the electrolyte abnormality?
3. Which single test would you request to confirm this?
4. What is the unifying diagnosis?

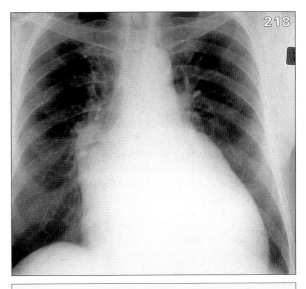

Hb	10 g/dl
WCC	6×10^9/l
Platelets	149×10^9/l
MCV	87 fl
Sodium	118 mmol/l
Potassium	5.3 mmol/l
Urea	3 mmol/l
Creatinine	69 µmol/l
Bilirubin	12 µmol/l
AST	20 iu/l
Alkaline phosphatase	100 iu/l
Albumin	36 g/l
Total protein	63 g/l
Chest X-ray (**218**)	
ECG	Normal rhythm and complexes

Question 219

A 69-year-old male was seen by his GP with pain in his wrist after a fall. He complained of generalized weakness and pains in his lower limbs over the past few months. Several investigations were ordered, the results of which are as follows:

1. Give two possible diagnoses.
2. Give three reasons to support the cause of this patient's raised IgG level.

Hb	13 g/dl	Phosphate	0.7 mmol/l
WCC	7×10^9/l	Alkaline phosphatase	240 iu/l
Platelets	350×10^9/l	IgG	23 g/l
ESR	55 mm/h	IgM	2 g/l
Sodium	136 mmol/l	IgA	2.4 g/l
Potassium	4 mmol/l	Paraprotein	6 g/l
Urea	6 mmol/l	X-ray of wrist	Fracture radius, small radiolucent area adjacent to fracture
Creatinine	90 µmol/l		
Calcium	2.0 mmol/l		

Answer 218

1. Postural hypotension.
2. Addison's disease.
3. Short synacthen test.
4. Polyendocrine deficiency type 2 (Schmidt's syndrome).

The postural hypotension and hyponatraemia suggest the diagnosis of Addison's disease. For causes and further details on Addison's disease, see Answer 273. The additional history of weight gain, croaky voice, and enlarged heart on the chest X-ray suggests coexistent hypothyroidism. (Note: in pure Addison's disease the heart is characteristically small owing to chronic hypovolaemia; however, if hypothyroidism is also present the heart may be enlarged owing to a consequent cardiomyopathy or a pericardial effusion.) Approximately 10% of cases of Addison's disease due to auto-immune adrenalitis are associated with other endocrine deficiencies (*Table*). The association of auto-immune adrenalitis with auto-immune hypothyroidism or insulin-dependent diabetes mellitus is termed Schmidt's syndrome or polyendocrine deficiency type 2.

The patient's confusion could be explained by either Addison's disease or hypothyroidism. Absent ankle jerks

The polyendocrine deficiency syndromes

Polyendocrine deficiency syndrome (type 2) comprises any two of the following
- Auto-immune hypoadrenalism
- Auto-immune hypothyroidism
- Insulin-dependent diabetes mellitus

Polyendocrine deficiency syndrome (type 1) comprises any two of the following
- Auto-immune hypoparathyroidism
- Auto-immune hypoadrenalism
- Mucocutaneous candidiasis, alopecia, pernicious anaemia

Vitiligo and hypogonadism may occur in both forms

are not uncommon in the elderly. In hypothyroidism, the ankle jerk characteristically demonstrates slow relaxation; however, there may be absent reflexes owing to a secondary peripheral neuropathy. Other neurological manifestations of hypothyroidism include cerebellar syndrome and coma.

Answer 219

1. i. Osteomalacia.
   ii. Monoclonal gammopathy of undetermined significance.
2. i. Not anaemic.
   ii. No evidence of immune paresis.
   iii. Paraprotein level below 20 g/l.

The diagnosis of osteomalacia is relatively straightforward on the bone biochemistry, which classically reveals hypocalcaemia, hypophosphataemia and a raised alkaline phosphatase, the latter being secondary to an increase in PTH release in response to hypocalcaemia. Skeletal manifestations of osteomalacia include Looser's zones, which are linear radiolucent areas seen most commonly in the bones of the forearms, scapulae, femurs and the pelvis. The raised ESR and IgG level associated with a very mild paraproteinaemia will confuse some readers, and commit

them to make the erroneous diagnosis of multiple myeloma. However, there are a few pointers to suggest that the cause for the raised IgG level is MGUS rather than myeloma.

MGUS affects a very small proportion of the elderly. It is characterized by benign monoclonal proliferation of lymphocytes, resulting in a modest increase in IgG levels and an associated paraprotein of <2 g/l (in myeloma, the paraprotein level is usually >20 g/l). In contrast with patients suffering from myeloma, these patients are not anaemic, they do not have immune paresis, i.e. the other immunoglobulins are not reduced because of monoclonal proliferation, Bence Jones proteins are classically absent (may be present in <10%), and the skeletal survey is normal. The condition was originally termed benign monoclonal gammopathy, but it is now recognized that 10% of patients develop multiple myeloma, hence the relatively new term, MGUS.

Question 220

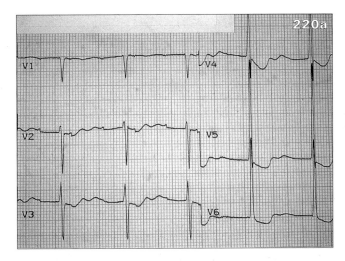

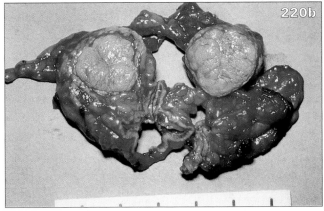

Sodium	142 mmol/l
Potassium	3.3 mmol/l
Urea	4.0 mmol/l
Creatinine	100 µmol/l
Bicarbonate	36 mmol/l
Chloride	107 mmol/l
ECG (**220a**)	

A 42-year-old male presented with a four-month history of headaches, generalized weakness and polyuria. On examination, the physical examination was normal with the exception of a blood pressure of 190/105 mmHg.

Initial investigations are shown.

The patient was treated with a calcium antagonist, and underwent further investigations which led to him having abdominal surgery to cure his hypertension. The full macroscopic specimen of the abnormality removed is shown (**220b**).

1. What is the electrolyte abnormality?
2. List four abnormalities on the ECG, and two inferences you would make from these abnormalities.
3. What was the cause of his hypertension?
4. Which two investigations would he have had to confirm the diagnosis before surgery?
5. With all of the above information at hand, which antihypertensive agent should he have been prescribed?

Answer 220

1. Hypokalaemic alkalosis (see Answer 275).
2. i. First-degree atrioventricular block. The PR-interval is much greater than 200 ms. There are many causes of first-degree atrioventricular block (*Table A*); however, in this case the most likely cause is hypokalaemia.
   ii. There is voltage criteria of left ventricular hypertrophy. The sum of the S-wave in V1 and the R-wave in V5 or V6 exceeds 0.35 mV (each small square on the ECG is 0.1 mV), which conforms with the Sokolow criteria for left ventricular hypertrophy.
   iii. There is ST-segment depression in the lateral leads which may be secondary to left ventricular hypertrophy or to hypokalaemia. Although myocardial ischaemia is also a recognized cause of ST-segment depression, it is unlikely in the context of this question.
   iv. There are prominent U-waves (upright waves immediately following the T-wave, **220c** arrowed) which are suggestive of hypokalaemia. Other ECG changes in relation to metabolic abnormalities are tabulated below (*Table B*).
3. Primary hyperaldosteronism or Conn's syndrome secondary to an adrenal adenoma. Conn's tumours are bright yellow as opposed to phaeochromocytomas, which are a greyish-purple colour (**220d**).
4. i. Lying and standing plasma renin and aldosterone levels.
   ii. High-resolution abdominal CT scan.
5. High doses of spironolactone, an aldosterone antagonist.

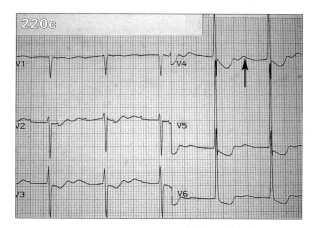

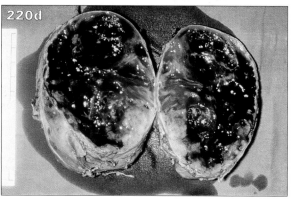

Hypokalaemic alkalosis and hypertension in the MRCP and similar examinations is highly suggestive of primary hyperaldosteronism, which is often referred to as Conn's syndrome. The syndrome is caused by excessive secretion of aldosterone by the adrenal gland. This leads to increased salt and water retention, causing hypertension and clinical symptoms of hypokalaemia which include muscle weakness, polyuria and polydipsia from nephrogenic diabetes insipidus, and paraesthesia. Accelerated hypertension may complicate primary hyperaldosteronism, and cardiac arrhythmias may result from hypokalaemia. The serum renin level in primary hyperaldosteronism is suppressed, whereas in conditions causing secondary hyperaldosteronism the renin is elevated. Primary hyperaldosteronism may be caused by an autonomous aldosterone-secreting adrenal adenoma or bilateral hyperplasia of the adrenal gland. Endocrine causes of hypertension are tabulated (*Table C*).

The diagnosis is made by simultaneous measurement of serum renin and aldosterone levels in the lying and standing positions. The renin is low, and the aldosterone level is high, in the supine position. On standing suddenly, there is a paradoxical drop in the aldosterone level in patients with an adenoma and an exaggerated rise in aldosterone levels in patients with hyperplasia. Imaging with CT scanning is very useful in distinguishing between adenoma and hyperplasia. Adrenal adenomas >0.5 cm in diameter can be diagnosed by high-resolution CT scan. Adrenal vein sampling is only useful when there is doubt about the existence of an adenoma.

Iodolabelled cholesterol scintiscan is not a very sensitive method for identifying Conn's tumours.

The management of adrenal adenoma is surgical excision, and the management of hyperplasia is with a high-dose aldosterone antagonist, such as spironolactone.

Table A Causes of first-degree atrioventricular block

- Ischaemic heart disease
- Cardiac conduction tissue disease (sinoatrial disease)
- Rheumatic fever
- Myocarditis
- Drugs
- Hypokalaemia
- Athlete's heart

Table B ECG changes in relation to metabolic abnormalities frequently encountered in the MRCP and similar examinations

Hypokalaemia
- Peaked P-waves
- Long PR-interval
- Increased duration of the QRS-complex
- U-waves
- Long QT-interval
- Flattened T-waves
- ST-segment depression

Hyperkalaemia
- Flat P-waves
- Peaked T-waves
- Increased duration of the QRS-complex
- Sinusoidal QRS-complexes (pre-arrest)

Hypocalcaemia
- Long QT-interval

Hypercalcaemia
- Short QT-interval

Table C Endocrine causes of hypertension

- Conn's syndrome
- Cushing's syndrome
- Phaeochromocytoma
- Acromegaly
- Thyrotoxicosis
- Hyperparathyroidism
- 11-β- and 17-β-hydroxylase deficiency

Question 221

A 15-year-old farmer's daughter was admitted to the infectious diseases unit with a five-day history of right upper quadrant pain. On examination, she was pyrexial with a temperature of 38.4°C (101.1°F). She appeared unwell and jaundiced.

Investigations are shown.

Hb	8 g/dl
WCC	18.8×10^9/l
Platelets	140×10^9/l
Reticulocyte count	20%
Blood film	No fragmented red cells seen
PT	36 s (control 12 s)
APTT	59 s (control 45 s)
Sodium	136 mmol/l
Potassium	4.9 mmol/l
Urea	26 mmol/l
Creatinine	400 µmol/l
Bilirubin	50 mmol/l
AST	900 iu/l
Alkaline phosphatase	300 iu/l
Albumin	33 g/l
Hepatitis B sAg	Absent
HCV Ab	Absent
CMV serology	Absent
Monospot test	Negative

1. Suggest at least two possible diagnoses.
2. Give three possible causes for the anaemia.

Answer 221

1. i. Leptospirosis (Weil's disease).
   ii. Acute hepatitis A infection.
   iii. Paracetamol overdose.
   iv. Iron overdose.
2. i. Blood loss from endothelial damage resulting in haemorrhage.
   ii. Haemolysis.
   iii. Disseminated intravascular coagulation causing blood loss.

The patient has evidence of hepatitis together with renal failure and a coagulation disorder. The clinical scenario which would fit this triad is fulminant hepatic failure complicated by the hepatorenal syndrome. The majority of cases are due to viral hepatitis (hepatitis A, B, C and D, although EBV, CMV, Coxsackie and herpes simplex virus have been implicated; Lassa fever, Ebola virus and Marburg virus should be considered in a patient who has recently returned from Africa), and drugs (paracetamol, iron, tetracycline, isoniazid, rifampicin, halothane). Other recognized causes include toxins (alcohol, carbon tetrachloride), leptospirosis (Weil's disease), Wilson's disease, and pregnancy. In a farmer's daughter leptospirosis causing hepatic and renal failure (Weil's disease) is a distinct possibility, but hepatitis A and drug overdose should also be borne in mind.

Leptospirosis is caused by the spirochaete *Leptospira icterohaemorrhagica*. Rodents, particularly rats, are the most important reservoir of infection. Other hosts include cattle, pigs, goats, hamsters, mice, hedgehogs, foxes and skunks. The organism is excreted in the urine and may survive in the soil for several weeks. Entry into the human host is through cuts and abrasions on the skin, or through intact mucous membranes. Occupations most susceptible are sewage workers, fishermen, vets and farmers. Replication occurs in the blood and tissue and multi-system involvement may occur. The kidneys and liver are most affected. Glomerular injury occurs first causing an acute interstitial nephritis and tubular necrosis. In the liver there is evidence of centrilobular necrosis in severe cases.

The incubation period is 7–12 days. The initial (septicaemic) phase is 4–7 days in duration. It is characterized by fever, headaches, myalgia, abdominal pain, vomiting, skin rash (macular, maculopapular or haemorrhagic) or conjunctival injection. Fever is high, myalgia is present in over 85% of cases and a major hallmark of the disease, and the headache may be severe. Persistent headache is suggestive of meningitis. Proteinuria and haematuria may be present during this phase, and renal failure is evident in just over 50% of patients. Jaundice and impairment of liver function are present only in severe cases. Some 90% of cases are anicteric. Hepatosplenomegaly is present in approximately 20%. Respiratory involvement is common, and manifests as a dry cough, haemoptysis and confluent shadow on the chest X-ray. The second phase of the disease (immune phase) varies between 4 and 30 days. The patient is afebrile. Antibody titres to *Leptospira* are rising. Deterioration in liver and renal function may continue. Meningism, uveitis and a rash are common. Haematological manifestations include thrombocytopenia, haemolytic uraemic syndrome characterized by fragmented red cells on the blood film and intravascular haemolysis. Endothelial injury may cause blood loss from the gastrointestinal tract and the lung.

Blood cultures are positive in the first week, and by the second week the urine culture is also positive. IgM antibodies to *Leptospira* are detectable in the first week. There is a rising titre in the second week. Treatment is with high-dose penicillin.

Brucellosis is also recognized in farmers. The bacterium (Gram-negative bacillus) infects mammals, particularly cows, and can be contracted from contact with infected urine or drinking unpasteurized milk. Acute brucellosis is also characterized by fever, headache and myalgia; however, it is unlikely in this case owing to the absence of a high fever, leucopenia, and assumed absence of hepatosplenomegaly, which is common in brucellosis. In addition, abnormal liver function or jaundice is extremely rare in brucellosis. Chronic brucellosis is associated with lassitude, headaches, depression, night sweats, skeletal, cardiovascular, neurological, genitourinary, pulmonary and intra-abdominal complications. Brucellosis has been eradicated in the UK owing to mandatory pasteurization of milk.

Question 222

A 60-year-old male was investigated for a two-year history of increasing breathlessness. He worked as a miner and smoked 20 cigarettes per day. His past medical history included psoriasis and rheumatoid arthritis. His medications included salbutamol inhaler, Becotide inhaler, methotrexate and folic acid.

Investigations are shown.

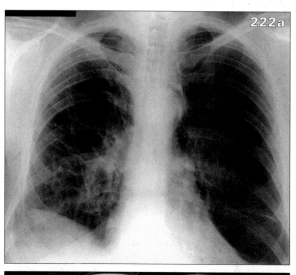

Hb	16 g/dl
WCC	$6.9 \times 10^9/l$
Platelets	$412 \times 10^9/l$
MCV	98 fl
Sodium	138 mmol/l
Urea	6 mmol/l
Calcium	2.31 mmol/l
Albumin	35 g/l
Bilirubin	18 mmol/l
Alkaline phosphatase	190 iu/l
AST	30 iu/l
Chest X-ray (**222a**)	
CT Thorax (**222b**)	

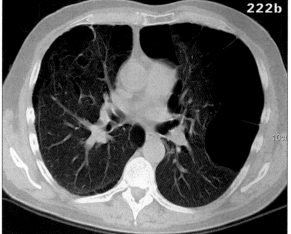

What is the diagnosis?
  a. Pleural fibrosis.
  b. Rheumatoid induced pulmonary fibrosis.
  c. Large pleural effusion.
  d. Emphysema.
  e. Caplan syndrome.

Question 223

A 70-year-old male developed atrial fibrillation 12 hours after thrombolysis for an anterior myocardial infarction. He did not have chest pain. He had a history of hypertension and chronic obstructive airways disease. The heart rate measured 122 beats/min. The blood pressure measured 130/80 mmHg and the chest was clear.

What immediate treatment is recommended for the management of the atrial fibrillation?
  a. IV digoxin.
  b. DC cardioversion.
  c. IV amiodarone.
  d. IV flecanide.
  e. IV metoprolol.

Question 224

A 44-year-old male was admitted to the Coronary Care Unit following an inferior myocardial infarction. He was a smoker and consumed up to 20 units of alcohol per day. On the third day of admission he became gradually clammy. He was aggressive towards the nursing staff. His heart rate was 130 beats/min. The blood pressure was 160/100 mmHg. Oxygen saturation on air was 96%.

What is the best management of this patient?
  a. Intravenous thiamine.
  b. Intravenous chlormethiazole.
  c. Oral diazepam.
  d. Intravenous midazolam.
  e. Intramuscular haloperidol.

Answer 222

> d. Emphysema.

In a patient with rheumatoid arthritis, a history of heavy smoking and an occupational history of mining there are several potential causes of dyspnoea, which include rheumatoid lung disease (see Answer 320), occupational dust induced fibrosis and obstructive airways disease. The chest X-ray shows reduced lung markings in the left upper and lower lobes and to some extent in the right upper lobe. The CT scan of the thorax demonstrates large emphysematous bullae in the left upper lobe and some emphysematous changes in the right upper lobe.

Answer 223

> a. IV digoxin.

The patient has developed rapid atrial fibrillation shortly after myocardial infarction. He is surprisingly asymptomatic. DC cardioversion is only indicated if there is ongoing myocardial ischaemia or heamodynamic compromise. In the absence of these features the aim is to control the ventricular rate to reduce myocardial oxygen consumption and to prevent systemic thromboembolism.

The most effective drugs to slow ventricular rate are beta-blockers, but these are relatively contraindicated in this patient, who also has COPD. Although diltiazem is effective, there have been recent reports suggesting that calcium channel antagonists may be associated with an increased mortality following myocardial infarction.

Digoxin is also highly effective and would be the drug of choice in this situation. In most cases AF following MI is transient, therefore chronic anti-arrhythmic therapy is not usually required. If the AF persists then elective cardioversion should be considered at a later date (usually after six weeks in the context of a recent myocardial infarction) ensuring that the patient has been anticoagulated throughout.

There are no trials assessing the effect of amiodarone in the management of AF following MI. Amiodarone should be reserved for patients who have several paroxysms of AF following MI (based on anecdotal evidence).

Flecanide is contraindicated after MI as it has been associated with an increased mortality in this particular situation.

Answer 224

> c. Oral diazepam.

The patient presents with features of delirium tremens (aggressive behaviour, sweating, tachycardia and hypertension), the best treatment for which is therapy with benzodiazepines. Short-acting agents such as lorazepam are usually not recommended because they have to be given relatively frequently. Chlormethiazole was commonly used in the 1980s but there have been adverse effects with respiratory suppression, therefore the drug is no longer recommended for alcohol withdrawal. Diazepam is advocated for use in DT but its long-acting duration may cause oversedation. The best treatment is a benzodiazepine with an intermediate effect such as chlordiazepoxide, but this is not one of the options given. Intravenous midazolam may cause marked sedation and is potentially harmful in this situation. Neuroleptic agents reduce the threshold for epileptic seizures. They should be avoided in DT. While all patients with alcohol dependence should be treated with thiamine to prevent Wernicke's encephalopathy, this particular scenario calls for specific management of delirium tremens.

Question 225

A 23-year-old male was admitted with a 24-hour history of cough, fever and confusion. He had a history of epilepsy that was well controlled on carbamazepine. Looking through his records there were several transient admissions for deliberate self-harm, including a history of Ecstasy abuse. According to a friend he consumed up to 70 units of alcohol per week.

On examination he was pale. The heart rate was 110/min and regular. The blood pressure measured 96/60 mmHg. There was reduced air entry over the anterior aspect of the right chest.

Investigations are shown.

Which antibiotic regime would you prescribe for the patient?
   a. IV cefuroxime.
   b. IV amoxycillin.
   c. IV clarithromycin.
   d. IV cefuroxime and clarithromycin.
   e. IV amoxycillin and metronidazole.

Hb	12 g/dl
WCC	14 × 10⁹/l
Platelets	200 × 10⁹/l
MCV	90 fl
Sodium	134 mmol/l
Potassium	3.8 mmol/l
Urea	7 mmol/l
Creatinine	120 μmol/l
Bilirubin	15 mmol/l
AST	140 iu/l
ALT	182 iu/l
Gamma GT	312 iu/l

Arterial blood gases on air:

pH	7.4
PaO_2	9.2 kPa
$PaCO_2$	4.8 kPa
Bicarbonate	21 mmol/l

Chest X-ray (**225a**, **b**)

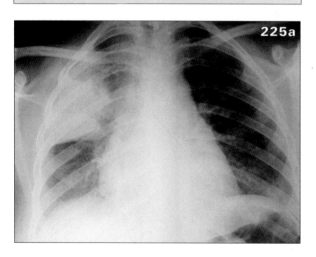

225a

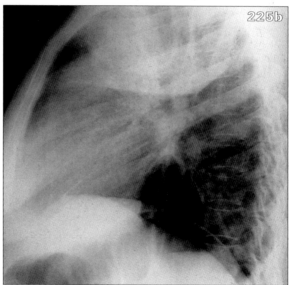

225b

Question 226

A 16-year-old girl was admitted with a 3-hour history of vomiting followed by collapse. She had recently split up from her boyfriend and was thought to have taken an overdose of digoxin that her father had been prescribed for atrial fibrillation.

On examination she was drowsy and confused. Her pulse was 36 beats/min. The blood pressure was 70 systolic.

Investigations are shown.

What is the immediate management of her condition?
   a. Activated charcoal via nasogastric tube.
   b. IV atropine.
   c. IV isoprenaline.
   d. IV dextrose 50% (50 ml).
   e. IV digoxin specific antibody fragments (Digibind).

Sodium	133 mmol/l
Potassium	4.8 mmol/l
Urea	5.6 mmol/l
Creatinine	100 μmol/l
Digoxin level	5 nmol/l
ECG	High second degree AV block; VR 36/min

Answer 225

> e. IV amoxycillin and metronidazole.

The patient has evidence of a right upper lobe consolidation, which would usually be treated conventionally with IV cefuroxime and IV clarithromycin in accordance with the guidelines set by the British Thoracic Society. However, he has several risk factors for aspiration, notably alcohol and recreational drug abuse. Aspiration pneumonia is caused by anaerobic bacteria that are not effectively treated with cephalosporins, macrolides, aminoglycosides or the quinolones.

Antibiotics of choice in the management of aspiration pneumonia include a combination of amoxycillin and metronidazole, or clindamycin or imipenem.

The coexistence of confusion and liver function tests may have led to a diagnostic dilemma between aspiration pneumonia and pneumonia due to *Legionella pneumophila*. However, the possibility of an unprotected airway (unconsciousness) in this individual means that aspiration pneumonia should be considered above the diagnosis of Legionnaire's disease.

Answer 226

> b. IV atropine.

Digoxin toxicity is characterized by gastrointestinal disturbance such as anorexia, nausea, vomiting and diarrhoea, blurred vision, xanthopsia, dizziness, confusion and delirium. Cardiac arrhythmias are usually the most serious complication and are the commonest cause of mortality in digoxin toxicity. Almost any arrhythmia is possible. Ventricular extra-systoles are the commonest rhythm disturbance. The presence of supraventricular tachyarrhythmias and atrioventricular block in a patient taking digoxin are highly suggestive of digoxin toxicity.

The management of digoxin therapy includes prevention of absorption of the drug, correction of electrolyte disturbances that promote digoxin toxicity or occur as a result of digoxin toxicity, and management of arrhythmias. A small proportion of patients may require digoxin specific antibody fragments (*Table*).

In severe digoxin toxicity, the inhibition of the Na^+/K^+ ATPase can result in hyperkalaemia that should be treated conventionally with 50 ml of 50% dextrose and 16–18 units of short-acting insulin. Severe bradyarrhythmias (HR <40 beats/min), as in this situation, should be treated with IV atropine. Temporary cardiac pacing is necessary in patients unresponsive to atropine. Isporenaline is contraindicated, as it may precipitate tachyarrhythmias.

Verapamil is the drug of choice in patients with supraventricular arrhythmias. Lignocaine and phenytoin are effective in the management of ventricular tachycardia. Electrical cardioversion is indicated in patients with haemodynamic compromise but with relatively low voltage DC shocks, e.g. 50 J, as there is a risk of asystole.

A small group of patients require the specific digoxin binding antibody fragments, which rapidly bind to circulating digoxin and prevent its effects on the heart. They are indicated in patients who have taken a large overdose (10 mg in adults; 4 mg in children), those with plasma digoxin >13 nmol/l, and in patients with K^+ level >5 mmol/l in the presence of life-threatening arrhythmias such as high AV block and VT/VF. They are given IV over 30 minutes but can be given as a bolus in the event of a cardiac arrest.

Digoxin binding antibody fragments are small molecules that pass through the glomerular basement membrane and are excreted via the kidneys. They can be safely given to patients with renal impairment including those who are dialysis dependent.

In this particular case the immediate management is atropine followed by temporary pacing if the heart block persists.

Management of digoxin toxicity

Action	Technique/drug
Prevent absorption of drug	Gastric lavage or ipecacuanha
	Activated charcoal if ingestion <6–8 hours
Correct electrolytes	Correct K^+ and Mg^{2+}
Manage bradyarrhythmias	Atropine
Temporary cardiac pacing	
Manage SVTs	Verapamil
Manage VT	Lignocaine
	Phenytoin
In very severe cases	Digoxin binding antibody fragments (see above)

Question 227

A 65-year-old smoker with exertional dyspnoea was investigated with a chest X-ray (**227**).

> What is the radiological diagnosis?
>   a. Left upper lobe consolidation.
>   b. Left upper lobe collapse.
>   c. Left lower lobe collapse.
>   d. Left-sided pneumothorax.
>   e. Left pleural effusion.

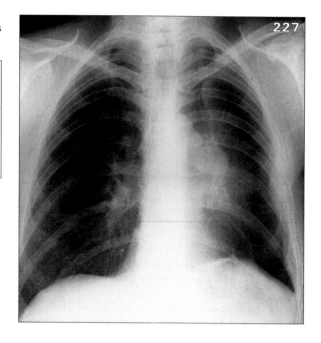

Question 228

A 30-year-old male with a family history of adult polycystic kidney disease wished to be screened for the condition. His mother was affected and a paternal aunt had recently suffered a subarachnoid haemorrhage as a result of a ruptured berry aneurysm.

> What is the standard screening investigation of choice?
>   a. CT scan abdomen.
>   b. Renal ultrasound.
>   c. CT scan brain.
>   d. Genotype for APCKD-1 gene.
>   e. Urinalysis.

Question 229

Below is an ECG (**229**) from a patient presenting with syncope.

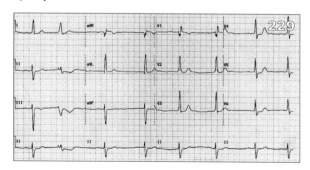

> What is the most likely cause of the syncope?
>   a. Complete heart block.
>   b. Torsades de pointes.
>   c. Posterior myocardial infarction.
>   d. Rapid atrial fibrillation.
>   e. Monomorphic ventricular tachycardia.

Answer 227

> b. Left upper lobe collapse.

There are three main features that are related to loss of lung volume: elevation of the left hemidiaphragm;

elevation of the left hilum; and reduction in the spaces between the ribs in the left upper zone. There is a veil-like shadow affecting the upper part of the lung, which represents a collapsed left upper lobe.

Answer 228

> b. Renal ultrasound.

The patient has adult polycystic kidney disease. 86% of patients with APCKD have an abnormality in a gene adjacent to the alpha globin gene in chromosome 16 (PKD-1 gene). The other patients with APCKD (PCKD-2) have an abnormal gene on chromosome 4. In PCKD-2 cysts and end-stage renal failure occur late (in the sixth or seventh decade), thus screening with ultrasound may miss young PCKD-2 patients. However, this is not felt to be particularly important since most patients with this genotype remain well throughout life.

With respect to APCKD-1, screening is based on the demonstration of cysts in one or both kidneys (depending upon age) using CT scan or renal ultrasound. In children CT scan of the abdomen is the screening test of choice as small cysts may be missed using ultrasound. By the age of 30–35 years all patients with APCKD-1 have visible cysts on renal ultrasound; therefore, for adults in or above this age group renal ultrasound is the screening test of choice. Even in patients aged 20, the false-negative rate with renal ultrasound is only 4%. See *Table* for ultrasound criteria for diagnosis of polycystic kidney disease.

Genetic testing for APCKD-1 is 99% accurate but is not widely available, and is currently reserved for screening children in whom CT scan may be normal and those who are potential transplant donors for their families.

APCKD is associated with intracranial aneurysms. Approximately 8% of patients with APCKD have intracranial aneurysms, which is four to five times higher than the general population. Ruptured aneurysms are responsible for around 6% of all deaths due to APCKD. Patients with APCKD and a family history of cerebral

Ultrasound criteria for the diagnosis of APCKD

Age	Criterion
<30	at least two cysts (unilateral or bilateral)
30–59	at least two cysts in each kidney
≥ 60	at least four cysts in each kidney

Algorithm for screening for intracranial aneurysms in patients with APCKD

haemorrhage should be offered screening with magnetic resonance angiography of the brain or spiral CT scan of the brain (see algorithm for screening for intracranial aneurysms in patients with APCKD).

Answer 229

> a. Complete heart block.

The patient has a bifascicular block (left anterior hemiblock and RBBB) and a prolonged PR interval.

There is a high probability that the syncopal episode is due to complete heart block resulting from impaired conduction through the third fascicle (the left posterior fascicle). Slow heart rates can also cause prolonged QT and torsades de pointes, but the QT interval is normal.

Question 230

A 48-year-old male, psychiatric patient, living in an institution, was witnessed to have a fit for the first time. He had been treated with chlorpromazine for the past four years. Three hours later the patient remained unconscious and was admitted to hospital where blood results were as follows:

Sodium	115 mmol/l
Potassium	3.4 mmol/l
Urea	1.1 mmol/l
Creatinine	60 μmol/l
Glucose	4.1 mmol/l
POsm	248 mOsm/l
Renin	90 pmol/l (NR 100–500 pmol/l)
Aldosterone	50 pmol/l (NR 100–500)
TSH	3 mu/l (NR 0.5–5.0 mu/l)
Urine sodium	10 mmol/l
Urine osmolality	90 mOsm/l

What is the diagnosis?
a. Chlorpromazine-induced ADH secretion.
b. Syndrome of inappropriate ADH secretion.
c. Lithium toxicity.
d. Diabetes insipidus.
e. Compulsive water drinking.

Question 231

A 56-year-old woman presented with a four-day history of breathlessness, cough and a high fever. She gave a long history of indigestion and intermittent dysphagia to solids and fluids. On several occasions undigested food would be regurgitated back shortly after she had eaten. She would often wake at night with episodes of coughing and spluttering. There was no history of weight loss.

On examination, she had a temperature of 39°C (102.2°F). The respiratory rate was 30/min, and the heart rate was 102 beats/min. Chest expansion was moderate and symmetrical. On auscultation of the lung fields there were coarse bilateral basal crackles.

The chest X-ray demonstrated bilateral lower lobe consolidation.

1. What is the cause of this patient's illness?
a. Hiatus hernia.
b. Benign oesophageal stricture.
c. Achalasia.
d. Pharyngeal pouch.
e. Bronchiectasis.

2. What investigation would be most useful in identifying the cause of her presentation?
a. Oesophagoscopy.
b. Barium swallow.
c. Oesophageal manometry.
d. Bronchoscopy.
e. CT scan of the thorax.

Answer 230

> e. Compulsive water drinking.

The patient has a very low serum sodium and low plasma osmolality (calculated 231 mOsmol/l). The main differential diagnoses are SIADH and primary polydipsia, although hypothyroidism and cortisol deficiency may also present with similar plasma biochemistry. In compulsive water drinking (primary polydipsia), ADH production is completely inhibited and urine osmolality is very low (<100 mOsm/l). In this particular case the very low urine osmolality is consistent with the diagnosis of compulsive water drinking. This is a relatively common problem in patients with schizophrenia.

Although chlorpromazine can cause SIADH, the low urine osmolality is against the diagnosis. Patients with SIADH have concentrated urine (high POsm) and urine sodium >40 mmol/l. Patients with diabetes inspidus have dilute urine but high plasma osmolality and plasma sodium. Patients with mineralocorticoid deficiency have low sodium, low plasma osmolality but high urine sodium and osmolality. In this case the renin and aldosterone levels are suppressed owing to the profound hyponatraemia caused by excessive water intake. Excess gastrointestinal fluid loss would cause dehydration and hyponatraemia resulting in salt and water retention by the kidneys and hence a high urine osmolality and low urine sodium (<20 mmol/l).

Diabetes insipidus is characterized by a normal or elevated plasma osmolality but a low urine osmolality (*Table*) (see Question 401).

Plasma sodium/osmolality, urinary sodium and urinary osmolality in various conditions			
	P Na/Osm	*U Na*	*U Osm*
Diabetes insipidus	Normal/high	Low	Low
SIADH	Low	High	High
Hypothyroidism	Low	High	High
Hypoadrenalism	Low	High	High
Effective volume depletion*	Low/normal	Low	High
Water intoxication	Low	Low	Low

*Includes dehydration from GI loss, excess perspiration, water loss, CCF, hypoalbuminaemic states.
Exceptions include renal failure due to interstitial nephritis, where sodium excretion is increased even in dehydration.

Answer 231

> 1. c. Achalasia.
> 2. b. Barium swallow.

A history of dyspepsia, dysphagia, oesophageal reflux and a possible aspiration pneumonia is consistent with the diagnosis of achalasia. Hiatus hernia may cause reflux and occasionally nocturnal cough and aspiration pneumonia; however, dysphagia is not a feature unless recurrent reflux has caused a peptic stricture. Peptic stricture may cause all the symptoms of achalasia; however, there is usually a long history of indigestion before the onset of dysphagia. Pharyngeal pouch does not cause retrosternal pain, although dysphagia and regurgitation are common.

A barium swallow is the best method of differentiating between achalasia, peptic stricture, hiatus hernia and pharyngeal pouch. Although it is relatively clear that the diagnosis is achalasia, oesophageal manometry scores fewer marks than barium swallow or oesophagoscopy because other causes of dysphagia – particularly oesophageal stricture – would have to be excluded before entertaining a diagnosis of achalasia. In achalasia, the barium demonstrates dilatation of the oesophagus and lack of peristalsis. The lower end gradually narrows owing to failure of the lower oesophageal sphincter to relax. Oesophageal manometry is useful for measuring motility.

Achalasia is a motility disorder affecting the oesophagus. It is characterized by lack of peristalsis and failure of the lower oesophageal sphincter to relax. Pathologically, there is degeneration of the ganglionic cells in the nerve plexus of the oesophageal wall. The aetiology is unknown. The disease often presents in middle age. There is a long history of retrosternal pain, intermittent dysphagia, oesophageal reflux and aspiration. Weight loss is unusual. Diagnosis is by a combination of barium swallow and oesophageal manometry. Treatment is by dilating the lower oesophagus by pneumatic inflation. In unsuccessful cases, surgical division of the lower end of the oesophagus (Heller's operation) is required.

Question 232

A 16-year-old girl who had undergone previous surgery for congenital heart disease presented with fatigue. On examination she had a heart rate of 40 beats/min. The blood pressure was 110/70 mmHg. There was no evidence of heart failure. The ECG showed complete heart block with a ventricular rate of 40/min.

What is the management?
   a. Dual chamber permanent pacemaker.
   b. Atrial pacemaker.
   c. Single chamber ventricular pacemaker.
   d. Reassure.
   e. Observe at six-monthly intervals.

Question 233

A 38-year-old man was investigated for lethargy and severe lower back pain. He had a past medical history of Hodgkin's lymphoma (stage 1A) which had been treated with radiotherapy one year previously. On examination he had a tender lumbar spine and palpable lymph nodes in the left axilla and both inguinal areas.

Investigations are shown.

Hb	9 g/dl
WCC	14 × 10⁹/l
Platelets	80 × 10⁹/l
MCV	88 fl
Reticulocyte count	0.4%
Blood film	Nucleated red cells; metamyelocytes and myeloblasts

What is the cause of the anaemia?
   a. Anaemia of chronic disease.
   b. Hypersplenism.
   c. Haemolysis.
   d. Marrow infiltration.
   e. Folate deficiency.

Question 234

A 15-year-old boy was admitted to the intensive care unit for the second time with meningococcal septicaemia.

Investigations on admission were as follows:

Hb	14.8 g/dl
WCC	18 × 10⁹/l (neutrophils 80%)
Platelets	190 × 10⁹/l

What investigation would you perform to identify the cause?
   a. White cell count.
   b. Neutrophil chemotactic factor.
   c. Serum complement level.
   d. Serum immunoglobulins.
   e. Neutrophil antibodies.

Question 235

Below is an ECG (**235**) from a 78-year-old patient with a slow pulse rate.

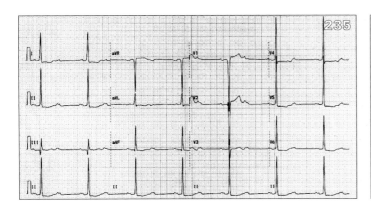

What are the two ECG diagnoses?
   a. Complete heart block.
   b. Left atrial enlargement.
   c. Mobitz II second degree AV block.
   d. 2:1 second degree AV block.
   e. Left ventricular hypertrophy.
   f. Left axis deviation.
   g. Inferior myocardial infarction.
   h. Anterior myocardial infarction.
   i. First degree AV block.
   j. Mobitz I second degree AV block.

Answer 232

> a. Dual chamber permanent pacemaker.

The patient has had prior cardiac surgery and presents with symptoms of fatigue and a heart rate of 40 beats/min secondary to third degree AV block. All forms of acquired third degree AV block should be paced. The annual mortality from acquired third degree block is 15% in the absence of cardiac pacing.

Congenital third degree heart block may not require pacing if the ventricular complexes are narrow and the rate is >50 beats/min. In the presence of broad ventricular complexes or a heart rate of <50 beats/min, pacing is indicated.

Answer 233

> d. Marrow infiltration.

The patient has a past history of Hodgkin's lymphoma and presents with back pain. There is evidence of a normochromic, normocytic anaemia. The blood film shows evidence of immature red and white cells, i.e. a leucoerythroblastic blood picture. In the context of this question, the most likely cause of the leucoerythroblastic blood picture is marrow infiltration (*Table*).

Causes of a leucoerythroblastic blood picture

- Bone marrow infiltration from malignant cells
- Myelofibrosis
- Marble-bone disease (osteopetrosis)
- Certain metabolic storage disorders, e.g. Gaucher's disease
- TB
- Septicaemia

Answer 234

> c. Serum complement level.

Patients with C5 to C9 complement deficiency are prone to recurrent *Neisseria* infections.

Hypocomplementaemia may be inherited or acquired. Inherited hypocomplementaemia is associated with a predisposition to auto-immune disorders and bacterial infections (*Table*). Acquired causes of hypo-complementaemia include glomerulonephritis, haemolytic uraemic syndrome and its variants, severe sepsis, pancreatitis, advanced renal disease and athero-embolic renal disease.

Hereditary causes of hypocomplementaemia

Deficiency	*Disorder*
C2 deficiency	Auto-immune diseases e.g. SLE
C1 q, r or s deficiency	SLE
C3 deficiency	Severe recurrent infections with encapsulated bacteria shortly after birth
C4 deficiency	Auto-immune disorders such as Henoch–Schönlein syndrome, membranous glomerulonephritis, scleroderma
C5–C9 deficiencies	Predisposition to *Neisseria* spp. infections (manifests in late teens usually)

Answer 235

> d. 2:1 second degree AV block.
> e. Left ventricular hypertrophy.

There are two P waves to every QRS complex. The patient also satisfies the Sokolow–Lyon voltage criteria for left ventricular hypertrophy.

Question 236

A 41-year-old schoolteacher was seen by a rheumatologist for intermittent painful blue fingers during exposure to the cold weather. She had also recently developed fixed flexion deformities of her fingers bilaterally and thickening on the dorsal aspects of the hands. She was subsequently commenced on penicillamine and a non-steroidal anti-inflammatory drug. Two months later she complained of breathlessness on exertion and retrosternal burning pain on stooping forward. On auscultation of the lung fields there were fine end-inspiratory crackles at both lung bases. Lung function tests revealed a restrictive defect with reduced transfer factor.

What is the most probable diagnosis?
a. Penicillamine-induced lung fibrosis.
b. Bronchiolitis obliterans.
c. Mixed connective tissue disease.
d. Systemic sclerosis.
e. Pulmonary fibrosis secondary to NSAID use.

Question 237

An 83-year-old woman was admitted with central chest pain radiating to her left arm while out shopping. She had never experienced chest pain previously. There was no history of smoking, hypertension or diabetes. The serum cholesterol was 8 mmol/l.

Physical examination was normal. The 12-lead ECG showed flattening of the T waves in leads I, V5 and V6. The troponin level 12 hours after the pain was not elevated. A diagnosis of angina was made. The patient remained stable and pain free over the next 48 hours. An exercise test performed on the third day of admission revealed ST segment depression >2 mm in leads V4–V6 after 4 minutes of exercise (HR 120 beats/min). The patient did not experience chest pain on the treadmill.

Which of the medications below is unlikely to alter her prognosis?
a. Atenolol.
b. Nifedipine.
c. Ramipril.
d. Aspirin.
e. Simvastatin.

Question 238

A 16-year-old female was referred with primary amenorrhoea and hirsutism. The patient had noticed excessive hair on her face, arms and legs since the age of 8 years. She had a past history of measles but had been well otherwise. She lived in a mountain hut with her father and aunt. She had two older siblings who were well. Her father was 1.8 m tall. On examination she had excessive acne and facial hair. The blood pressure was 105/65 mmHg. On inspection of the genitalia, there was evidence of pubic hair up to the umbilical region and moderate cliteromegaly.

What is the diagnosis?
a. Congenital adrenal hyperplasia secondary to 21-hydroxylase deficiency.
b. Testosterone secreting adrenal tumour.
c. Arrhenoblastoma.
d. Polycystic ovarian syndrome.
e. Cushing's syndrome.

Answer 236

> d. Systemic sclerosis.

The patient has scleroderma and associated Raynaud's phenomenon as well as other organ involvement, notably the lungs (pulmonary fibrosis) and the oesophagus (dysmotility/lower oesophageal sphincter dysfunction). The best diagnosis is systemic sclerosis. 90% of patients with systemic sclerosis have gut involvement (50% are symptomatic). Oesophageal dysmotility is the most frequent visceral complication of systemic sclerosis. 70% have pulmonary involvement. Renal, cardiac and musculoskeletal involvement is well recognized. Renal involvement is characterized by hypertension that may be acute and severe; cardiac involvement comprises pericarditis and its complications, restrictive cardiomyopathy and myocardial fibrosis. Myocardial fibrosis is responsible for fatal ventricular arrhythmias causing sudden death in some cases of systemic sclerosis.

The sera of patients with scleroderma may display one of the hallmark antibodies of scleroderma: anti-centromere, antitopoisomerase-1 (Scl-70), anti-RNA polymerase, or U3-RNP antibodies. ANCAs are present in scleroderma syndromes.

Treatment is aimed at management of Raynaud's phenomenon (keep hands warm, calcium channel blockers, alpha-blockers). Specific therapy is based on immune modulating drugs. Several treatments have been used with varying degrees of efficacy and include cyclophosphamide, ciclosporin, azathioprine, methotrexate and interferons. Steroids should be used with extreme caution as they have been shown to precipitate renal failure.

Answer 237

> b. Nifedipine.

All patients with angina should be prescribed an anti-thrombotic drug. The antithrombotic drug of choice is aspirin, which has been shown to significantly reduce mortality following myocardial infarction (ISIS 2 trial). No other antithrombotic drug has been shown to be superior to aspirin, although clopidogrel is equally effective. Beta-blockers reduce myocardial oxygen demand and are prognostically useful in the event of myocardial infarction (ISIS 1). In patients with coronary artery disease, ACE inhibitors prevent future myocardial infarction and mortality (EUROPA and HOPE studies). Cholesterol lowering with statins has been shown to reduce mortality in patients with established coronary artery disease (4S and LIPID studies) even in patients with mildly elevated or borderline levels of total cholesterol (CARE and REGRESS studies). Nifedipine, on the other hand, has been shown to exacerbate myocardial ischaemia (in the absence of a beta-blocker) and in one trial was associated with increased mortality.

Answer 238

> a. Congenital adrenal hyperplasia secondary to 21-hydroxylase deficiency.

The differential diagnosis of hirsutism and virilism includes congenital adrenal hyperplasia, polycystic ovary syndrome, androgen secreting adrenal tumour, Cushing's syndrome, arrhenoblastoma (ovarian tumour secreting androgens) and anabolic drug abuse. The patient has presented with primary amenorrhoea and had evidence of virilism at a relatively young age, which would be consistent with 21-hydroxylase deficiency congenital adrenal hyperplasia. PCOS rarely presents with primary amenorrhoea. Androgen secreting tumours of the ovary are malignant and would not have such a long history. Furthermore, they usually present at an older age. Androgen secreting adrenal tumours are also usually malignant and usually also produce cortisol, therefore affected females are virile and have features of Cushing's syndrome.

The diagnosis of congenital adrenal hyperplasia secondary to 21-hydroxylase deficiency can be established by demonstrating high levels of 17-hydroxyprogesterone in the blood and an increased concentration of keto-steroids in the urine. (See Question 334.)

Questions 239, 240 and 241

A 23-year-old female student consulted her GP for constant headaches for several weeks, which were worse in the mornings. She also found that her vision had become blurred recently and she had developed diplopia two days ago. She had no past medical history of note. The patient was taking the oral contraceptive pill.

On examination the blood pressure measured 125/80 mmHg. Her body mass index was 27. Her pupils were equal and reactive to light. Visual field testing revealed enlarged blind spots bilaterally. She has diplopia on looking to the right and impaired abduction of the right eye. Fundoscopy revealed bilateral papilloedema. All other cranial nerves were normal, as was the examination of the cerebellar and peripheral nervous system.

Investigations were as follows:

ESR	8 mm/h
CT scan of the brain without contrast	Normal
Lumbar puncture and CSF analysis:	
Opening pressure	29 cmH$_2$O
Protein	0.4 g/l
Glucose	4.5 mmol/l
Microscopy	Lymphocytes 4/mm^3

Question 239

What is the next investigation of choice?
 a. Contrast enhanced CT scan.
 b. MRI scan of the brain with MR venography.
 c. CSF analysis.
 d. Skull X-ray.
 e. Serum retinoic acid level.

Question 240

What would your next management step be?
 a. Anticoagulation.
 b. Corticosteriods.
 c. Stop the oral contraceptive pill.
 d. Neurosurgical referral.
 e. Nimodipine.

Question 241

The patient is seen again 48 hours later with significant reduction in visual acuity. What is the best management?
 a. Acetazolamide.
 b. Dexamethasone.
 c. Intravenous mannitol.
 d. Neurosurgical referral for optic nerve fenestration.
 e. Lumbo-peritoneal shunt.

Question 242

A 46-year-old obese woman was recently diagnosed as having diabetes mellitus. Investigations on presentation are shown.

Sodium	132 mmol/l
Potassium	4.6 mmol/l
Urea	12 mmol/l
Creatinine	190 μmol/l
Fasting glucose	13 mmol/l
Fasting cholesterol	8.2 mmol/l
Fasting triglycerides	8 mmol/l
HbA1c	9.4%
Urinalysis	Protein ++
	Glucose ++
	Microscopy normal

What is the best management for her diabetes?
 a. Gliclazide.
 b. Insulin.
 c. Stringent diabetic diet.
 d. Metformin.
 e. Insulin and metformin.

Answers 239, 240 and 241

Answer 239
b. MRI scan of the brain with MR venography.

Answer 240
c. Stop the oral contraceptive pill.

Answer 241
d. Neurosurgical referral for optic nerve fenestration.

The presentation of benign intracranial hypertension may simulate that of a cerebral tumour, hence it is also known as 'pseudotumour cerebri'. Patients present with symptoms of raised intracranial pressure, which comprise headache, transient visual obscurations and diplopia. The most significant physical finding in these patients is bilateral disc oedema. The diplopia is due to unilateral or bilateral sixth nerve palsies and resolves on lowering the intracranial pressure.

The diagnostic criteria include the following:
- Symptoms and signs restricted to those of elevated intracranial pressure.
- Normal neuroimaging studies (excluding non-specific findings of raised intracranial pressure).
- Increased cerebrospinal fluid pressure with a normal composition.

The pathophysiology of this disorder is unclear. It is widely presumed that a relative resistance to the absorption of cerebrospinal fluid across the arachnoid villi is present. The disease commonly occurs in individuals who are overweight. There is a strong predilection for women, with a female-to-male ratio of up to 10:1 (*Table A*).

The morbidity of BIH is mainly related to the effects of papilloedema. If left untreated, long-standing disc oedema results in an irreversible optic neuropathy with accompanying constriction of the visual field and loss of colour vision. In end-stage papilloedema, central visual acuity also is involved. Permanent visual loss occurs in 10% of patients.

A patient with bilateral disc swelling should undergo urgent neuroimaging to rule out an intracranial mass or a dural sinus thrombosis (**239a**). Although CT scan of the brain is adequate in most instances, MRI is most effective in ruling out both a mass lesion and a potential dural sinus thrombosis.

In the setting of BIH, neuroimaging will be either normal or demonstrate small, slit-like ventricles, enlarged optic nerve sheaths and occasionally an empty sella.

The treatment goal for these patients is to preserve optic nerve function while managing their increased intracranial pressure. Optic nerve function should be monitored carefully with the assessment of visual acuity, colour vision, optic nerve head observation and perimetry. For an overview of management see *Table B* and (**239b**, overpage).

Despite careful follow-up care and maximum medical treatment, some patients develop deterioration of visual function. In this situation, surgical intervention should be considered. The two procedures that can be performed are optic nerve sheath fenestration and lumbo-peritoneal shunting procedure. Treatment of this disorder by repeated lumbar punctures is considered to be of historic interest.

Table A Causes of benign intracranial hypertension

Endocrinal risk factors
- Female sex
- Reproductive age group
- Menstrual irregularity
- Obesity – recent weight gain
- Adrenal insufficiency
- Cushing's disease
- Hypoparathyroidism
- Hypothyroidism
- Excessive thyroxine replacement in children

Miscellaneous risk factors
- SLE
- Chronic renal failure

Pharmacological risk factors
- Cimetidine, corticosteroids
- Danazol
- Isotretinoin (Accutane)
- Levothyroxine
- Lithium
- Minocycline
- Nalidixic acid
- Nitrofurantoin
- Tamoxifen
- Tetracycline
- Trimethoprim-sulfamethoxazole
- All-trans-retinoic acid (ATRA)
- Ciclosporine
- Levonorgestrel implant
- Pancreatin recombinant human growth hormone
- Vitamin A in infants

Investigation of bilateral papilloedema

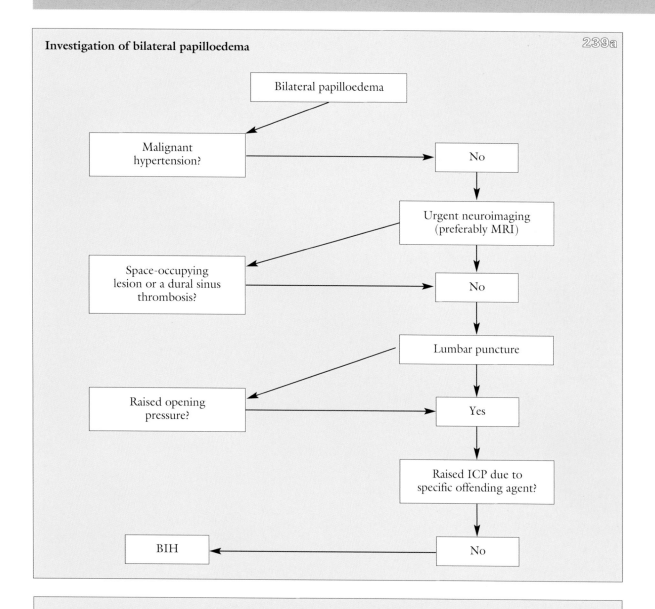

Table B Medical management of benign intracranial hypertension

- Weight control. Weight loss is a cornerstone in the management of patients.
- Treatment of related underlying diseases
- Cessation of exogenous agents related to increased intracranial pressure
- Treatment of headache
- Reduction of the intracranial pressure in order to protect optic nerve function.
- Diuretics. Acetazolamide appears to be the most effective diuretic in lowering the intracranial pressure.
- Corticosteroids are used as a supplement to acetazolamide to hasten recovery in patients who present with severe papilloedema. Significant adverse effects preclude long-term use in such patients

---

Patients with lateral sinus thrombosis may present with a pseudotumor cerebri-like syndrome. The scenario describes a patient whose sex, history of smoking and oral contraceptive use put her at risk of developing cerebral venous sinus thrombosis, which typically presents with a short history of headache, vomiting and papilloedema. If venous infarction supervenes, focal neurology will be seen.

CT may show the characteristic delta sign – a filling defect within the sinus after contrast administration. Magnetic resonance venography is the investigation of choice as it is an excellent method of visualizing the dural venous sinuses and larger cerebral veins.

(Continued over page)

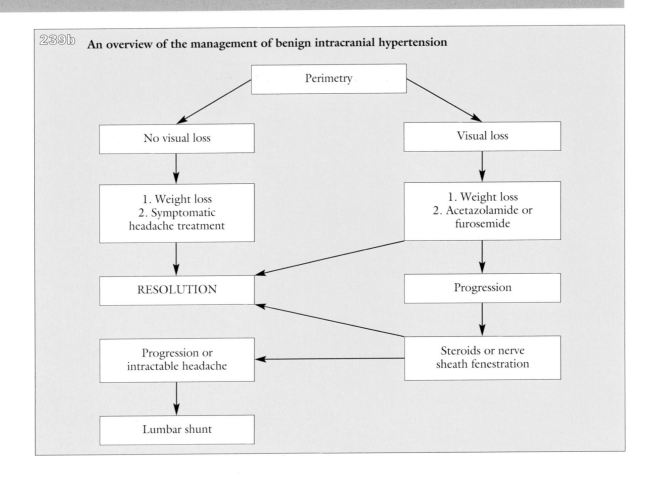

239b **An overview of the management of benign intracranial hypertension**

Answer 242

b. Insulin.

The three main goals in the management of diabetes are:
1. Good glycaemic control, which has been shown to reduce microvascular complications.
2. Treatment of nephropathy, retinopathy and diabetic foot disease.
3. Aggressive treatment of risk factors for atherosclerosis to reduce morbidity and mortality from macro-vascular disease (*Table*).

This particular question tests the candidate on management of hyperglycaemia. Glycaemic control involves dietary modification, weight loss, regular exercise and pharmacological therapy.

The patient in question has evidence of nephropathy and has a mixed hyperlipidaemia. There is good evidence that meticulous glycaemic control will retard progression of renal impairment and have a beneficial effect on lipid profile. Weight loss and stringent diabetic diet should always be implemented in overweight diabetics as increased body mass index is linked with insulin resistance. However, this patient has nephropathy, an unsatisfactory HbA1c and

hyperlipidaemia, which necessitate additional pharmacological measures to improve glycaemic control.

Gliclazide, a sulphonylurea, promotes release of insulin and potentiates its effects in the periphery. Unfortunately it is associated with weight gain. Furthermore, sulphonylureas only reduce blood sugar by 20%. Metformin is an ideal drug in obese diabetics because it promotes weight reduction and aids hyperlipidaemia; however, its use is contraindicated in patients with a serum creatinine >150 mmol/l. The safest option here is insulin therapy.

Goals in diabetes mellitus management to prevent cardiovascular/cerebrovascular mortality

- Achieve BMI 28
- Cessation of smoking
- Regular exercise*
- HbA1c ≤ 7%
- BP ≤ 130/80 mmHg
- Total cholesterol ≤ 5 mmol/l
- LDL cholesterol ≤ 2.2 mmol/l

*30 minutes of aerobic exercise five times per week.

Question 243

A 60-year-old woman attended the Accident and Emergency Department with central chest pain radiating to the jaw. Risk factors for coronary artery disease included hypercholesterolaemia and a family history of ischaemic heart disease. The 12-lead ECG revealed ST segment depression in leads V2–V6. Troponin T 12 hours after admission was 0.4 ng/l (NR <0.1ng/l).

What is the diagnosis?
  a. Acute infero-lateral myocardial infarction.
  b. Musculoskeletal chest pain.
  c. Stable angina.
  d. Non-ST elevation myocardial infarction.
  e. Unstable angina.

Questions 244 and 245

A 64-year-old male presented with sudden onset of breathlessness. He had experienced a transient ischaemic attack three months previously and had a history of intermittent claudication. The chest X-ray on admission was consistent with pulmonary oedema. He was taking nifedipine and atenolol for hypertension. He was treated with intravenous diuretics and glyceryl trinitrate for 48 hours with good effect. He was subsequently switched to oral furosemide 40 mg od. The atenolol was stopped and substituted with an ACE inhibitor.

Blood tests on admission are shown.

Sodium	137 mmol/l
Potassium	3.6 mmol/l
Urea	8.2 mmol/l
Creatinine	137 μmol/l

Blood tests one week later:

Sodium	135 mmol/l
Potassium	4.6 mmol/l
Urea	15 mmol/l
Creatinine	220 μmol/l

Question 244

What is the most likely cause for the patient's deterioration?
  a. Initiation of furosemide.
  b. Initiation of an ACE inhibitor.
  c. Hypertensive nephropathy.
  d. Relative hypotension.
  e. Left ventricular dysfunction.

Question 245

What is the next best investigation to ascertain the cause of the abnormal renal function?
  a. Renal biopsy.
  b. Renal angiography.
  c. Renal isotope scan.
  d. Captopril renogram.
  e. Echocardiogram.

Answer 243

d. Non-ST elevation myocardial infarction.

The patient presents with chest pain, non-ST elevation ECG changes and a raised troponin level (specific for myocardial damage). The triad is consistent with the diagnosis of NSTEMI. Since the widespread use of troponin in the investigation of chest pain, there has been some confusion with respect to the diagnosis of myocardial infarction. As a result, acute coronary syndromes have been divided into three categories:
1. Classic ST elevation myocardial infarction.
2. NSTEMI (where patient may or may not have classic chest pain associated with ST segment depression or T wave inversion and raised troponin*).
3. Unstable angina (troponin-negative chest pain with or without non-ST elevation ECG changes).
*Troponin T >0.05 mg/l; troponin I >0.3 mg/l.
STEMI is managed with urgent thrombolysis or primary angioplasty if the patient presents within 12 hours and had no contraindications to thrombolysis. Patients who have failed thrombolysis, or have on-going myocardial ischaemia, should have in--patient coronary angiography. Patients with a positive exercise stress test following STEMI should also have early coronary angiography.

The immediate prognosis in STEMI is worse than that in NSTEMI; nevertheless over the following six months patients with NSTEMI have a 16% mortality. Therefore patients presenting with NSTEMI should undergo early coronary angiography with a view to revascularization (co-morbidities, quality of life and cognitive state allowing).

The differentiation between NSTEMI and unstable angina is retrospective and based on a troponin result performed 12 hours after admission. The management is essentially the same, comprising of aspirin, clopidogrel, heparin, glycoprotein IIb/IIIa receptor inhibitor, GTN and beta-blocker therapy. Aggressive management of risk factors for coronary artery disease is important. In unstable angina early angiography is recommended in patients with chest pain associated with ST segment depression or T wave inversion.

A raised troponin is specific for myocyte necrosis but does not always indicate myocardial damage secondary to coronary artery occlusion. Myopericarditis, tachycarrhythmias, DC cardioversion, the cardiomyopathies, and large pulmonary embolus are all recognized causes of a raised troponin level. Septicaemia may also be associated with raised troponin levels in up to 80% of cases. Chronic renal impairment is associated with raised troponin levels due to accumulation of cardiac troponin fragments in the blood, which are identified as raised troponins by current assays (Table).

Troponin I assays are less likely to identify these troponin fragments than troponin T assays; therefore, troponin I measurements may be more accurate than troponin T measurements in patients with chronic renal failure. However, it is well established that patients with chronic renal failure and raised troponin measurements have a higher risk of morbidity/mortality than patients without raised troponin levels.

A raised cardiac troponin should be interpreted in the context of the presentation and the ECG. For example, a patient with meningococcal septicaemia and a raised troponin is not necessarily an indication for anti-thrombotic therapy and subsequent coronary angiography.

Causes of raised cardiac troponins

- Myocardial infarction
- Myopericarditis
- Dilated and hypertrophic cardiomyopathy
- DC cardioversion
- Tachyarrhythmias
- Pulmonary embolus
- Exacerbation of chronic obstructive airways disease
- Chemotherapy
- Chronic renal impairment
- Septicaemia
- Subarachnoid haemorrhage
- Marathon running

Answers 244 and 245

Answer 244
b. Initiation of an ACE inhibitor.

Answer 245
b. Renal angiography.

Sudden onset of pulmonary oedema in a patient with generalised arteriosclerosis raises the diagnosis of renal artery stenosis in which rapid onset of pulmonary oedema, sometimes termed 'flash pulmonary oedema' is recognized.

An abnormal baseline creatinine (>140 μmol/l) is usually suggestive of the diagnosis in patients with flash pulmonary odema. In this case, however, the diagnosis becomes clear because initiation of an ACE inhibitor results in deterioration of renal function, a finding that is so characteristic of renal artery stenosis. Remember ACE inhibitors cause a profound drop in GFR by causing afferent vasodilatation of the glomerular tuft.

The gold standard test for diagnosing renal artery stenosis is direct renal angiography, contrast CT scan of the renal arteries or magnetic resonance imaging of the renal arteries.

Question 246

The following are cardiac catheter data on a 40-year-old male with heart failure.

Chamber	Pressure (mmHg)	Oxygen saturation (%)
Superior vena cava		60
Inferior vena cava		61
Right atrium	15	65
Right ventricle	105/40	64
Pulmonary artery	102/50	68
Left ventricle	98/36	95
Ascending aorta	98/60	95
Descending aorta	98/60	80

What two conclusions can be drawn from these data?
a. Atrial septal defect.
b. Ventricular septal defect.
c. Primary pulmonary hypertension.
d. Coarctation of the aorta.
e. Patent ductus arteriosus.
f. Chronic obstructive airways disease.
g. Eisenmenger's syndrome.
h. Pulmonary stenosis.
i. Fallot's tetralogy.
j. Patent foramen ovale.

Question 247

A 31-year-old pregnant woman in her third trimester complained of pain and tingling affecting her right hand, forearm and shoulder. The symptoms were worse at night but were relieved by shaking the hand. Her hand felt weaker than usual. On examination there was no wasting of the hand muscles. Abduction of the right thumb was difficult. There was impaired touch sensation affecting the palmar aspects of the first three digits in the right hand. The biceps, triceps and supinator reflexes were intact.

What is the diagnosis?
a. Carpal tunnel syndrome.
b. C6,7 radiculopathy.
c. Ulnar nerve lesion.
d. Thoracic inlet syndrome.
e. Radial nerve palsy.

Question 248

A 19-year-old woman presented with lethargy and constipation. Her appetite had increased. On examination the heart rate was 100 beats/min and there was a soft systolic murmur at the left lower sternal edge. She was not taking any medication. Her mother and sister had hypothyroidism.

Investigations are shown.

Haemoglobin	11.4 g/dl	
WCC	$4 \times 10^9/l$	
Platelets	$179 \times 10^9/l$	
MCV	80 fl	
Sodium	138 mmol/l	
Potassium	3.6 mmol/l	
Urea	6 mmol/l	
Total T_4	190 nmol/l	(NR 60–160 nmol/l)
Total T_3	3.5 nmol/l	(NR 1.2–3.1 nmol/l)
Free T_4	20 pmol/l	(NR 20–30 pmol/l)
Free T_3	Normal	
TSH	3.5 mu/l	(NR 0.5–5.0 mu/l)

What is the diagnosis?
a. Choriocarcinoma.
b. Factitious hyperthyroidism.
c. Pregnancy.
d. Sick euthyroid syndrome.
e. Amiodarone therapy.

Answer 246

> e. Patent ductus arteriosus.
> g. Eisenmenger's syndrome.

There is evidence of a right-to-left shunt after the ascending aorta. The most likely diagnosis is a patent ductus arteriosus allowing communication between the aorta (just distal to the left subclavian artery usually) and the pulmonary artery. The left-to-right shunt leads to a hyperkinetic pulmonary circulation and an elevated right ventricular pressure. If the defect is large the right ventricular pressure may subsequently become high enough to exceed that of the left ventricle resulting in shunt reversal (right-to-left shunt). This phenomenon of shunt reversal with cardiac defects is sometimes termed Eisenmenger's syndrome.

Answer 247

> a. Carpal tunnel syndrome.

The patient has the classic symptoms of carpal tunnel syndrome, which is caused by compression of the median nerve beneath the transverse carpal ligament. It is usually bilateral and more common in females than males (*Table*).

Pregnancy is a recognized cause, presumably owing to fluid retention. Symptoms include pain in the first three digits of the hand that may also affect the arm and shoulder. There is tingling and pain in the palmar aspects of the first three digits that may be relieved by shaking the hand. The symptoms are worse at night but may be present in the day when carrying out actions that involve repetitive flexion of the hand.

Clinical examination reveals reduced sensation affecting the first three digits. There is weakness affecting the first lumbrical muscle, opponens pollicis and abduction pollicis brevis. Wasting of abductor pollicis brevis causes wasting of the thenar eminence. Tinel's sign (precipitation of symptoms by flexing the wrist) and Phelan's signs (provoking symptoms by flexion of the wrist) are unreliable. Nerve conduction studies are essential. Slow sensory velocity and reduced amplitude of the median nerve action potential are diagnostic. Treatment involves that of the underlying cause in some circumstances. Carpal tunnel steroid injection may prevent symptoms in patients with arthritis, but surgical decompression is the treatment of choice in most patients with symptoms.

Causes of carpal tunnel syndrome

- Pregnancy
- Oral contraceptive pill
- Acromegaly
- Amyloidosis
- Hypothyroidism
- Rheumatoid arthritis
- Tight plaster casts
- Repetitive wrist movements

Answer 248

> c. Pregnancy.

Lethargy, weight gain, constipation and increased appetite are consistent with pregnancy in a young woman. Raised total T_3 and T_4 but normal free T_3 and T_4 suggest high concentrations of thyroid binding globulin, which are present in pregnancy. It is important to note that high concentrations of HCG in early pregnancy may result in subclinical hyperthyroidism since HCG has a common beta subunit to TSH.

Choriocarcinoma or a hydatidiform mole produce high concentrations of HCG that induce profuse vomiting. Both choriocarcinoma and hydatidiform mole can result in severe biochemical hyperthyroidism. The diagnosis should always be considered in a pregnant woman with hyperemesis, very high T_3/T_4 and low TSH. In this case the TSH is normal, therefore the patient is clinically euthyroid. Factitious thyrotoxicosis would be associated with a high free T_4. The biochemical picture is against sick euthyroid syndrome.

Questions 249 and 250

A 30-year-old male presented with severe pain in his right flank radiating to the groin. He was diagnosed with severe Crohn's disease five years ago and had a terminal ileal resection three years ago. He also had a history of hypertension that was well controlled on a low-salt diet and amlodipine 5 mg daily.

An intravenous urogram was performed which confirmed findings consistent with a right ureteric stone. The serum calcium, phosphate and urate levels were normal.

Question 249

What is the most probable consistency of the ureteric stone?
  a. Calcium phosphate.
  b. Calcium oxalate.
  c. Uric acid.
  d. Magnesium ammonium sulphate.
  e. Cystine.

Question 250

What initial treatment is required to prevent further episodes?
  a. Thiazide diuretic.
  b. Chronic antibiotic therapy.
  c. High fluid intake.
  d. Calcium carbonate supplements.
  e. Potassium citrate therapy.

Question 251

A 63-year-old patient who had a cadaveric renal transplant six months ago was admitted to the dialysis unit with nausea, vomiting and deteriorating renal function. He also complained of headache.

On examination he was tremulous. The heart rate was 90 beats/min and regular. The blood pressure measured 200/110 mmHg. The temperature was 37°C (98.6°F). The JVP was not raised. Both heart sounds were normal. Inspection of the fundi revealed grade II hypertensive retinopathy. There were no focal neurological signs. The renal graft was non-tender.

Investigations are shown.

The patient was commenced on dialysis but had a grand mal seizure while he was being dialysed.

Sodium	131 mmol/l
Potassium	5.6 mmol/l
Urea	20 mmol/l
Creatinine	400 μmol/l
Bicarbonate	15 mmol/l
Chloride	111 mmol/l

What is the diagnosis?
  a. Hypertensive encephalopathy.
  b. Ciclosporin toxicity.
  c. Subarachnoid haemorrhage.
  d. Disseminated CMV infection.
  e. Meningitis.

Answers 249 and 250

Answer 249
b. Calcium oxalate.

Answer 250
c. High fluid intake.

Patients with Crohn's disease are prone to nephrolithiasis. The renal stones in Crohn's disease are most commonly composed of calcium oxalate, primarily owing to enteropathic hyperoxaluria. Terminal ileal disease is associated with reduced free fatty acid absorption. The free fatty acids bind intraluminal free calcium, allowing increased oxalate reabsorption. Furthermore, the presence of bile salts in the colon increases colonic permeability to small molecules such as oxalic acid. The condition is exacerbated by low fluid intake and metabolic acidosis.

The management of renal stones due to enteropathic hyperoxaluria is as follows (*Table*):
- Increased fluid intake to enable urine volumes of 2 l or more per day.
- Reduced fat and oxalate in diet
- Calcium carbonate supplements (increase intraluminal calcium and enable excretion of oxalate by the gut).
- Cholestyramine is very effective at preventing enteropathic hyperoxaluria, but its use is limited by its side-effect profile.

Dietary calcium should not be reduced. Thiazide diuretics are only useful in patients who have renal stones due to hypercalcuria.

Management of renal stones

General measures
1. Increase fluid intake to enable a diuresis of at least 2 litres per day.
2. Low-salt, low-oxalate, low-protein diet.
3. Consider drug therapy if there is evidence of active stone disease or stone enlargement despite 3–6 months of dietary modification. The specific drug therapies depend on the conditions predisposing to the stones and the urine calcium and urate concentrations.

Specific measures for the five main types of renal stones

Composition of stone	Predisposing condition	Specific management
1. Calcium phosphate	Hypercalcuria	Thiazide diuretics
	Distal (type 1) RTA	Potassium citrate/thiazide diuretics (if hypercalcuria)
2. Calcium oxalate	Hypercalcuric states	Thiazide diuretic
	Enteropathic hyperoxaluria	Calcium carbonate
	Hyperuricosuria	Potassium citrate
3. Uric acid stones	Gout/hyperuricosuria	Allopurinol or potassium citrate
4. Struvite stones	Recurrent UTI*	Surgical removal
5. Cystine stones	Cystinuria	Penicillamine
		Captopril
		Tiopronin

*Due to *Proteus* or *Klebsiella* species

Answer 251

b. Ciclosporin toxicity.

Deteriorating renal function (usually due to interstitial fibrosis with chronic therapy or arteriolar vasoconstriction in the early treatment), headache, rising BP and an epileptic seizure are all in keeping with ciclosporin toxicity. Acute ciclosporin toxicity is reversible by transiently stopping the drug and re-introducing it at lower doses. Treatment of chronic nephrotoxicity is more difficult. Options include reduction of the dose of ciclosporin or switching to an alternative immuno-suppression regime.

Question 252

This 40-year-old male had a long history of recurrent lower respiratory chest infection that required aggressive treatment with intravenous antibiotics. He had a recent appendicectomy that proved to be technically difficult. He was a non-smoker and married with three children. A chest X-ray performed after surgery is shown.

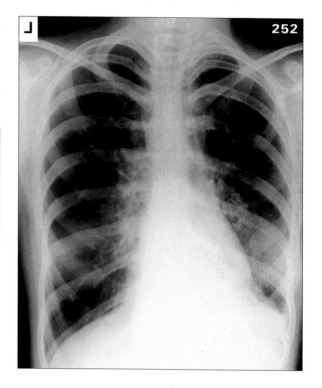

252

What is the diagnosis?
- a. Cystic fibrosis.
- b. Bronchiectasis.
- c. Kartagener's syndrome.
- d. Immotile ciliary syndrome.
- e. Right lower lobe collapse.

Question 253

A 32-year-old woman, who had recently seen her GP for a chest infection, visited her GP again complaining of being clumsy and dropping things. Her husband had also noticed that her speech was slurred in the evening when he saw her after work. There was no previous medical history or family history of note. She was on no medication. She appeared well and there was nothing to find on general examination. Her pupillary reflexes, visual fields and fundoscopy were normal. She had diplopia on looking left and upwards to the right. All cranial nerves were normal. Tone, power and reflexes were all normal as were coordination and sensation.

What is the most likely diagnosis?
- a. Guillain–Barré syndrome.
- b. Myasthenia gravis.
- c. Motor neurone disease.
- d. Miller–Fisher syndrome.
- e. Multiple sclerosis.

Question 254

A 54-year-old non-insulin-dependent diabetic is seen in the diabetic control clinic. His blood pressure is 130/80 mmHg. HbA1c measures 9.6%. The creatinine is 160 μmol/l. Urinalysis reveals protein ++ and glucose ++.

What is the best treatment for preventing deterioration of renal function?
- a. Insulin.
- b. Metformin.
- c. Irbesartan.
- d. Atenolol.
- e. Gliclazide.

Answer 252

> c. Kartagener's syndrome.

The chest X-ray reveals thickened and dilated bibasal bronchioles, consistent with bronchiectasis, which are most prominent in the right lower lobe. Looking carefully at the left/right annotation on the chest X-ray one notices that the X-ray has been switched the wrong way round (left side is on the right side). Therefore, the patient also has dextrocardia. The difficulty with the appendicectomy suggests that the appendix must have been in the left iliac fossa. The combination of situs inversus and bronchiectasis is consistent with a diagnosis of Kartagener's syndrome.

Cystic fibrosis is not associated with dextrocardia and there is no mention of gastrointestinal complications – that would normally relate to cystic fibrosis – in this patient. Furthermore, males with cystic fibrosis are infertile as a rule.

Immotile ciliary syndrome is a genetic disorder that is inherited as an autosomal recessive trait. It is characterized by abnormal ciliary motility in the upper and lower respiratory tracts. Common manifestations include sinusitis, nasal polyps and bronchiectasis. Headaches and hydrocephalus are recognized. While dextrocardia is present in 50% of cases, patients with this disorder are invariably infertile, unlike the patient in question. The diagnosis is made by demonstrating abnormal ciliary function. Treatment of lower respiratory tract infections requires aggressive antibiotic treatment.

Answer 253

> b. Myasthenia gravis.

The patient has evidence of fatiguability (slurred speech in the evenings and extraocular muscle weakness) which helps make the diagnosis. There are no neurological signs on examining the limbs, therefore all the other options provided are excluded. Weakness is exacerbated by pregnancy, hypokalaemia, infection, over-treatment of myasthenia gravis, a change in climate, emotion, exercise and certain drugs, for example aminoglycosides.

The incidence of myasthenia gravis has two age peaks: the second and third decades (F > M) and the sixth and seventh decades (M > F). Acetylcholine receptor antibodies are detectable in 90% of patients. A thymoma is associated in 10% of cases and thymus abnormalities in 75%. There is a high incidence of myasthenia gravis in patients with thyrotoxicosis, RA, SLE and DM. The disease may never progress beyond an ophthalmoplegia. Periods of remission up to three years occur. Thymectomy improves the outlook unless a thymoma is present and achieves remission in up to 30% of patients. The survival rate in the presence of a thymoma is 30%.

Miller–Fisher syndrome, which is a variant of Guillain–Barré syndrome, is characterized by ophthalmoplegia, sensory ataxia and a descending (predominantly motor) neuropathy.

(See Answers 65, 200.)

Answer 254

> c. Irbesartan.

The patient has evidence of overt diabetic nephropathy, i.e. impaired renal function and frank proteinuria. Urine dipsticks only become positive for protein once urine protein concentration is between 0.3 and 0.5 g/day.

The UKPDS study showed that aggressive glycaemic control prevented microvascular complications. However, the vast majority of patients studied had either no microvascular complications or mild microvascular complications. There is currently a lack of good evidence regarding the effect of tight glycaemic control on the progression of diabetic nephropathy in patients with advanced microvascular complications. On the other hand trials using ACE inhibitors and more recently angiotensin receptor blocking agents have shown retardation of diabetic nephropathy in patients with type 1 and type 2 diabetes mellitus respectively who have established renal disease. (See Question 154.)

Questions 255 and 256

A 60-year-old male presented with sudden onset of reduced visual acuity in the right eye. Six months prior to the presentation the patient had experienced a three-day episode of ataxia that had resolved spontaneously. The patient had a history of diabetes mellitus that was well controlled on insulin. There was no family history of note. The patient consumed 12 units of alcohol per week.

On examination he was in sinus rhythm. The blood pressure measured 130/80 mmHg. Neurological examination was normal with the exception of markedly reduced visual acuity in the right eye. Fundoscopy was normal.

Question 255

What is the most probable diagnosis?
   a. Central retinal artery occlusion.
   b. Leber's hereditary optic neuropathy.
   c. Multiple sclerosis.
   d. B_{12} deficiency.
   e. Ischaemic optic neuropathy.

Question 256

What is the treatment of choice?
   a. B_{12} injections.
   b. Aspirin.
   c. High-dose folic acid.
   d. IV methylprednisolone.
   e. No treatment required.

Question 257

A 14-year-old girl was investigated for abdominal pain. Abdominal examination was normal.

Hb	10.8 g/dl
WCC	8×10^9/l
	(normal differential)
Platelets	200×10^9/l
MCV	75 fl
Sodium	136 mmol/l
Potassium	3.8 mmol/l
Urea	6 mmol/l
Creatinine	100 μmol/l
Amylase	100 iu/l (NR <220 iu/l)
Serum Iron	33 μmol/l (NR 13–32 μmol/l)
TIBC	49 μmol/l (NR 42–80 μmol/l)
Urinary coproporphyrins	640 nmol/24h (NR 50–350 nmol/24h)

Investigations are shown.

What is the diagnosis?
   a. Acute intermittent porphyria.
   b. Porphyria cutanea tarda.
   c. Haemochromatosis.
   d. Lead poisoning.
   e. Hereditary coproporphyria.

(See Question 213.)

Question 258

A 24-year-old woman presented with severe menorrhagia. There were several bruises on her arms and legs.

Hb	6.2 g/dl
WCC	29×10^9/l
Platelets	32×10^9/l
Marrow aspirate	Metamyelocytes Promyelocytes ++++ Myelomonocytes and myeloblasts
D-dimer	Massively elevated

Investigations are shown.

What is the most likely chromosomal abnormality accounting for this disorder?
   a. Monosomy 17.
   b. Translocation (9,22).
   c. Translocation (15,17).
   d. Translocation (4,11).
   e. Trisomy 12.

Answers 255 and 256

> **Answer 255**
> c. Multiple sclerosis.
>
> **Answer 256**
> d. IV methylprednisolone.

The patient presents with sudden onset of reduced visual acuity in one eye and fundoscopy suggests the possibility of optic neuritis. The preceding history of transient ataxia six months previously is highly suggestive of an underlying diagnosis of multiple sclerosis.

The diagnosis of multiple sclerosis is usually clinical and should be considered in any patient who has neurological episodes that are scattered in time (two or more separate episodes) and space (two or more separate locations) (*Table*). There is no single test that can confirm the diagnosis, although the use of MRI scanning in conjunction with clinical findings has improved diagnostic accuracy. CSF analysis for oligoclonal bands continues to remain useful.

Optic neuritis and all other acute episodes in multiple sclerosis that are serious enough to cause distress or increase limitation of activities should be treated with a course of high-dose steroids as soon as possible after the onset of symptoms. The therapy of choice is intravenous or oral methyprednisolone for 3–5 days.

> **Diagnostic criteria for suspected multiple sclerosis (McDonald criteria)**
>
> - If the patient has two or more clinical attacks with two or more objective lesions then MS is diagnosed clinically although many neurologists still request an MRI scan of the brain to help confirm MS or exclude other diagnoses
> - If the patient has two or more attacks with one objective lesion then further information is required from MR brain or CSF analysis. There are two possible approaches:
>   (1) The following findings on brain MRI showing dissemination in space confirm the diagnosis:
>   One gadolinium-enhancing lesion or Nine T2 hyperdense lesions if no gadolinium-enhancing lesion *plus*
>   (a) one or more infratentorial lesions *plus*
>   (b) one or more juxtacortical lesions *plus*
>   (c) three or more periventricular lesions
>   (2) Alternatively positive CSF for oligoclonal bands and brain MRI showing two or more lesions consistent with MS is sufficient to make the diagnosis
>
> NB: One cord lesion can substitute one brain lesion. If a patient with two or more attacks but only one objective lesion goes on to have a further attack involving a different site while awaiting further investigation, the diagnosis of MS becomes more probable.

Answer 257

> d. Lead poisoning.

Abdominal pain and raised serum coproporphyrin levels are indicative of either lead poisoning or hereditary coproporphyria. The most probable answer is lead poisoning since lead poisoning is much more common than hereditary coproporphyria and there is a history of patient exposure to lead through his occupation.

Hereditary coproporphyria is inherited as an autosomal dominant trait and is due to a partial deficiency in the enzyme coproporphyrinogen oxidase. The condition is rare and has a prevalence of 2 per million. The symptoms are identical to those of lead poisoning although photosensitivity may also be an additional feature. In patients with hereditary coproporphyria, faecal and urinary coproporphyrin levels are hugely elevated. In contrast, coproporphyrin levels are only modestly elevated in lead poisoning.

While acute intermittent porphyria also presents with abdominal pain, faecal and urinary coproporphyrin levels in AIP are low. (See Question 213.)

Answer 258

> c. Translocation (15,17).

The blood film and coagulation profiles are consistent with AML type 3 (promyelocytic leukaemia). AML 3 is associated with disseminated intravascular coagulation. The genetics of AML 3 are understood. Reciprocal translocation of the long arms of chromosomes 15 and 17 is the basic genetic defect. The break point on chromosome 17 has been mapped to the retinoic acid receptor alpha (RAR-alpha). The translocation creates a fusion gene known as PML-RAR-alpha, which impairs apoptosis in promyelocytes. This particular form of AML is amenable to treatment with all-trans retinoic acid. Karyotyping is important in AML type 3 as another rarer variant t (11-17) does not respond to all-trans retinoic acid.

More urgently, the patient requires fresh-frozen plasma and a platelet transfusion to treat the DIC. In the absence of active bleeding platelet transfusion is considered only if the platelet concentration falls below $20 \times 10^9 /l$.

Question 259

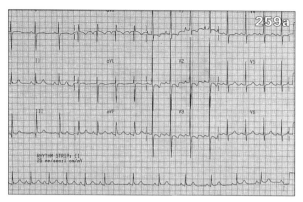

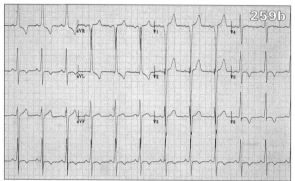

These ECG traces are from 40-year-old men. One is breathless on exertion (**259a**) and the other has a systolic murmur (**259b**).

Question 259a

1. What information does the ECG give you with respect to cardiac morphology?
2. Give four acquired causes and three inherited causes for the ECG abnormalities.

Question 259b

1. List two abnormalities.
2. Suggest two possible diagnoses.

Question 260

A 17-year-old male was referred to the local paediatrician because his mother was concerned that he was considerably shorter than his peers. He was well in himself. He had never required to shave, and had just recently noticed some pubic hair in his genital area. On examination, he measured 1.58 m. He had slight bilateral gynaecomastia. His voice had not broken. There was no facial hair. There was scanty pubic hair in the genital region and his testes were small. His father and mother were 1.83 m and 1.68 m tall, respectively.

Results of dynamic pituitary function testing with 0.2 units/kg insulin, 100 µg of LHRH and 200 mg of TRH were as follows:

Time (min)	Glucose (mmol/l)	GH mu/l	Cortisol (nmol/l)	TSH (mu/l)	LH (iu/l)	FSH (iu/l)	Testosterone (nmol/l)
0	4.0	1.4	400	2.0	29	16	34
20	2.8	12.0	860	5.2	40	24	60
30	1.6	28	1270	-	-	-	-
40	1.5	32	1450	-	-	-	-
60	2.2	20	1120	8	34	20	60

What is the most probable diagnosis?
  a. Prader–Willi syndrome.
  b. Kleinfelter's syndrome.
  c. Recent onset of puberty.
  d. Kallman's syndrome.
  e. Testicular feminization syndrome.

Answer 259

Answer 259a
1. The ECG demonstrates voltage criteria for right atrial enlargement and right ventricular hypertrophy.
2. Acquired causes include:
   i. Fibrotic lung disease.
   ii. Bronchiectasis.
   iii. Thromboembolic pulmonary disease.
   iv. Chronic obstructive airways disease.
   Inherited causes:
   i. Cystic fibrosis.
   ii. α-1 antitrypsin deficiency.
   iii. Ostium secundum atrial septal defect (may be inherited as an autosomal dominant trait).

Answer 259b
1. i. Voltage criteria for left atrial enlargement.
   ii. Left ventricular hypertrophy (see explanation).
2. i. Aortic stenosis.
   ii. Hypertrophic cardiomyopathy.

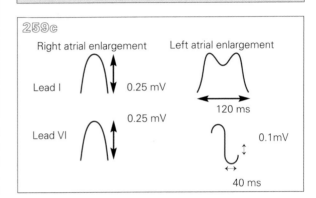

259c

Information regarding atrial enlargement is gained from leads II and V1 (**259c**). Right atrial enlargement is characterized by a tall P-wave in both II and V1 that exceeds 0.25 mV (or two-and-a-half small squares). Voltage criteria for left atrial enlargement are a little more complicated. In lead II, the P-wave has a bifid appearance and the duration of the P-wave is 120 ms (three small squares). In V1, the P-wave is biphasic with a terminal (negative) portion of the P-wave exceeding or equal to 40 ms in duration (one small square) and more than or equal to –0.1 mV (one small square) in depth. The presence of a biphasic P-wave in V1 which does not satisfy these criteria cannot be diagnosed as left atrial enlargement on the ECG.

Information regarding voltage criteria for ventricular hypertrophy is gained from leads V1 and V5, particularly if the Sokolow's criteria (most commonly used) are to be applied. Right ventricular enlargement is suggested by the sum of the R-wave in V1 and the S-wave in V5 or V6 exceeding 1.25 mV (12.5 small squares). In addition, there may be ST-segment depression and T-wave inversion in leads V1–V3 and right axis deviation. Left ventricular hypertrophy is characterized by the sum of the S-wave in V1 and the R-wave in V5 or V6 exceeding 40 mm. The additional presence of ST-segment depression and/or T-wave inversion in V5 and V6 is more suggestive of the diagnosis.

Answer 260

c. Recent onset of puberty.

The findings are consistent with recent onset of puberty. The basal gonadotrophin and testosterone levels are generally high during puberty. The patient has scanty pubic hair and gynaecomastia, both markers of puberty. Prader–Willi and Kleinfelter's syndrome are recognized causes of primary hypogonadism; however, the high testosterone level is against this. Testicular feminization syndrome would be associated with a similar testosterone and gonadotrophin level; however, patients affected with the testicular feminization syndrome are phenotypically female (see Answer 397). Kallman's syndrome is rare and often inherited as an X-linked recessive trait. It is characterized by deficient gonadotrophin production by the pituitary, anosmia, cleft palate and colour blindness. These patients may also have congenital renal

Causes of primary hypogonadism in the male
- Testosterone biosynthetic enzyme deficiencies
- Kleinfelter's syndrome
- Prader–Willi syndrome
- Lawrence–Moon–Biedel syndrome
- Noonan's syndrome
- Rubella
- Mumps orchitis
- Castration
- Cystic fibrosis
- Sickle cell anaemia
- Cirrhosis
- Chemotherapy
- Alcohol

and cerebral defects. Other causes of primary hypogonadism in males are given (*Table*).

Question 261

A 47-year-old female visited her GP to request hormone replacement therapy. She had been amenorrhoeic for four months, and had complained of sweating excessively and fatigue. She had also noticed an increase in the size of her hands such that her wedding ring was very tight, her shoe size had increased recently and her head appeared larger. Three years ago she had an episode of haemoptysis, following which she had a chest X-ray (**261**) that revealed a small opacity in the right lung. She was subsequently lost to follow-up.

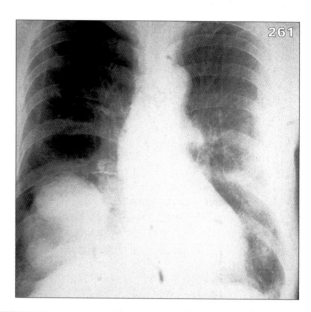

On examination, she had large, spade-shaped hands and broad feet. There was a palpable smooth thyroid goitre. The heart rate was 96 beats/min and the blood pressure was 160/90 mmHg. On examination of the respiratory system there was dullness and reduced air entry at the right lung base.

The patient was referred to an endocrinologist for further investigations.

Initial investigations are shown.

Hb	13 g/dl	Calcium	2.5 mmol/l
WCC	9×10^9/l	Phosphate	1 mmol/l
Platelets	210×10^9/l	Albumin	40 g/l
MCV	89 fl	Alkaline phosphatase	100 iu/l
Sodium	135 mmol/l	Bilirubin	10 µmol/l
Potassium	4 mmol/l	AST	20 iu/l
Urea	6 mmol/l	ALT	25 iu/l
Creatinine	98 µmol/l	Chest X-ray (**261**)	
CT scan of thorax	Bulky mediastinum due to lymphadenopathy (mediastinal views)		
MRI of pituitary	Normal		
TSH	3 mu/l (normal range 0.5–5.0 mu/l)		
Thyroxine	110 nmol/l		
FSH	60 iu/l		
LH	30 iu/l		

Oral glucose tolerance test with 75 g glucose after an overnight fast:

Time (min)	0	30	60	120
Blood glucose (mmol/l)	8	15	20	10.5
GH (mu/l)	60	64	94	58

Insulin tolerance test: 0.3 units/kg:

Time (min)	0	30	45	60	90	120
Blood glucose (mmol/l)	8	4	1.8	3	8	11
Cortisol (nmol/l)	180	260	700	620	500	400

Serum calcitonin	Normal	Serum PTH	Normal
Serum glucagon	Normal	Serum noradrenaline	Normal
Serum VIP	Normal	Urinary VMA	Normal

---

1. List two inferences you can make from the oral glucose tolerance test.
2. Comment on the insulin tolerance test.
3. Comment on the abnormal gonadotrophin levels, and give the most likely explanation.
4. Comment on the chest X-ray.
5. What is the connection between the chest X-ray and the endocrine abnormality?

Answer 261

1. The patient has diabetes mellitus and acromegaly. The fasting blood glucose is over 6.7 mmol/l and the 2-hour blood glucose level is 10.5 mmol/l. Impaired glucose tolerance is diagnosed when fasting blood glucose is above 6.7 mmol/l and the 2-hour blood glucose is under 10 mmol/l. The resting growth hormone level of above 4 mu/l is highly suggestive of acromegaly. In normal people, growth hormone secretion is suppressed to below 2 mu/l with hyperglycaemia; however, in acromegaly there is failure of growth hormone secretion suppression and there may be a paradoxical rise in growth hormone levels with hyperglycaemia.

2. There is adequate hypoglycaemia (blood glucose falls to under 2.2 mmol/l after 45 min) and there is an appropriate rise in serum cortisol (>550 nmol/l), suggesting adequate pituitary ACTH reserve.

3. The patient is aged 47 and has amenorrhoea. The grossly elevated gonadotrophin reflects menopause. The low circulating oestrogen level (lack of negative feedback of oestrogen on the pituitary) is the stimulus for hypersecretion of the gonadotrophins.

4. The chest X-ray demonstrates a large, well-defined circular mass situated in the lower lobe of the right lung which may be consistent with a carcinoma, adenoma or a large secondary metastasis.

5. The endocrine tests are suggestive of acromegaly. The most common cause of acromegaly is autonomous secretion of growth hormone by an acidophil adenoma in the pituitary. In this case, the pituitary appears normal on the MRI scan and there is no other pituitary endocrine abnormality. It is highly possible that the cause of acromegaly is due to ectopic growth hormone or GHRH secretion. Ectopic growth hormone or GHRH secretion is a very rare but recognized characteristic of certain tumours, particularly those affecting the lung, pancreas or ovary. Small-cell lung carcinoma or bronchial carcinoid, and ovarian teratomas are capable of growth hormone or GHRH secretion. More common examples of ectopic hormone production include ACTH (small-cell carcinoma lung), ADH (small-cell carcinoma lung), PTH-related peptide (hypernephroma, squamous-cell lung carcinoma), erythropoietin (hepatocellular carcinoma, hypernephroma) and 5-HIAA (carcinoid tumours).

Question 262

A 29-year-old male living in a hostel presented with a three-week history of reduced visual acuity and a six-week history of watery diarrhoea. There was no history of headaches or abdominal pain. On further questioning, he mentioned he had a sore mouth and throat, and found it difficult to swallow. He had not been on any medications in the past six months.

On examination, he was thin. Inspection of his tongue and oral cavity are shown (**262a, b**). Examination of his fundi is shown (**262c**). Examination of the abdomen and central nervous system was normal.

Investigations are shown.

Hb	10 g/dl
WCC	4 × 10⁹/l
Platelets	170 × 10⁹/l
Sodium	134 mmol/
Potassium	4.1 mmol/l
Urea	4 mmol/l
Creatinine	67 µmol/l
Glucose	4 mmol/l
Chest X-ray	Clear
Upper gastrointestinal endoscopy	Oesophagitis
Oesophageal washings (**262d**)	
Stool microscopy (**262e**)	
Rectal biopsy (**262f**)	

1. What is the cause of his reduced visual acuity?
2. Why does he have dysphagia?
3. What is the cause of the abnormality on his tongue?
4. Give two possible explanations for his diarrhoea.
5. What two drugs should the patient take for his diarrhoea and reduced visual acuity?

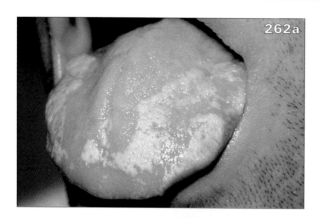

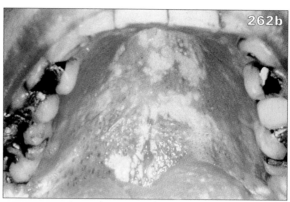

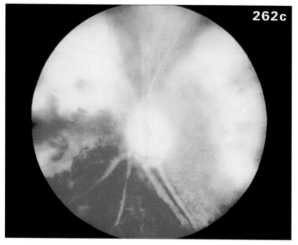

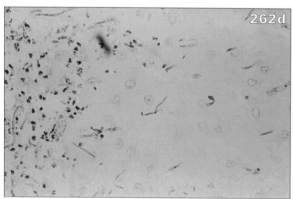

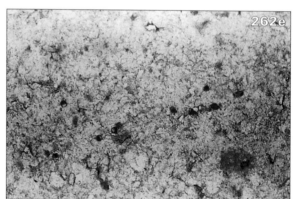

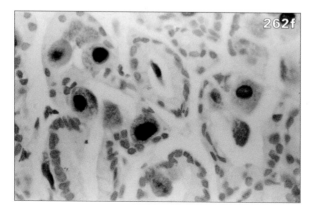

Answer 262

1. CMV retinitis.
2. Oesophageal candidiasis.
3. Oral hairy leukoplakia.
4. i. Cryptosporidial infection.
   ii. CMV colitis.
5. i. Ganciclovir.
   ii. Paromomycin.

The patient has evidence of several AIDS-defining conditions. The fundal appearance is consistent with CMV retinitis, which is the most common cause of visual impairment in these patients. The diagnosis is clinical. Early retinal changes include narrowing of the lumen of the retinal vessels. This is followed by vascular occlusion and perivascular haemorrhages (red areas), resulting in retinal ischaemia (white areas). Without therapy, the condition progresses to bilateral blindness. Treatment is with intravenous ganciclovir, followed by oral maintenance therapy. CMV may also cause encephalitis, colitis and cholangitis, all of which are best treated by the same drug. In the gastrointestinal tract CMV is diagnosed histologically by the demonstration of round intranuclear inclusion bodies within epithelial cells of the intestinal mucosa, as shown in the rectal biopsy (**262f**).

Oral candidiasis is common in patients with HIV and is treated with nystatin or fluconazole. Gastric washings in this patient reveal *Candida* hyphae. Oesophageal *Candida* may cause severe dysphagia, but responds to the same treatment. Hairy leukoplakia affects the lateral borders of the tongue. Unlike *Candida*, it cannot be scraped off the tongue with ease. The condition is painless and is due to infection with EBV. Its presence is highly suggestive of HIV infection. Acyclovir may be of some benefit in its management.

The stool reveals evidence of *Cryptosporidium*, which is the most common cause of diarrhoea in patients with HIV infection. The diarrhoea may be transient or persistent, and may be mild or profuse. The diagnosis is made by staining stool with modified Ziehl–Neelsen stain (**262e**) to demonstrate red cysts of *Cryptosporidium*. Treatment may be difficult and usually involves anti-diarrhoeal agents and fluid replacement. Definitive drugs in the management of cryptosporidial infection include spiramycin and paromomycin.

The neurological complications of HIV are discussed in Answer 277. Other complications are shown (*Table*).

Complications of HIV

Respiratory
- *Pneumocystis carinii* pneumonia
- CMV pneumonia
- Cryptococcal pneumonia
- TB (including *Mycobacterium avium* intracellulare)
- Histoplasmosis
- Lymphoma
- Kaposi's sarcoma

Skin
- Seborrhoeic dermatitis
- Molluscum contagiosum
- Folliculitis
- TB
- *Candida* infection
- *Tinea* infection
- Pityriasis versicolor
- Kaposi's sarcoma

Gastrointestinal
- HIV enteritis
- CMV colitis
- Giardiasis
- *Cryptosporidium*
- *Isospora belli*
- *Salmonella enteritidis*
- *Shigella* dysentery
- *Candida* infection

Mouth
- Herpetic stomatitis
- Aphthous ulcers
- Kaposi's sarcoma

Question 263

A 16-year-old Nigerian male presented to hospital with severe pain affecting his left knee and right elbow. He required admission to another hospital with similar pain three years ago, and was treated with painkillers. He had experienced milder pains at home for which he had required paracetamol. He was one of four siblings and had an older sister who was known to have a form of anaemia.

On examination, he was distressed with pain. His temperature was 38°C (100.4°F). The left knee and right elbow joints were extremely painful, but joint movement was not restricted. The rest of the physical examination was normal.

Investigations are shown.

Hb	10.2 g/dl
WCC	11×10^9/l
Platelets	190×10^9/l
MCV	69 fl
MCHC	29 g/dl
Reticulocyte count	7.7%
Blood film	Numerous target cells and polychromasia
Sodium	135 mmol/l
Potassium	3.7 mmol/l
Urea	6 mmol/l
Aspartate aminotransferase	48 iu/l
Bilirubin	40 µmol/l
Alkaline phosphatase	130 iu/l

1. What is the mechanism of joint pain in this patient?
2. List two investigations you would perform to help with the diagnosis.
3. What is the underlying diagnosis?

Question 264

A 35-year-old Irish nurse returns from Baltimore and is admitted with sharp right lower chest pain which is worse on inspiration. The following day she develops similar pain in the left lower chest. On examination, she has a temperature of 39°C (102.2°F) and reduced air entry at the base of the right lung. There are pleural rubs at the base of both lungs.

Investigations are shown.

Hb	12 g/dl
WCC	3.5×10^9/l
Platelets	300×10^9/l
ESR	33 mm/h
Chest X-ray	Normal lung fields and cardiac size
Arterial gases:	
pH	7.4
PaO_2	11.5 kPa
$PaCO_2$	4.5 kPa
Bicarbonate	25 mmol/l

1. List two possible diagnoses which account for all her symptoms and signs.
2. List at least two tests you would perform to confirm each diagnosis.

Answer 263

> 1. Bone infarction.
> 2. i. Hb electrophoresis.
>   ii. Family screening.
> 3. Sickle cell anaemia. It is also possible that he may have another sickle syndrome such as HbSC disease or HbS/β-thalassaemia trait.

Complications of sickle cell anaemia

- Hand and foot syndrome. Usually seen in infancy
- Painful bony crises. Seen later in life. Precipitated by cold, dehydration, fever or hypoxia
- Aplastic crises. May follow infection from parvovirus B19
- Splenic sequestration. Common in infancy. Severe anaemia and splenic enlargement
- Hepatic sequestration. As with splenic sequestration
- Pulmonary syndromes (thrombotic and sequestration)
- Cerebral syndromes (usually thrombotic)
- Infections from capsulated organisms (autosplenectomy)
- Gall stones (pigment). Usually in adults
- Progressive renal failure (papillary necrosis). Usually in adults
- Chronic leg ulcers. Usually in adults
- Recurrent priapism
- Avascular necrosis of femoral heads
- Salmonella osteomyelitis

Sickle cell anaemia (HbSS) is the most common sickling disorder and it is inherited as an autosomal recessive trait. It is due to a point mutation in both β-globin genes, which results in the substitution of the amino acid glutamine for valine at position 6. Other sickling disorders include HbSC disease (where one β-globin chain is similar to that seen in HbSS and the other β-globin chain is similar to that seen in HbC, another haemoglobin variant), and HbS/β-thalassaemia trait. Patients with HbSC make equal quantities of HbS and HbC, whereas those with HbS/β-thalassaemia trait make predominantly HbS. The amino acid substitution in HbS causes red cell sickling during deoxygenation, leading to increased rigidity and aggregation in the microcirculation. This results in a haemolytic anaemia and episodic tissue infarction – 'the sickle cell crises' (*Table*).

The sickle cell gene is spread widely throughout Africa, some Mediterranean countries, the Middle East and parts of India. It confers protection to malaria.

Patients with sickle cell anaemia are anaemic (Hb 6–10 g/dl) and have a high reticulocyte count (10–20%). The blood film demonstrates polychromasia, target cells and variable numbers of sickle cells. In general, patients with HbSC disease have a less severe form of anaemia, more target cells and fewer sickle cells. They have fewer crises; however, retinal damage, aseptic necrosis of neck of femur and recurrent haematuria are important complications. Pulmonary emboli may occur, particularly during and after pregnancy. Individuals who are carriers, i.e. those with just one abnormal β-globin gene (sickle cell trait) are not anaemic and do not have clinical abnormalities, but may rarely develop a sickling crisis in conditions of extreme hypoxia. Renal papillary necrosis and an inability to concentrate urine is recognized in a very small proportion of individuals with sickle cell trait.

The diagnosis is made by Hb electrophoresis. A definitive diagnosis requires the demonstration of sickle cell trait in both parents.

Answer 264

> 1. i. Systemic lupus erythematosus.
>   ii. Bornholm's disease (Coxsackie virus).
> 2. i. Double-stranded DNA antibody.
>   ii. Antinuclear antibody.
>   iii. CRP.
>   iv. Serum complement.

The patient has symptoms suggestive of polyserositis (pleurisy and pericarditis), a high temperature, a slightly elevated ESR and a relative leucopenia. The most probable diagnosis is SLE, although epidemic myalgia or Bornholm's syndrome due to Coxsackie virus (A or B) infection may present in a similar fashion. The patient has returned from Baltimore, where there may have been an epidemic of Coxsackie virus infection. Familial Mediterranean fever is also characterized by polyserositis and a fever; however, her place of origin is against the diagnosis.

SLE is a multi-system disorder due to a vasculitic process. The disease is thought to have a genetic and auto-immune basis, although a viral aetiology has been proposed by some. It usually affects patients below 40 years, is more common in Negroes, and has a female-to-male ratio of 10:1. The disease often presents with fatigue, arthralgia and arthritis. Pyrexia is common. In addition, there may be renal, pulmonary, cardiac, neurological, haematological and cutaneous involvement. Renal disease is either due to acute diffuse, diffuse proliferative, membranous or focal segmental glomerulonephritis. Pleurisy, pleural effusions and fibrotic lung disease are well recognized (30–40%). Pericarditis is the most common cardiological manifestation of the condition, affecting 30% of patients.

Pericardial constriction and tamponade are rare complications. Non-infective endocarditis (Libmann–Sacks endocarditis) is extremely rare and is rarely of clinical significance. It is usually a post-mortem finding. Neurological manifestations include peripheral and cranial neuropathy, aseptic meningitis, seizures, chorea, neuropsychiatric disorders and a syndrome resembling multiple sclerosis. Haematological manifestations are common, especially in active disease, and include mild normochromic, normocytic anaemia, leucopenia, thrombocytopenia and auto-immune haemolysis. Leucopenia occurs in 65% of patients, which is in contrast with the other vasculitides where the WCC is elevated. Skin manifestations include the characteristic malar butterfly rash on the face in acute SLE or chronic discoid lesions in areas exposed to sunlight. Livedo reticularis, vasculitic skin nodules, alopecia and Raynaud's phenomenon may also occur.

The collection of symptoms affecting different systems should raise suspicion in a young woman, and the diagnosis is confirmed by detection of antibodies to double-stranded DNA, which is relatively specific for SLE. However, the test is positive in only 60% of patients. Antinuclear antibody is present in 90% of patients. It is less specific for SLE and may be present in other vasculitides. The ESR is usually high and may exceed 100 mm/h. The CRP is characteristically normal unless there is underlying infection, a feature common to patients taking immunosuppressant medication for management of disease. Complement levels, particularly C3, are depressed. Circulating lupus anticoagulant, an antiphospholipid antibody, is detected in 30–40% of patients.

Management includes NSAIDs for musculoskeletal problems. Chloroquine is useful where cutaneous manifestations predominate. Corticosteroids and other immunosuppressants (azathioprine, cyclophosphamide and chlorambucil) are used when disease is severe.

Epidemic myalgia due to Coxsackie A or B (Bornholm's disease) is also possible. Despite the name, sporadic cases do exist. Children and young adults are affected most commonly. The symptoms are usually sudden and comprise abdominal or thoracic pain. Myalgia affecting the chest muscles, fever and headaches are usually present. Pleurisy and pericarditis are recognized features, and both pleural and pericardial rubs may be present. The diagnosis is clinical, but the virus may be isolated in faeces. Acute and convalescent sera for Coxsackie virus antibodies will confirm the diagnosis if there is a four-fold rise in antibody titres between the two samples.

Question 265

An 8-year-old male with a known history of haemophilia A presented with a ten-hour history of pain in the left groin, which radiated to the back. He described this as a dull pain which was constant in nature. He was given Factor VIII concentrate and admitted for observation; however, the pain persisted and a few hours later was radiating into the anterior aspect of the left thigh.

On examination, he appeared unwell. He was afebrile. The heart rate was 90 beats/min and the blood pressure was 100/55 mmHg. The patient's left hip was held in flexion. Power testing revealed that he was unable to extend his left hip from the flexed position and knee extension on the left side was weak. The left knee jerk was absent, and sensory testing demonstrated reduced sensation in the anterior and medial aspect of the left thigh. Examination of the abdomen was normal.

1. Which of the following cannot explain why he failed to respond?
   a. Inadequate dose of factor VIII.
   b. Antibodies to factor VIII.
   c. Factor VIII may have expired.
   d. Factor VIII stored at 4°C (39.2°F).
   e. Deficiency of other clotting factor owing to chronic active hepatitis.

2. What is the cause of the neurological signs?
   a. Occlusion of the femoral artery.
   b. Allergic reaction to Factor VIII.
   c. Femoral nerve compression.
   d. Prolapsed L3/L4.
   e. Spinal cord tumour.

3. What is the diagnosis?
   a. Psoas abscess.
   b. Psoas haematoma.
   c. Necrosis of the quadriceps muscle.
   d. Haemarthrosis affecting the left hip joint.
   e. Spinal cord arachnoiditis.

4. Which investigation would be least useful in the management of this patient?
   a. CT scan of the abdomen.
   b. Factor VIII antibody level.
   c. Factor VIII estimation.
   d. APTT.
   e. Bleeding time.

Answer 265

1. d. Factor VIII stored at 4°C (39.2°F).
2. c. Femoral nerve compression.
3. b. Psoas haematoma.
4. e. Bleeding time.

Haemophilia A is inherited as an X-linked recessive condition. The incidence is between 30 and 120 per million. It is due to the deficiency or low levels of Factor VIII, which results in abnormal clotting and a tendency to spontaneous bleeding or bleeding after minor injury. Important sites of bleeding are the joints, the psoas muscle, sublingual and pharyngeal areas, renal and gastrointestinal tract. Cerebral haemorrhage is an important cause of death.

The question requires knowledge regarding important bleeding sites in haemophilia and the management of such an emergency. The presentation comprises pain in the left groin, hip held in flexion, absent knee jerk (L3,L4) and reduced sensation in the anterior and medial aspect of the thigh (L2,L3). All these features are typical of femoral nerve compression (L2–L4). A femoral nerve lesion actually causes weakness of hip flexion, and therefore in this case the flexed hip implies irritation of the nerve. In the context of the history of haemophilia this almost certainly represents a psoas haematoma. (The femoral nerve crosses the iliac fossa between the psoas muscle and the iliacus muscle before entering the thigh deep to the inguinal ligament.) A psoas abscess may present with similar neurological signs; however, the absence of fever or rigors is against this. Haemarthrosis is common in haemophilia, and although it is possible for a patient to have haemorrhage into the hip bone, this would not explain the sensory signs or the absence of the knee reflex. Spinal cord arachnoiditis generally presents with root pain and gradual paraplegia. Muscle haematomas may cause necrosis, but in this case the muscle at risk is the psoas, not the quadriceps muscle. Femoral artery thrombosis would be most unusual in a haemophiliac, and the presentation would consist of sudden onset of pain and paralysis of the left lower limb.

Failure to manage the bleed may be owing to a variety of reasons, which have been listed in the items in the first part of the question. Patients with Factor VIII antibodies are those who are completely deficient in Factor VIII, or have very low (<5%) levels. In this case, possible therapeutic remedies are very high doses of Factor VIII, purified porcine Factor VIII, Factor IX concentrates or activated prothrombin complex (contains activated X). An inadequate dose of Factor VIII is a very important cause of continued bleeding. Factor VIII which has been held at a temperature exceeding 4°C (39.2°F) for more than a couple of hours is not very effective. In the past, up to 50% of patients had CAH, and it is possible that underlying chronic liver disease may prevent early haemostasis owing to several other clotting factor deficiencies.

Further useful investigations should consist of a CT scan of the abdomen to confirm the psoas haematoma. The APTT is an indicator of the severity of the clotting abnormality and a good guide to adequate replacement of Factor VIII levels. Factor VIII levels are useful in determining the amount of Factor VIII which should be replaced to correct the APTT. Estimation of Factor VIII antibodies is very useful because it calls for other therapeutic applications which have been mentioned above. The BT is of no use because it is unchanged in haemophilia, but is elevated in von Willebrand's disease (*Table*).

Clotting abnormalities

	PT	APTT	TT	BT
Haemophilia A	N	↑	N	N
Haemophilia B	N	↑	N	N*
Von Willebrand's disease	N	↑	N	↑
Vitamin K deficiency	↑	N	N	N
Heparin therapy	↑	↑	↑	(↑)**
DIC	↑	↑	↑	(↑)**

* Can be differentiated from haemophilia A, by measuring Factor VIII and IX levels. In haemophilia A, Factor VIII is low, and in haemophilia B, Factor IX is low.

** Increased if the platelet count is low.

Question 266

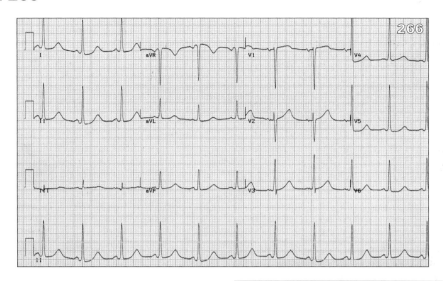

This is an ECG (**266**) from an 18-year-old male with a single episode of syncope. He had no past medical history of note. His mother died suddenly while swimming at the age of 29, but no obvious cause was found at post-mortem examination.

What is the ECG diagnosis?
  a. Wolff–Parkinson–White syndrome.
  b. Brugada's syndrome.
  c. Long QT syndrome.
  d. Arrhythmogenic right ventricular cardiomyopathy.
  e. Commotio cordis.

Question 267

A 37-year-old man was admitted to hospital with a three-day history of a generalized headache and photophobia. He gave a five-day history of a dry cough before the onset of headache. On examination, he was unwell. The temperature was 37.7°C (99.9°F). Kernig's sign was absent. There was no evidence of papilloedema or any neurological deficit. There was no history of travel abroad. He was married with two children. He was a non-smoker and consumed 4–8 units of alcohol per week. The following day his condition deteriorated. He became drowsy and developed weakness in his lower limbs.

On examination, he was drowsy and his temperature was 38°C (100.4°F). He had a left facial nerve palsy and had failure of lateral gaze on the same side. The upper limbs were normal. The lower limbs had diminished power. Lower-limb reflexes were brisk. The left plantar was upgoing and the right plantar was equivocal. Abdominal reflexes were diminished.

Investigations are shown.

CSF analysis:
Cells	White cells 80/mm³ (40% lymphocytes) Red cells Absent
Protein	0.8 g/l
Glucose	3 mmol/l (blood glucose 4.4 mmol/l)
Gram stain	Negative
EEG	Slow waves

What is the diagnosis?
  a. Viral encephalomyelitis.
  b. *Listeria* meningoencephalitis.
  c. Tuberculous meningitis.
  d. Lyme disease.
  e. Cortical vein thrombosis.

Answer 266

c. Long QT syndrome (see Question 368). Brugada's syndrome is discussed in Answer 353 and ARVC in Answer 362.

Commotio cordis is a term used to describe the onset of ventricular fibrillation after being struck in the precordium by a highly projectile object. It is a recognized cause of death in ice hockey. Post-mortem examination reveals a normal heart.

Answer 267

a. Viral encephalomyelitis.

The most likely diagnosis is viral encephalomyelitis. There is a prodrome of dry cough in an otherwise fit, relatively young healthy male with no past history or history of travel, followed by drowsiness and signs consistent with brainstem involvement. Most cases of viral encephalitis are self-limiting and may present as a febrile illness associated with headache and photophobia. In a small proportion of patients the illness is more severe and is accompanied by progressive drowsiness, coma, seizures and focal neurological signs, particularly affecting the brain and spinal cord. Demyelination of the spinal cord and brainstem is characteristic. The patient has left-sided 6th and 7th cranial nerve palsies, which are suggestive of pontine involvement. In addition, he has brisk lower-limb reflexes, upgoing plantars, and absent abdominal reflexes suggestive of spinal cord involvement. The CSF reveals a modestly elevated WCC with a significant number of lymphocytes and a modestly elevated protein count. The CSF sugar content is normal, which excludes tuberculous and bacterial meningitis. Other causes of high lymphocyte count and elevated protein are shown in *Table A*. The EEG demonstrates the characteristic slow waves seen in viral encephalitis, although this appearance may also be seen in metabolic encephalopathies and cortical vein thrombosis. The most commonly implicated viruses in viral encephalitis are measles, herpes, influenza and pertussis.

Lyme disease may also cause neurological involvement. It is caused by the spirochaete *Borrelia burghdorferi*, which is transmitted by tick bites. The initial illness (stage 1) is characterized by a fever and a typical erythematous indurating rash at the site of the tick bite, known as erythema chronicum migrans. The second stage of the disease occurs between two and three weeks afterwards, and is characterized by cardiac and neurological involvement. Cardiac manifestations include pericarditis, myocarditis and heart block of varying degrees. Neurological involvement is characterized by symptoms of meningitis, focal neurological signs including cranial nerve palsies and a radiculopathy. There is no history of tick bites or travel to North America; however, the history of tick bites is not always elicited. It is only remotely possible that the patient may have been in contact with ticks. CSF findings include lymphocytosis and a modestly elevated protein count (*Table B*). The CSF sugar is normal. The diagnosis is made by demonstrating elevated titres of IgG to the spirochaete.

The diagnosis of *Listeria* meningoencephalitis is less likely for several reasons. First, listerosis usually affects neonates, elderly patients, pregnant women and the immunosuppressed. Second, the CSF usually demonstrates features of a bacterial meningitis (high neutrophil count, high protein and low sugar), but Gram stain is positive in a very few cases. The condition is characterized by a febrile illness. Cerebral involvement is characterized by features of meningitis and drowsiness. Focal neurological signs and cranial nerve palsies are recognized features.

Cortical vein thrombosis is characterized by rapid onset of headache, drowsiness and focal neurological signs and epilepsy. The EEG reveals slow waves. The CSF is characterized by a high content of neutrophils and lymphocytes and a high protein content. It may complicate bacterial meningitis or tuberculous meningitis. It usually occurs in young children following serious illness and dehydration. It is a recognized complication of myeloproliferative disorders, pregnancy and the

---

Table A Causes of lymphocytosis and elevated CSF protein

Infections
- Viral meningitis
- Tuberculous meningitis
- *Listeria* meningoencephalitis
- Neurosyphilis
- Leptospirosis
- Lyme disease
- Brucellosis
- Toxoplasmosis
- Cryptococcal meningitis
- Partially treated bacterial meningitis
- Cerebral abscess

Non-infectious
- Cerebral lymphoma/leukaemia
- Sarcoidosis
- SLE
- Behçet's disease
- Multiple sclerosis
- Cortical vein thrombosis

Table B CSF findings in infectious meningitis

	Pressure	WCC (mm3)	Protein g/l	Sugar
Viral meningitis or encephalitis*	Normal Slightly raised	10–100 (lymphocytes)	0.4–0.8	>1/2 blood glucose
Bacterial meningitis**	Raised	200–3,000 (neutrophils)	0.5–2.0	<1/3 blood glucose
TB meningitis	Raised	50–500 (lymphocytes)	0.5–3.0	<1/3 blood glucose
Lyme disease	Normal Slightly raised	50–500 (lymphocytes)	0.4–0.8	>1/2 blood glucose
Cryptococcal meningitis	Normal Slightly raised	50–300 (lymphocytes)	0.5–3.0	Usually low

* Similar findings may be seen in cerebral toxoplasmosis, leptospiral meningitis, brucellosis, *Listeria* meningitis.
** In partially treated bacterial meningitis there may be evidence of a pleiocytosis (presence of both lymphocytes and neutrophils) where the predominant cells are lymphocytes. The sugar content of the CSF may be only slightly reduced.

contraceptive pill. There is a possibility that the sudden deterioration in the patient's condition may be due to this complication. However, CSF features are not in keeping with bacterial or tuberculous meningitis, the prodromal illness was short and did not seem severe, and his past good health is against a coexisting disorder that may have predisposed to cortical vein thrombosis.

Question 268

A 20-year-old female is admitted to hospital with a 12-hour history of weakness in her arms and legs. This was accompanied by paraesthesia in her hands and feet. Five days before admission she experienced severe pain between her shoulder blades, and shortly afterwards developed blurred vision. The back pain had persisted but was less severe on admission. There was no history of headaches or nausea, but she had been constipated for two days and had intermittent lower abdominal pain. At the age of eight years she suffered a bout of viral meningitis for which she was in hospital for a week. At the age of 15 years she took an overdose of sleeping tablets while her parents were undergoing a divorce. She had enjoyed good health otherwise.

On examination, the patient was not distressed but had an expressionless face and found it difficult to close her eyes. She was afebrile. Examination of her fundi demonstrated blurred discs but no haemorrhages. Power in all her limbs was markedly diminished. She found it difficult to raise her arms above her shoulders, and could not move her legs. The tone in the legs was diminished and the reflexes in all her limbs were absent. Abdominal reflexes were present and the plantar response was normal. On examination of the abdomen she had a smooth palpable mass just above the symphysis pubis.

Investigations were as follows:

Hb	13 g/dl
WCC	7×10^9/l
Platelets	300×10^9/l
CT scan of brain	Normal

1. What two investigations (apart from CSF examination) would affect your immediate management?
   a. Forced vital capacity.
   b. Muscle biopsy.
   c. Serum creatinine phosphokinase.
   d. CSF analysis.
   e. Urinary porphobilinogen estimation.
   f. MRI scan brain.
   g. Tensilon test.
   h. Arterial blood gases.
   i. Stool culture.

2. What is the diagnosis?
   a. Myasthenia gravis.
   b. Acute polymyositis.
   c. Acute intermittent porphyria.
   d. Multiple sclerosis.
   e. Guillain–Barré syndrome.

Answer 268

1. a. Forced vital capacity.
   h. Arterial blood gases.
2. e. Guillain–Barré syndrome.

The patient presents with generalized muscle weakness following severe pain in the mid-thoracic area. She also complained of diplopia before the weakness, and has evidence of papilloedema and generalized motor neuropathy on examination. The patient has no sensory level to suggest spinal cord compression, therefore the constipation and the palpable bladder indicate an underlying autonomic neuropathy. The diagnosis which fits best with the symptoms and signs is Guillain–Barré syndrome or post-infectious polyneuropathy.

Guillain–Barré syndrome is a polyneuropathy which may develop over a few days or even a few weeks after an infectious illness, usually involving the respiratory tract. Enterovirus, EBV, *Mycoplasma, Campylobacter jejuni* and *Chlamydia* have been implicated, but the condition may occur following surgical conditions. In the majority of cases the underlying cause is never identified. The onset is often heralded by severe lumbar or interscapular pain, as in this case, and is followed by proximal, distal or generalized muscle weakness due to a motor neuropathy; however, some sensory loss is also present. Sensory loss commonly manifests as distal paraesthesiae and loss of vibration and positional sensation. The latter results in a sensory ataxia.

The cranial nerves may also be involved, particularly those innervating the extraocular muscles of the eye. In the context of the history above, the diplopia is almost certainly due to cranial nerves supplying the extraocular muscles. Bulbar involvement is also recognized. Autonomic neuropathy may complicate some cases, and may present as accelerated hypertension, tachyarrhythmias, abdominal pain, and bladder atony. Death may occur from respiratory failure due to respiratory muscle paralysis, or from arrhythmias and haemodynamic instability due to autonomic neuropathy. Aspiration may also cause death in patients with bulbar muscle involvement. The differential diagnosis and prognostic markers of the disease are listed below (*Tables A* and *B*).

The disease is characterized by a significantly elevated protein content in the CSF in the presence of a normal WCC. However, cases due to infectious mononucleosis may be associated with a mild pleiocytosis. The differential diagnosis of a high CSF WCC and a high protein content is tabulated below (*Table C*). Papilloedema may develop due either to accelerated hypertension or to impaired CSF resorption because of the elevated CSF protein content. The presence of papilloedema in this case makes it mandatory to measure the blood pressure. Histologically, there is segmental demyelination – possibly due to a cell-mediated delayed hypersensitivity. In the form of Guillain–Barré which accompanies *Campylobacter jejuni* infection there is an acute, purely axonal motor neuropathy with rapid progression and a mortality rate as high as 5%.

Management of the disease is by intravenous immunoglobulin or plasmapharesis. There is no role for corticosteroids in the management of Guillain–Barré syndrome.

A variant of Guillain–Barré is the Miller–Fisher syndrome, which comprises external ophthalmoplegia, ataxia and areflexia. The condition is highly suggested by the presence of antibodies to the sphyngomyelin component GQ1b.

Table A Differential diagnoses of Guillain–Barré syndrome

- Acute polymyositis
- Myaesthenia gravis
- Acute intermittent porphyria (motor and autonomic neuropathy)
- Lead poisoning
- Hypokalaemic periodic paralysis

Table B Poor prognostic markers in Guillain–Barré syndrome

- FVC <1.1 litres
- Arterial blood oxygen <8 kPa
- Arterial blood carbon dioxide >6 kPa
- Coexistent lower respiratory tract infection
- Coexistent pulmonary oedema
- Accelerated hypertension
- Arrhythmias
- Bulbar muscle involvement
- Guillain–Barré syndrome following *Campylobacter* infection

Table C Causes of a high CSF protein in the presence of a normal CSF cell count

- Guillain–Barré syndrome
- Spinal cord tumour causing spinal block (Froin's syndrome)
- Acoustic neuroma
- Lead encephalopathy
- Subacute sclerosing panencephalopathy

Question 269

This pedigree chart (**269a**) is from a family with a bleeding disorder.

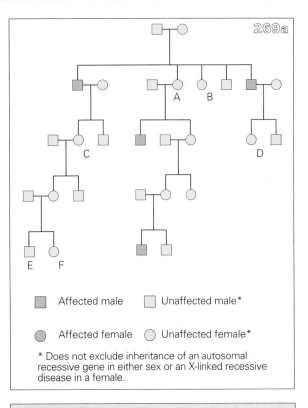

269a

Affected male ■   Unaffected male* □

Affected female ●   Unaffected female* ○

* Does not exclude inheritance of an autosomal recessive gene in either sex or an X-linked recessive disease in a female.

1. What is the mode of inheritance?
   a. X-linked recessive.
   b. Autosomal dominant.
   c. X-linked dominant.
   d. Autosomal recessive.
   e. Autosomal dominant with incomplete penetrance.

2. What is the most probable diagnosis?
   a. von Willebrand's disease.
   b. Haemophilia A.
   c. Antithrombin III deficiency.
   d. Dysfibrinogenaemia.
   e. Factor VII deficiency.

3. What are the chances of A being a carrier?
   a. 0%. b. 25%. c. 50%. d. 75%. e. 100%

4. What are the chances of B being affected?
   a. 0%. b. 25%. c. 50%. d. 75%. e. 100%

5. What are the chances of C being affected?
   a. 0%. b. 25%. c. 50%. d. 75%. e. 100%

6. What are the chances of D being a carrier?
   a. 0%. b. 25%. c. 50%. d. 75%. e. 100%

7. What are the chances of E being affected?
   a. 0%. b. 25%. c. 50%. d. 75%. e. 100%

8. What are the chances of E being a carrier?
   a. 0%. b. 25%. c. 50%. d. 75%. e. 100%

9. What are the chances of F being a carrier?
   a. 0%. b. 25%. c. 50%. d. 75%. e. 100%

Question 270

The following are cardiac catheter data from an 18-year-old female with breathlessness on exertion.

Chamber	Pressure (mmHg)	Oxygen saturation (%)
Superior vena cava	–	68
Inferior vena cava	–	67
Right atrium	a = 14	
	v = 20	
		(high) 68
		(mid) 69
		(low) 83
Right ventricle	92/20	83
Pulmonary artery	94/42	82
PCWP	a = 14	
	v = 22	
Left ventricle	106/20	96
Aorta	100/70	96

1. List at least four physical signs that you would elucidate on examination of this patient.
2. List at least three abnormalities which may be seen on the ECG.
3. What is the diagnosis?

Answer 269

1. a. X-linked recessive.	5. a. 0%.
2. b. Haemophilia A.	6. c. 100%.
3. e. 100%.	7. b. 25%.
4. a. 0%.	8. a. 0%.
	9. b. 25%.

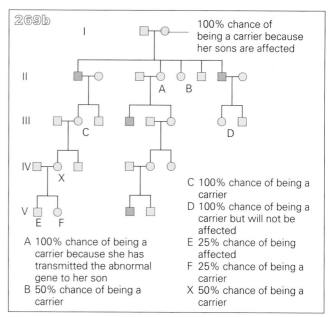

The answer is illustrated (**269b**). In this pedigree, only males are affected. Therefore, the condition must be X-linked recessive. In X-linked recessive conditions, only males will be affected; females will be carriers. In this pedigree, the female in generation I is a definite carrier because she has two affected sons (who have inherited the X-chromosome with the abnormal gene from their mother). Female A in generation II is also a definite carrier because she has an affected son. There is a 50% chance that female B is a carrier because a female carrier (her mother) will transmit the abnormal gene to 50% of her sons and 50% of her daughters. A female harbouring an X-linked recessive genetic abnormality will not be affected – assuming her other X-chromosome is free of the genetic mutation. Female C is a definite carrier because her father is affected. In X-linked conditions the male passes his X-chromosome (with the abnormal genetic mutation) to all his daughters. In contrast none of the sons receive the abnormal gene from the father because they inherit his Y chromosome. For the same reasons, female D is also a definite carrier.

There is a 50% chance that female X in generation IV is a carrier, therefore half of her sons will be affected and half of

her daughters will be carriers, that is, there is a 25% chance of male E being affected and a 25% chance of female F being a carrier.

The underlying diagnosis is haemophilia A. The other possibility is haemophilia B, which is also inherited as an X-linked recessive trait and is due to abnormally low Factor IX levels. Dysfibrinogenaemia is inherited as an autosomal dominant or recessive trait. Factor V deficiency is inherited as an autosomal recessive trait and most cases of von Willebrand's disease are inherited as an autosomal dominant trait.

Answer 270

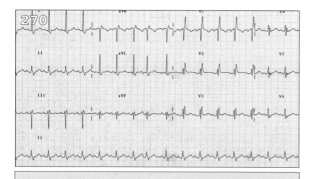

A step up in oxygen saturation in the upper right atrium would indicate a sinus venosus defect, and a step up in the mid right atrium would indicate an ostium secundum ASD. (See Interpretation of Cardiac Catheter Data, page 418.)

1. i. A right ventricular heave. The right ventricle must have hypertrophied to generate such a high systolic pressure.
   ii. A pansystolic murmur of mitral regurgitation at the apex. The large 'v'-wave in the PCWP suggests mitral regurgitation.
   iii. Fixed splitting of second heart sound from ASD.
   iv. Pansystolic murmur of tricuspid regurgitation at the left sternal edge. The large 'v'-wave in the right atrial pressure suggests tricuspid regurgitation.
   v. Systolic flow murmur in the pulmonary area.

2. i. Partial RBBB.
   ii. Right ventricular hypertrophy.
   iii. Left atrial enlargement.
   iv. Right atrial enlargement.
   v. Left axis deviation. The ECG in ostium primum defects characteristically reveals partial or complete RBBB and left axis deviation (**270**). In contrast, patients with ostium secundum defects have partial RBBB and right axis deviation.

3. There is a step up in the oxygen saturation in the low right atrium, suggesting an ostium primum ASD. The defect is associated with mitral and tricuspid ring defects, causing both mitral and tricuspid regurgitation.

Question 271

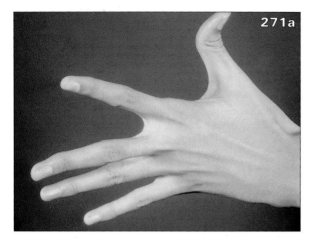

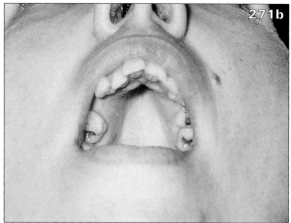

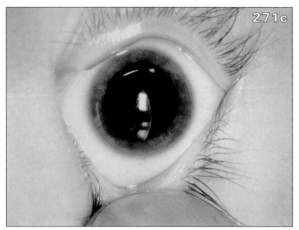

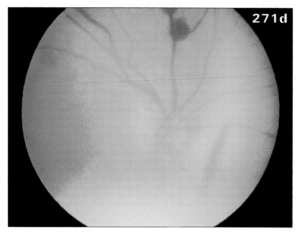

A 19-year-old dustman was admitted to hospital with severe retrosternal chest pain associated with belching and vomiting. He was a non-smoker. He had been celebrating a friend's birthday and had consumed a considerable amount of alcohol the night before. He was diagnosed as having epilepsy 12 years ago and was on regular anticonvulsant medication. There was no family history of ischaemic heart disease or epilepsy. He had an older brother who was fit and well. He had been in hospital eight months previously with an axillary vein thrombosis which had been treated with warfarin for six months. He wore glasses for being short-sighted.

On examination, he was thin and tall, measuring 1.9 m. He had a kyphoscoliotic spine. Examination of his hands, oral cavity and left eye is shown (**271a–c**, respectively). The findings on fundoscopy are also shown (**271d**). A cardiovascular examination was normal. The patient had pectus excavatum; the chest was clear on auscultation. An abdominal examination revealed mild tenderness in the epigastrum.

Investigations are shown.

Hb	11 g/dl
AST	60 iu/l
WCC	5×10^9/l
Bilirubin	11 μmol/l
Platelets	160×10^9/l
Alkaline phosphatase	112 iu/l
MCV	105 fl
Albumin	43 g/l
U&E	Normal
Chest X-ray	Kyphoscoliosis
	Clear lung fields
	Normal heart size
ECG	Normal
Gastroscopy	Gastro-oesophagitis

1. What is the diagnosis?
2. Give two explanations for the raised MCV.
3. How would you confirm the diagnosis?
4. How is the condition inherited, and where is the chromosomal defect?

Answer 271

1. Homocystinuria.
2. i. Phenytoin therapy. Phenytoin is thought to interfere with folate absorption. Other anticonvulsants causing folate deficiency include primidone and barbiturate therapy.
   ii. The conversion of homocystine to methionine requires large amounts of the enzyme 5-methyl tetrahydrofolate methyltransferase, which utilizes folate as a cofactor. During the enzyme reaction some of the folate is degraded, and folate deficiency can occur.
3. The urine gives a positive nitroprusside test. Raised levels of plasma methionine and homocystine are more reliable because the nitroprusside test is also positive in cystinuria.
4. Autosomal recessive inheritance. The gene is located on chromosome 21.

The chest pain due to oesophagitis has no connection with the underlying diagnosis. The examiner expects the reader to pick up on the skeletal, ocular and neurological abnormalities to come to a diagnosis of homocystinuria.

Homocystinuria is due to cystathionine deficiency. As a result, there is accumulation of homocysteine which in turn is oxidized to homocystine. There is no production of cystine. Plasma and urinary levels of homocystine are elevated. Homocystine is thought to affect cross-linking of collagen, leading to skeletal, ocular, neurological and vascular abnormalities.

Skeletal: The patients have the same skeletal abnormalities as in Marfan's syndrome. These include tallness, kyphoscoliosis, arachnodactyly, high-arched palate, pectus excavatum and flat feet. The ligaments are lax, and muscular development weak. Osteoporosis is a feature and classically affects the vertebrae. These patients need to be distinguished from Marfan patients, who have a strong family history, and often have evidence of cardiovascular involvement in the form of mitral valve prolapse and aortic root dilatation, but do not have associated neurological abnormalities. Osteoporosis is not a feature of Marfan's syndrome.

Ocular: The suspensory ligaments of the lens are weakened, causing lens dislocation which is usually downward. This is complicated by glaucoma, iridodonesis, myopia and cataracts. Optic atrophy and retinal detachment are also recognized ocular problems.

Neurological: Mental handicap occurs in approximately 50% of patients and 10–20% of patients have epilepsy. The degree of mental retardation can be mild or severe. There is a form of homocystinuria which responds to pyridoxine. Patients with this form are less severely affected.

Vascular: Both venous and arterial thromboses occur and are thought to be due to the effects of methionine causing vascular damage, and increased platelet adherence. This has important therapeutic implications in patients undergoing surgery for correction of skeletal abnormalities, because there is a risk of deep-vein thrombus, and prophylactic heparin should be given following surgery. The oestrogen-containing oral contraceptive pill is contraindicated in women with homocystinuria. Recent studies have shown that homocystinuria is also associated with premature coronary artery disease.

Treatment is with dietary restriction of methionine and cystine supplements. Pyridoxine should be given immediately after the diagnosis has been made and is beneficial in some cases.

Question 272

A 59-year-old farmer was referred to a chest unit with an 18-month history of progressive breathlessness. Over the past four years, he had noticed a dry cough in the afternoons and evenings. His effort tolerance three years previously was very good, allowing him to work on the farm for almost 12 hours per day. Since then he had resolved to work only two days a week owing to fatigue and breathlessness, and had asked both his sons to take over his farm.

His GP diagnosed asthma, but his condition had continued to deteriorate despite the use of steroid and salbutamol inhalers. He was now breathless after walking just 200 metres. He was a non-smoker. There was no family history of lung disease. He had never worked with asbestos, and did not keep pets.

On examination, he was cyanosed and tachypnoeic. He had evidence of early clubbing. The JVP was not raised, and heart sounds were normal. On auscultation of the lung fields there were bilateral fine end-inspiratory crackles in both lungs.

Investigations are shown.

Hb	12 g/dl	
WCC	5×10^9/l	
Platelets	400×10^9/l	
ESR	54 mm/h	
Chest X-ray	Diffuse reticulonodular shadowing in both apices and midzones	
FEV_1 (%)	50	Blood gases on air:
FVC (%)	52	pH 7.45
FEV_1/FVC (%)	89	$PaCO_2$ 3.5 kPa
TLC (%)	56	pO_2 6.4 kPa
KCO (%)	60	Bicarbonate 22 mmol/l

1. What is the diagnosis?
2. List at least two tests that would help to confirm the diagnosis.

Question 273

A 78-year-old male presented with a several weeks' history of weakness, lethargy, weight loss and vomiting.

On examination, the blood pressure (standing) was 80/50 mmHg.

Blood results are shown.

Sodium	124 mmol/l
Potassium	4.9 mmol/l
Urea	15 mmol/l
Bicarbonate	15 mmol/l
Blood glucose	4.0 mmol/l

List three possible causes for this biochemical picture.

Question 274

A 51-year-old dentist presented to his GP because he had difficulty lifting his right arm for over one week. For the past few days he could not hold the razor to his face with his right arm while shaving. About two weeks previously he received a hepatitis B booster vaccine which was associated with pain over his deltoid and shoulder region for almost 48 hours.

On examination there was wasting over the deltoid region. There was reduced power on abduction, flexion and internal rotation of the right arm and flexion of the right elbow. The right biceps and supinator reflexes were absent. All other examinations were normal.

Investigations are shown.

Hb	14.3 g/dl
WCC	5×10^9/l
Platelets	199×10^9/l
ESR	11 mm/h
Biochemistry	Normal
X-rays of chest and cervical spine	Normal

What is the diagnosis?
  a. Radiculopathy secondary to Lyme disease.
  b. Neuralgic amyotrophy.
  c. Syringomyelia.
  d. Cervical myelopathy.
  e. Motor neurone disease.

Answer 272

1. Extrinsic allergic alveolitis.
2. i. Precipitins from *Micropolyspora faenii*.
   ii. High-resolution CT scan.
   iii. Bronchoalveolar lavage.
   iv. Bronchoscopy with transbronchial lung biopsy.

Extrinsic allergic alveolitis is a cell-mediated allergic reaction that occurs in response to inhalation of a variety of agents. It is characterized by interstitial inflammation and progressive lung fibrosis. Patients typically present with fever and dyspnoea several hours after inhaling the antigen. In this case, the farmer who has been working in the morning will not develop symptoms until late afternoon. During the reaction the patient will be tachypnoeic, febrile and have widespread coarse crackles throughout the lung. Continuing exposure and inflammation results in interstitial fibrosis, leading to progressive dyspnoea and functional limitation. The chest X-ray reveals nodular shadows in the upper zones that eventually involve the mid-zones. In severe cases the lung will have a honeycomb appearance on the X-ray owing to severe fibrosis. Several antigens are recognized and several occupations are at risk. In farmers, the culprit antigen is commonly the spores of the fungus *M. faenii* that are inhaled while forking mouldy hay. Malt workers may be affected by inhalation of products of the fungus *Aspergillus clavatus* while turning germinating barley, and pigeon keepers may develop the condition after inhaling avian proteins from feathers of the birds.

The diagnosis relies on an abnormal chest X-ray, and the demonstration of antibodies to the culprit antigens. High-resolution CT scan of the thorax will reveal the extent of parenchymal involvement. Formal spirometry is useful in assessing lung reserve in patients with fibrosis. The KCO is reduced owing to interstitial lung damage. Transbronchial lung biopsy is rarely required to make the diagnosis unless the cause of lung fibrosis is unclear. Bronchoalveolar lavage reveals increased cells that are predominantly lymphocytes.

Management is to remove the patient from the antigen. In the early stages of the disease, high-dose prednisolone will cause regression of the condition.

Answer 273

i. Addison's disease/primary hypoadrenalism.
ii. Diuretic therapy.
iii. Salt-losing nephritis.

The combination of lethargy, weight loss, vomiting, hypotension, hyponatraemia and hyperkalaemia is suggestive of Addison's disease. Addison's disease is caused by destruction of the adrenal glands, resulting in deficiency of glucocorticoid and mineralocorticoid hormones. The most common cause of Addison's disease is auto-immune adrenalitis. Other causes are listed (*Table*). The condition has an insidious presentation in the majority of cases, but may present as a crisis. Lethargy, anorexia, nausea, vomiting, abdominal pain and symptoms of postural hypotension are common. Some patients are misdiagnosed as having depression. In the elderly, the condition may present as a confusional state. On examination, there may be evidence of pigmentation which is prominent in skin creases, scars and the buccal mucosa. The supine blood pressure may be normal, but there is a marked drop in systolic pressure on standing (>25 mmHg).

Acute Addisonian crisis is characterized by coma, profound hypotension and hypoglycaemia. The electrolytes are usually abnormal (as above) but may also be normal. Acute adrenal failure or Addisonian crisis is a medical emergency which should be aggressively treated with intravenous hydrocortisone and saline. Dextrose is used in hypoglycaemic cases.

Long-term treatment is with oral hydrocortisone, prednisolone or dexamethasone (glucocorticoids) and fludrocortisone (mineralocorticoid).

Addison's disease is diagnosed by performing the synacthen test. Serum cortisol is measured before and 30 min after intramuscular ACTH (synacthen). In normal individuals, the serum cortisol rises to above 600 nmol/l, or is increased by 300 from the basal level. Patients with Addison's disease will not demonstrate this level of rise.

Causes of Addison's disease (primary hypoadrenalism)

- Autoimmune adrenalitis
- TB
- Carcinomatous infiltration of adrenal glands (bronchial carcinoma)
- Adrenal haemorrhage or infarction (Waterhouse–Friedrichson syndrome)
- Infiltration disorders:
  - haemochromatosis
  - amyloidosis
  - granulomatous disorders
- Metyrapone therapy
- Schilder's disease
- Wolman's disease (hepatosplenomegaly and steatorrhoea)

Adrenal antibodies are present in cases of auto-immune adrenalitis. In cases of tuberculous adrenal gland destruction there may be obvious calcification of the adrenal gland on the plain abdominal X-ray. Alternatively, the demonstration of an inappropriately raised serum ACTH and a low simultaneous serum cortisol level is diagnostic.

Diuretic therapy with spironolactone (aldosterone antagonist) or combined loop diuretic and potassium-sparing diuretic preparations will produce the same biochemical picture. Dehydration from diuresis may lead to pre-renal failure, reflected by rising urea and a low bicarbonate. The serum aldosterone is elevated in dehydration due to diuretics. This is in direct contrast to Addison's disease, where the aldosterone level will be low. Salt-losing nephritis is characterized biochemically by hyponatraemia and impaired renal function.

Answer 274

> b. Neuralgic amyotrophy.

The diagnosis is neuralgic amyotrophy. This is an inflammatory process affecting the roots of C5 and C6 and occasionally C7. It usually follows an infective illness or trauma to the deltoid region. It is preceded by pain over the shoulder and arm followed by weakness and wasting of the muscles supplied by the affected roots. Spontaneous recovery is usual but may take several months. The differential diagnosis is cervical cord compression, but the absence of lower limb signs is against this. Lyme disease may produce a similar radiculopathy but in this case there is no history of a skin rash, tick bite, cardiac involvement or arthropathy. Furthermore, the history of immunization into the deltoid is more in keeping with amyotrophy. Syringomyelia is unlikely in the absence of sensory signs. Although motor neurone disease may present with pure lower motor neurone signs as in this case, the rapid onset of neurological signs in just one limb does not favour the diagnosis.

Question 275

A 28-year-old obese female was admitted to the ward for further investigation after presenting with lethargy. She did not give any further history of significance. Her blood pressure in clinic was 128/85 mmHg. Blood results are shown.

After these blood results, the patient was questioned further about her bowel habit and medication. She denied having diarrhoea or taking any medication. She was observed on the ward for 48 hours, during which time her blood pressure did not fluctuate.

A repeat serum renin level was 1,600 pg/ml/h.

Sodium	135 mmol/l
Potassium	2.2 mmol/l
Urea	7.3 mmol/l
Creatinine	60 μmol/l
Bicarbonate	36 mmol/l
Renin	1,500 pg/ml/h (NR [lying supine] 300–1,300 pg/ml/h)
24-h urine output	500 ml
24-h urine potassium	10 mmol/l

1. Comment on the initial results.
2. Suggest a possible cause for the abnormalities, given the results of the tests performed while she was observed in hospital.

Answer 275

1. The patient has a hypokalaemic alkalosis and an appropriate hypokaluria. Patients with a serum potassium of <3.5 mmol/l conserve potassium and excrete <20 mmol/l of potassium in the urine. The urea is modestly elevated, as is her serum renin, both of which suggest hypoperfusion of the afferent glomerular vessels. This may occur in dehydration, shock, glomerular and renal parenchymal disease. However, in primary renal disease the serum creatinine is also elevated, and in this history the blood pressure is not suggestive of shock.

2. In the context of this history the most probable cause for the hypokalaemia is loss of potassium from the gastrointestinal tract. This is also causing dehydration and hence the elevated urea and renin. There is no history of diarrhoea or vomiting, but given her obesity there is a chance that she is abusing laxatives or has self-induced vomiting in order to try and lose weight (**275**).

Potassium may be lost via the GI tract (diarrhoea, vomiting, intestinal fistulae, villous adenoma, nasogastric aspiration) or the kidneys (primary and secondary hyperaldosteronism, Cushing's syndrome, Liddle's syndrome, renal tubular disorders or drugs). Loss of potassium from the GI tract is associated with conservation of potassium by the kidneys.

Hypokalaemia is generally associated with a metabolic alkalosis with the exception of RTA.

Many conditions associated with renal loss of potassium also cause hypertension. The most common cause of hypertension, hypokalaemia and alkalosis encountered in the MRCP and similar examinations is primary hyperaldosteronism (Conn's syndrome). However, other recognized causes include Cushing's, Liddle's syndrome (pseudohyperaldosteronism), accelerated hypertension, renal artery stenosis or hypertensive therapy with diuretics (*Table*). Liddle's

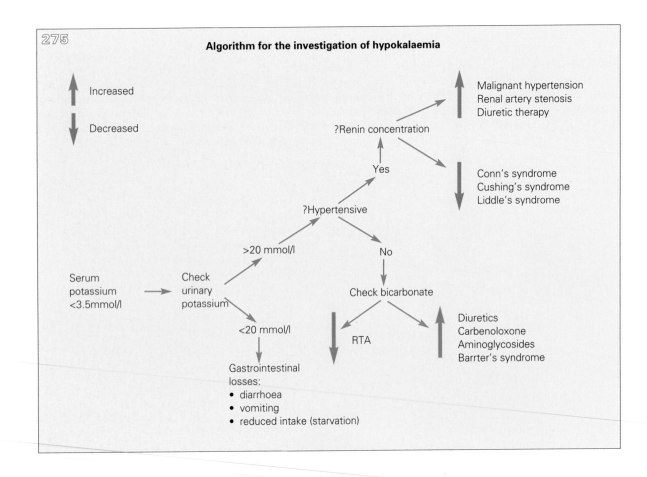

275 Algorithm for the investigation of hypokalaemia

Causes of hypokalaemic alkalosis and hypertension

- Primary hyperaldosteronism (Conn's syndrome)
- Cushing's syndrome
- Liddle's syndrome
- Accelerated hypertension
- Hypertension treated with diuretics
- Renal artery stenosis
- Carbenoxolone therapy
- Liquorice abuse
- Congenital adrenal hyperplasia (11-β-hydroxylase deficiency)*

*In 11-β-hydroxylase deficiency, the aldosterone levels are low; however, there is excessive production of deoxycorticosterone which has strong mineralocorticoid effects and causes both hypertension and hypokalaemia.

---

syndrome is a tubular defect characterized by excessive sodium absorption and increased potassium excretion. The biochemistry is identical to that of Conn's syndrome, but there is no abnormality of the renin–angiotensin–aldosterone axis.

In the absence of hypertension, other causes of hypokalaemic alkalosis include carbenoxolone therapy, liquorice abuse, aminoglycosides, and Bartter's syndrome – which is due to hyperplasia of the juxtaglomerular apparatus. In Bartter's syndrome, affected children present with nocturia, muscle weakness and failure to thrive. It is important to note that carbenoxolone therapy and liquorice abuse may cause hypertension.

Question 276

A 17-year-old female was referred to the gynaecologist with primary amenorrhoea. She had been relatively well throughout her life. Her mother was concerned that she was not gaining any weight, despite eating well. She had been investigated for diabetes by the GP and was found to have a normal blood glucose. Apart from complaining of intermittent headaches and feeling tired at the end of the day, there were no other symptoms. She was still at college. She had two brothers and a sister who were well. Her sister was aged 14 and had just started menstruating.

On examination, the patient measured 1.5 m and weighed 40 kg. She was pale, and had scanty axillary and pubic hair. Breast development had just begun.

Investigations are shown.

Hb	9.8 g/dl
WCC	5×10^9/l
Platelets	190×10^9/l
MCV	104 fl
Blood film	Target cells, anisocytosis, macrocytes, poikilocytosis
Sodium	137 mmol/l
Potassium	4.1 mmol/l
Urea	3 mmol/l
Creatinine	78 μmol/l
Calcium	2.0 mmol/l
Phosphate	0.75 mmol/l
Albumin	37 g/l
AST	20 iu/l
Alkaline phosphatase	300 iu/l
Bilirubin	11 μmol/l
Thyroxine	100 nmol/l
TSH	2.0 mu/l

1. What is the cause of the patient's amenorrhoea?
2. What is the most probable underlying diagnosis?
3. Give two possible explanations for the alkaline phosphatase level.
4. Give two tests you would perform to confirm the diagnosis.

Answer 276

1. Underweight owing to malabsorption (malabsorption syndrome).
2. Coeliac disease.
3. i. Osteomalacia.
   ii. Patient in a growth spurt.
4. i. Duodenal biopsy or jejunal biopsy.
   ii. Antiendomyosium, antigliadin or antireticulin antibodies.

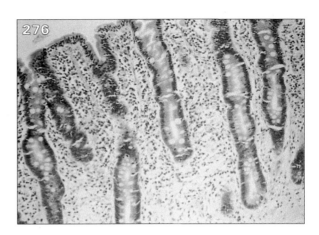

The patient is short for her age. She has a macrocytic anaemia. The blood film reveals hypochromasia, macrocytosis and target cells, suggesting either isolated folate (or possibly B_{12}) deficiency or combined iron and folate deficiency. The bone biochemistry is in keeping with vitamin D deficiency. The slightly low albumin level is indicative of poor nutritional status in this context. Failure to grow, or weight loss despite a normal appetite, plus a combination of nutritional deficiencies should always raise the question of a malabsorption syndrome. The lack of secondary sexual characteristics and delayed menstruation in this patient may be explained by the fact that she has yet to reach puberty, either because of a constitutional delay or because puberty has been delayed owing to a malabsorption syndrome.

Malabsorption syndromes are a recognized cause of primary and secondary amenorrhoea in girls and young women, predominantly as a result of poor nutrition causing profound weight loss. Readers may fall into the trap of diagnosing hypopituitarism in this case, given the short stature and absent secondary sexual characteristics. However, the diagnosis of hypopituitarism fails to explain the normal thyroid function tests and the abnormal bone biochemistry. Anaemia is a recognized feature of hypopituitarism. It is usually normochromic normocytic, but may be macro- or microcytic.

A variety of conditions produce malabsorption syndromes (*Table*), but the most common cause by far in the Western world is coeliac disease. This affects 1 in 2,000 patients in the UK, and is even more common in Ireland, affecting 1 in 300. The disorder is characterized by total villous atrophy in the small intestine as a result of ingestion of gluten-containing food. The majority (80%) of patients have the haplotype HLA A1, B8, DR7 or DQW2, suggesting a genetic basis. There is 30% disconcordance among identical twins, which suggests that non-genetic factors may also be involved. Small bowel injury occurs as a result of gluten ingestion. Gluten is a high-molecular weight compound which contains various gliadins. α-gliadin damages small bowel mucosa in these patients, probably through an immune-mediated mechanism. Antigliadin antibodies are strong evidence for this postulation. Small bowel damage produces malabsorption which manifests as weight loss, abdominal pain, diarrhoea and nutritional deficiencies. Diarrhoea may be absent in up to 20% of patients. The disease can present at any age. In children, it occurs soon after weaning and presents as failure to thrive. In adults, it presents with abdominal symptoms, weight loss and fatigue. Ankle oedema may complicate albumin deficiency. Mouth ulcers may occur as a result of iron deficiency. Osteomalacia, tetany and muscle weakness may be present owing to vitamin D deficiency.

Anaemia is present in 50% of cases. Macrocytosis is invariably due to folate deficiency. Iron deficiency is common, but B_{12} deficiency is rare. Hypochromia and target cells may be present on the blood film.

Howell–Jolly bodies may be seen on the blood film in patients who develop splenic atrophy. The diagnosis is made by sampling small bowel from the second portion of the duodenum (D2 biopsy) via endoscopy or a jejunal biopsy (**276**). Antiendomyosium antibodies are detected in almost 50% of all cases of coeliac disease, and are highly specific for the disorder. Antigliadin antibodies and antireticulin antibodies are found in the serum of the majority of patients.

Treatment is with a gluten-free diet. Gluten is present in the cereals wheat, rye, barley and oats, all of which should be excluded from the diet.

Associations of coeliac disease include auto-immune thyroid disorders, chronic liver disease, fibrosing alveolitis, ulcerative colitis and insulin-dependent diabetes mellitus. Complications include small bowel lymphoma and adenocarcinoma and splenic atrophy.

Small bowel malabsorption syndromes

Disorder	Additional comments
Coeliac disease	High antigliadin or antireticulin antibodies Antiendomyosium antibodies highly specific
Dermatitis herpetiformis	Gluten-sensitive enteropathy. Associated subepidermal blistering rash
Bacterial overgrowth	Low B_{12} but normal or high serum folate. Previous gastric surgery (Billroth II), jejunal diverticuli
Giardiasis	May be detected on stool microscopy. Travel abroad or immunosuppressed
Whipple's disease	Associated locomotor/neurological/cardiac features HLA B27 PAS-positive macrophages which contain the bacillus *Tropheryma whipelli* on small bowel biopsy
Tropical sprue	History of living in an endemic area for >3 months
Radiation enteritis	Previous history of abdominal irradiation
Crohn's disease	Abdominal pain/diarrhoea predominate. May have isolated B_{12} deficiency which is not corrected with intrinsic factor
Hypogammaglobulinaemia	Very similar to cystic fibrosis. Gut, respiratory and locomotor involvement. Low globulins. *Giardia* infections common
Zollinger–Ellison syndrome	History of recurrent peptic ulceration predominates
Intestinal lymphangiectasia	Hypoproteinaemia as a result of protein-losing enteropathy and steatorrhoea. Associated immunoglobulin deficiency. Congenital dilatation of small bowel lymphatics. May occur secondary to pericardial constriction or severe heart failure. Primary lymphatic abnormalities elsewhere may lead to chylous pleural effusions and chylous ascites

Question 277

A 30-year-old sailor was admitted to the navy hospital with a seven-day history of increasing confusion, malaise, fever and reduced visual acuity in his left eye. Two weeks previously he had developed weakness affecting his left arm and left lower limb. He had a past history of Hodgkin's lymphoma which was successfully treated with chemotherapy five years ago.

On examination, he was confused. His temperature was 40°C (104°F). There was evidence of cervical lymphadenopathy on palpation of the neck. On examination of the fundi, there was widespread retinal scarring in both eyes, the right eye being more affected than the left. There was no obvious papilloedema. The left-sided limbs demonstrated marked weakness.

Investigations are shown.

Hb	11 g/dl
WCC	6×10^9/l
Platelets	190×10^9/l
ESR	80 mm/h
EEG	Diffuse slow wave activity

1. Suggest at least two possible diagnoses.
2. Give one investigation which would help make the diagnosis in each case.
3. What treatment would you institute for each of your diagnoses?

Answer 277

1. i. Cerebral toxoplasmosis.
   ii. Tuberculous meningitis.
   iii. Cryptococcal meningitis.
   iv. Cerebral lymphoma.
2. i. CT scan brain (**277**). Multiple ring-enhancing lesions may suggest cerebral toxoplasmosis, TB abscesses or lymphoma.
   ii. CSF IgM levels or Sabin–Feldman dye test for *Toxoplasma gondii*.
   iii. CSF staining with auramine or Ziehl–Neelsen stain may detect TB and staining with Indian ink will identify cryptococcal meningitis.
   iv. Brain biopsy.
3. i. Pyrimethamine and sulphadiazine for toxoplasmosis.
   ii. Ansamycin and clofazimine for TB (particularly effective for atypical TB).
   iii. Amphotericin for cryptococcal meningitis.
   iv. Radiotherapy to the skull for cerebral lymphoma.

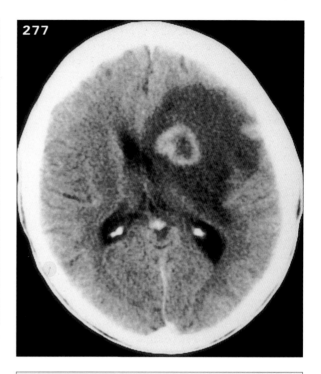

277

The patient is a sailor. In MRCP and similar examinations questions, sailors are associated with a high level of promiscuity and high risk for HIV infection. This patient is confused, has focal neurological signs, and evidence of bilateral scarring of the retina. The confusion may be the manifestation of an encephalitis, meningitis, cerebral abscess or cerebral metastases in the context of the question.

Focal neurological signs may be caused by all of the above. The presence of chorioretinitis and focal neurological signs favours the diagnosis of cerebral toxoplasmosis, TB or cryptococcal meningitis. Cerebral lymphoma *per se* does not cause chorioretinitis; however, it is possible that the patient has both cerebral lymphoma and a CSF infection causing chorioretinitis. Other recognized causes of chorioretinitis in patients with HIV include CMV and syphilitic infection. The slow waves on the EEG are suggestive of an encephalitic process, which may be part of the cerebral effect of the HIV itself, or as a result of opportunistic infections such as CMV, herpes virus, toxoplasmosis, atypical mycobacteria or lymphomatous infiltration.

The diagnosis and management for each condition are outlined above. It may be difficult to differentiate between cerebral lymphoma and toxoplasmosis in this

Cerebral manifestations of HIV

- HIV dementia
- Progressive multifocal leucoencephalopathy
- Tuberculous meningitis/tuberculoma
- Toxoplasmosis
- Lymphoma
- Herpes encephalitis
- Peripheral neuropathy

particular case. The usual management policy would be to treat for cerebral toxoplasmosis in the first instance and repeat the CT scan in two weeks, which should reveal resolution of the ring-enhancing lesions if they are due to toxoplasmosis. If the lesions persist, then a tissue diagnosis using brain biopsy may become necessary.

The cerebral manifestations of HIV infection are listed (*Table*).

Question 278

A 15-year-old girl presented with a 48-hour history of a sore throat and dark urine. On examination she appeared relatively well at rest. The blood pressure was 100/60 mmHg.

Investigations are shown.

HB	12.5 g/dl
WCC	11×10^9/l
Platelets	240×10^9/l
Sodium	136 mmol/l
Potassium	4.1 mmol/l
Urea	4.2 mmol/l
Serum creatinine	80 μmol/l
Urinalysis	Microscopic haematuria

Which of the following antibodies is likely to be raised in the blood?
a. ASO.
b. ANA.
c. Anti-GBM.
d. ANCA.
e. None of the above.

Question 279

A 55-year-old man was seen by a respiratory physician for daytime somnolence. According to his wife he snored loudly in his sleep. He was a life-long heavy smoker. He took salbutamol intermittently for breathlessness. On examination he weighed 88 kg and was 1.72 m tall. There was an expiratory wheeze heard throughout his lung fields.

Investigations are shown.

Arterial blood gases:	
pH	7.35
$PaCO_2$	7.0 kPa
PaO_2	8.2 kPa
Bicarbonate	35 mmol/l
O_2 saturation	85%
FEV_1	45% predicted
FVC	55% predicted
FEV_1/FVC	50%

What is the most appropriate therapy?
a. Nocturnal oxygen therapy.
b. Uveoplasty.
c. Nocturnal continuous positive-pressure airway ventilation.
d. Steroid therapy.
e. Protryptiline.

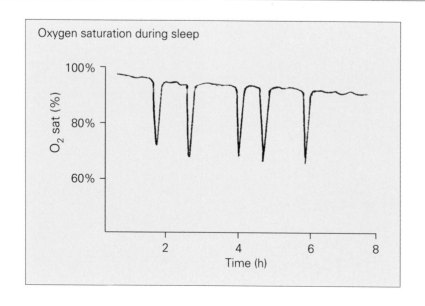

Answer 278

> e. None of the above.

Causes of haematuria after an upper respiratory tract infection include IgA nephropathy, post-streptococcal glomerulonephritis and non-specific mesangioproliferative glomerulonephritis. IgA nephropathy is probably the most common cause of glomerulonephritis after a URTI. Patients present with recurrent episodes of gross haematuria one to three days after a URTI. The haematuria resolves within a few days. Some patients develop acute renal failure. The serum IgA may be raised in 50% of cases but there are no other specific auto-antibodies to help make the diagnosis.

Post-streptococcal glomerulonephritis is induced by infection with specific strains of group A, ß-haemolytic streptococci (such as type 12 and type 49). This can occur in sporadic cases or during an epidemic. The clinical presentation can vary from asymptomatic, microscopic haematuria to the full-blown acute nephritic syndrome and renal failure. Although the presentation may be similar to that seen with IgA nephropathy, the following can be used to differentiate between these disorders (*Table*). Renal biopsy is not required in most cases.

	Post Strep GMN	IgA nephropathy
Onset of haematuria	10 days after sore throat	5 days after sore throat
Recurrent haematuria	Rare	Common
Throat culture	Positive	Negative
ASO titre	Positive	Negative
Haematuria after 6 months	Rare	Common

Answer 279

> c. Nocturnal continuous positive-pressure airway ventilation.

The patient has features of obstructive sleep apnoea. He snores and has daytime somnolence. He also appears to be overweight. The sleep study shows marked oxygen desaturations throughout the night. These desaturations represent apnoeic episodes due to airway obstruction. The fact that he also has respiratory failure suggests that he must also have underlying parenchymal lung disease, since pure obstructive sleep apnoea syndrome does not usually cause respiratory failure unless the patient has low tidal volumes due to gross obesity, as seen in the Pickwickian syndrome.

Obstructive sleep apnoea is usually due to an abnormality in the size or collapsibility of the pharynx. During sleep there is a combination of factors (reduced tone input into the upper airways, diminished reflexes to protect the pharynx from collapse) that cause upper airway obstruction. The resulting apnoea eventually wakes the patient. Airway obstruction manifests as loud snoring with apnoeic episodes.

Since sleep is disturbed the patients complain of tiredness and daytime somnolence. Early morning headaches due to CO_2 retention are a recognized feature. The sympathetic response to the apnoeic episodes results in systemic hypertension and left ventricular hypertrophy. There is some anecdotal evidence that OSA is associated with a higher cardiovascular mortality.

Treatments include weight reduction, avoidance of alcohol or sedatives. Protryptiline (a respiratory stimulant) is not particularly effective. The most effective therapy is nocturnal continuous positive-pressure ventilation, which keeps the upper airways patent. Reduced tolerance and compliance with nocturnal CPAP are the main issues.

Question 280

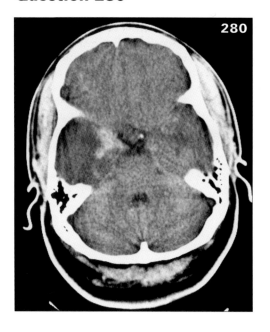

A 34-year-old Nigerian male presented with a 48-hour history of fever and headache. According to his wife he became confused two hours prior to admission and was talking nonsense. The patient underwent a CT scan of the brain (**280**).

What is the management?
a. IV cefotaxime.
b. Neurosurgical referral.
c. IV acyclovir.
d. IV amphotericin.
e. IV dexamethasone.

Question 281

A 62-year-old asymptomatic female had the following thyroid function tests as part of a health screen. She was not taking any medication and had always enjoyed good health:

Serum T4 20 iu/l
Serum TSH 8 iu/l
Antithyroid myoperoxidase antibodies: absent

What is the management of her abnormal thyroid function tests?
a. Start thyroxine.
b. No treatment. Repeat thyroid function tests in six months.
c. Reassure. No further follow up required.
d. Perform a radio-iodine scan and treat only if there is reduced uptake in the gland.
e. Start triiodothyronine.

Question 282

A 64-year-old male presented with reduced visual acuity. He had a long history of hypertension.

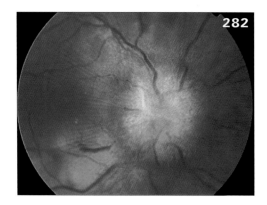

What is the ophthalmological diagnosis (**252**)?
a. Central retinal vein occlusion.
b. Central retinal artery occlusion.
c. Optic atrophy.
d. Myelinated nerve fibre.
e. Papilloedema.

Answer 280

> c. IV acyclovir.

Herpes simplex encephalitis is most usually due to HSV 1 and presents with headache, fever and drowsiness. The virus may complicate HSV infecting the oropharyngeal area or may be due to reactivation of latent virus in the CNS. It affects the inferior aspects of the frontal lobes and the medial aspects of the temporal lobes. Olfactory and gustatory hallucinations and impairment of memory are recognized. The patient may exhibit multiple cranial nerve palsies and ataxia. Some patients develop hypomania or the Kluver–Bucy syndrome ('psychic blindness', loss of fear and anger response and increased sexual activity). Untreated patients develop seizure and lapse into a comatosed state. The mortality is high. CT scan may reveal hypodense medial temporal lobes that enhance with contrast. The diagnostic investigation of choice is CSF analysis for PCR for HSV. Treatment comprises early treatment with IV acyclovir for 14–21 days in total.

Answer 281

> b. No treatment. Repeat thyroid function tests in six months.

The patient has very mild subclinical hypothyroidism. She does not have raised antithyroid microsomal peroxidase antibiodies to indicate chronic auto-immune thyroiditis. Only a small proportion of such patients progress to overt hypothyroidism per year. Treatment of all patients in this group has cost implications and commits patients to lifelong therapy early; therefore, the current recommendation is to observe and perform thyroid function tests every six months.

In asymptomatic patients, the presence of antithyroid peroxidase antibodies is an indication to treat since approximately 5% of patients with antithyroid peroxidase antibodies progress to overt hypothyroidism each year. In asymptomatic patients without circulating antithyroid peroxidase antibodies, treatment is recommended once the TSH reaches 15 iu/l (algorithm). Treatment of hypothyroidism at this level improves lipid profile and blood pressure and may have an impact on reducing cardiovascular morbidity from hypothyroidism.

Patients with clinical (symptomatic) hypothyroidism should be treated irrespective of the TSH concentration.

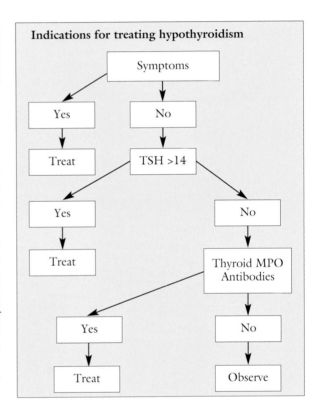

Indications for treating hypothyroidism

Answer 282

> e. Papilloedema.

The patient had blurred disc margins with a few haemorrhages around the disc. The diagnosis is papilloedema, which is a feature of raised intracranial pressure. Causes of papilloedema are tabulated.

Causes of papilloedema

- Malignant or accelerated hypertension
- Benign intracranial hypertension
- Intracranial mass lesions
- Intracerebral haemorrhage
- Meningitis, encephalitis
- Cavernous sinus thrombosis
- Severe hypoxia
- Severe hypercapnia
- Severe anaemia
- Lead poisoning

Question 283

A 62-year-old female with a two-year history of non-insulin-dependent diabetes mellitus was admitted with nausea and vomiting. Her diabetes was usually well controlled on a combination of chlorpropamide 500 mg and metformin 500 mg bd. One week previously she was seen by her GP with general malaise and noted to have a BM stix reading of 19 mmol/l, and the dose of metformin was doubled.

On examination she was drowsy (Glasgow coma score 10) but clinically well perfused. The heart rate was 120 beats/min and regular. The pulse was bounding. The blood pressure was 100/60 mmHg. The temperature was 36.8°C (98.2°F). All other physical examination was normal.

Investigations are shown.

Hb	15.2 g/dl
WCC	16.4 × 10^9/l
Platelets	284 × 10^9/l
Sodium	134 mmol/l
Potassium	5.0 mmol/l
Urea	30.5 mmol/l
Creatinine	160 μmol/l
Chloride	106 mmol/l
Blood sugar	9 mmol/
Arterial blood gases:	
pH	7.3
PaCO$_2$	2.6 kPa
PaO$_2$	9.6 kPa
HCO$_3$	11 mmol/l

Urinalysis: Protein + 1   Blood – negative
            Glucose + 1   Ketones – negative

What is the diagnosis?
a. Renal tubular acidosis.
b. Diabetic ketoacidosis.
c. Lactic acidosis secondary to sepsis.
d. Hyperosmolar non-ketotic diabetic coma.
e. Acute pancreatitis.

Question 284

A 39-year-old woman with depression presented with nausea, vomiting, tremor and convulsions.

Investigations are shown.

Sodium	149 mmol/l
Potassium	3.9 mmol/l
Urea	18 mmol/l
TSH	14 mu/l

What is the diagnosis?
a. Lithium toxicity.
b. Hypothyroidism.
c. Chronic renal failure.
d. Tricyclic antidepressant overdose.
e. Hyperthyroidism.

Question 285

A 32-year-old woman had had persistently raised BP measurements over the past six months. Her systolic blood pressure readings had ranged from 158 to 170 mmHg and the diastolic blood pressure readings had ranged between 90 and 98 mmHg. She was asymptomatic. She was not on any medications (including the oral contraceptive pill). There was no past medical history of note or any family history of hypertension. Physical examination did not reveal any abnormalities other than a BP reading of 160/96 mmHg. Blood urea and electrolytes were normal.

What is the most probable cause for the raised blood pressure?
a. Essential hypertension.
b. Primary hyperaldosteronism.
c. Cushing's syndrome.
d. Renal artery stenosis.
e. Adult polycystic kidney disease.

Answer 283

> c. Lactic acidosis secondary to sepsis.

The patient has features of septicaemia and a metabolic acidosis. Overproduction of lactic acid secondary to diminished organ perfusion as a result of hypotension is the most probable cause of the acidosis. Lactic acidosis usually occurs in states where there is increased pyruvate production due to excessive anaerobic metabolism, for example in shock states, excessive exercise, grand mal seizures, cyanide toxicity, and carbon monoxide poisoning. Renal failure and liver disease cause lactic acidosis primarily owing to decreased utilization of the substrate. Biguanide drugs and malignancy cause lactic acidosis but the mechanisms by which acidosis occurs are unclear (*Table*).

The diagnosis can be confirmed by measuring the plasma lactate concentration. Concurrent treatment with metformin is probably contributing to the lactic acidosis.

Metformin causes lactic acidosis in conditions associated with shock or in the presence of coexisting renal or liver failure.

The most important step is to stop metformin and to restore circulation with intravenous saline. The efficacy of and indications for alkali administration in hypoperfusion-induced lactic acidosis remain unresolved.

Causes of lactic acidosis

- Shock (hypovolaemic or septic)
- Severe hypoxia
- Renal failure
- Liver failure
- Drugs – phenformin, metformin
- Leukaemia
- Total peripheral nutrition
- Glucose-6-phosphate dehydrogenase deficiency

Answer 284

> a. Lithium toxicity.

The patient has a history of depression therefore it is possible that her presentation is secondary to drug overdose. Overdose with neuroleptic agents, tricyclic antidepressant drugs or lithium may present with a reduced conscious level and convulsions. However, the biochemistry in this case is highly suggestive of lithium overdose. The raised serum sodium and urea indicate severe water loss, as may occur in diabetes insipidus. Lithium is a recognized cause of nephrogenic diabetes insipidus. The patient also has biochemical evidence of hypothyroidism. Chronic use also interferes with iodine uptake in the thyroid and may result in hypothyroidism.

Lithium has a narrow therapeutic–toxic range. While a plasma level of between 0.6 and 1.2 mmol/l is therapeutic, a plasma level of 2.5 mmol/l or more is toxic. Toxicity is precipitated by conditions causing sodium depletion or a reduction in glomerular filtration rate, therefore diarrhoea, vomiting, diuretics, ACE inhibitors and NSAIDs may all cause Li toxicity. Features of toxicity include tremor, cerebellar signs, drowsiness, convulsions, hyperpyrexia, nephrogenic diabetes insipidus, long QT/ventricular arrhythmias and hyperpyrexia.

Treatment involves fluid repletion and forced diuresis. Haemodialysis is necessary when plasma Li levels exceed 4 mmol/l in patients with normal renal function but the indications for dialysis is much lower (2.5 mmol/l) in patients with known renal insufficiency.

Answer 285

> a. Essential hypertension.

The patient is relatively young but does not have symptoms to suggest a secondary cause such as headaches, hyperhidrosis, palpitation or nocturia. She has not been described to be cushingoid and the absence of hypokalaemia makes a primary hyperaldosteronism or Cushing's disease unlikely. Adult polycystic kidney rarely presents with hypertension before the fifth decade, and renal artery stenosis is uncommon in young females. Essential hypertension accounts for over 90% of all cases of hypertension even in this particular age group.

Question 286

A 29-year-old male with Marfan's syndrome had a prolonged stay in hospital following a subarachnoid haemorrhage, which rendered him with a residual left hemiparesis. A right posterior communicating artery aneurysm was clipped. On discharge the patient had normal speech and was able to carry out basic domestic tasks. During his hospital stay he had been made redundant from his job as a postman. Following discharge he had been placed in a warden-controlled flat. His friends had seen very little of him for the past month.

His GP had treated him for reactive depression. He was admitted after being found collapsed by the warden one evening.

On arrival at hospital he was deeply comatosed and had a Glasgow coma scale of 5. The heart rate was 130 beats/min and regular. The blood pressure was 110/70 mmHg. The respiratory rate was 14/min and temperature was 36.8°C (98.2°F).

Both pupils were 9 mm in diameter and reacted sluggishly to light. All reflexes were brisk and both plantars were upgoing. Examination of his fundi demonstrated temporal pallor of his optic discs. There were no retinal haemorrhages. Heart sounds were normal and his chest was clear. Abdominal examination revealed dullness over the suprapubic area. During his admission he suffered two epileptic seizures, which were short lived.

Routine investigations were as follows:

Hb	14 g/dl
WCC	12×10^9/l
Platelets	175×10^9/l
Sodium	136 mmol/l
Potassium	4.6 mmol/l
Urea	6.0 mmol/l
Creatinine	107 μmol/l
HCO_3	18 mmol/l
Glucose	6.1 mmol/l
ECG	Sinus tachycardia; QRS duration 110 msec
CXR	Cardiac size normal. Normal lung fields
CT scan brain	Old left-sided infarction

What is the most common cause of mortality in this situation?
  a. Overwhelming septicaemia.
  b. Cardiac tamponade.
  c. Status epilepticus.
  d. Ventricular arrhythmias.
  e. Cerebral oedema.

Question 287

A 75-year-old woman was admitted with an anterior myocardial infarction for which she received thrombolysis. Within 6 hours of admission she became confused. The blood pressure was 80/36 mmHg. The JVP was raised. Both heart sounds were normal and there was an added third heart sound; there were no audible murmurs. Auscultation of the chest revealed fine crackles in the mid- and lower-zones in both lungs.

Subsequent investigations were as follows:

Which of following therapeutic options is most likely to improve outcome?
  a. Further thrombolytic therapy.
  b. IV noradrenaline.
  c. NIPPV.
  d. Intra-aortic balloon counterpulsation.
  e. Early invasive coronary revascularization.

Hb	12 g/dl
WCC	15×10^9/l
Platelets	200×10^9/l
Sodium	136 mmol/l
Potassium	3.9 mmol/l
Urea	17 mmol/l
Creatinine	140 μmol/l
Glucose	16 mmol/l
Chest X-ray	Bilateral alveolar shadows and small bilateral pleural effusions
ECG	Sinus tachycardia; ST elevation and q waves in V1–V6
Echocardiography	Dilated left ventricle with akinetic anterior wall and apex. No evidence of VSD. Functional mitral regurgitation. No pericardial effusion

Answer 286

> d. Ventricular arrhythmias.

The patient has features consistent with the diagnosis of tricyclic antidepressant overdose. Ventricular arrhythmias are the most common cause of death in TCAD overdose.

Intravenous sodium bicarbonate is the single most effective intervention for the management of TCAD cardiovascular toxicity. This agent can reverse QRS prolongation, ventricular arrhythmias and hypotension. Because acidosis aggravates TCAD toxicity, the beneficial action of sodium bicarbonate may be partly due to correction of acidosis. It is clear, however, that sodium bicarbonate administration is effective even when the arterial pH is normal.

This beneficial effect appears to be mediated by increases in both pH and the plasma sodium concentration. Alkalinization to an arterial pH of 7.5, for example, appears to reduce the incidence of cardiac arrhythmias, and intravenous sodium bicarbonate (in a dose of 1–2 mEq/kg) is the treatment of choice for sudden-onset ventricular tachycardia, ventricular fibrillation or cardiac arrest. Class Ia and Ic antiarrhythmic agents should be avoided as they block sodium ion channels and may increase the prevalence of ventricular arrhythmias.

To maintain an arterial pH of 7.5, an intravenous infusion of two 50 ml ampoules of sodium bicarbonate (containing approximately 90 mEq of sodium bicarbonate) in 1 litre of 5% dextrose in water is started in all comatosed patients following TCAD poisoning, particularly those with a QRS duration above 0.10 sec (100 msec).
(See Answers 28,209,366.)

Answer 287

> e. Early invasive coronary revascularization.

The patient has hypotension, oliguria, raised JVP and pulmonary oedema following an extensive anterior myocardial infarction. Clinically she has evidence of cardiogenic shock, which is associated with a poor prognosis (50–80% mortality within 48 hours). In the context of the clinical circumstances, the differential diagnosis is between severe left ventricular dysfunction due to loss of a large amount of myocardium, acute VSD, papillary muscle rupture causing severe mitral regurgitation or cardiac tamponade. The patient does not have any obvious murmurs but the echocardiogram proves useful in resolving the cause of cardiogenic shock. Echocardiography is an important investigative tool in a patient with cardiogenic shock and should be employed whenever possible.

There is no evidence that further thrombolytic therapy would be useful. Insulin is recommended in patients with a blood sugar >11 mmol/l after myocardial infarction, but insulin is unlikely to influence the immediate prognosis in this particular situation, where cardiac embarrassment is the main problem. NIPPV is contraindicated in cardiogenic shock because it may cause a further drop in blood pressure. Noradrenaline and other inotropes are transiently useful in improving cardiac contractility and blood pressure but have not been shown to improve outcome. Similarly balloon counterpulsation may be transiently effective at resting the left ventricle until invasive revascularization is carried out, but has not been shown to reduce mortality on its own. Indeed the only treatment that has been shown to improve prognosis in randomized controlled trials is early invasive revascularization. Early revascularization is key to improving prognosis in a patient with cardiogenic shock.

Question 288

A 17-year-old male presented with blurring of vision followed by total loss of vision in the left eye. A few days later he developed total blindness in the other eye. There were no other neurological symptoms. There was no past medical history of significance or any history of alcohol abuse. The patient was not taking any medications. He had a maternal uncle who had become blind before the age of 18 years. On examination there was evidence of bilateral optic atrophy and a mild tremor.

Investigations are shown.

FBC	Normal
U&E	Normal
Liver function	Normal
Vitamin B screen	Normal
Serum lead	Not elevated
CT scan brain	Normal
CSF analysis	Normal

What is the diagnosis?
- a. Multiple sclerosis.
- b. Ischaemic optic atrophy.
- c. Toxic optic neuritis.
- d. Leber's hereditary optic neuropathy.
- e. Cerebellar syndrome.

Question 289

A patient was brought into the Accident and Emergency Department in ventricular fibrillation. After prolonged resuscitation he was admitted to the Intensive Care Unit and developed oliguric renal failure. Serum and urine electrolytes were as follows:

Serum electrolytes	Sodium	132 mmol/l
	Potassium	5 mmol/l
	Urea	30 mmol/l
	Creatinine	400 μmol/l
	Osmolality	320 mOsmol
Urine electrolytes	Sodium	90 mmol/l
	Potassium	30 mmol/l
	Urea	120 mmol/l
	Creatinine	7 μmol/l
	Osmolality	300 mOsmol

Which two comments below suggest that the patient has developed acute tubular necrosis?
- a. Increased urine urea:serum urea.
- b. Increased urine creatinine:serum creatinine.
- c. Increased urine sodium:serum sodium.
- d. Post-cardiac arrest renal failure.
- e. Increased urinary sodium excretion.
- f. Relatively low urine osmolality.
- g. Urine osmolality:plasma osmolality 1:1.1.
- h. Increased urine potassium.
- i. Reduced urine potassium.
- j. Increased serum creatinine.

Question 290

A 70-year-old patient was admitted in a drowsy state after being found collapsed by his neighbour. On admission the Glasgow coma score was 9. A CT scan (**290**) of the brain was performed as an emergency.

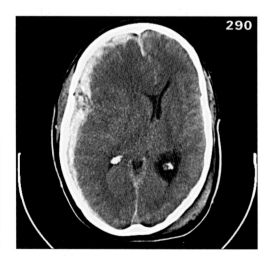

What is the diagnosis?
- a. Subarachnoid haemorrhage.
- b. Intracerebral haematoma.
- c. Epidural haematoma.
- d. Subdural haematoma.
- e. Herpes simplex encephalitis.

Answer 288

> d. Leber's hereditary optic neuropathy.

This young male presents with bilateral blindness in a relatively short space of time. There are no obvious acquired precipitating factors such as drugs or toxins. The patient does not have diabetes and has normal B_{12} levels. He does not have any symptoms or other indications to suggest an ischaemic optic neuropathy. Optic neuropathy is a common feature of multiple sclerosis but it is usually unilateral. The presence of bilateral optic neuropathy should raise the possibility of a toxic neuropathy or the rarer Leber's hereditary optic neuropathy.

The family history of premature blindness in a maternal uncle indicates a hereditary aetiology and provides a vital clue to the underlying diagnosis. Leber's hereditary optic neuropathy is an inherited disorder of mitochondrial DNA encoding the electron transport chain that is characterized by bilateral subacute optic neuropathy. Three specific mutations – at positions 3460, 11778 and 14484 – account for over 90% of all recognized mutations responsible for the disorder. All male offspring of affected females are affected (mitochondrial gene inheritance pattern).

LHON produces severe and permanent visual loss in young males. The time interval between affected eyes may be very short. Tremor and a multiple sclerosis type illness are recognized features. Young children may also have extrapyramidal symptoms, and epilepsy, ataxia, spasticity, mental retardation and peripheral neuropathy may also be present.

The diagnosis is made on muscle biopsy, which reveals abnormal mitochondria on electron microscopy with defective respiratory enzymes within the mitochondria. The demonstration of point mutations on genetic analysis of mitochondrial DNA using white blood cells is diagnostic.

Answer 289

> e. Increased urinary sodium excretion.
> g. Urine osmolality:plasma osmolality 1:1.1.

Acute tubular necrosis is caused by renal ischaemia and may be precipitated by a variety of insults including hypovolaemia and septicaemia (causing reduced renal perfusion), drugs and rhabdomyolysis. It is usually characterized by oliguric renal failure that is often reversible. Ischaemia typically affects the medullary area, therefore (unlike pre-renal failure), the concentrating ability of the urine is diminished and sodium excretion is inappropriately increased (*Table*).

Pre-renal failure versus ATN

Measure	Pre-renal failure	ATN
Urine output	Low	Low
Urine osmolality	>500	<350
U/P osmolality	1.5:1	1.1:1
Ucreat/Pcreat	>20:1	<20:1
Urine sodium	<20 mmol/l	>50 mmol/l

Answer 290

> d. Subdural haematoma.

There is a collection of fresh blood in the right subdural space (bright white) with significant mass effect. The treatment involves neurosurgical intervention.

Question 291

A 68-year-old male was brought into the Accident and Emergency Department with severe chest pain and an ECG consistent with a recent anterior myocardial infarction. According to his wife he had been experiencing pain for three days but over the previous three hours the pain had become very intense. He was diabetic. On arrival at hospital he received IV tenectoplase. Two hours after thrombolysis he dropped his blood pressure and became very breathless. On examination the heart rate was 120 beats/min and regular. The blood pressure was 80 mmHg systolic. Auscultation over the precordium revealed a pansystolic murmur. Auscultation of the lungs revealed widespread inspiratory crackles.

What is the immediate investigation of choice to ascertain the cause of the deterioration?
 a. Transoesophageal echocardiography.
 b. Transthoracic echocardiogram.
 c. Swann–Ganz right heart catheter.
 d. Chest X-ray.
 e. 12-lead ECG.

Question 292

A 44-year-old male presented to his GP with a two-day history of severe boring intermittent pain just below the supraorbital ridge of the right eye. The pain had awoken the patient from his sleep in the early hours of the morning and lasted 3 hours before subsiding. The pain recurred again in the afternoon and persisted for 4 hours despite the patient having taken paracetamol. In 48 hours he had experienced five episodes of similar pain. The patient had also noticed that he had a blocked nose and therefore made a self-diagnosis of sinusitis. He recalled having two similar episodes of pain two and four months previously that he attributed to sinusitis and treated himself with steam inhalations for four days. On examination the patient was distressed with pain. His right eye was red and watering. He had a partial ptosis and miosis affecting the right eye. His blood pressure was 160/90 mmHg. All other physical examination was normal.

1. What is the most probable diagnosis?
 a. Tension headache.
 b. Hemiplegic migraine.
 c. Migrainous neuralgia.
 d. Ophthalmoplegic migraine.
 e. Posterior communicating artery aneurysm.

2. Choose two therapeutic steps from the following list for treating his symptom rapidly:
 a. IV verapamil.
 b. Ergotamine.
 c. Atenolol.
 d. IM sumatriptan.
 e. High-concentration inhaled oxygen.
 f. High-dose oral augmentin.
 g. Oral gabapentin.
 h. Carbamazepine.
 i. Lithium.
 j. Oral verapamil.

Question 293

Hb	10 g/dl
WCC	5 × 10⁹/l
Platelets	200 × 10⁹/l
ESR	12 mm/h
Sodium	135 mmol/l
Potassium	3.6 mmol/l
Urea	2 mmol/l
AST	21 iu/l
Alkaline phosphatase	160 iu/l
Albumin	37 g/l
Calcium	2.0 mmo/l
Phosphate	0.7 mmol/
Glucose	8 mmol/l
HbA1c	7.2%

A 17-year-old girl with insulin-dependent diabetes mellitus was investigated for weight loss and amenorrhoea.
  Investigations are shown.

What is the most probable cause for the weight loss?
 a. Poorly controlled diabetes mellitus.
 b. Anorexia nervosa.
 c. Coeliac disease.
 d. Crohn's disease.
 e. Addison's disease.

Answer 291

> b. Transthoracic echocardiogram.

The patient has developed severe pulmonary oedema after a myocardial infarction. He also has a pansystolic murmur, indicating that he may have mitral regurgitation due to papillary muscle rupture or a ventricular septal defect.

Echocardiography would be the most practical method of differentiating between the possibilities. As the patient is so unstable, a transthoracic echocardiogram is preferable to transoesophageal echocardiogram. In general transthoracic echo is better at visualizing a VSD than transthoracic echo. The indications for transoesophagel echocardiography in routine clinical practice are listed in the table below. Swan–Ganz right heart catheterization may also help but it is invasive and requires the patient to lie supine. Mitral regurgitation is diagnosed by demonstrating a high PCWP with large v-waves. VSD is diagnosed by demonstrating a left-to-right shunt at the level of the ventricles (step up in oxygen saturation in the right ventricle).

Indications for transoesophageal echocardiography

- Patients who have poor transthoracic echo windows
- Identification of thrombi in the left atrial appendage in atrial fibrillation
- Assessment of prosthetic valve endocarditis
- Assessment of complications of native and prosthetic valve endocarditis
- Diagnosis of aortic dissection
- Evaluation of atrial septal defect

Answer 292

> 1. c. Migrainous neuralgia.
> 2. d. IM sumatriptan.
>   e. High-concentration inhaled oxygen.

The features are typical of migrainous neuralgia (*Table*). High-concentration inhaled oxygen (10–12 l/min) and the triptan drugs are very effective at aborting an acute attack. Verapamil is the drug of choice at preventing frequent recurrence, although lithium, methysergide, sodium valproate, ergotamine and prednisolone are all useful therapies in this respect. Methysergide is no longer used owing to its association with retroperitoneal fibrosis.

Characteristic features of migrainous neuralgia

- Frequency 0.1%; M:F ratio 3:1
- Unilateral pain, often around the ocular orbit; severe
- Periodic, usually every 1–3 months; 1–2 attacks daily for 8–10 weeks per year
- Pain lasts between 15 min and 3 hours at a time
- Patient well inbetween bouts of pain
- Associated unilateral watering eye, miosis, ptosis, nasal congestion or rhinorrhoea
- Acute attacks are best treated by 100% oxygen inhalation at 10–12 l/min for 15 min
- Sumatriptan is very useful in some patients but not effective above 6 mg
- Preventative therapy includes verapamil in high doses (up to 720 mg per day)

Answer 293

> c. Coeliac disease.

The commonest cause of weight loss in a patient with insulin-dependent diabetes is poor glycaemic control. The HbA1c of 7.2% is not suggestive of recent poor control. Furthermore the calcium level is at the lower limit of normal, the phosphate is low and the alkaline phosphatase is high, indicating biochemical osteomalacia. The haemoglobin is also low. Low haemoglobin and low serum calcium should raise the suspicion of malabsorption in the absence of renal failure. The most likely diagnosis is coeliac disease. Coeliac disease is associated with type 1 diabetes mellitus, IgA deficiency, inflammatory bowel disease, hyperthyroidism, fibrosing alveolitis and primary biliary cirrhosis.

Question 294

Hb	10 g/dl
WCC	$3.5 \times 10^9/l$
Neutrophils	$1.1 \times 10^9/l$
Lymphocytes	$2.4 \times 10^9/l$
Eosinophils	$0.03 \times 10^9/l$
Basophils	$0 \times 10^9/l$
Monocytes	$0.1 \times 10^9/l$
Platelets	$140 \times 10^9/l$
ESR	100 mm/h
Sodium	130 mmol/l
Potassium	5.5 mmol/l
Chloride	87 mmol/l
Bicarbonate	24 mmol/l
Urea	9 mmol/l
Creatinine	133 μmol/l
Glucose	6 mmol/l
Urine output	45 ml/h
Urinary microscopy	NAD
ECG	Sinus tachycardia

A 35-year-old patient with type 1 diabetes presented three months following a renal transplant with fever, night sweats and malaise. He had experienced two episodes of transplant rejection, which were successfully reversed with corticosteriods. He was currently maintained on prednisolone and ciclosporin. On examination he had a temperature of 39°C (102.2°F). The heart rate was 120 beats/min and blood pressure was 110/65 mmHg. The respiratory rate was 40/min. Precordial examination revealed a soft systolic murmur at the apex. The chest was clear. The abdomen including the graft was non-tender.

Investigations are shown.

What is the most likely diagnosis?
a. Acute renal transplant rejection.
b. CMV infection.
c. Endocarditis.
d. Gram-negative sepsis.

Question 295

A 36-year-old nurse with two children, aged 8 and 14 years of age, went to see her GP, concerned that her maternal aunt had recently had a pulmonary embolus and was heterozygous for the Factor V Leiden mutation. The patient was taking the combined oral contraceptive pill and was adamant that she did not want any more children. Her own mother had never had thrombotic tendencies and had normal pregnancies except for varicose veins during her second pregnancy. The patient herself had never experienced any thrombotic episodes and was a non-smoker.

What is the best advice for the patient?
a. Finish the current monthly packet and stop taking the contraceptive pill.
b. Referral to a gynaecologist to discuss sterilization.
c. Suggest alternative methods of contraception.
d. Risk of thrombotic tendencies low; therefore reassure.
e. Screen her blood for Factor V Leiden mutation. Stop pill if positive.

Question 296

A 62-year-old male presented with acute dyspnoea. He had clinical and radiological evidence of pulmonary oedema that responded well to intravenous nitrates and

Hb	13 g/dl
WCC	$8 \times 10^9/l$
Platelets	$200 \times 10^9/l$
Sodium	138 mmol/l
Potassium	4.2 mmol/l
Urea	6 mmol/l
Creatinine	100 μmol/l
Echocardiography	Dilated left ventricle with poor left ventricular function
Coronary angiography	Normal coronary arteries

diuretics. He was discharged on furosemide 40 mg od and ramipril 5 mg od. Since discharge he had been relatively well. He could walk unlimited distances on the flat and could negotiate inclines without dyspnoea. The heart rate was 80 beats/min. The pulse rate was regular. The blood pressure measured 105/70 mmHg. Both heart sounds were normal and the chest was clear.

Investigations were as follows:

Which drug would you initiate next?
a. Digoxin.
b. Spironolactone.
c. Atenolol.
d. Bisoprolol.
e. Candesartan.

Answer 294

> b. CMV infection.

The neutropenia and mild hepatitis in a patient a few months after renal transplantation favour CMV infection. The raised creatinine level may reflect dehydration; if acute, however, concomitant allograft rejection (a feature of CMV infection) and ciclosporin toxicity could also explain the raised creatinine level.

Infections are the leading cause of morbidity and mortality in the early post-transplant period, as more than 80% of recipients suffer at least one episode of infection in the first year. Infection and allograft dysfunction caused by rejection are closely interrelated through the use of immunosuppressive therapy (see below).

CMV is the most important infection in renal transplant recipients. More than two-thirds of donors and recipients have detectable IgG anti-CMV antibodies in the plasma prior to transplantation. It is therefore common for the donor and/or recipient to be CMV-positive at the time of transplantation. The virus can be transmitted from the donor either by blood transfusion or by the transplanted kidney; the concurrent administration of immunosuppressive drugs to prevent rejection further increases the risk of clinically relevant CMV disease.

Symptomatic CMV infections typically occur one to four months after transplantation, but can develop later. Typically, the onset of disease usually follows the period of maximal immunosuppression (associated with neutropenia) for the prevention and treatment of acute rejection. Clinical features include fever, deteriorating renal function and a tender graft. However, the latter feature is rarely present as it is masked by immunosuppressive therapy. CMV infection in transplant patients may affect other organs causing hepatitis, pneumonitis, pancreatitis, gastroenteritis, meningo-encephalitis and rarely myocarditis.

Patients with organ involvement benefit from a 2–3 week course of ganciclovir. Since the immune system may be directly suppressed because of CMV infection, modification of the immunosuppressive regimen is also required.

Marked leucopenia is a cardinal feature of CMV disease among patients treated with azathioprine or monoclonal antilymphocyte preparations. Increasing use of mycophenolate instead of azathioprine and effective prophylactic antiviral therapy in most patients means that fever and leucopenia may not be as prominent a feature of CMV disease as it used to be.

Infections in post-transplant patients
Month 1
The usual post-operative surgical infections, similar to those seen in non-immunosuppressed patients undergoing similar surgical procedures, are most common, e.g. wound infections, line sepsis, urinary tract infection and pneumonia.
Months 2–6
Infections with immunomodulating viruses, particularly CMV, are most important. In addition to the clinical syndromes induced by these viruses, their immunomodulating properties predispose to opportunistic infections with organisms such as *Pneumocystis carinii*, *Listeria monocytogenes* and *Aspergillus fumigatus*. Other infections commonly occurring during this period include hepatitis, herpes simplex, herpes zoster, *Mycobacterium tuberculosis* and Epstein–Barr virus, which can be complicated by the development of lymphoproliferative disorders. Recurrence or relapse of UTI can also occur.
Month 6 onwards
Community-acquired infections, for example, influenza, bacterial infections (pneumococcus) and recurrence of inadequately treated opportunistic infections.

Answer 295

> e. Screen her blood for Factor V Leiden mutation. Stop pill if positive.

The risk of venous thromboembolism is approximately 3–4 times higher in patients who are heterozygous for the Factor V Leiden mutation. The risk is increased to 30–40 fold in women who are smokers or on the contraceptive pill. Even though population screening for Factor V Leiden mutation is not cost effective, since only a small proportion of patients with it will suffer from systemic thromboembolism, the patient cannot be advised accurately without screening for this mutation (screening for Factor V Leiden mutation is reserved only for patients with multiple family members with a history of venous thromboembolism). One could argue that even if she was heterozygous for the Factor V Leiden mutation the risk of venous thromboembolism is lower than the risk of an unwanted pregnancy. However, the patient is worried about her risk of venous thromboembolism, and estimation of that risk is not possible without knowing her Factor V Leiden status.

Answer 296

d. Bisoprolol.

The patient has a dilated, poorly contracting left ventricle and therefore has dilated cardiomyopathy. There are no obvious reversible causes in this case such as B_{12} deficiency, anaemia, haemochromatosis, thyroid dysfunction or coronary artery disease. The treatment of dilated cardiomyopathy aims to improve symptoms and prognosis.

The low cardiac output resulting from dilated cardiomyopathy offsets the renin–angiotensin–aldosterone system and the sympathetic nervous system in an attempt to restore circulation. Unfortunately activation of both systems has a detrimental effect on the heart, causing volume overload, progressive deterioration of cardiac function owing to adverse remodelling, cardiac arrhythmias and sudden death.

The goals in the management of heart failure are to improve symptoms and prognosis. Therapeutic modalities in chronic heart failure include lifestyle modification, pharmacotherapy, device therapy and surgery (*Table A*).

Loop diuretics are very effective at improving symptoms of pulmonary and peripheral congestion rapidly but do not have an impact on prognosis. Digoxin is particularly effective at providing symptomatic relief in patients with atrial fibrillation, but has also been shown to be effective in patients in sinus rhythm through its weakly inotropic effects. Interestingly it is the only inotropic agent used in heart failure that has not been shown to cause sudden death. Like loop diuretics, digoxin does not have an impact on prognosis.

The prognosis of dilated cardiomyopathy has been improved significantly by the use of pharmacological agents that inhibit the renin–angiotensin–aldosterone system and beta-blockers. ACE inhibitors improve symptoms in patients with left ventricular systolic dysfunction, irrespective of their functional capacity, and should be used in all patients with heart failure provided there are no contraindications and they are tolerated. Impaired baseline renal function is not a contraindication to initiating ACE inhibitor therapy although caution needs to be exercised in patients with a serum creatinine of >265 mmol/l. An increase in serum creatinine of more than 25% after starting an ACE inhibitor may be an indication that the patient has underlying reno-vascular disease, which should be excluded before continuing ACE inhibitor therapy. ACE inhibitor therapy may be initiated in patients with a systolic blood pressure reading as low as 90 mmHg.

AIIRBs have also been shown to provide symptomatic and prognostic benefit. While one major trial (the CHARM study) has shown that AIIRBs provide additive prognostic benefit when they are used in patients already taking ACE inhibitors, the use of AIIRBs is currently reserved for patients who develop side-effects on ACE inhibitors. The AIIRBs used in heart failure are losaran, candesartan and valsartan.

Spironolactone, used in relatively small doses, is prognostically beneficial when used in patients who are in NYHA functional class III or IV despite taking ACE inhibitors, AIIRBs or beta-blockers. In this particular question the patient is in NYHA functional class I, i.e. he is not functionally limited when performing usual daily tasks, therefore spironolactone is not indicated.

Certain β_1 receptor specific beta-blockers have been shown to improve symptoms and prognosis in patients with systolic left ventricular dysfunction. Beta-blockers currently licensed for use in heart failure include carvedilol, bisoprolol, metoprolol and more recently nebivolol. Atenolol has not been evaluated and acebutalol has not been shown to improve symptoms or prognosis in heart failure patients. Beta-blockers improve

---

Table A Therapeutic modalities in the chronic management of dilated cardiomyopathy

Lifestyle modification	Restrict salt consumption
	Restrict fluid intake to 1.5 litres per day
	Aerobic exercise for 30 min three times per week
	Reduce alcohol consumption to a minimum
Pharmacological therapy	Loop diuretics and digoxin to treat pulmonary and peripheral congestion
	ACE inhibitors, beta-blockers, AIIRBs and spironolactone to improve symptoms and prognosis
	Amiodarone to treat ventricular tachycardia
Device therapy	ICD to prevent arrhythmogenic death
	Biventricular pacing to improve symptoms
Surgery	Coronary revascularization, valve surgery to improve cardiac function
	Cardiac transplantation

(Continued over page)

cardiac status via many mechanisms (*Table B*). The overall effect of beta-blocker therapy is to improve stroke volume and cardiac ejection fraction. Beta-blocker therapy in heart failure is associated with better functional capacity, lower rehospitalization rates and lower mortality. Initially beta-blockers were recommended only in patients in NYHA functional classes I and II. However, further studies showed that they can be used cautiously in patients in NYHA classes III and IV, where they also provided significant symptomatic and prognostic benefit. Beta-blockers are recommended in all patients with systolic heart failure provided there are no contraindications. Owing to the negatively inotropic effect of beta-blockers they should be used at the lowest possible doses (*Table C*) and the dose is gradually maximized over a period of two months. Ideally beta-blockers should be commenced once symptoms and signs of pulmonary congestion have resolved on a loop diuretic and ACE inhibitor. A practical algorithm for the management of chronic heart failure is provided below.

Table B Mechanisms of action of beta-blockers

- Reduce myocardial ischaemia
- Increase diastolic filling time and improve stroke volume
- Inhibit cardiotoxic effects of catecholamines such as apoptosis
- Inhibit down-regulation of β_1 receptors
- Prevent adverse cardiac remodelling
- Prevent arrhythmias

Table C Beta-blocker dose

Beta-blocker	Initiation dose
Bisoprolol	1.25 mg od
Carvedilol	3.125 mg od
Metoprolol	6.25 mg tds
Nebivolol	1.25 mg od

Management algorithm for chronic heart failure

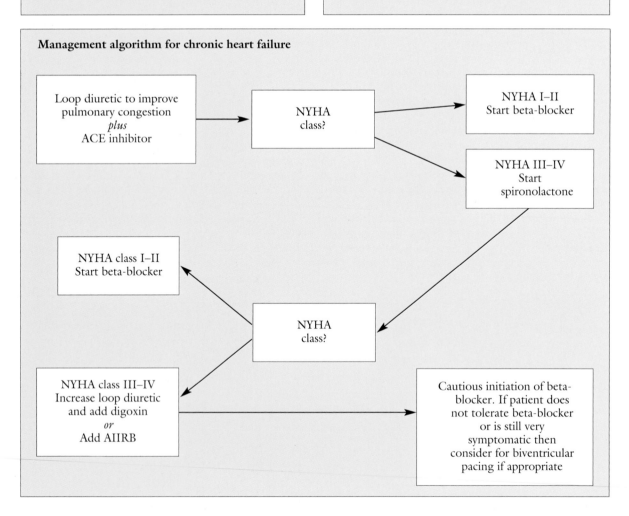

Question 297

A 75-year-old woman with a long history of atrial fibrillation was seen in the anticoagulant clinic and noted to have an INR of 8.2. She had been on warfarin for three years without any complications. One week previously she had received a course of erythromycin for a lower respiratory tract infection. There was no history of blood loss from the respiratory and gastrointestinal tracts or the genito-urinary system. There was no history of alcohol abuse. The INR two weeks previously was 2.3. On examination she appeared well but had multiple bruises on her arms.

Investigations are shown.

Hb	12 g/dl
WCC	5.2 × 10⁹/l
Platelets	180 × 10⁹/l
Urea	6 mmol/l
Creatinine	92 µmol/l
AST	20 iu/l
Alkaline phosphatase	30 iu/l
Albumin	39 g/l

What is the management of her anticoagulation?
a. Stop warfarin and repeat the INR in three days.
b. Stop warfarin, give intravenous fresh-frozen plasma and 5 mg intravenous vitamin K.
c. Stop warfarin and give 5 mg oral vitamin K.
d. Stop warfarin and give 0.5 mg intravenous vitamin K.
e. Stop warfarin and give fresh-frozen plasma.

Question 298

A 40-year-old male consulted his GP at the end of the year for wheeze and dyspnoea. He was given a bronchodilator with good effect. Two weeks later he had an exacerbation of his symptoms, which responded well to a one-week course of steroids. Following this his symptoms were stable and completely resolved when he went to the Caribbean for a two-week holiday, only to return within a few days when he came back to England. He had no history of atopy and did not keep any pets. He did not smoke. He was married with two children and had been working as a solderer for a car manufacturing company for the past 14 months. Apart from a bronchodilator inhaler, the patient was not taking any other medications.

1. What is the diagnosis?
a. Adult-onset asthma.
b. Occupational asthma.
c. Allergic bronchopulmonary aspergillosis.
d. Extrinsic allergic alveolitis.
e. Chronic obstructive airways disease.

2. What is the most practical test for making the diagnosis?
a. Peak flow monitoring at work and home.
b. Allergen skin testing.
c. CT thorax.
d. *Aspergillus* precipitins.
e. Formal pulmonary function tests.

Question 299

Hb	11 g/dl
WCC	30 × 10⁹/l
Platelets	160 × 10⁹/l
PCV	44 l/l
MCV	100 fl
Blood film	Spherocytes, red cell agglutination
Bilirubin	78 µmol/l
AST	40 iu/l
Alkaline phosphatase	100 iu/l
Albumin	39 g/l

A patient on treatment with prednisolone and chlorambucil for chronic lymphatic leukaemia over a five-year period presented with a two-day history of jaundice.

Investigations are shown.

What is the cause of her jaundice?
a. Folate deficiency.
b. Auto-immune haemolytic anaemia.
c. Acute hepatitis.
d. Chlorambucil therapy.
e. Cholestasis secondary to steroids.

Answer 297

> a. Stop warfarin and repeat the INR in three days.

The answer to this question is based upon guidelines provided by the British Society of Haematology for anticoagulation reversal with warfarin, which are as follows:

- In the event of major bleeding stop warfarin and give 5 mg IV vitamin K slowly and IV fresh-frozen plasma or prothrombin concentrate.

- INR >8 with no major bleeding or minor bleeding then stop warfarin and re-start when INR has fallen below 5. If the presence of risk factors for bleeding such as renal failure, hepatic dysfunction or low platelets, give either 0.5 mg of IV vitamin K slowly or 5 mg oral vitamin K. The INR should be checked after 24 hours and the dose of vitamin K repeated if it is still too high.
- INR 6–8 with no major bleeding or minor bleeding, then stop warfarin and re-start when the INR has fallen below 5.
- INR <6 but more than 0.5 units above target, then reduce dose or stop warfarin and re-start once INR is below 5.

Answer 298

> 1. b. Occupational asthma.
> 2. a. Peak flow monitoring at work and at home.

The patient has been complaining of cough and wheeze for the past year that has responded to a bronchodilator inhaler and then a steroid trial. The history would be consistent with reversible bronchospasm. While adult-onset asthma can occur at this age, there appears to be a relationship between the onset of his symptoms and the time he has worked as a car solderer. Further evidence for this comes from the fact that his symptoms resolved while he was away on holiday only to return a few days after he arrived back to the country (and presumably returned to work). These findings indicate that the patient is exposed to an allergen at work that causes bronchospasm. Soldering material contains colophony, which is a large molecular weight allergen that induces bronchospasm by hypersensitivity immune reactions.

The diagnosis of occupational asthma is made by demonstrating improvement of peak expiratory flow rate or lung volumes when the patient is away from the allergen. Indicators of bronchospasm reversibility are the same as those for non-occupational asthma and include an increase in PEFR of 20% (or at least 60 ml) or an increase in FEV1 by 15% (or at least 200 ml) when the patient is away from the allergen. A PEFR is the most practical method of making the diagnosis of occupational asthma; however, there is the potential problem of honesty of the subject.

Allergen skin testing is not practical, as skin test reagents are not available for most allergens that cause occupational asthma. The technique may be able to identify asthma due to certain high molecular weight allergens such as animal or plant proteins.

Management is to remove the patient from or reduce exposure to the allergen.

Answer 299

> b. Auto-immune haemolytic anaemia.

Chronic lymphatic leukaemia is associated with a warm auto-immune haemolytic anaemia. In this case the presence of spherocytes and red cell agglutination, raised MCV and bilirubin suggests haemolysis. The other cause of raised macrocytosis in lymphoma is folate deficiency (see Question 204).

Question 300

This is a chest X-ray (**300**) from a 50-year-old patient who was investigated for cough and dyspnoea.

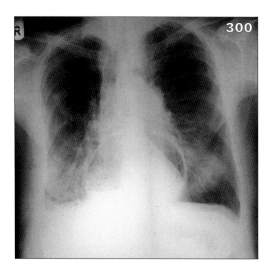

What is the radiological diagnosis?
  a. Hiatus hernia.
  b. Thoracic aortic aneurysm.
  c. Left lower lobe abscess.
  d. Pericardial calcification.
  e. Achalasia.

Question 301

A 67-year-old Afro-Caribbean patient was being followed up in clinic for hypertension. He had been adhering to a low-salt diet. He was currently taking bendroflumetha-zide 2.5 mg od. The blood pressure measured 160/90 mmHg. Blood pressure prior to the initiation of bendroflumethazide was 180/96 mmHg.

Investigations are shown.

Sodium	138 mmol/l
Potassium	3.3 mmol/l
Urea	6 mmol/l
Creatinine	150 μmol/l
Glucose (fasting)	13 mmol/l
12-lead ECG	Left ventricular hypertrophy
Urinalysis	No blood pre protein
	Glucose +

Which one of the following is the best therapeutic option in the management of his blood pressure?
  a. Increase dose of thiazide diuretic.
  b. Add beta-blocker.
  c. Add losartan.
  d. Add calcium channel blocker.
  e. Add doxasosin.

Question 302

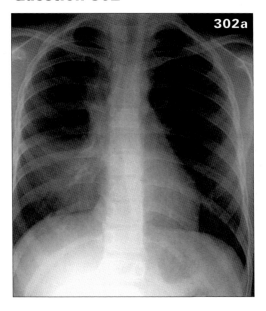

A 30-year-old clerical worker presented with a cough, fever and rash. The chest X-ray is shown (**302a**).

What is the radiological diagnosis?
  a. Right middle lobe consolidation.
  b. Right lower lobe consolidation.
  c. Right-sided empyema.
  d. Right-sided lung abscess.
  e. Right-sided pleural effusion.

Answer 300

a. Hiatus hernia.

The patient has a localised air-filled cavity with a fluid level behind the heart which is highly characteristic of a hiatus hernia. In achalasia the whole oesophagus is dilated so there is wide mediastinum with an air fluid level in the upper chest.

Answer 301

c. Add losartan.

Hypertension is very common among black patients and affects 1 in 2 individuals aged >40 years. Hypertension in black patients usually occurs at a younger age, is more severe and associated with a higher rate of stroke, heart failure and renal failure than in white patients. Hypertension in black patients is salt-sensitive and associated with an expanded vascular volume. It responds well to low salt intake and to pharmacological agents that promote urinary sodium excretion and to vasodilators. Thiazide diuretics or calcium channel blockers are the first-line drugs of choice. Since plasma renin levels are generally low in black patients, agents affecting the renin–angiotensin–aldosterone system (i.e. ACE inhibitors, angiotensin II receptor blockers and beta-blockers) are not particularly effective when used as first-line agents (see Answer 123). However any of these three drugs is effective when added to a thiazide or a calcium channel blocker. Adding a calcium channel blocker to a thiazide diuretic or *vice versa* is not particularly effective, as both drugs work predominantly by increasing urinary sodium excretion.

The theory is to use a diuretic or calcium channel blocker to increase sodium loss. This should offset the renin–angiotensin–aldosterone system and make the addition of an ACE inhibitor, AIIRB or beta-blocker more effective. In this particular case losartan is the drug of choice since the patient is diabetic and has evidence of diabetic nephropathy and LVH. Losartan has been shown to specifically reduce mortality in hypertensive diabetics (LIFE study). It has also been shown to cause regression of LVH (LIFE study) and to retard nephropathy (RENAAL study). (See Answer 125).

Doxasosin should only be used when other (more prognostically useful) options have been explored. The only condition where there is a compelling indication for the use of doxasosin in hypertension.

Answer 302

a. Right middle lobe consolidation.

There is loss of the contour of the right heart border on the PA film. There is also evidence of a slight increase in the opacification of the right lower lung and a slight reduction in overall lung volume compared with the left lung. These features are consistent with right middle lobe collapse/consolidation.

The right middle lobe accounts for just 10% of the total lung volume and is more prone to collapse than the other lung lobes because of decreased collateral ventilation. Owing to its small size, collapse of the right middle lobe has little impact on the appearance of the surrounding structures. In the PA film there may be a triangular opacity pointing laterally. In some patients an absent contour of the right heart border is the only indicator of right middle lobe collapse/consolidation. The diagnosis can be confirmed on a lateral film, which demonstrates an oblique triangular opacity with its apex pointing towards the hilum (**302b**, *arrows*). This appearance results from the antero-superior displacement of the major fissure and the postero-inferior displacement of the minor fissure.

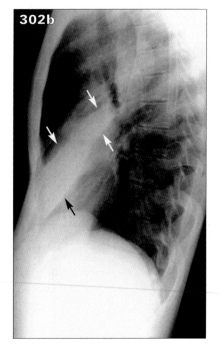

302b

Question 303

Hb	15 g/dl
WCC	11×10^9/l
Neutrophils	8×10^9/l
Lymphocytes	1.5×10^9/l
Eosinophils	1.5×10^9/l
Platelets	200×10^9/l
ESR	80 mm/h
CRP	100 g/l
Urea	13 mmol/l
Creatinine	178 µmol/l
ANA	Negative
ANCA	Negative
C3	Low
C4	Low
Blood culture	Sterile
Urinalysis	White cells ++
	Protein ++

A 70-year-old male underwent coronary angiography after presenting with unstable angina. The angiogram revealed that three-vessel coronary artery disease resulting in deployment of stents in the left anterior descending and right coronary arteries. The following day he developed general malaise and a fever. On examination he had a vasculitic rash on his hands and feet.

The patient had a past history of asthma. His medications included aspirin, clopidogrel, simvastatin and heparin.

Investigations are shown.

What is the diagnosis?
a. Infective endocarditis.
b. Cholesterol atheroemboli.
c. Churg–Strauss syndrome.
d. Polyarteritis nodosa.
e. Contrast nephropathy.

Question 304

Hb	7.5 g/dl
MCV	76 fl
WCC	8×10^9/l
MCH	28 pg
Urea	15 mmol/l
Creatinine	136 µmol/l
Chest X-ray	Bilateral alveolar shadowing
Renal ultrasound	Normal-sized echogenic kidneys
Urinalysis	>50 rbc, red cell casts seen

Lung function:	Actual	Predicted
FEV$_1$ (l)	2.6	3.0
FVC (l)	2.9	4.2
TLC (l)	5.1	6.5
KCO	2.8	2.2

A 30-year-old garage mechanic presented with a one-week history of generalized malaise, fever, cough and intermittent haemoptysis.

Investigations are shown.

What are the two best investigations that would establish the diagnosis?
a. Serum IgE specific for *Aspergillus*.
b. Serum angiotensin-converting enzyme level.
c. Antistreptococcal antibodies.
d. Lupus anticoagulant.
e. Serum cryoglobulin.
f. Antiglomerular basement membrane antibodies.
g. Antineutrophil cytoplasmic antibodies.
h. Serum IgA.
i. Serum complement.
j. Urinary *Legionella* antigen.

Question 305

Which of the following drugs have an impact on the prognosis in heart failure?
a. Atenolol.
b. Digoxin.
c. Furosemide.
d. Carvedilol.
e. Bumetanide.

Answer 303

> b. Cholesterol atheroemboli.

The history of renal failure and cutaneous manifestations after coronary angiography is most consistent with cholesterol atheroemboli.

Cholesterol atheroemboli may complicate manipulation of atheromatous arteries, such as during angiography, angioplasty or vascular surgery. Embolization of cholesterol crystals results in fever, raised inflammatory markers, eosinophilia, hypocomplementaemia, cutaneous manifestations and renal failure. Cholesterol atheroemboli lodge in small capillaries in the skin, producing livedo reticularis and occasionally a vasculitic rash. The distal extremities may appear blue. The emboli may also cause ischaemia of the renal cortex leading to cortical atrophy and a progressive decline in renal function that persists for over two weeks. Urinalysis usually reveals white cells in the urine and mild proteinuria; however, proteinuria in the nephritic range and haematuria have also been described. Baseline renal function may never return to normal in severe cases.

In patients developing renal failure after coronary angiography the differentiation between contrast nephropathy and cholesterol atheroemboli can be difficult. However, in contrast nephropathy cutaneous manifestations are uncommon. Furthermore, renal function usually returns to baseline after approximately one week whereas renal failure secondary to cholesterol atheroemboli may persist for several weeks, and renal function may never normalize.

The diagnosis of cholesterol emboli is confirmed by the demonstration of cholesterol crystals on skin or renal biopsy. Treatment is supportive. Anticoagulation should be stopped, since it is thought that it prevents healing of the atheromatous lesions.

Although Churg–Strauss syndrome may present with vasculitis and haematuria in an individual with a history of asthma (asthma may predate the vasculitic manifestations of Churg–Strauss syndrome by several years), the temporal relationship between coronary angiography and the onset of the illness favours cholesterol atheroemboli. Polyarteritis nodosa is also unlikely for similar reasons. Renal involvement in Churg–Strauss syndrome and polyarteritis nodosa would also be associated with microscopic haematuria or red cell casts.

Answer 304

> f. Antiglomerular basement membrane antibodies.
> g. Antineutrophil cytoplasmic antibodies.

The patient presents with an acute renal–pulmonary syndrome characterized by pulmonary haemorrhage and an acute nephritis. The differential diagnosis (in decreasing frequency) is between antiglomerular basement membrane (anti-GBM) disease (Goodpasteur's syndrome), Wegener's granulomatosis, microscopic polyangiitis, polyarteritis nodosa, SLE and post-streptococcal glomerulonephritis. In individuals with a coexistent purpuric rash the diagnosis of Henoch–Schönlein purpura may also be considered, although pulmonary vasculitis is a very rare complication of the disorder.

The most probable diagnosis in this particular case is anti-GBM disease followed by a vasculitis. The first two diagnostic investigations should include anti-GBM antibodies and serum antineutrophil cytoplasmic antibodies. The presence of anti-GBM antibodies in this context is virtually diagnostic of anti-GBM disease. The presence of ANCA is highly suggestive of Wegener's granulomatosis or a related disorder. SLE classically presents with constitutional symptoms such as lethargy and malaise together with arthralgia and mild haematological features. Pulmonary haemorrhage is a recognized complication but is a relatively rare manifestation of the disorder.

Answer 305

> d. Carvedilol.

Prognostically useful drugs in heart failure are tabulated below. In Afro-Caribbean patients the combination of isosorbide dinitrate or mononitrate and hydralazine has been shown to improve prognosis in symptomatic patients when added to conventional heart failure therapy that includes ACE inhibitors, beta-blockers and spironolactone (see Answer 296).

Prognostically useful drugs in heart failure	
Class of drug	*Examples*
ACE inhibitors	Captopril, enalapril, lisinopril, ramipril, trandolapril
Beta-blockers	Carvedilol, bisoprolol, metoprolol, nebivolol
ARII receptor blockers	Losartan, valsartan, candesartan
Spironolactone	

Question 306

A 49-year-old male with alcohol-related liver disease presented with burning epigastric pain and loss of appetite. An upper gastrointestinal endoscopy revealed gastritis and he had very small oesophageal varices that had not bled. There was no previous history of haematemesis or malena. The patient was haemodynamically stable.

What is the most effective prophylactic therapy to prevent a variceal bleed in this particular situation?
  a. Enalapril.
  b. Atenolol.
  c. Banding the varices.
  d. Propranolol.
  e. Octreotide.

Question 307

A 70-year-old female presented with sudden onset of expressive dysphasia and a right hemiparesis. She had a long-standing history of hypertension and had been investigated for an episode of amurosis fugax five years ago. There was no history of diabetes mellitus and the patient was a non-smoker. The patient was taking bendroflumethiazide 2.5 mg for hypertension. She was not on any other medication.

On examination she had a heart rate of 100 beats/min, which was irregularly irregular. The blood pressure measured 170/100 mmHg. There was clear evidence of an expressive dysphasia and a left-sided hemiparesis. Auscultation of the heart revealed normal heart sounds without any murmurs. There were no carotid bruits.
Investigationsare shown.

12-lead ECG	Atrial fibrillation
CT scan brain	Cerebral infarction affecting the territory supplied by the left middle cerebral artery

What is the immediate treatment of choice?
  a. Aspirin.
  b. Warfarin.
  c. Heparin.
  d. Add ACE inhibitor.
  e. DC cardioversion.

Question 308

This is a blood film (**308**) from a young male who presented with severe lower back pain.

What is the haematological diagnosis?
  a. Hereditary spherocytosis.
  b. Microangiopathic haemolytic anaemia.
  c. Hereditary elliptocytosis.
  d. Sickle cell anaemia.
  e. Leucoerythroblastic anaemia secondary to bone marrow infiltration.

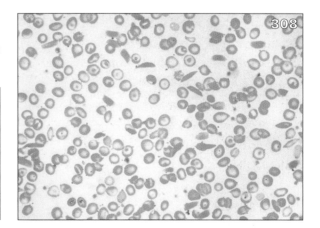

Question 309

A 67-year-old male with a mechanical aortic valve is admitted with a dense left hemiparesis. CT scan of the brain reveals evidence of cerebral infarction but no haemorrhage. The INR on admission is 2.1.

What is the best step in managing his anticoagulation?
  a. Stop warfarin.
  b. Reverse anticoagulation with Vitamin K.
  c. Reverse anticoagulation with FFP.
  d. Increase dose of warfarin.
  e. Stop warfarin and switch to intravenous heparin.

Answer 306

> d. Propranolol.

All patients with cirrhosis of the liver should undergo upper gastrointestinal endoscopy to evaluate the presence of varices. Prevention of bleeding of varices reduces mortality.

There is good evidence from large trials that beta-blockers, particularly propranolol and nadolol, are highly effective agents at controlling portal hypertension and preventing variceal bleeds. Beta-blockers are recommended as prophylactic therapy in patients with mild to moderate oesophageal or gastric varices to prevent bleeding. Sclerotherapy is not recommended for primary prophylaxis, as the risk of causing haemorrhage from the procedure outweighs the benefits. While band endoscopic ligation is the treatment of choice following acute or recurrent variceal haemorrhage, the role of endosopic ligation as primary prophylactic therapy is not entirely clear and should be reserved for patients with large varices at high risk of bleeding who are intolerant of beta-blockers.

Octreotide, transjugular intrahepatic portosystemic shunt and surgery do not have a role in primary prophylaxis for variceal bleeding. Drugs inhibiting angiotensin production have been evaluated in small trials, but they have not convincingly reduced the risk of variceal haemorrhage.

Answer 307

> a. Aspirin.

The patient has suffered a recent cerebrovascular accident. In this particular case the CVA may be secondary to thrombosis of the middle cerebral artery due to atherosclerotic plaque rupture or due to an embolus arising from the carotid arteries or the left atrium. The probability of embolism from left atrial thrombus is high since the patient is in atrial fibrillation. A cerebral haemorrhage has been excluded by CT scan; therefore, treatment with an antithrombotic agent such as aspirin or clopidogrel is relatively safe. Both drugs will be effective in preventing further thrombotic episodes. In relation to AF, the most effective method for preventing systemic thrombo-embolism is anticoagulation. However, anticoagulation early after a thrombotic or embolic CVA increases the risk of haemorrhage into the infarcted area. Current guidelines recommend withholding anticoagulation for at least two weeks following a CVA in the context of AF. The anticoagulation agent of choice in chronic AF is warfarin, which may be safely started after two weeks. Persistently elevated blood pressure should be treated after 72 hours. (See explanation and algorithm in Answer 103.)

Answer 308

> d. Sickle cell anaemia.

The blood film reveals multiple sickle cells and target cells. Bone crisis is the most common type of sickle-related crisis in patients with sickle cell anaemia. The management includes pain relief with opiates, rehydration, oxygen and antibiotics if there is evidence of infection. (See Question 263.)

Answer 309

> e. Stop warfarin and switch to intravenous heparin.

It is very difficult to stop anticoagulation completely in this situation and there is a high risk of prosthetic valve obstruction with thrombus. Furthermore, it is likely that the embolic cerebrovascular accident in this patient was due to under anticoagulation for the mechanical valve. Patients with mechanical valve prostheses are usually maintained on an INR of 3–4. Although continued anticoagulation increases the risk of a cerebral haemorrhage into the infarcted area, the aim here would be to cautiously achieve therapeutic anticoagulation to prevent further embolic strokes. At the same time the patient should be observed carefully for neurological deterioration in the event of a cerebral haemorrhage. Switching to heparin enables more rapid anticoagulation and also more rapid reversal of anticoagulation compared to using warfarin alone.

Question 310

A 20-year-old male was investigated for a six-year history of blistering of the forehead and the hands that was worse during the summer. He was not on any medications. He had been investigated for several episodes of severe central abdominal pain over the past two years for which no obvious cause had been identified. He admitted to binge drinking and consumed up to 100 units of alcohol per week. Abdominal examination was normal. Investigations are shown.

Hb	13.8 g/dl
WCC	8 × 10⁹/l
	(normal differential)
Platelets	200 × 10⁹/l
Blood film	Normal
Amylase	100 iu/l
	(NR <220 iu/l)
Serum iron	33 mmol/l
	(NR 13–32 mmol/l)
TIBC	49 mmol/l
	(NR 42–80 mmol/l)
Serum ferritin	300 iu/l
Urinary coproporphyrins	1640 nmol/24h
	(NR 50–350 nmol/24h)
Faecal coproporphyrin	1900 nmol/24h
Urinary protoporphyrin	400 nmol/24h
	(slightly raised)
CT scan abdomen	Normal

What is the diagnosis?
a. Acute intermittent porphyria.
b. Porphyria cutanea tarda.
c. Haemochromatosis.
d. Variegate porphyria.
e. Hereditary coproporphyria.

Question 311

A 65-year-old male presented with pain in his wrists (**311a**). There was no history of trauma or joint pains elsewhere. He had a past history of hypertension and gout. He smoked 20 cigarettes per day and consumed 24 units of alcohol per week.

What investigation would you perform next?
a. Chest X-ray.
b. Serum parathyroid hormone level.
c. Bone scan.
d. Auto-antibody screen.
e. Serum ACE.

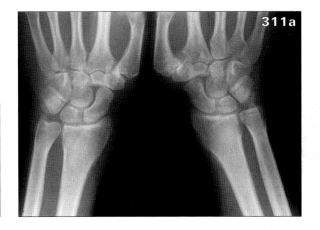
311a

Question 312

An alcohol-dependent patient was admitted with asterixis and jaundice. Blood results are shown.

Hb	10g/dl
MCV	102 fl
WCC	14 × 10⁹/l
Platelets	80 × 10⁹/l
Sodium	131 mmol/l
Potassium	3.2 mmo/l
Urea	2 mmol/l
Glucose	4.2 mmol/l

The patient was given IV thiamine and prescribed diazepam 10 mg six-hourly. Over the next 24 hours his condition deteriorated. He became drowsy and collapsed. The BM stix reading was 6 mmol/l.

What is the definitive treatment?
a. IV flumazenil.
b. IV dextrose 50% (50 ml).
c. IV hydrocortisone.
d. IV naloxone.
e. IV acyclovir.

Answer 310

> e. Hereditary coproporphyria.

Hereditary coproporphyria is an autosomal dominant porphyria caused by deficiency of the enzyme coproporphyrinogen oxidase. The disorder results in increased excretion of coproporphyrin in the urine and faeces and is characterized by a combination of neurovisceral features that are similar to but less severe than those seen in acute intermittent porphyria, and photosensitivity. Patients experience blistering, scarring and hypertrichosis of the skin exposed to sunlight that is identical to that seen in porphyria cutanea tarda. HC has been reported mainly in the UK, Europe and North America. HC is precipitated by the same factors that precipitate acute intermittent porphyria.

The disorder can be differentiated clinically from acute intermittent porphyria by the fact that photosensitivity is not a feature of acute intermittent porphyria. In patients who do not have photosensitivity, the differentiation from acute intermittent porphyria is based on the identification of high concentrations of urinary and faecal porphyrins in HC.

Another porphyria that causes both neurovisceral symptoms and photosensitivity is variegate porphyria. VP is also an autosomal dominant-type hepatic porphyria caused by deficiency of the haem biosynthetic enzyme protoporphyrinogen oxidase. It is common in the South African white population. The disorder is differentiated from HC by measuring urinary and faecal coproporphyrins and protoporphyrins. Both are characterized by high concentrations of faecal and urinary coproporphyrins; however, in VP the concentration of protoporphyrins is considerably higher than that seen in HC.

The management of neurovisceral symptoms in both VP and HC is similar to that of acute intermittent porphyria (Answer 147). There is no effective therapy for photosensitivity other than avoidance. Unlike porphyria cutanea tarda, the photosensitivity does not respond to chloroquine.

Answer 311

> a. Chest X-ray.

The patient has a symmetrical periosteal bone reaction (**311b** periostitis, arrows). The differential diagnosis of symmetrical periostitis is tabulated below. Hypertrophic pulmonary osteoarthropathy, a recognized cause of a symmetrical periostitis, may complicate bronchial carcinoma therefore, the next investigation should be a chest X-ray.

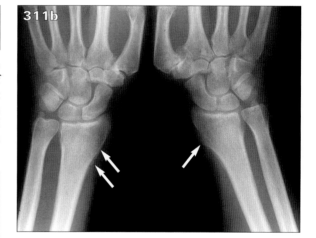

Causes of a symmetrical periostitis
• Hypertrophic pulmonary osteoarthropathy
• Vascular insufficiency
• Thyroid acropathy
• Fluorosis
• Pachydermoperiostitis

Answer 312

> a. IV flumazenil.

The patient has become encephalopathic owing to diazepam. Patients with advanced cirrhosis may be particularly sensitive to benzodiazepines because of an increased concentration of benzodiazepine receptor ligands in the brain. Flumazenil has been shown to be helpful for encephalopathic patients who have received benzodiazepines.

Question 313

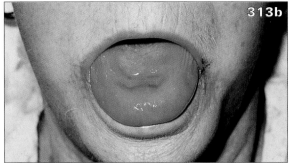

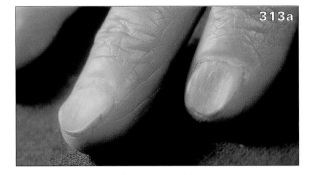

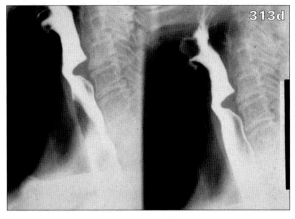

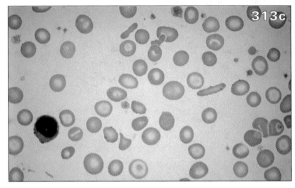

A 60-year-old female presented with a two-month history of lethargy and dysphagia for solid food. Her appetite was slightly reduced, but there was no history of indigestion or weight loss. The examination of her hands and tongue are shown (**313a, b**). There was no lymphadenopathy, or any other palpable masses in the neck. Examination of all the major systems was normal.

Investigations are shown.

Hb	8.8 g/dl
WCC	$6 \times 10^9/l$
Platelets	$170 \times 10^9/l$
Blood film (**313c**)	
Barium study (**313d**)	

1. What is the probable cause of the appearance of the hands and the tongue?
2. Comment on the blood film.
3. What is the abnormality on the barium study?
4. List two possible diagnoses.
5. Which single investigation would you perform?

Question 314

A 14-year-old female was referred to a specialist because she had difficulty in walking over the past eight months. She tripped easily. Her feet had adopted a strange shape and she had problems fitting her shoes. Her father had weakness affecting his legs and was under regular review by a neurologist.

On examination, she appeared well and a general examination was normal. There was wasting of the small muscles of the hand, but upper-limb tone was normal and the reflexes were preserved. On examination of the lower limbs she had bilateral pes cavus. The calf muscles were wasted and exhibited fasciculation. There was mild weakness of dorsiflexion, plantar flexion and eversion at the ankle joint. Examination of the thighs was normal. Both the ankle and knee reflexes were absent. Proprioception was impaired at the level of the first metatarsal joint. Two-point discrimination sense was also impaired in both feet but pain, temperature and pressure sense was normal.

1. What is the diagnosis?
2. What three tests would you perform to confirm the diagnosis?

Answer 313

1. The woman has koilonychia and glossitis, which are features of iron-deficiency anaemia.
2. Anaemia with microcytosis, anisocytosis, poikilocytosis and hypochromia. The features are consistent with iron-deficiency anaemia.
3. Stricture in the upper oesophagus consistent with an oesophageal web (Paterson–Brown–Kelly or Plummer–Vinson syndrome).
4. The differential diagnosis is between oesophageal web and carcinoma of the upper oesophagus.
5. Oesophagoscopy and biopsy of stricture for histological analysis.

This woman has the features of oesophageal web, which is a rare condition characterized by submucosal inflammation, usually in the post-cricoid region, although any part of the oesophagus can be affected. The inflammation produces a 'web' or a concentric stenosis. The condition affects women in their fourth to sixth decade. The classic features are dysphagia, iron-deficiency anaemia, koilonychia and other stigmata of iron deficiency, such as glossitis. It is a pre-malignant condition, and can predispose to carcinoma of the oesophagus, which needs to be excluded by endoscopy and biopsy of the stricture.

Answer 314

1. Charcot–Marie–Tooth disease (hereditary sensorimotor neuropathy (HSMN)/peroneal muscular atrophy).
2. i. Nerve conduction studies.
   ii. Sural biopsy.
   iii. Family screening.

The patient presents with difficulty in walking. On physical examination, she has pes cavus, weakness of the distal aspects of the upper and lower limbs. The lower-limb reflexes are absent and proprioception and two-point discrimination sense are impaired. These are the features of HSMN. A family history is not given, but this should be an important part of the investigation.

HSMN is divided into Types I, II and III. Type I is the classic, familial type in which there is a diffuse demyelinating neuropathy which usually presents in the first two decades. Distal wasting of the lower limbs produces peroneal muscular atrophy and the characteristic 'inverted champagne bottle' appearance. Deformities of the feet and scoliosis are common. The sensory fibres of proprioception are affected, producing a sensory ataxia. Linkage studies on families with this neuropathy have localized the condition to a genetic defect on the long arm of chromosome 1. Nerve conduction is very reduced.

Type II HSMN is similar, but much milder. In this condition, nerve conduction is only very slightly reduced or normal.

HSMN III – also known as Dejerine–Sottas disease – is inherited as an autosomal recessive trait. It is a slow, progressive mixed sensory and motor neuropathy that starts in the first decade and is typically associated with enlargement of the peripheral nerves, which are easily palpable on examination. Differential diagnosis of thickened or enlarged peripheral nerves is listed below. Recently, the classification of the HSMNs has been extended to include types IV and V. Descriptions of the latter are beyond the scope of this book.

Causes of thickened peripheral nerves

- HSMN type III
- Acromegaly
- Tuberculoid leprosy
- Neurofibromatosis
- HIV syndrome

Question 315

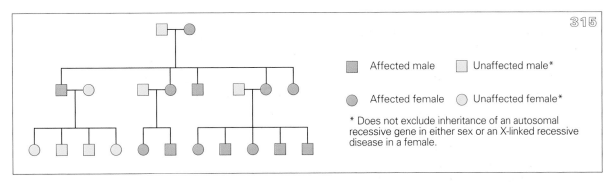

A family pedigree suffering from a very rare condition is shown (**315**).

1. What is the mode of inheritance?
2. Give one example of a condition inherited in this way.

Question 316

A 59-year-old female was referred to the out-patient clinic with lethargy and chest pain consistent with angina. She was on a gluten-free diet and on long-standing treatment for a skin rash (**316**). On examination, she was thin and had pale conjunctivae. She appeared cyanosed. The heart rate was 110 beats/min, with good volume; the blood pressure was 130/75 mmHg. The heart sounds were normal and the chest was clear.

Investigations are shown.

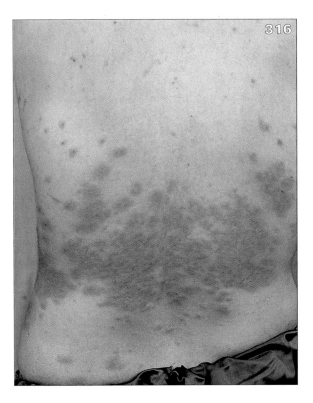

Hb	8 g/dl
WCC	11×10^9/l
Platelets	240×10^9/l
MCV	110 fl
PCV	0.34
Reticulocytes	10%
Blood film	Polychromasia, macrocytosis, target cells, a few fragmented red cells
Serum B_{12}	470 ng/l
Red cell folate	65 µg/l
Serum folate	1.8 µg/l

1. Give two possible explanations for the folate levels.
2. What is the most likely cause for the blood picture?
3. What additional morphological feature in the blood film would be diagnostically helpful?
4. What test would you request to determine the cause of the cyanosis?
5. Give three reasons for the patient's chest pain.

Answer 315

1. Inheritance of maternal mitochondrial genetic abnormality.
2. Conditions inherited in this way are listed (*Table*).

Syndromes associated with mitochondrial gene mutations

- MERRF: myoclonic epilepsy, ragged red fibres (mutation in t-RNA Lys)
- MELAS: mitochondrial encephalomyopathy, lactic acidosis, stroke (mutation in t-RNA Leu)
- NARP: neuropathy, ataxia, retinitis pigmentosa (mutation at nucleotide 8893; coding for ATPase 6)
- LHON: Leber's hereditary, optic neuropathy (mutation in NADH dehydrogenase Subunit 4)
- Kearnes–Sayer syndrome: progressive external ophthalmoplegia, retinitis pigmentosa, heart block, myopathy, diabetes
- Usher's syndrome: deafness, retinitis pigmentosa, myopathy

During conception, all the mitochondria inherited by the zygote come from the ovum because the spermatozoon is relatively depleted of mitochondria by the time it reaches the ovum; therefore, abnormalities in mitochondrial DNA can only be transmitted by a female. An affected female will transfer the abnormal gene and the abnormal phenotype to all offspring; however, a male does not transfer the disease.

Mitochondrial DNA contains a limited number of genes that may be subject to point mutations, deletions or duplications. Abnormalities in mitochondrial DNA result in a variety of abnormalities, including easy fatigue, myopathy, epilepsy, diabetes, optic atrophy, deafness, retinitis pigmentosa and cardiomyopathy. Calcification of basal ganglia is well recognized with mitochondrial disease. The most common mutation is an A to G mutation at nucleotide 3243. Most recognized mutations occur in transfer RNA or genes encoding the proteins involved in the oxidative phosphorylation pathway. The serum lactate/pyruvate ratio is elevated, indicating impaired aerobic glycolysis. CSF lactate may be elevated even when serum lactate is normal. Muscle biopsy may reveal red ragged fibres (increased fibre staining with stain for succinate dehydrogenase) representing abnormal mitochondria.

Answer 316

1. i. Malabsorption.
   ii. Dapsone-induced haemolysis.
2. Dapsone-induced haemolytic anaemia.
3. The presence of Heinz bodies (oxidative haemolysis).
4. Serum methaemoglobin level.
5. i. Anaemia.
   ii. Reduced delivery of oxygen to the heart due to leftward shift of the oxygen dissociation curve resulting from methaemoglobinaemia.
   iii. Tachycardia.

The patient is on a gluten-free diet, suggesting that she has a gluten-sensitive enteropathy. She is on treatment for a long-standing rash (316) which is characteristic of dermatitis herpetiformis. The association between dermatitis herpetiformis and gluten-sensitive enteropathy is well recognized. Dermatitis herpetiformis is effectively treated with dapsone. An important side-effect of dapsone is haemolytic anaemia because of its oxidant effect on Hb. This effect is severe in patients with glucose-6-phosphate dehydrogenase deficiency, but may also occur in some individuals as an idiosyncratic reaction, particularly with chronic use of the drug. Iron within the haem molecule of haemoglobin is oxidized from the ferrous state (Fe^{2+}) to the ferric state (Fe^{3+}), resulting in methaemoglobin (*Table A*). This leads to depletion of the red cell NADPH (which is utilized to try and maintain iron in the ferrous form) and consequent reduction in the integrity of the red cell membrane. Patients with glucose-6-phosphate dehydrogenase deficiency have lower cellular levels of NADPH than normal individuals, and are more severely affected. Methaemoglobin has a very high affinity for oxygen molecules, resulting in a leftward shift in the oxygen dissociation curve and impaired unloading of oxygen to the tissues (*Table B*). Methaemoglobin has a bluish colour, therefore patients with significant methaemoglobinaemia appear cyanosed even when the arterial oxygen tension is normal. Pulse oximetry shows low oxygen saturations because it does not register oxymethaemoglobin. A normal arterial oxygen tension and a low oxygen saturation should raise the suspicion of methaemoglobinaemia in a patient who appears cyanosed. This contrasts with carbon monoxide poisoning, in which oxygen saturation on the pulse oximeter is normal but arterial oxygen tension may be

Table A Causes of methaemoglobinaemia

Genetic
NADPH diaphorase deficiency
Hb M

Acquired
Drugs: Sulphonamides
           Primaquin
           Phenacetin

Toxins: Ferric cyanide
            Chlorate
            Aniline dyes

Table B Causes of left-shift of O_2 dissociation curve

- Methaemoglobinaemia
- Sulphaemoglobinaemia
- Fetal Hb
- 2,3 diphosphoglycerate deficiency
- Alkalosis
- Hypocapnia
- Hypothermia

normal because the pulse oximeter cannot differentiate between oxyhaemoglobin and carboxyhaemoglobin.

Methaemoglobin levels exceeding 20% are associated with dyspnoea and headaches. Patients may develop angina, despite normal coronary arteries, owing to reduced delivery of oxygen to myocardial cells. Collapse and sudden death may occur when levels exceed 60%. The blood film will demonstrate features of intravascular haemolysis (polychromasia, macrocytes, red cell fragmentation) and Heinz bodies, which are small red cell inclusions of denatured Hb. These are scarce on the peripheral blood film unless the spleen has been removed. Other causes of methaemoglobinaemia are shown (*Table A*). Dapsone-induced chronic haemolysis may lead to depletion of folate.

Question 317

A 76-year-old female was admitted to hospital with malaise, weakness, nausea and anorexia. She had been relatively well until two weeks previously when she developed a painful left calf for which she was prescribed 'some tablets' by her GP. On examination, she appeared dehydrated and her blood pressure was 90/50 mmHg. She had clinical evidence of a deep-vein thrombosis in her left calf. All other physical examination was normal.

Investigations are shown.

Hb	13 g/dl
WCC	8×10^9/l
Platelets	300×10^9/l
MCV	88 fl
Sodium	128 mmol/l
Potassium	6.2 mmol/l
Chloride	88 mmol/l
Bicarbonate	13 mmol/l
Urea	24 mmol/l
Creatinine	297 μmol/l
Blood glucose	10 mmol/l
Urinalysis	24-hour sodium 68 mmol/l

What is the cause of this patient's low sodium?
a. Addison's disease.
b. Diuretic excess.
c. Acute tubulointerstitial nephritis secondary to NSAIDs.
d. Diabetic ketoacidosis.
e. Vomiting.

Answer 317

> c. Acute tubulointerstitial nephritis secondary to NSAIDs.

All five suggested answers can be responsible for hyponatraemia, but in a woman who has recently been treated for a painful calf it is most likely that she was prescribed some form of pain killer. She has subsequently presented with anorexia, malaise and vomiting and has deranged renal function. Urinalysis reveals a 24-hour urine of over 20 mmol/l sodium, which suggests a salt-losing state when one considers her low serum sodium. The most probable cause of her presentation is an acute nephritis secondary to prescription of an NSAID.

The biochemistry is partly consistent with Addison's disease; however, the diagnosis is less likely in the context of the history and the presence of a raised blood sugar. Diuretic excess is also possible. One could assume that she was prescribed a diuretic; this has resulted in dehydration and pre-renal failure, but the serum bicarbonate and the potassium levels suggest that this is unlikely. Diuretics used to treat ankle swelling alone comprise thiazides or loop diuretics, which result in a hypokalaemic alkalosis. Potassium-sparing drugs such as amiloride alone or spironolactone are not the drugs of choice to treat ankle swelling. Vomiting is also a recognized cause of hyponatraemia, but there is no mention of it in the history, and the raised potassium is unlikely to explain profuse vomiting, which usually results in low sodium, potassium and chloride levels because gastric fluid contains high concentrations of all these ions.

Diabetic ketoacidosis would be lowest in the differential diagnosis because the blood sugar is relatively low. The hyponatraemia resulting from ketoacidosis is a result of osmotic diuresis from the very high blood sugar. A random blood sugar of 10 mmol/l could represent impaired glucose tolerance or mild non-insulin-dependent diabetes, but is against diabetic ketoacidosis.

NSAIDs may cause acute tubular necrosis or an acute tubulointerstitial nephritis (*Table*). Acute tubular necrosis is an increasing problem with NSAID prescription. NSAIDs inhibit cyclo-oxygenase activity and decrease prostaglandin synthesis. Prostaglandins have a number of functions in the kidney, one of which is to stimulate renin production and thus activate the angiotensin–aldosterone system. With NSAIDs, there is a state of hyporeninanaemic hypoaldosteronism causing hyperkalaemia, hyponatraemia, increased urinary sodium loss and dehydration. In patients with pre-existing renal disease, or in diabetics, this may be significant enough to produce acute renal failure. Such patients usually have a significant hyperkalaemia. Acute tubulointerstitial nephritis is often due to a hypersensitivity reaction to drugs (*Table*). NSAIDs and the penicillins are most commonly implicated in the UK. Patients may present with malaise, arthralgia and/or acute renal failure. Many patients have eosinophilia or eosinophiluria.

Treatment of both forms of renal failure involves withdrawal of the offending drug. The treatment of acute tubular necrosis is supportive, and involves careful fluid balance, correction of hyperkalaemia and hypovolaemia, and dialysis if necessary. Acute interstitial nephritis is treated in the same way, but in addition high-dose prednisolone is prescribed to reduce the acute inflammatory response in the kidney.

Causes of acute interstitial nephritis

- Penicillins
- NSAIDs
- Sulphonamides
- Allopurinol
- Phenindione
- Acute pyelonephritis
- Sickle cell crisis
- Lead poisoning

Renal manifestations of NSAIDs

- Acute tubular necrosis
- Acute interstitial nephritis
- Minimal change glomerulonephritis

Question 318

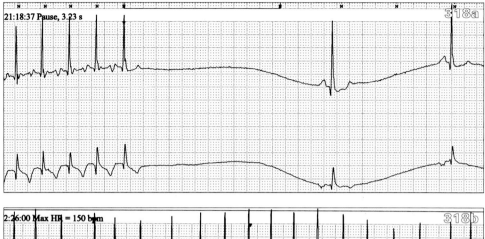

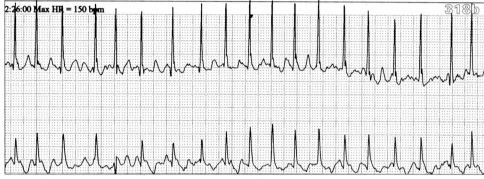

The above (**318a, b**) are two rhythm strips from a 24-hour ECG in a 70-year-old male with dizziness and palpitation.

1. What is the diagnosis?
2. What is the management?

Question 319

A 40-year-old dentist presented with a five-month history of weight loss. He had recently become jaundiced.
   Blood results are shown.

AST	40 iu/l
Alkaline phosphatase	165 iu/l
Bilirubin	80 µmol/l
Albumin	32 g/l
α-fetoprotein	40 ng/l
Serum ferritin	450 µg/l
Hepatitis serology	Hep B sAg positive
	Hep B eAg positive
	Hep B cAb positive

1. What is the diagnosis?
2. Which four tests would you perform next?
3. What is the management?

Answer 318

1. Sick sinus syndrome. Rhythm strip **318a** reveals sinus tachycardia followed by sinus arrest or sinus pause of 2.5 seconds. Rhythm strip **318b** reveals atrial fibrillation with a rapid ventricular rate.
2. Symptomatic patients should be paced.

The diagnosis is consistent with sick sinus syndrome, which is a degenerative condition affecting the sino-atrial node and the atrial myocardium. It is characterized by long sinus pauses and paroxysmal atrial arrhythmias comprising atrial tachycardia, flutter and fibrillation. These patients are at increased risk of systemic emboli. Many go on to develop atrioventricular nodal disease.

Patients in sinus rhythm are implanted with an atrial pacemaker as they have effective atrial transport; however, those with atrial fibrillation are treated with ventricular pacing. Unlike atrioventricular block, pacing for sick sinus syndrome does not save lives.

Answer 319

1. Chronic active hepatitis B infection.
2. i. Hepatitis B e antibody (Hep B eAb)/hepatitis s antibody (Hep B sAb).
   ii. Liver ultrasound.
   iii. Liver biopsy (if platelets and clotting not severely deranged).
   iv. HIV antigen.
3. α-interferon.

The differential diagnosis of weight loss and jaundice is wide, but the presence of Hep B eAg and Hep B sAg narrows this down to active hepatitis B infection. (Note: dentistry is a high-risk occupation for hepatitis B.)

The symptoms have been present for five months, suggesting that there is a chronic active infection. Investigations should be based on confirming the extent of hepatic damage and determining the patient's infectivity and immune status. The α-fetoprotein is modestly elevated in severe viral hepatitis and active cirrhosis. Levels exceeding 1,000 ng/l are strongly suggestive of hepatocellular carcinoma. Liver biopsy will reveal a ground-glass appearance of infected hepatocytes and evidence of balloon degeneration. Serological markers such as Hep B eAb and Hep B sAb will determine infectivity and immune response. Liver ultrasound may be useful in determining the extent of liver damage when clotting and platelets are very abnormal. Hepatitis B-positive patients in high-risk occupations should also be offered HIV testing, because both conditions are acquired in the same manner from the same type of patients. There is evidence that treatment with α-interferon in patients with circulating Hep B sAg and Hep B eAg will reduce viral replication and infectivity.

Some 2% of patients with hepatitis B infection develop fulminant hepatitis, while 10% of patients become carriers after the initial infection. Some carriers are positive for Hep B sAb, but have normal liver histology, while others have chronic active or chronic persistent hepatitis. Chronic active hepatitis may progress to cirrhosis of the liver. Patients with cirrhosis of the liver as a result of hepatitis B infection are more prone to hepatocellular carcinoma.

Hep B sAg appears in the circulation 1–5 weeks before the onset of symptoms. It is no longer detectable when the infection has resolved, but its presence six months after infection indicates chronic infection.

Hep B eAg appears in the circulation shortly before or 1–3 weeks after the onset of symptoms. Its presence indicates active viral replication, either in acute or in chronic infection, and high infectivity. Its disappearance is suggestive of resolution of infection. Hepatitis B virus DNA also appears at around the same time and its presence also indicates active viral replication. Disappearance of Hep B virus DNA correlates with resolution of infection. Hep B cAg is only seen within hepatocytes, and does not circulate in the serum.

IgM anti-Hep B cAb appears at the time of onset of symptoms. It is a marker of recent hepatitis B infection and may be the only marker of hepatitis B infection before the appearance of Hep B sAg. IgG anti-Hep B cAb is present lifelong after hepatitis B infection. It does not indicate immunity. Hep B eAb appears after the cAb. Its presence indicates reduced infectivity. Hep B sAb is the last antibody to appear. Its presence indicates immunity.

Interferon therapy will reduce Hep B e and sAg levels (40% and 10%, respectively). All patients with circulating e and sAg are offered treatment with interferon unless there is evidence of gross hepatic decompensation. Interferon has the effect of exacerbating coexisting auto-immune conditions, and is contraindicated in these situations.

Question 320

A 62-year-old female with rheumatoid arthritis was referred to an ophthalmologist with a three-day history of a painful left eye. The visual acuity was normal. She had a similar problem three years ago which required therapy with oral steroids. She was diagnosed with rheumatoid arthritis 21 years ago after presenting with pain in her hands, feet and elbows. Initial treatment comprised NSAIDs, then chloroquine, but over the past five years she was successfully managed on a combination of NSAIDs and penicillamine. On further questioning, she complained of a slightly reduced appetite, lethargy and breathlessness on trying to negotiate inclines, and swollen ankles. There was no other past medical history. She was a non-smoker. She was married and her husband worked as an architect.

On examination, the appearance of the eye was as shown (**320a**). The anterior chamber was clear and the pupils reacted normally to light. Visual acuity was 6/6 in the left eye, and 6/12 in the right eye. Examination of the fundi was normal. Examination of her hands and feet revealed evidence of a generalized, symmetrical deforming arthropathy. The heart rate was 90 beats/min and regular. The blood pressure was 140/90 mmHg. The jugular veins were not distended. The heart sounds were normal. Auscultation of the lung fields revealed fine inspiratory crackles at both bases, which persisted after coughing. On examination of the abdomen, there was a palpable spleen 3 cm below the costal margin. The liver was not palpable, and there was no ascites. Examination of the lower limbs revealed multiple bruises and pitting ankle oedema to the shins.

Investigations are shown.

Hb	7.4 g/dl
WCC	3×10^9/l
Platelets	45×10^9/l
MCV	78 fl
ESR	56 mm/h
Sodium	134 mmol/l
Potassium	4.4 mmol/l
Urea	13 mmol/l
Creatinine	168 µmol/l
Calcium	2.0 mmol/l
Phosphate	1.2 mmol/l
Alkaline phosphatase	200 iu/l
Albumin	29 g/l
IgM	2.0 g/l
IgG	19 g/l
IgA	1.9 g/l
Immunoelectro-phoresis	Increased gamma-globulin band No paraproteinaemia Rheumatoid factor positive 1 in 460
Chest X-ray	Normal
Urine dipstick	Protein ++ Blood 0

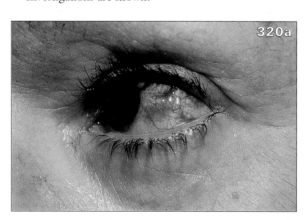
320a

1. What is the most probable cause of the painful eye?
2. Give two possible explanations for the FBC.
3. List two tests you would perform to ascertain the cause of the abnormal FBC.
4. List two possible causes for the ankle swelling?
5. What is the most likely cause of the breathlessness?
6. Which two investigations would you perform to ascertain the cause of the breathlessness?

Answer 320

1. Scleritis.
2. i. Penicillamine-induced marrow suppression.
   ii. Hypersplenism (Felty's syndrome).
3. i. Bone marrow aspirate/trephine.
   ii. Red cell sequestration study.
4. i. Penicillamine-induced membranous glomerulonephritis and secondary nephrotic syndrome.
   ii. Renal amyloidosis.
5. Interstitial lung fibrosis or fibrotic lung disease.
6. Formal spirometry and transfer factor.

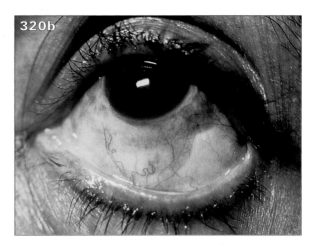

320b

This woman with long-standing rheumatoid arthritis presents with a second attack of unilateral painful red eye, which has previously required systemic steroids. The most probable diagnosis is scleritis. Other causes of a red eye in rheumatoid arthritis include episcleritis and keratitis secondary to Sjögren's syndrome. The former is painless, and the latter is bilateral. It is important to note that the only definitive method of differentiating scleritis from episcleritis without a history is by slit-lamp examination of the eye. Recurrent episodes of scleritis may result in perforation of the sclera (scleromalacia perforans) (**320b**).

In addition to the scleritis, she has other problems commonly seen in patients with rheumatoid arthritis which include anaemia, Felty's syndrome (which itself may be responsible for the anaemia), renal and respiratory involvement. Drugs used in the treatment of rheumatoid arthritis may themselves cause many of the complications seen in rheumatoid arthritis, and a knowledge of the drugs used – and their complications – is essential in the management of a patient with rheumatoid arthritis.

The anaemia is part of pancytopenia which, in the context of this question, is due to either penicillamine-induced marrow aplasia or hypersplenism resulting in Felty's syndrome. The former may be diagnosed by histological examination of the marrow, and the latter by demonstrating increased red cell uptake and destruction by the spleen.

The low albumin, swollen ankles and proteinuria are indicative of nephrotic syndrome, which may be due to a penicillamine-induced membranous glomerulonephritis or renal amyloid complicating chronic inflammation. Other causes of renal involvement in patients with rheumatoid arthritis are tabulated below. The fine inspiratory crackles at both lung bases probably represent interstitial lung disease, and require investigation with formal spirometry and KCO. Early interstitial fibrosis may not be identified on a chest X-ray, but respiratory function tests will reveal reduced lung volumes and reduced KCO. The haematological, ocular, renal, and respiratory complications of rheumatoid arthritis are tabulated (*Tables A–D*).

Table A Causes of anaemia in rheumatoid arthritis

- Iron deficiency secondary to NSAIDs
- Marrow suppression from drugs such as penicillamine and gold
- Hypersplenism seen as part of Felty's syndrome
- Anaemia of chronic disease
- Folate deficiency resulting from increased cell turnover in chronic inflammation
- Auto-immune haemolysis
- Associated pernicious anaemia

Table B Causes of ocular involvement in rheumatoid arthritis

- Episcleritis/scleritis/scleromalacia
- Sjögren's syndrome
- Cataracts secondary to steroid therapy
- Retinopathy secondary to chloroquine
- Extraocular muscle tendon synovitis
- Extraocular muscle paralysis secondary to penicillamine-induced myaesthenia
- Extraocular muscle paralysis secondary to a mononeuritis multiplex

Table C Causes of renal involvement in rheumatoid arthritis

- Acute tubulointerstitial nephritis secondary to NSAIDs
- Renal papillary necrosis secondary to analgesic abuse
- Renal amyloid
- Membranous nephropathy secondary to gold or penicillamine
- Minimal change glomerulonephritis complicating NSAIDs

Table D Causes of respiratory involvement in rheumatoid arthritis

- Cricoarytenitis
- Pleural effusion
- Pulmonary fibrosis
- Bronchiolitis obliterans
- Pneumonitis
- Pulmonary nodules
- Caplan's syndrome (nodules plus progressive massive fibrosis in coal worker's disease)

Question 321

An 11-year-old male was referred to the local paediatrician after his mother complained that he was unusually short for his age. His appetite was normal, and there was no history of recent diarrhoea or weight loss. He was performing well at school and enjoyed a relatively active life. His mother was short, measuring 1.48 m, but his father measured 1.81 m. There were no siblings.

On examination, the boy measured 0.97 m. There was no evidence of pallor, cyanosis or oedema. The heart sounds were normal and the chest was clear. The abdomen was soft, and there was no palpable organomegaly. The lower limbs appeared bowed. Neurological examination was normal.

Investigations are shown.

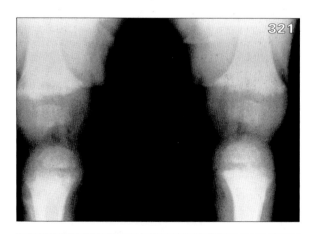

Hb	11 g/dl
WCC	5 × 10⁹/l
Platelets	180 × 10⁹/l
Sodium	135 mmol/l
Potassium	4 mmol/l
Urea	4 mmol/l
Calcium	2.2 mmol/l
Phosphate	0.3 mmol/l
Albumin	39 g/l
Alkaline phosphatase	500 iu/l
X-ray of knees (**321**)	

1. What is the abnormality on the X-ray?
2. What is the diagnosis?
3. What tests would you perform to confirm the diagnosis?
4. What is the management?

Answer 321

1. Splaying of the metaphyses and widening of the epiphyseal plate, indicating rickets.
2. Hypophosphataemic rickets; X-linked dominant hypophophataemic rickets; vitamin D resistant rickets.
3. i. Urinary phosphate excretion (elevated).
   ii. Renal tubular reabsorption rate of phosphate.
4. High-dose vitamin D and oral phosphate supplements.

Both the boy and his mother are short. There is radiological evidence of rickets and a hypophosphataemia, but the serum calcium level is normal. The findings are consistent with the diagnosis of hypophosphataemic rickets or vitamin D resistant rickets. The condition is inherited as an X-linked dominant condition. The fundamental abnormality is failure of phosphate reabsorption by the kidney. The diagnosis is confirmed by the demonstration of a high urinary phosphate excretion rate.

Unlike vitamin D dependent rickets, myopathy does not occur. The main features of the condition are short stature and radiological evidence of rickets. Ossification of the ligamentum flavum is recognized and may cause paraplegia. The serum calcium and active metabolites of vitamin D are usually normal.

Correction of the disorder is by a combination of high-dose vitamin D and oral phosphate supplements. Vitamin D alone aids resolution of biochemical rickets, but does not promote growth of height. Untreated patients are short and rarely measure more than 1.53 m.

Other causes of renal rickets are proximal RTA and Fanconi's syndrome (*Table A*). Vitamin D dependent rickets is very rare. Two forms are recognized, the characteristics of which are listed (*Table B*).

Table A Causes of rickets and osteomalacia

- Vitamin D deficiency due to poor nutrition, malabsorption
- Chronic renal failure (failure to synthesize 1α-hydroxycholecalciferol)
- Renal tubular disorders (see above)
- Anticonvulsants (rapid metabolism of 25-hydroxycholecalciferol to inactive derivatives)
- Tumours (certain mesenchymal tumours; cause unknown; associated profound myopathy)
- Vitamin D dependent rickets (*Table B*)

Table B Characteristics of vitamin D dependent rickets

	Type 1	Type 2
Mode of inheritance	Autosomal recessive	Autosomal recessive
Defect	Reduced 1α-hydroxycholecalciferol	Resistance to 1,25-dihydroxycholecalciferol
1,25-dihydroxycholecalciferol level	Reduced	Elevated
Myopathy	Present	Present
Associations		Alopecia
Treatment	Very high doses of 1,25-dihydroxycholecalciferol	Very high doses of 1,25-dihydroxycholecalciferol and i.v. calcium. Spontaneous resolution with advancing age is recognized

Question 322

CD4 count	300×10^6/l
Viral load	1,000 copies/ml
CT scan	Normal
CSF pressure	10 cmH$_2$O
CSF analysis:	
White cells	580/mm^3 (90% lymphocytes)
Red cells	3/mm^3
Protein	0.9 g/l
Glucose	1.5 mmol/l
Gram stain	Negative
Ziehl–Neelsen stain	Negative
Blood glucose	5 mmol/l

A 25-year-old homosexual male presented with an epileptic seizure.

Investigations are shown.

1. List at least three possible diagnoses.
2. List three investigations you would perform on the CSF to help make the diagnosis.

Question 323

A 57-year-old male was admitted to the coronary care unit with a two-hour history of crushing central chest pain radiating to his jaw. On examination, he was sweating. His heart rate was 90 beats/min, and regular, and blood pressure was 160/90 mmHg. He had a 12-lead ECG (**323**), after which he was given recombinant tissue plasminogen activator. Two hours later he complained of feeling dizzy and unwell. On examination, he was pale, but not cyanosed. His heart rate was 110 beats/min, and regular. His systolic blood pressure was 80 mmHg. The JVP was elevated 7 cm above the sternal angle. The heart sounds were normal and the chest was clear.

Investigations are shown.

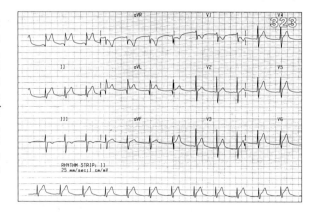

Sodium	136 mmol/l	Hb	13 g/dl
Potassium	4.0 mmol/l	WCC	17×10^9/l
Urea	8 mmol/l	Platelets	159×10^9/l
Creatinine	90 µmol/l	Chest X-ray	Normal
Glucose	6 mmol/l		

1. What is the ECG diagnosis?
   a. Acute anterior myocardial infarction.
   b. Acute inferior myocardial infarction.
   c. Acute inferior myocardial infarction complicated by third degree atrioventricular block.
   d. Acute posterior myocardial infarction.
   e. Acute posterolateral myocardial infarction.

2. What is the cause of his symptoms two hours after thrombolysis?
   a. Complete heart block complicating myocardial infarction.
   b. Acute pulmonary embolus.
   c. Acute mitral regurgitation following papillary muscle rupture.
   d. Acute VSD complicating myocardial infarction.
   e. Right ventricular hypokinesia.

Answer 322

1. i. Tuberculous meningitis.
   ii. Cryptococcal meningitis.
   iii. Listeria meningitis.
   iv. Cerebral lymphoma or leukaemia.
   v. Brucellosis.
2. i. Ziehl–Neelsen stain or PCR on the CSF for tuberculous meningitis.
   ii. Indian ink stain on CSF to identify Cryptococcus neoformans.
   iii. CSF analysis by the cytology department to look for malignant cells.

Causes of CSF lymphocytosis, raised CSF protein and CSF sugar less than half of blood sugar

- Tuberculous meningitis
- Brucellosis*
- Fungal meningitis
- Cerebral lymphoma
- Leukaemic infiltration into the brain
- Metastatic brain disease
- Cerebral abscess

*This may be similar to that seen in viral meningitis.

This homosexual male with a low CD4 count presents with an epileptic seizure. The CD4 count suggests that he has advanced HIV infection. The CSF reveals a lymphocytosis, high protein and a sugar concentration less than half of the blood sugar. The differential diagnosis of these CSF findings is listed (*Table*). The normal CT scan is against the diagnosis of a cerebral abscess, and metastatic brain disease; however, all the other diagnoses listed are possible.

Answer 323

1. e. Acute posterolateral myocardial infarction.
2. e. Right ventricular hypokinesia.

The ECG on admission reveals ST-segment elevation of more than 2 mm in leads I and aVl. This is consistent with a limited lateral myocardial infarction. The J-point in leads II and V3–V6 is elevated, but there is no pathological ST-segment elevation in these leads. There is also evidence of a dominant R-wave in leads V1–V3 which, in the context of the history, represents posterior extension of the infarct. Posterior infarction gives the opposite appearance of an acute anterior infarction; therefore instead of Q-waves (which would be seen in the case of an anterior infarction) there are prominent R-waves. The full diagnosis is acute posterolateral myocardial infarction.

There are several possible causes of hypotension in this man; however the only real possibility in this clinical scenario is right ventricular infarction and secondary right ventricular hypokinesia. This is a recognized complication of inferior and posterior myocardial infarction, and is characterized by a reduced cardiac output from the right heart causing hypotension and a raised JVP. Treatment is with a careful fluid challenge of 100 ml at a time to increase the PCWP to approximately 10 cmH$_2$O, which should be monitored using a Swan–Ganz catheter. Haemorrhage is unlikely with a raised JVP unless the patient has bled into his pericardial space. However, in this rare event one would expect an increased heart size on the chest X-ray.

While allergic reactions are relatively common with non-human thrombolytic agents such as streptokinase, they are rare with recombinant human tissue plasminogen activator. In any case, allergic shock occurs during infusion of the drug rather than two hours afterwards. Although pulmonary embolism is a recognized complication of myocardial infarction and could explain the raised JVP, low blood pressure and normal chest X-ray, it does not occur for at least three days after myocardial infarction. Both papillary muscle rupture and ventricular septal perforation, which usually occur 72 hours following myocardial infarction, are usually associated with an acute fall in cardiac output and pulmonary oedema. Complete heart block may cause hypotension, but is most unlikely in a patient with a heart rate of 110 beats/min.

Question 324

A 5-year-old male was admitted with a one-week history of fever, general malaise and pain in his hands and feet. Two weeks previously he had had a bout of tonsillitis which required a course of antibiotics. On the day of admission he complained of intermittent chest pain radiating into his back and his arms. He was born at 41 weeks' gestation via a normal vaginal delivery. He had achieved his milestones normally. He was the only child. His father was a businessman, and his mother a teacher. He had been seen by the GP two days earlier and diagnosed as having a viral illness for which he was prescribed paracetamol syrup.

On examination, he appeared unwell. He had a fever of 40°C (104°F). His heart rate was 140 beats/min and regular. His lips appeared oedematous, and examination of his mouth revealed a white-coated tongue with prominent papillae. On examination of the neck there was widespread, tender, cervical lymphadenopathy. Examination of the pharynx and tonsillar area was normal. The palms of his hands and feet were red, and there was evidence of early desquamation of the skin on the palmar surface of both hands. There was tenderness over the metacarpophalangeal joints of both hands. The interphalangeal joints in both feet were tender. Cardiovascular and respiratory examination was normal.

Investigations are shown.

Hb	10.5 g/dl
WCC	15 × 10⁹/l
Platelets	490 × 10⁹/l
ESR	90 mm/h
CRP	80 g/l
Biochemistry	Normal
Blood cultures	Normal
Chest X-ray	Normal
ECG	Sinus tachycardia
	Inverted T- waves V1–V6

1. What is the diagnosis?
2. What other important investigation would you perform?
3. List two important therapeutic steps in his management.

Question 325

A 33-year-old single male was admitted with a one-week history of fever, sore throat, a maculopapular rash on the trunk and cervical lymphadenopathy. His only past medical history consisted of treatment for urethritis one year previously following a trip abroad. His most recent sexual contact was eight weeks ago. Four months previously, he expressed the wish for HIV testing, which was negative.

Investigations are shown.

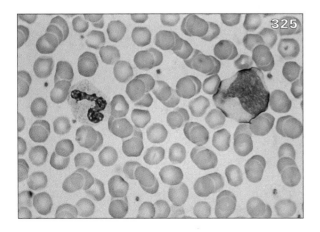

Hb	11 g/dl
WCC	6 × 10⁹/l
Platelets	180 × 10⁹/l
Blood film (**325**)	
Paul Bunnell test	Negative
CMV titre	Increased IgG at a titre of 1/16
Toxoplasma titres	Negative
VDRL	Negative
FTA IgG	Positive
Hep B sAg	Absent
HCV Ab	Absent

1. What is the cause of this patient's symptoms?
2. What further definitive investigation is required?

Answer 324

> 1. Kawasaki's disease.
> 2. Transthoracic echocardiography to visualize the coronary arteries on the short-axis views of the aorta.
> 3. i. Oral aspirin.
>   ii. Intravenous human immunoglobulin.

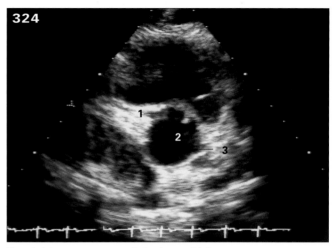

Key: 1 right coronary artery 2 Aortic root 3 left coronary artery

The combination of mucocutaneous, rheumatological and dermatological involvement in a young boy shortly after a sore throat could be due to scarlet fever, Stevens–Johnson syndrome complicating streptococcal infection, an idiosyncratic reaction to antibiotics, or a systemic reaction to a general viral illness. The rash is not typical of Stevens–Johnson syndrome. The description of the tongue and the generalized erythema fit well with scarlet fever; however, the additional chest pain and abnormal ECG should raise the possibility of Kawasaki's disease.

Kawasaki's disease has been very topical, and it is only a matter of time before it appears in general examinations. It is an acute multi-system vasculitis which affects medium-sized arteries. It appears to be endemic in Japan, where there have been more than 100,000 cases since 1991. In contrast, the incidence in Britain is 35 per million. The disorder is thought to be due to a severe immune reaction following streptococcal or staphylococcal infections, although other organisms have also been implicated. The condition is almost confined to children below the age of six years.

Characteristic features include:
- Fever for more than five days.
- Erythematous palms and soles followed by desquamation of skin from these areas.
- Conjunctival congestion.
- Strawberry tongue and swollen lips.
- Polymorphous rash.
- Non-purulent cervical lymphadenopathy.

Vasculitis commonly affects the coronary arteries causing micro-aneurysms, coronary thrombosis and myocardial infarction. Death is usually from cardiac failure following infarction. Features of cardiac involvement include tachycardia, prolonged PR interval, ST-segment elevation and T-wave inversion.

Other organs which may be affected include the lungs (pulmonary infiltrates), the brain (convulsions, cranial nerve palsies, deafness, CVA) and the gastrointestinal tract (abdominal pain from ischaemia). The small joints of the body may be affected in approximately 30% of cases.

The diagnosis is clinical. There are no specific tests, but inflammatory markers such as the ESR, CRP and platelets are elevated. The WCC is also elevated, as are the immunoglobulins. The haemoglobin may fall rapidly. Coronary involvement may be detected non-invasively by viewing the origins of the coronaries by echocardiography (324). This is not difficult in young children because they are thin.

The mainstay of treatment is oral aspirin and intravenous Sandoglobulin (c globulin). These reduce the mortality of the condition from more than 30% to less than 1%.

Differential diagnosis of Kawasaki's disease is streptococcal infection (scarlet fever), staphylococcal infection (scalded skin or toxic shock syndrome), Stevens–Johnson syndrome, juvenile chronic arthritis, leptospirosis, rickettsial infection and a generalized drug reaction.

Answer 325

> 1. The diagnosis is HIV seroconversion.
> 2. Repeat HIV antibody test.

HIV seroconversion occurs 2–6 weeks after HIV infection. The illness resembles infectious mononucleosis, comprising fever, pharyngitis, lymphadenopathy and a rash. The patient may have a mild anaemia, relative lymphopenia and thrombocytopenia. The blood film may reveal atypical lymphocytes (325). Other differential diagnoses include CMV infection, *Toxoplasma* infection and secondary syphilis.

Although secondary syphilis produces an identical syndrome to HIV seroconversion, the syphilis serology is

Positive syphilis serology in relation to the various stages of syphilis			
Test	*Primary syphilis (%)*	*Secondary syphilis (%)*	*Tertiary syphilis (%)*
VDRL	70	99	77
FTA	55	100	96
TPHA	80	99	95

suggestive of previous syphilis infection rather than secondary syphilis. In secondary syphilis, reagin antibodies become positive in almost 100% of cases, as do the more specific antibodies such as the FTA and the TPHA. However, the VDRL test becomes negative in over one-third of patients following therapy or in tertiary and quaternary syphilis, whereas the more specific antibodies persist in almost every patient, even after successful treatment (*Table*). In this case, the negative VDRL in a patient with a pharyngitis and a rash is against secondary syphilis, the more likely diagnosis being HIV

seroconversion. Persistent FTA suggests previous syphilis infection.

HIV IgG antibodies are detectable six weeks after infection with the virus. The detection of HIV antibody using a Western blot technique or ELISA is the most widely performed test if HIV infection is suspected. In the case of a negative HIV antibody test (usually in very early infection), the diagnosis may be confirmed by measuring HIV p24 antigen, a viral capsid protein which is detectable within 24 hours of the onset of illness. Alternatively, PCR methods may be used to detect viral RNA.

Question 326

A 39-year-old male presents with a three-month history of lower back pain. Over the past two years he has experienced three episodes of severe right lower quadrant pain.

Investigations are shown.

Sodium	138 mmol/l
Potassium	3.5 mmol/l
Chloride	119 mmol/l
Bicarbonate	13 mmol/l
Urea	7 mmol/l
Creatinine	112 µmol/l
Calcium	2.1 mmol/l
Phosphate	0.7 mmol/l

1. What is the diagnosis?
2. What single investigation would you perform to confirm the diagnosis?
3. What is the cause of his back pain?
4. List two simple investigations that may help to confirm the cause of his back pain.
5. What is the cause of his abdominal pain?
6. List two radiological tests that may help to confirm the cause of his abdominal pain.

Answer 326

1. Distal (type I) RTA.
2. Early morning urinary pH measurement or measurement of urine pH after ammonium chloride infusion.
3. Osteomalacia.
4. i. X-ray of the lumbar spine may reveal osteopenia or Looser's zones in osteomalacia.
   ii. Serum alkaline phosphatase level, which is characteristically raised in osteomalacia.
5. Renal colic.
6. i. Plain abdominal X-ray may identify a radio-opaque renal stone.
   ii. Intravenous urography is the investigation of choice to identify stones in the renal tract.

The biochemical results reveal a hypokalaemic, hyperchloraemic acidosis. In addition, there are low calcium and phosphate levels. These are features of RTA, which is characterized by abnormalities in urinary acidification. RTA may be divided into type 1 (distal RTA) and type 2 (proximal RTA). The causes and associations of renal tubular acidosis are tabulated below. Distal RTA is due to defective excretion of H+ in the distal convoluted tubule, and proximal RTA is due to failure of H+ secretion by the proximal convoluted tubule. In both cases there is hypokalaemia and hypercalcuria. Hypokalaemia can be explained as follows.

In distal RTA the defective H+ excretion means that the absorption of sodium requires increased potassium excretion. In proximal RTA there is excessive bicarbonate loss, which in turn results in excessive sodium loss. The resulting hypotension activates the renin–angiotensin–aldosterone system to aid sodium and water retention, but at the expense of potassium loss. Hypercalcuria is more common in distal RTA. Osteomalacia is common to both, but nephrocalcinosis and nephrolithiasis are confined to distal RTA.

Patients with distal RTA may present at any age. In children, the condition presents with failure to thrive. In adults, it presents with renal colic or muscle weakness from hypokalaemia. Patients with proximal RTA present with symptomatic acidosis, polydipsia, polyuria, hypokalaemic myopathy and rickets or osteomalacia. The diagnosis should be suspected if an individual has a hyperchloraemic acidosis, and can be confirmed by demonstrating an early morning urinary pH of >5.5. In some individuals in whom the diagnosis is suspected, but there is no evidence of systemic acidosis, an acid load test using ammonium chloride is required. This involves measuring urinary pH on samples collected hourly for 6 hours after the administration of intravenous ammonium chloride. Failure to acidify the urinary pH below 5.5 indicates RTA.

Treatment is with sodium bicarbonate and potassium citrate. The latter reduces calcium excretion and provides supplementary potassium.

Causes of RTA

Distal (Type 1)	Proximal (Type 2)
Inherited	Inherited
	Part of Fanconi's syndrome
Acquired	Acquired
Primary biliary cirrhosis	Hyperparathyroidism
CAH	Heavy metal poisoning (lead, arsenic)
Obstructive nephropathy	Myeloma
Vitamin D intoxication	Acetazolamide
Tetracycline	

Question 327

A 64-year-old female was admitted to hospital with a three-month history of increasing breathlessness and swollen ankles. She had been well until two-and-a-half years ago, when she experienced sudden onset of breathlessness while walking. She was observed in hospital overnight but was much improved the following day and allowed home. She had a further similar episode four months later, and then again a year later. On each occasion she improved within 24–48 hours. In between the two most recent episodes she had noticed that she was unable to exert herself as much without becoming breathless. There was no history of chest pain or a cough. Physical examination performed by the senior house officers during each hospital admission had been normal, with the exception of a sinus tachycardia of 110 beats/min. A chest X-ray performed on the admission one year ago is shown (**327a**). The patient had a past medical history of hysterectomy aged 43 years for menorrhagia due to uterine fibroids. Three years ago she had surgery for varicose veins of the lower limbs. She was a non-smoker. She was not taking any medication. She was a receptionist in a doctor's surgery for 20 years before retiring 20 years ago. She was married and lived with her husband. The couple had a dog and a parrot as pets.

On examination, she was breathless at rest and cyanosed. There was no clubbing. She had marked pitting lower-limb oedema up to her thighs. The heart rate was 102 beats/min and blood pressure 105/60 mmHg. The JVP was elevated to the level of the mastoid. Closer inspection revealed prominent c-v waves. On examination of the precordium, the apex was displaced to the anterior axillary line. There was a marked left parasternal heave. On auscultation of the precordium there was a soft systolic murmur and a loud fourth heart sound at the left lower sternal edge. The chest was clear. Abdominal examination demonstrated ascites and a pulsatile liver edge 5 cm below the costal margin. The ECG performed on admission is shown (**327b**).

Respiratory function tests performed on this admission are shown.

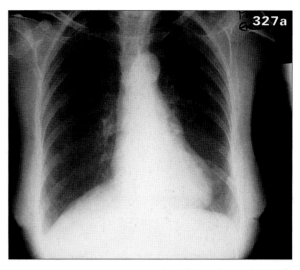

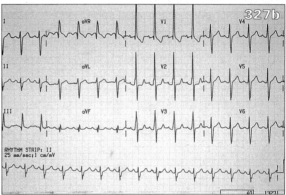

	Actual	Predicted
FEV$_1$ (l/min)	0.94	1.26–2.94
FVC (l/min)	1.12	1.82–3.81
TLC (l)	2.1	4.38–6.8
Transfer factor	3.4	4.2–8.8
Corrected transfer factor	0.4	0.7–1.62

What investigation is most likely to provide the diagnosis?
   a. Echocardiography.
   b. CT pulmonary angiography.
   c. High-resolution CT scan of the lungs.
   d. Arterial blood gases.
   e. Right heart catheter plus pulmonary angiography.

Answer 327

> e. Right heart catheter plus pulmonary angiography.

The patient has a history of progressive breathlessness, and now presents with ECG evidence of right ventricular hypertrophy and a clinical picture of severe right heart failure. Lung function tests demonstrate a restrictive defect and a low transfer factor. She has cor pulmonale complicating multiple pulmonary emboli, extrinsic allergic alveolitis, or CFA. The latter two diagnoses are unlikely in the absence of chest signs on three hospital admissions and the normal chest X-ray one year previously. In contrast the chest X-ray in multiple pulmonary emboli may appear relatively normal, the only evidence of pulmonary emboli being oligaemic lung fields. Another possible diagnosis is right heart failure due to chronic pulmonary hypertension from an ostium secundum ASD; however, the chest X-ray in this condition would reveal cardiomegaly. Investigations to confirm the diagnosis of multiple pulmonary emboli should include arterial blood gases (which will show low PaO_2 and $PaCO_2$ due to severe ventilation/perfusion mismatch) and a ventilation–perfusion scan to demonstrate perfusion defects. A right heart catheter combined with pulmonary angiography would provide the most diagnostic information and would be useful in assessing the severity of pulmonary hypertension. Spiral CT scan of the thorax is an increasingly popular method of identifying peripheral pulmonary emboli, which may be difficult to detect with angiography. Echocardiography is useful in excluding an ASD with shunt reversal or tight mitral stenosis. Echo-Doppler may be useful in quantifying pulmonary artery pressure; however, it has no direct role in the diagnosis of multiple pulmonary emboli.

Question 328

A 42-year-old, insulin-dependent diabetic was investigated further after he was noted to have a positive dipstick for protein on urine analysis. He was diagnosed with diabetes at the age of 23 years after presenting with ketoacidosis. Initial management with porcine insulin was good; however, he was switched to human insulin 10 years ago because of severe lipoatrophy at sites of injection. Over the past three years blood glucose control had been suboptimal, and the dose of insulin had been increased on five occasions. He was married with two children. He owned a grocer's shop which was open seven days a week and was staffed by the patient and his wife at all times. He smoked five cigarettes per day. He did not consume alcohol.

On examination, he had bilateral corneal arcus. His heart rate was 80 beats/min and regular; blood pressure was 150/90 mmHg. There was no evidence of cardiac enlargement or cardiac failure. The peripheral pulses were all palpable, and there were no audible bruits over the carotid arteries or in the abdomen. Examination of his fundi is shown (328a).

Investigations are shown below.

Hb	12.8 g/dl	Glycosylated Hb	9% (normal range 3.8–6.4%)
WCC	6 × 10⁹/l	Cholesterol	8.2 mmol/l
Platelets	212 × 10⁹/l	Triglycerides	8 mmol/l
MCV	89 fl	24-hour urinalysis	Volume 2.7 l
Sodium	136 mmol/l		Protein 0.7 g/l
Potassium	3.4 mmol/l	Renal US	Two kidneys, 12 cm each
Urea	6.8 mmol/l		Normal parenchymal texture
Creatinine	117 µmol/l		
Glucose	11 mmol/l	Renal biopsy (328b [haematoxylin and eosin stain])	

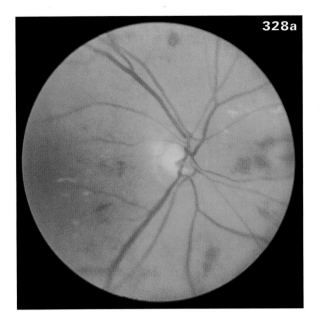

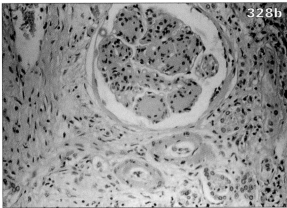

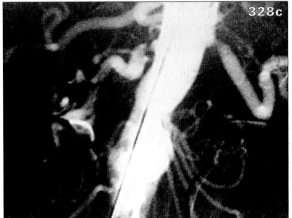

The patient was commenced on captopril, the dose of which was gradually increased to 50 mg, three times daily. Three months later, the patient was admitted with vague abdominal discomfort, nausea and anorexia. On examination, he appeared euvolaemic. The blood pressure was 120/65 mmHg.

Investigations are shown.

Another investigation was performed, which is shown (**328c**).

Sodium	133 mmol/l
Potassium	6.4 mmol/l
Urea	32 mmol/l
Creatinine	500 µmol/l
Glucose	10 mmol/l

1. What is demonstrated on the examination of the fundi?
2. What is shown on the renal biopsy?
3. What is the cause of his proteinuria?
4. What was the cause of the marked deterioration in renal function?
5. List six management strategies to help ameliorate the renal function and the rate of future deterioration in renal function.

Question 329

A 16-year-old female was brought into the Accident and Emergency Department with shortness of breath.

Blood gases on inspiring room air are shown.

pH	7.49
$PaCO_2$	2.4 kPa
PaO_2	15.5 kPa
Bicarbonate	12 mmol/l
O_2 saturation	96%

1. What is the acid–base disturbance?
2. What is the underlying cause?
3. What is the management?

Answer 328

> 1. Small retinal haemorrhages, and micro-aneurysms consistent with background diabetic retinopathy.
> 2. There is evidence of eosin staining (pink) fibrotic (hyaline) nodules characteristic of diabetic glomerulosclerosis, sometimes known as Kimmelsteil–Wilson nodules.
> 3. Diabetic nephropathy. Other causes of protein in the urine in diabetics include a urinary tract infection.
> 4. Angiotensin-converting enzyme inhibitor-induced glomerular hypoperfusion in a patient with bilateral renal artery stenosis.
> 5. i. Stop ACE inhibitor.
>   ii. Bilateral renal angioplasty.
>   iii. Improve diabetic control.
>   iv. Control hyperlipidaemia.
>   v. Ensure blood pressure below 140/85 mmHg.
>   vi. Advise against smoking.

Overt diabetic nephropathy is based on the demonstration of over 0.5 mg of protein on a 24-hour urinary collection. A protein content of this level is easily detected on a urine dipstick. More recently, it has been noted that some patients pass small amounts of albumin in the urine (0.02–0.3 mg/24 h) before the development of a positive dipstick test. Such patients are said to have 'micro-albuminuria' or incipient diabetic nephropathy.

The prevalence of diabetic nephropathy in the UK is 4–8%. The pathological basis for this is diabetic glomerulosclerosis, as shown in the renal biopsy (328b).

Patients with diabetic nephropathy have an increased mortality from cardiovascular and renal causes. Poor glycaemic control, raised blood pressure and smoking expedite the development and progression of nephropathy. In patients with early nephropathy the GFR is increased, and the associated hyperinfiltration is thought to damage glomeruli by increasing the intraglomerular capillary blood pressure. Patients with nephropathy very often also have retinopathy, and *vice versa*.

The management includes good glycaemic control, maintaining blood pressure below 135/85 mmHg (this slows the rate of fall in the GFR rate by 60%). ACE inhibitors reduce albumin excretion in patients with micro-albuminuria. In diabetic rats, ACE inhibitors reduce intraglomerular capillary pressure and prevent a decline in GFR. Whether they have the same effect in humans is currently under investigation. Renal function should be observed carefully after the initiation of an ACE inhibitor because they may precipitate renal failure in patients with silent renal artery stenosis, as in this case. Renal failure is precipitated by reduction in the pressure within the afferent arteriole, which causes a significant decrease in glomerular perfusion pressure in the presence of renal artery stenosis (328c).

Answer 329

> 1. There is a respiratory alkalosis and a metabolic acidosis.
> 2. Aspirin toxicity (see also Answer 172).
> 3. The management is dependent on the serum salicylate level. Levels below 500 mg/l are treated with intravenous saline to promote renal clearance. Levels between 500 and 750 mg/l are treated with intravenous bicarbonate but may require forced alkaline diuresis on a high-dependency unit. Levels between 750 and 1,000 mg/l are best treated with haemodialysis.

There is a low $PaCO_2$ and a high pH, suggesting a respiratory alkalosis. The serum bicarbonate is very low, indicating a coexistent metabolic acidosis. In chronic respiratory alkalosis there would be increased excretion of bicarbonate ions in an attempt to lower the arterial pH; however, the bicarbonate concentration is only modestly reduced. (See Acid-base Disturbance, page 426.)

Question 330

A 46-year-old garage mechanic was investigated in a medical clinic for weight loss. Six months previously he had commenced a voluntary diet to reduce weight. He lost 4 kg over two months, following which he stopped his diet. Despite a normal appetite he continued to lose another 4 kg in weight over the next four months. He had also noticed that he tired easily, and was finding it difficult to perform heavy manual work as part of his profession. His arms felt weak. He was breathless on strenuous effort and found heavy lifting increasingly difficult. More recently, he had developed lower back pain which was worse when he sat upright and was associated with pain and numbness of his left calf and left foot. The pain was worsened by movement and he was forced to stop working. His appetite remained good. He had moved his bowels twice daily ever since he could remember. The stool was of normal consistency and did not contain blood. He was married with three children. He stopped smoking 15 years ago after an attack of bronchitis. He consumed 2–3 units of alcohol per week.

On examination, he was of relative heavy build. There was no evidence of pallor or clubbing. The heart rate was 102 beats/min and irregularly irregular. The blood pressure was 130/80 mmHg. The JVP was not raised. On examination of the upper limbs there was no muscle tenderness, but there was wasting of the proximal muscles of the upper limb with weakness of abduction and adduction. The upper limb reflexes were brisk. Sensory testing was normal. On examination of the lower limbs, there was wasting of the muscles of the thighs. Power testing demonstrated weakness of plantar flexion on the left side. Reflexes were brisk with the exception of the left ankle jerk, which was absent. Plantar responses were normal. Sensory testing demonstrated reduced pin-prick sensation affecting the anterolateral aspect of the left foot.

Investigations are shown.

Hb	14 g/dl
WCC	6×10^9/l
Platelets	210×10^9/l
ESR	10 mm/h
Chest X-ray	Normal
Sodium	135 mmol/l
Potassium	3.4 mmol/l
Urea	5 mmol/l
Calcium	2.4 mmol/l
Phosphate	1 mmol/l
Albumin	40 g/l

1. What is the cause of the absent ankle jerk?
   a. Paraneoplastic syndrome.
   b. Prolapsed intervertebral disc between L4/L5.
   c. Prolapsed intervertebral disc between L5/S1.
   d. Peripheral neuropathy.
   e. Mononeuritis multiplex.
2. What is the diagnosis?.
   a. Polymyositis.
   b. Polymyalgia rheumatica.
   c. Thyrotoxic myopathy.
   d. Eaton–Lambert syndrome.
   e. Paraneoplastic syndrome.

Question 331

This ECG (**331**) is from a 35-year-old male with sudden onset of expressive dysphasia and right upper-limb weakness. On examination, he was apyrexial. The heart rate was 100 beats/min and regular; blood pressure was 110/80 mmHg. He had a soft systolic murmur. There were no carotid bruits. He had been well and asymptomatic all his life, and was a non-smoker.

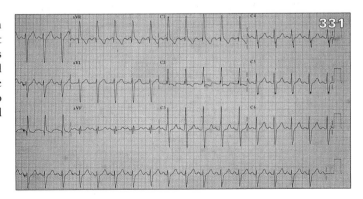

1. List three abnormalities.
2. What is the most likely cause of his murmur?
3. What is the most probable cause of his neurological signs?

Answer 330

> 1. c. Prolapsed intervertebral disc between L5/S1.
> 2. c. Thyrotoxic myopathy.

The patient has weight loss, despite a normal appetite. The differential diagnosis for this scenario is malabsorption, diabetes mellitus, phaeochromocytoma and thyrotoxicosis. He has atrial fibrillation, which is most consistent with thyrotoxicosis. He also has proximal muscle wasting of his limbs, a well-known feature of thyrotoxic myopathy. A paraneoplastic syndrome is unlikely because there is no immediate evidence of an underlying neoplastic process. For similar reasons, he is unlikely to have Eaton–Lambert syndrome, which is a myasthenic syndrome associated with malignancy. Proximal myopathy is a feature, but reflexes are absent. In contrast to myasthenia, weakness improves with repetitive muscular stimulation. Both polymyalgia rheumatica and polymyositis are associated with muscle tenderness and a raised ESR, which are absent in this patient. Furthermore, polymyalgia rheumatica is a disorder that affects the elderly rather than young patients.

The chronic back pain worsened by movement and radiating to his left calf is consistent with a lumbar radiculopathy. A lateral disc protrusion is most likely. An absent ankle jerk (S1), weakness of dorsiflexion of the left side, and impaired sensation of the anterolateral aspect of the foot (L5 and S1) is consistent with an L5/S1 disc prolapse. In the case of an L4/L5 lesion the knee jerk would be absent. A peripheral neuropathy or mononeuritis multiplex cannot explain the root symptoms (back pain radiating to calf and made worse with movement) or the lack of neuropathy elsewhere (all other reflexes preserved).

Answer 331

> 1. i. Right axis deviation.
>   ii. RBBB.
>   iii. Voltage criteria for right ventricular hypertrophy.
> 2. Ostium secundum ASD.
> 3. Paradoxical embolus from the systemic veins.

The combination of right axis deviation and RBBB in a young, previously asymptomatic man with a soft systolic murmur is suggestive of an underlying ostium secundum ASD. Ostium primum defects are associated with left axis deviation and RBBB. Although both pulmonary stenosis and VSDs can produce similar ECG changes, a soft murmur in a patient with a VSD is suggestive of a large defect which would almost certainly cause symptoms of cardiovascular dysfunction before the third decade. Mild pulmonary stenosis is characterized by lack of symptoms and a soft systolic murmur, heard best in the left second intercostal space, but this is not usually enough to cause right ventricular hypertrophy. Moreover, it does not explain the neurological defect in this case, which has resulted from a paradoxical embolus of thrombus within the systemic veins to the brain via a defect in the interatrial septum. Paradoxical embolism is a rare but well-recognized complication of all septal defects. Thrombus from the systemic veins may result in emboli to the brain, limbs and gastrointestinal tract. Paradoxical embolus may be the presenting feature in a patient with a cardiac septal defect.

The differential diagnosis is a mycotic embolus complicating infective endocarditis involving an ASD; however, the patient is not febrile and infective endocarditis very rarely involves an ASD.

Question 332

A 22-year-old basketball player presented with sudden onset of severe left-sided chest pain radiating into his neck four hours before he was due to play in a large tournament. He had never experienced any previous chest pain, and was extremely fit, according to his team coach.

On examination, he was distressed with chest pain. His heart rate was 70 beats/min and blood pressure 190/110 mmHg. Examination of the precordium and the chest was normal. An ECG was performed immediately (332), and he was subsequently admitted to the Coronary Care Unit. The following day he was asymptomatic and his blood pressure was normal. Examination of his fundi did not demonstrate any fundal changes of hypertension, and general examination did not reveal any peripheral stigmata of hyperlipidaemia. He denied any previous history of hypertension, diabetes mellitus or a family history of coronary artery disease. He had never smoked previously.

Investigations following admission are shown.

An echocardiogram performed three days later demonstrated minor apical hypokinesia, but satisfactory overall systolic function. Coronary angiography before discharge was entirely normal.

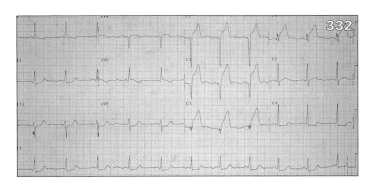

Hb	13 g/dl
WCC	12×10^9/l
Platelets	204×10^9/l
Sodium	139 mmol/l
Potassium	3.9 mmol/l
Glucose	4.2 mmol/l
Creatinine kinase	560 iu/l

1. What important piece of information should be elicited in the history to help ascertain the cause of his chest pain?
2. Which drug would you use in the management of his hypertension?

Question 333

A 66-year-old male with a long history of breathlessness presented with a three-day history of profound breathlessness and a cough productive of yellow sputum.

Arterial blood gases are shown.

pH	7.33
$PaCO_2$	8.8kPa
PaO_2	6.5kPa
Bicarbonate	36 mmol/l
Base excess	+11

What is the acid–base abnormality?
   a. Acute respiratory acidosis.
   b. Metabolic alkalosis.
   c. Partially compensated respiratory acidosis.
   d. Compensated respiratory acidosis.
   e. Compensated metabolic alkalosis.

Answer 332

> 1. A history of amphetamine abuse.
> 2. A calcium channel blocker such as amlodipine or verapamil.

The clinical scenario is that of an elite athlete presenting with an acute myocardial infarction but subsequently he has normal coronary arteries, although the echocardiogram is indicative of myocardial damage. While there are several causes of myocardial ischaemia despite normal coronary arteries (*Table A*), the possibility of cocaine (an amphetamine) abuse should be considered.

Cocaine abuse has reached epidemic proportions in some groups of elite athletes; however, the incidence of cardiac complications remains low. Cocaine inhibits re-uptake of the catecholamine neurotransmitter noradrenaline, which is a potent vasoconstrictor. By this mechanism it may induce coronary artery spasm and myocardial infarction. The drug has also been implicated in causing myocarditis through direct effects on the heart. In addition, its local anaesthetic properties block the fast inward sodium and slow calcium currents within myocardial cells, thereby predisposing to lethal ventricular arrhythmias. Cocaine also prolongs the QT-interval and increases the risk of torsades de pointes-type polymorphic ventricular tachycardia. Arrhythmias are best treated by antiarrhythmic agents which do not prolong the QT-interval. Beta-blockers are contraindicated in the management of cocaine-induced cardiac problems because they would result in unopposed alpha activity, causing profound vasoconstriction. Cocaine is a relatively rare cause of sudden death in young elite athletes. Relatively more common causes are shown (*Table B*).

Non-cardiac causes of mortality from cocaine include CVA, status epilepticus and rhabdomyolysis.

Table A Myocardial ischaemia/infarction with normal coronary arteries

- HCM
- Aortic stenosis
- Hypertensive heart disease
- Coronary arteritis, particularly polyarteritis nodosa
- Coronary artery embolus secondary to intramural thrombus or vegetation
- Severe anaemia
- Thyrotoxicosis
- Phaeochromocytoma
- Cocaine
- Amphetamines

Table B Causes of sudden cardiac death in young elite athletes

- HCM (almost 50% of all cases)
- Coronary artery anomalies
- Arrhythmogenic right ventricular cardiomyopathy
- Myocarditis
- Mitral valve prolapse
- Wolff–Parkinson–White syndrome
- LQTS
- Drug abuse
- Sarcoidosis
- Rhabdomyolysis
- Heatstroke
- Commotio cordis

Answer 333

> c. Partially compensated respiratory acidosis.

The high $PaCO_2$ and low pH is diagnostic of respiratory acidosis. The arterial bicarbonate is high, indicating that there is increased absorption of bicarbonate ions by the kidney in an attempt to normalize the pH. As the pH is still slightly lower than normal, this is most accurately termed partial compensation. (See Acid–base Disturbance, page 426.)

Question 334

A 16-year-old Turkish female was referred to the gynaecological outpatient clinic with a 14-month history of amenorrhoea. She started menstruating at the age of 13 years. She had almost regular periods until the age of 14 and after this had three scanty periods and none for the past year. She was born in Turkey and had only recently come to England. At the age of nine years she had been commenced on hydrocortisone 15 mg in the morning and 10 mg in the evening for an illness about which both parents were very vague. Apart from occasional dizziness on standing suddenly, and infrequent headaches, there was no other past history of note. She had an 18-year-old sister who was well. Her parents were first cousins. Her father worked as a tailor and her mother was a housewife. None of them spoke much English.

Examination was declined by the patient, but the height and weight were recorded (1.52 m (under 50th centile) and 42 kg (less than 3rd centile)), and the blood pressure measured (90/60 mmHg).

Investigations are shown.

Hb	13 g/dl	17-hydroxyprogesterone	23 nmol/l
WCC	7×10^9/l		(NR <5 nmol/l)
Platelets	200×10^9/l	Androstenedione	16 nmol/l
Sodium	138 mmol/l		(NR 5–12 nmol/l)
Potassium	4.0 mmol/l	Dihydroepiandrostenedione	21 nmol/l
Urea	4 mmol/l		(NR <12 nmol/l)
Creatinine	60 µmol/l	Recumbent plasma renin	9 pmol/l/ml/h
Blood sugar	5 mmol/l		(NR 0.2–2.2 pmol/l/ml/h)
Calcium	2.4 mmol/l	Ambulant plasma renin	12 pmol/l
Phosphate	1.0 mmol/l		(NR 1.2–4.4 pmol/l)
AST	22 iu/l	Prolactin	385 mu/l
Alkaline phosphatase	179 iu/l		(NR <450 mu/l)
Thyroxine	18 pmol/l	Urinary pregnantetriol	Elevated +++
TSH	3.1 mu/l	US ovaries	Normal-sized ovaries
FSH	5 u/l (NR 1–7 iu/l)		containing multiple
LH	8 u/l (NR 2–20 iu/l)		cysts
Oestradiol	90 pmol/l		Small uterus
	(NR 40–92 pmol/l)		
Testosterone	9 nmol/l (NR 1–3 nmol/l)		

1. What is the diagnosis?
2. Which other drug should this patient be given?
3. Suggest at least three possible causes for the amenorrhoea.

Question 335

A 75-year-old male was investigated for increasing dyspnoea.

Results of investigations are shown.

Chamber	Pressure (cmH$_2$O)	Oxygen saturation (%)
Right atrium	6	65
Right ventricle	25/6	67
Pulmonary artery pressure	25/18	67
PCWP (mean)	16	
Left ventricle	210/18	98
Aorta	210/55	98

What sign would you ascertain on auscultation of the precordium?
   a. Ejection systolic murmur in the aortic area.
   b. Prominent right ventricular in pulse.
   c. Fixed splitting of the second heart sound.
   d. Long early diastolic murmur at left lower sternal edge and in the aortic area.
   e. Soft mid-diastolic rumbling murmur in the mitral area.

Answer 334

1. Congenital adrenal hyperplasia (21-hydroxylase deficiency).
2. Fludrocortisone.
3. i. Underweight.
   ii. Inadequate treatment for congenital adrenal hyperplasia.
   iii. Elevated testosterone.
   iv. Coexistent polycystic ovary syndrome.

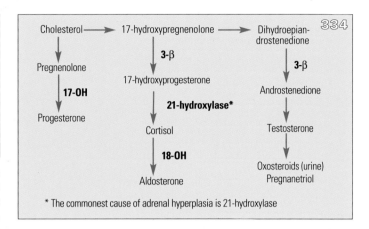

334

* The commonest cause of adrenal hyperplasia is 21-hydroxylase

The presenting complaint of amenorrhoea has a wide differential diagnosis (*Table A*); however, the endocrine tests are most compatible with the diagnosis of congenital adrenal hyperplasia. Congenital adrenal hyperplasia may be caused by a number of enzyme defects in the biosynthetic pathway for steroid hormone synthesis within the adrenal gland. The deficiencies are inherited as an autosomal recessive trait. The most common abnormality by far is 21-hydroxylase deficiency, the gene for which is on chromosome 6 (adjacent to the HLA B locus). The enzyme is responsible for the conversion of 17-hydroxyprogesterone to cortisol (**334**).

21-hydroxylase deficiency leads to elevated 17-hydroxyprogesterone, which is metabolized to adrenal androgens. These ketosteroids (particularly pregnanetetriol) are found in high concentrations in the urine. The patients are cortisol-deficient, and some may also have aldosterone deficiency. Patients with severe 21-hydroxylase deficiency present in infancy with vomiting and failure to thrive. Ambiguous genitalia are common. Males may have hypospadias and females may have fusion of the labia. Males with mild deficiency may present with precocious puberty and females with primary amenorrhoea, hirsutism and virilism. Hirsutism occurring before menarche is suggestive of congenital adrenal hyperplasia. Lack of cortisol is responsible for high ACTH levels, which continue to drive the biosynthetic pathway.

Laboratory investigations reveal an elevated plasma 17-hydroxyprogesterone and ACTH. Urinary pregnanetriol (ketosteroid) levels are also elevated. Treatment is with hydrocortisone replacement. The dose is similar to that used in Addison's disease. The therapeutic response is judged by suppression of the urinary pregnanetriol levels to the upper limit of normal. Considerable care should be taken not to give a very high dose of hydrocortisone, as this may stunt growth. Patients with aldosterone deficiency as judged by an elevated renin level and postural hypotension should receive fludrocortisone.

In this patient there are several potential causes of amenorrhoea. The most obvious cause is her very low weight (*Table A*). Another important cause is the raised testosterone levels caused by an inadequate dose of hydrocortisone. The dose should be enough to inhibit ACTH secretion and suppress androgen synthesis. In this case, the adrenal androgen levels (dihydroepiandrostenedione) are very high. The patient also has evidence of polycystic ovaries, which are themselves a cause of primary amenorrhoea but may coexist with hyperandrogenic states such as congenital adrenal hyperplasia and Cushing's syndrome. The differential diagnoses of congenital adrenal hyperplasia are shown (*Table B*).

Differentiating congenital adrenal hyperplasia from arrhenoblastoma is usually easy because in the former cortisol levels are low and dihydroepiandrosterone sulphate is high. Similarly, congenital adrenal hyperplasia can easily be distinguished from Cushing's syndrome by measuring serum cortisol and ACTH.

Table A Causes of amenorrhoea

- Physiological (pregnancy)
- Systemic disease (e.g. coeliac disease)
- Weight loss
- Anorexia nervosa
- Excessive stress
- Hypopituitarism
- Prolactinoma
- Primary ovarian failure
- Congenital adrenal hyperplasia
- PCOS
- Cushing's syndrome
- Androgen-secreting adrenal tumour
- Arrhenoblastoma

Table B Differential diagnoses of mild 21-hydroxylase deficiency

- Polycystic ovaries
- Androgen-secreting adrenal tumour
- Arrhenoblastoma
- Cushing's syndrome

Differentiation from an adrenal androgen-secreting tumour is possible by performing a low-dose dexamethasone suppression test, which will reduce urinary pregnanetriol levels in congenital adrenal hyperplasia, but not in an adrenal androgen-secreting tumour.

The differentiation from PCOS is possible by measuring 17-hydroxyprogesterone levels and dihydroepiandrosterone sulphate, both of which are high in congenital adrenal hyperplasia. Alternatively, a synacthen test may be performed which is associated with a normal cortisol response in PCOS, but not in congenital adrenal hyperplasia.

Answer 335

> d. Long early diastolic murmur at left lower sternal edge and in the aortic area.

The only abnormality is the very wide pulse pressure in the ascending aorta, which would be consistent with the diagnosis of aortic regurgitation. (See Interpretation of Cardiac Catheter Data, page 418.)

Question 336

A 58-year-old male presented with nausea and pain in his right upper quadrant. On examination he had tender hepatomegaly with an irregular edge.

Investigations are shown.

Hb	8 g/dl
WCC	$18 \times 10^9/l$
Platelets	$100 \times 10^9/l$
Neutrophils	68%
Normoblasts	8%
Myeloblasts	8%
Myelocytes	4%
Metamyelocytes	6%
Lymphocytes	15%

1. What is the cause of his anaemia?
   a. Chronic myeloid leukaemia.
   b. Marrow infiltration by malignant cells.
   c. Aplastic anaemia.
   d. Myelofibrosis.
   e. Hydatid disease.

2. What investigation would you perform to confirm the diagnosis?
   a. Bone marrow trephine.
   b. Bone scan.
   c. Ultrasound of the liver.
   d. Blood analysis for Philadelphia chromosome.
   e. Leucocyte alkaline phosphatase level.

Question 337

A 13-year-old male was admitted to hospital with complete loss of vision in his right eye. He had been placed in a juvenile offenders' residential home six months ago for stealing on several occasions. His parents had separated a few months previously, and before that he had been living with his father, who was an alcohol abuser, and had three dogs. Two weeks before admission he had complained of reduced visual acuity in his right eye, which had progressively become worse.

On examination, he appeared well. He had generalized lymphadenopathy, and was clinically blind in the right eye. Examination of the fundus in the right eye revealed two large, raised white lesions situated adjacent to the optic disc and in the macular region. He was apyrexial and all other physical examinations were normal.

Investigations are shown.

Hb	11.4 g/dl
WCC	$6.6 \times 10^9/l$ (differential below)
Platelets	$180 \times 10^9/l$
Neutrophils	$4.1 \times 10^9/l$
Lymphocytes	$1.2 \times 10^9/l$
Eosinophils	$1.1 \times 10^9/l$
Monocytes	$0.11 \times 10^9/l$
Basophils	$0.09 \times 10^9/l$
ESR	25 mm/h
Biochemistry	Normal

1. What is the diagnosis?
2. List two investigations useful in confirming the diagnosis.

Answer 336

1. b. Marrow infiltration by malignant cells.
2. a. Bone marrow trephine.

Causes of a leucoerythroblastic anaemia

- Malignant infiltration of any type
- Storage disorders, e.g. Gaucher's disease
- Myelosclerosis
- Marble bone disease (osteopetrosis)
- Leukaemoid reaction secondary to severe infections

The patient has a leucoerythroblastic anaemia (*Table*), which is characterized by immature granulocytes and red cells (normoblasts) in the peripheral blood film. This characteristically occurs when the marrow is replaced by malignant cells, cells containing metabolic products of storage disorders, fibrous tissue and bone. Leukaemias, lymphoma, adenocarcinoma, myeloma and myeloproliferative disease are all capable of malignant infiltration. In this case, the patient has a 'knobbly' liver, suggesting liver metastases most probably from a primary lung carcinoma. Carcinoma of the lung also metastasizes to the bone and may result in marrow infiltration by malignant cells. Other causes of a leucoerythroblastic anaemia are tabulated above. In marble bone disease bony replacement of the marrow causes the leucoerythroblastic anaemia. In myelosclerosis the cause is extensive fibrosis within the marrow space, and in Gaucher's disease the cause is large white cells laden with glucocerebrosides.

Answer 337

1. Ocular *Toxocara* infection or ocular larva migrans.
2. i. IgM antibodies to *Toxocara* in the aqueous or vitreous humour of the eye.
   ii. IgM antibodies to *Toxocara* in the blood.

The patient has contracted *Toxocara* infection from the dogs. Toxocariasis is due to migrating larvae of the parasite *T. canis*. The disease occurs where there is a large dog or cat population. It is well-recognized in the Western world, and it is estimated that approximately 2–3% of the population carry antibodies to the parasite. The parasite is carried in dogs (*T. canis*) and cats (*T. cati*). Embryonated eggs are passed into faeces and may be ingested by humans, particularly children in close contact with cats and dogs (ingestion of contaminated fur or soil). The larvae from the eggs hatch out into the small intestine and migrate to liver, lungs and brain, where they stimulate local granuloma formation by the immune system. They do not mature into adult worms.

Toxocariasis can produce two distinct clinical patterns; the classical visceral larva migrans syndrome, and ocular toxocariasis. Most children who develop the classical larva migrans remain asymptomatic. The minority develop myalgia, cough and anorexia. An urticarial rash is not uncommon. Physical examination may reveal lymphadenopathy and hepatosplenomegaly. The blood picture comprises a neutrophil leucocytosis and a significant eosinophilia. The acute illness is of 2–3 weeks' duration, following which complete recovery is usual. In some individuals complete recovery may take as long as two years. The diagnosis is made by demonstrating positive antibodies to the secretory or excretory products of *Toxocara*. Liver biopsy may demonstrate granulomas with eosinophilic infiltration.

Ocular toxocariasis is characterized by granuloma formation in the eye. If the macular area is involved, blindness may occur. The general manifestations of classical visceral larva migrans and accompanying eosinophilia may be absent. Physical examination reveals a round swelling near the optic disc. The diagnosis is made by the demonstration of IgM antibodies to *Toxocara* in the aqueous or vitreous humour.

Treatment of the classical visceral larva migrans is with thiabendazole or diethylcarbamazine. Ocular toxocariasis is treated with laser photocoagulation. Local or intraocular steroids may be used as adjunct therapy.

Question 338

A 58-year-old man presented with recent onset of epigastric burning that was precipitated by hunger or after a heavy meal. His appetite was unchanged and his weight was stable. He was a non-smoker and did not consume alcohol. The patient took paracetamol only for a painful left hip.

Investigations are shown.

Hb	11 g/dl
MCV	70 fl
Ferritin	20 iu/l
Colonoscopy	Normal
H. pylori urease test	Positive
Upper gastrointestinal endoscopy showed small duodenal ulcer	

The patient was treated with *H. pylori* eradication therapy and was completely asymptomatic when reviewed six weeks later. The Hb was 13 g/dl.

What is the next management step?
a. Reassure and discharge. Review again if he becomes symptomatic.
b. Continue with proton pump inhibitor indefinitely.
c. Repeat upper gastrointestinal endoscopy to ensure the ulcer has healed.
d. Repeat urease breath test to ensure eradication therapy is successful.
e. Cimetidine therapy indefinitely.

Question 339

A 72-year-old woman underwent upper gastrointestinal endoscopy for epigastric discomfort, which revealed mild antral gastritis. She had a history of transient ischaemic attacks for which she was taking aspirin 75 mg daily. The patient also took regular diclofenac for arthritis. The urease breath test for *H. pylori* was negative.

What is the best management of her epigastric symptoms?
a. Start omeprazole 20 mg daily.
b. Switch patient from aspirin to clopidogrel.
c. Switch patient from diclofenac to rofecoxib.
d. Start ranitidine 300 mg daily.
e. Start misoprostil.

Question 340

A 68-year-old woman presented with lethargy, mild weight loss, weakness, and progressive pain and stiffness of her shoulders and thighs. On examination, she had tender shoulder and thigh muscles and a fever of 38°C (100.4°F).

Investigations are shown.

Hb	11 g/dl
WCC	13×10^9/l
Platelets	160×10^9/l
ESR	85 mm/h
Rheumatoid factor	1/640
AST	86 iu/l
ALT	296 iu/l
Alkaline phosphatase	100 iu/l
Bilirubin	12 μmol/l
LDH	1500 iu/l

What is the diagnosis?
a. Polymyositis.
b. Polymyalgia rheumatica.
c. Rheumatoid arthritis.
d. Primary biliary cirrhosis.
e. SLE.

Answer 338

> a. Reassure and discharge. Review again if he becomes symptomatic.

This patient with dyspepsia had iron deficiency anaemia, which is an indication for upper gastrointestinal endoscopy. He has a duodenal ulcer and has evidence of *H. pylori* infection. His symptoms have been successfully treated with eradication therapy. He does not warrant any further investigation unless he has a recurrence of symptoms. Over 90% of duodenal ulcers secondary to *H. pylori* infection heal following eradication therapy. (See Answer 369.)

Answer 339

> e. Start misoprostil.

Gastroduodenal toxicity secondary to non-steroidal anti-inflammatory drugs (NSAIDs) is relatively common. The patient takes two NSAIDs, namely diclofenac and aspirin. The best treatment would be to stop both drugs, but she needs diclofenac for the treatment of her arthritis and aspirin to reduce the risk of transient ischaemic attacks. Until recently patients experiencing intolerable gastroduodenal side-effects from NSAIDs used for arthritis were switched from NSAIDs to COX II inhibitors such as rofecoxib; however, the latter group of drugs have been associated with an increased frequency of adverse cardiovascular events and have been withdrawn from the market.

The patient requires aspirin to prevent adverse cardiovascular and cerebrovascular events. Although clopidogrel has fewer gastroduodenal side-effects than aspirin, it is not free from gastroduodenal toxicity itself. Proven therapies that prevent gastroduodenal toxicity resulting from NSAIDs include treatment with misoprostil, a prostaglandin E analogue, or lansoprazole, a proton pump inhibitor. None of the other proton pump inhibitors have been proven or tested (in large trials) to be effective in this situation. H2 blockers are not effective in preventing gastroduodenal toxicity. Instead of stopping both diclofenac and aspirin, the best treatment would be to add misoprostil.

Answer 340

> a. Polymyositis.

The differential diagnosis is between polymyalgia rheumatica and polymyositis (*Table*). Both present with lethargy and weakness, and both may cause a polyarthropathy and tender muscles; however, elevated muscle enzymes and positive serology for rheumatoid arthritis are more characteristic of polymyositis. In 20%, anti-jo-1 antibodies may be present.

Polymyositis versus polymyalgia rheumatica		
	Polymyositis	*Polymyalgia rheumatica*
Muscle tenderness	Common	Common
Muscle wasting	Common	May occur
Proximal myopathy	Present	Recognized
Headaches	Absent	May be present
Skin involvement	Present (30%)	Absent
Raised enzymes	Present (usually)	Absent
ANA	Present (30%)	Absent
Rh factor	Present	Absent
Anti-jo-1 Abs	Present (20%)	Absent

Question 341

A 74-year-old male presented with sudden onset of dyspnoea. There was no preceding history of a cough or chest trauma. He was a smoker. Four weeks previously he had had a right knee replacement. There was a past history of prostatic carcinoma, which was being controlled with antiandrogen therapy. On examination he was not cyanosed. The heart rate was 90 beats/min and blood pressure was 140/88 mmHg. The JVP was not raised. Both heart sounds were normal. Auscultation of the lungs revealed decreased air entry at the left lung base. The lower limbs appeared normal.

Investigations are shown.

Arterial blood gases (air):
pH	7.45
$PaCO_2$	3.4 kPa
PaO_2	9.1 kPa
HCO_3	21 mmol/l
Chest X-ray	Left lower lobe shadowing
ECG	Non-specific T wave flattening in leads V5 and V6
	Inverted T waves in III and aVf

What is the diagnostic investigation of choice?
 a. Ventilation–perfusion lung scan.
 b. Serum cardiac troponin level.
 c. Echocardiography.
 d. CT pulmonary angiography.
 e. Serum d-dimer assay.

Question 342

A 70-year-old patient presented with dizziness (**342**).

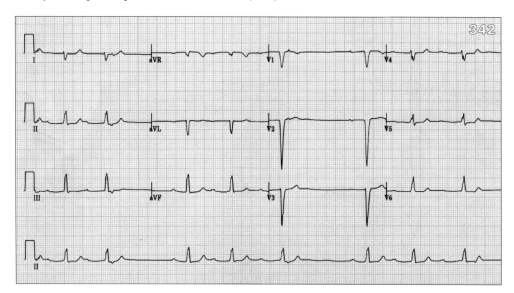

What is the ECG diagnosis?
 a. Third degree AV block.
 b. Mobitz type II second degree AV block.
 c. First degree AV block.
 d. Nodal bradycardia.
 e. Mobitz type I second degree AV block.

Answer 341

> d. CT pulmonary angiography.

The patient presents with sudden onset of dyspnoea in the absence of a lower respiratory tract infection or pulmonary oedema. He has a major risk factor for venous thromboembolism, having had a recent knee replacement. A coexisting history of prostatic carcinoma may also contribute to his risk of venous thromboembolism. Therefore the clinical probability of the presentation being secondary to pulmonary embolism is high. The probability of PE is calculated by (a) demonstrating the absence of another reasonable clinical explanation of the presentation and (b) the presence of a major risk factor (*Table*). If both (a) and (b) are present the probability of PE is high; if either (a) or (b) is present the probability is intermediate; and if neither (a) nor (b) is present the probability is low.

In patients where the clinical probability of PE is high, the investigation of choice is CT pulmonary angiography, (**341**) which has superseded ventilation–perfusion scanning in the investigation of PE. It is superior to ventilation–perfusion scanning in diagnosing and excluding PE. It is quicker to perform, easier to arrange urgently out of hours, and rarely needs to be followed up by further imaging. Furthermore, CT pulmonary angiography may identify an alternative diagnosis when PE has been excluded.

Ventilation–perfusion scan may only be considered as a first-line investigation if all of the following criteria are satisfied:
- Facilities to perform the test are available on site.
- The chest X-ray is normal.
- There is no significant cardio-pulmonary disease.
- Standardized reporting criteria are used.
- A non-diagnostic test is always followed by further imaging.

A normal ventilation–perfusion scan reliably excludes PE, but an intermediate scan should be followed up by CT pulmonary angiography.

In patients who have an intermediate probability of PE on clinical grounds alone, a d-dimer assay should be performed. A negative d-dimer assay reliably excludes PE and the need for imaging to diagnose PE. There are currently three commercially available d-dimer assays (SimpliRED, Vidas and MDA). A SimpliRED is only effective in excluding PE in patients with low probability whereas the Vidas and MDA are useful in intermediate and low probability cases (algorithm).

Echocardiography is only diagnostic in massive PE and may reveal right heart dilatation and dysfunction as well as thrombus in the inferior vena cava, right atrium or right ventricle. Our patient does not have any features to suggest massive PE such as circulatory collapse, acidosis or clinical signs of right heart strain.

In patients with symptoms of PE and clinical features of a lower-limb DVT, the confirmation of deep-vein thrombosis on Doppler ultrasonography of the deep leg veins obviates the need for pulmonary imaging.

Major risk factors for thromboembolism

Risk factor	Examples
Surgery	Major abdominal, pelvic, hip or knee
Obstetrics	Late pregnancy, Caesarean section, puerperium
Lower limb problems	Fracture, varicose veins
Malignancy	Abdominal/pelvic, advanced metastatic
Reduced mobility	
Previous DVT	

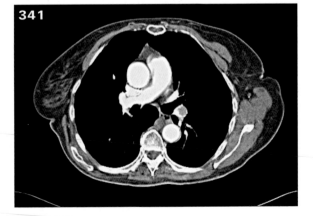

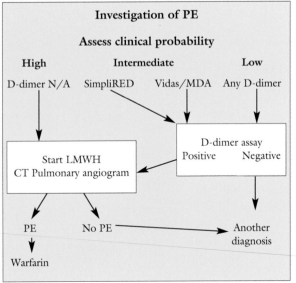

Answer 342

> e. Mobitz type I second degree AV block.

There is failure of some P-waves to conduct that is preceded by progressive prolongation of the PR interval, which is typical of Mobitz type I second degree AV block. The conduction disturbance is due to an abnormality at the level of the AV node. In the presence of symptoms the treatment is implantation of a permanent pacemaker.

Question 343

A 68-year-old Caucasian male complained of a four-year history of increasing breathlessness on exertion. There were no other respiratory symptoms. There was no history of smoking. The patient had a history of hypertension and had been taking an ACE inhibitor for over six years. He was a retired clerk.

On examination he appeared well and was not cyanosed. There was evidence of early clubbing. Auscultation of the lungs revealed fine end inspiratory crackles. All other aspects of physical examination were normal.

Investigations are shown.

Hb	13 g/dl
WCC	6×10^9/l
Platelets	200×10^9/l
ESR	28 mm/h
CRP	32 g/l
Arterial blood gases:	
pH	7.4
$PaCO_2$	4.3 kPa
PaO_2	8.3 kPa
Bicarbonate	26 mmol/l
Chest X-ray (**343**)	

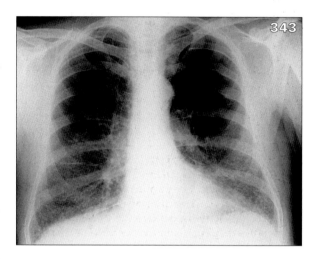

What is the most probable diagnosis?
a. ACE inhibitor related alveolitis.
b. Bronchiectasis.
c. Cryptogenic fibrosing alveolitis.
d. Sarcoidosis.
e. Asbestosis.

Question 344

A 44-year-old male who was receiving haemodialysis three times weekly complained of fatigue, night sweats and a dry cough and was found to have a haemoglobin of 8.5 g/dl. His haemoglobin two months previously had been 11.4 g/dl on regular erythropoietin and intermittent intravenous iron supplements. There was no history of haematemesis or malena.

Investigations are shown.

Hb	8.5 g/l
MCV	87 fl
WCC	11×10^9/l
Serum ferritin	580 mg/l
Serum B_{12}	260 ng/l
Serum folate	7 mg/l
Serum aluminium	6 mg/l
Plasma PTH	15 pmol/l (NR 0.9–5.4 pmol/l)
C-reactive protein	110 mg/l (NR <10 mg/l)

What is the most likely cause for the resistance to erythropoietin therapy?
a. Aluminium toxicity.
b. Hyperparathyroidism.
c. Chronic sepsis.
d. Red cell aplasia.
e. Iron deficiency.

Answer 343

c. Cryptogenic fibrosing alveolitis.

There is no obvious cause for the increasing breathlessness in the history. Although the patient has been taking an ACE inhibitor for six months, there is no association between ACE inhibitors and pulmonary fibrosis. The physical findings and the chest X-ray are consistent with cryptogenic fibrosing alveolitis. There is reticulonodular shadowing of both lung bases. The differential diagnosis for bibasal lung shadowing is shown (*Table*). Although sarcoidosis is listed in the potential choices, there is no previous history of acute sarcoid nor any evidence of multi-system involvement.

Causes of lower lung fibrosis

- Cryptogenic fibrosing alveolitis
- Asbestosis
- Aspiration pneumonia
- Rheumatoid arthritis
- Drug-related pulmonary fibrosis
- Systemic sclerosis
- Sarcoidosis

Answer 344

c. Chronic sepsis.

The patient has resistance to erythropoietin – despite satisfactory iron stores – the causes of which are tabulated below. Iron deficiency is by far the commonest cause of anaemia despite erythropoietin. Erythropoeitin should not be started until iron stores are replenished as evidenced by a serum ferritin ≥ 150 mg/l, or the transferrin saturation is $\geq 20\%$.

The data provided in the question are against folate or B_{12} deficiency or aluminium toxicity. The patient has a mildly raised serum PTH, as one would expect in a patient with chronic renal failure. In general erythropoietin resistance is only seen in bone disease due to severe hyperparathyroidism. The history of malaise and night sweats together with the raised serum CRP, indicates that the most probable cause for failure to respond to erythropoietin is chronic sepsis. The identification and treatment of the source of sepsis should help resolve the anaemia.

Treatment with erythropoietin in patients with chronic renal failure has significantly improved the quality of life and well-being of patients. Erythropoietin prevents the development of cardiac enlargement and high output heart failure. For unexplained reasons treatment with erythropoietin has also been shown to improve sleep pattern, sexual function, and increase cognitive function. Erythropoietin is usually administered subcutaneously two or three times per week. It is well tolerated but complications include hypertension, headache (15%) and flu-like symptoms (5%). A specific brand of recombinant erythropoietin alpha, termed Eprex, has been associated with pure red cell aplasia owing to the development of erythropoietin-specific antibodies.

Causes of resistance to erythropoietin in patients with renal failure

- Inadequate iron stores
- Blood loss
- Folate or B_{12} deficiency
- Inadequate dialysis
- Chronic inflammation
- Sepsis
- Severe hyperparathyroidism
- Aluminium toxicity

Question 345

A 38-year-old male with HIV presented with confusion and ataxia and reduced visual acuity in the left eye. A brain MRI scan is shown (**345a**).

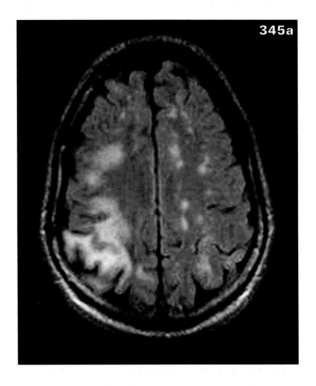

345a

What is the diagnosis?
  a. Multiple sclerosis.
  b. Progressive multifocal leucoencephalopathy.
  c. Cerebral toxoplasmosis.
  d. Cerebral lymphoma.
  e. Cerebral tuberculosis.

Question 346

A 72-year-old male presented with anorexia, nausea and intermittent falls secondary to dizziness. The BP measured 110/60 mmHg when lying and 70/30 mmHg on standing (accompanying dizziness). The JVP was raised. Cardiac auscultation revealed a loud third heart sound. There was mild pitting ankle oedema.

Investigations were as follows:

Hb	8.9 g/dl
WCC	9×10^9/l
Platelets	170×10^9/l
ESR	89 mm/h
Sodium	131 mmol/l
Potassium	3.8 mmol/l
Urea	14 mmol/l
Calcium	2.8 mmol/l
Phosphate	1.9 mmol/l
AST	26 iu/l
Alkaline phosphatase	140 iu/l
Albumin	19 g/l
Total protein	70 g/l
24-hour urinalysis:	
Protein	5 g/l
Sodium	7 mmol/l

What is the cause of his dizziness?
  a. Hypoadrenalism.
  b. Postural hypotension secondary to dehydration.
  c. Autonomic neuropathy secondary to amyloidosis.
  d. Anaemia.
  e. Syndrome of inappropriate ADH secretion.

Answer 345

> b. Progressive multifocal leucoencephalopathy.

The MRI scan reveals multiple bilateral, asymmetrical confluent high intensity signals without any evidence of raised intracranial pressure or mass effect. This is the characteristic finding in progressive multifocal leucoencephalopathy. The lesions usually involve the periventricular areas and subcortical white matter. The spinal cord is rarely affected in PMLE.

In contrast, most patients with HIV syndrome develop cerebral disorders associated with cerebral oedema and mass effect on CT scan or MR scan of the brain (345b).

Multiple sclerosis may have similar findings on the MRI scan; however, confusion and multifocal abnormalities occurring simultaneously in an immuno-compromised patient are more consistent with the diagnosis of PMLE.

PMLE is characterized by rapidly progressive focal neurological deficit without evidence of raised intracranial pressure. The disorder affects immunocompromised patients who become infected with the human polyoma virus, JC virus. Manifestations are due to cerebral white matter involvement but cerebellar and brainstem involvement also occur. Clinical features include cognitive impairment, visual field defects, and hemiparesis. Aphasia, ataxia and cortical blindness are also recognized. The severity of the clinical findings is disproportionate to the abnormalities identified on brain scans. Patients with advanced disease go on to develop severe dementia and coma. In most patients death usually occurs within a year of diagnosis. The diagnosis is usually made on clinical and radiological grounds. Definitive diagnosis requires brain biopsy. The identification of JC virus on PCR of CSF specimens supports the diagnosis in patients with clinical features to suggest PMLE; however, many immunocompromised patients without PMLE and some healthy individuals have positive PCR results for JC virus, therefore the investigation cannot be relied upon to make the diagnosis in isolation.

Other infections caused by JC virus in immuno-compromised patients include haemorrhagic cystitis in bone marrow transplant patients and interstitial nephritis in renal transplant patients.

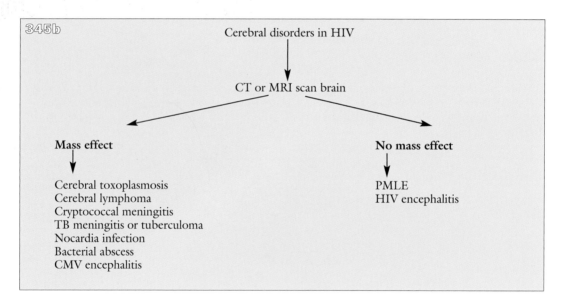

345b

Cerebral disorders in HIV

↓

CT or MRI scan brain

Mass effect

Cerebral toxoplasmosis
Cerebral lymphoma
Cryptococcal meningitis
TB meningitis or tuberculoma
Nocardia infection
Bacterial abscess
CMV encephalitis

No mass effect

PMLE
HIV encephalitis

Answer 346

> c. Autonomic neuropathy secondary to amyloidosis.

The patient has anaemia, a raised ESR, and hypercalcaemia, which are all consistent with the diagnosis of multiple myeloma. The heart failure and nephrotic syndrome in a patient with myeloma is highly suggestive of primary amyloidosis complicating the multiple myeloma. Primary amyloidosis is a recognized cause of autonomic neuropathy, which would explain the falls and the postural hypotension. The low sodium in the context of postural hypotension may lead some candidates to opt for the diagnosis of Addison's disease, but in this particular case it is most likely to represent pseudohyponatraemia due to increased protein in the plasma rather than true hyponatraemia. (The causes of autonomic neuropathy are discussed in the Answer 395).

Question 347

A 78-year-old female patient presented with acute abdominal pain and vomiting. A plain abdominal film is shown (**347a**).

What is the diagnosis?
  a. Large bowel obstruction.
  b. Nephrolithiasis.
  c. Gallstone ileus.
  d. Acute chronic pancreatitis.
  e. Acute colitis.

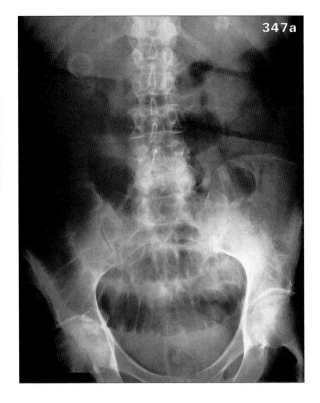

347a

Question 348

A 30-year-old female presented with malaise, nausea, vomiting and right upper quadrant pain in the last week of her pregnancy. She had tolerated the pregnancy very well prior to the event. Her blood pressure control throughout the pregnancy had been good, with the last reading measuring 96/60 mmHg two weeks previously. There was no history of headache or diarrhoea.

On examination she appeared pale. There was no obvious evidence of jaundice. There was marked right upper quadrant tenderness. The blood pressure measured 130/86 mmHg.

Investigations are shown.

Hb	10 g/dl
WCC	12 × 10⁹/l
Platelets	33 × 10⁹/l
PT	12 sec
APTT	43 sec
Sodium	137 mmol/l
Potassium	3.4 mmol/l
Urea	12 mmol/l
Creatinine	223 μmol/l
Bilirubin	20 μmol/l
AST	250 iu/l
ALT	298 iu/l
Alk Phos	200 iu/l
LDH	800 iu/l
Albumin	33 g/l
Amylase	150 iu/l (NR <220 iu/l)
Urinalysis	Protein +
Hepatobiliary ultrasound	Normal

What is the definitive treatment?
  a. IV cefuroxime and metronidazole.
  b. Start methyldopa.
  c. Deliver the baby urgently.
  d. Exploration laparoscopy.
  e. IV hydrocortisone.

Answer 347

c. Gallstone ileus.

There is evidence of small bowel obstruction and three visible gallstones (in right upper quadrant, adjacent to the head of the right femur and in the left upper quadrant, **347b**). The patient has gallstone ileus, which is a rare complication of gallstones that results from mechanical small bowel obstruction following ulceration of a gallstone through the common bile duct directly into the small bowel. Most patients who develop gallstone ileus have previously had cholecystitis. As the stone enters the small bowel it becomes bigger owing to sedimentation of the gut contents. The vast majority of obstructing stones are >2 cm in diameter. Obstruction characteristically occurs in the ileum, which is the narrowest part of the small bowel.

The diagnosis requires erect and supine plain abdominal films. The presence of small bowel obstruction, visible gallstones in the small bowel and air in the biliary tree (arrows) is diagnostic. In many instances, however, the gallstones in the bowel are not visible on plain abdominal films, and abdominal ultrasound and CT scan are more specific investigations. Initial treatment involves resting the bowel and restoring fluids. Definitive treatment is surgical.

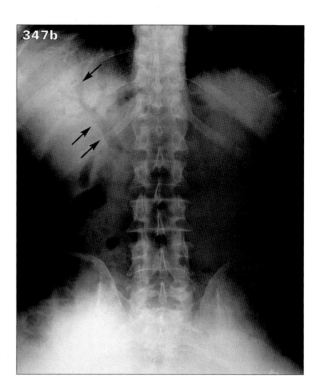

Answer 348

c. Deliver the baby urgently.

The patient presents with nausea, vomiting and right upper quadrant discomfort towards the end of her pregnancy. Her blood pressure is at the upper limit of normal and considerably higher than it was two weeks previously. The patient also has proteinuria, a micro-angiopathy as characterized by the fragmented red cells on the blood film, abnormal liver enzymes and low platelets. The diagnosis is consistent with the HELLP syndrome (haemolysis, elevated liver enzymes and low platelets. The condition affects approximately 1 per 1000 pregnancies. It is more common in multiparous women. Some authorities believe that it is a manifestation of severe pre-eclampsia; however, approximately 15% of affected females do not have hypertension and proteinuria, which are the classical hallmarks of pre-eclampsia, causing other authorities to postulate that it may be a completely separate disorder.

HELLP syndrome usually occurs in the last trimester of pregnancy or within the first week of parturition. A few cases may have been reported to occur in the second trimester. Patients often present with malaise, nausea, vomiting and right upper quadrant tenderness. The condition may mimic several other medical conditions such as viral hepatitis and cholecystitis. Hypertension and proteinuria are often present. The blood film shows evidence of a micro-angiopathic haemolytic anaemia associated with a platelet count, and liver enzymes are raised. The hepatic transaminase concentrations are elevated but there is no recognized diagnostic limit. In general the presence of schistocytes on the blood film, a platelet count <100 × 10^9/l, an AST >70 iu/l and an LDH >600 iu/l are highly suggestive of the HELLP syndrome. Clotting is normal unless HELLP is complicated by disseminated intravascular coagulation.

The differential diagnosis includes TTP, HUS and fatty liver. In TTP and HUS a history of preceding hypertension or proteinuria is usually absent and the only haematological abnormalities are micro-angiopathy and low platelets. DIC does not complicate HUS and TTP. Fatty liver may be difficult to differentiate from HELLP as it presents in a similar fashion; however, the

---

Management of HELLP

1. Deliver the foetus as soon as possible.
2. Intravenous corticosteroids in females <34 weeks' gestation to defer early delivery.
3. Treat hypertension.
4. Platelet and blood transfusion if there is bleeding.
5. Magnesium sulphate for epileptic seizures.
6. Dialysis for rapidly deteriorating renal function.

transaminase levels are usually in the thousands and the clotting screen is frequently abnormal in fatty liver.

Patients may develop severe hypertension, epileptic seizures and bleeding complications. The mainstay of treatment is to deliver the foetus as soon as practical. In females >34 weeks' gestation this is the definitive treatment. In females <34 weeks' gestation it may be possible to defer delivery with intravenous corticosteroids while the foetal lungs mature.

Question 349

A 30-year-old male presented with sudden onset of left-sided weakness. The was no history of headache. He had experienced transient weakness of his right arm three years previously, which resolved spontaneously after 5 hours and did not receive medical attention. He had a past history of multiple episodes of epistaxis which had not been investigated. Eight months previously he had experienced a cough associated with fever and intermittent haemoptysis, which improved after a course of amoxicillin, but he had been more breathless than usual since the episode. There was no family history of premature atherosclerosis. His father was fit and well but his mother was anaemic and had been investigated on numerous occasions for gastrointestinal haemorrhage. The patient smoked 20 cigarettes per day.

On examination he had a left-sided hemiparesis. The pulse was regular. The blood pressure measured 120/70 mmHg. Auscultation of the heart was normal. All peripheral pulses were easily palpable; there was no clinical evidence of bruits over the carotid arteries. The chest was clear. Apart from small red cutaneous lesions around the inner aspect of the left nostril there were no other abnormalities on examination.

Investigations are shown.

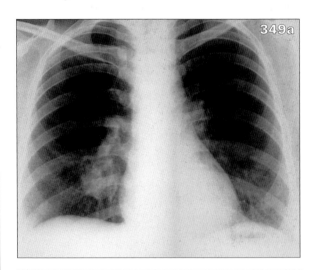

349a

Hb	18 g/dl
WCC	11×10^9/l
Platelets	206×10^9/l
PCV	0.58
CRP	9 g/l
Total cholesterol	5.2 mmol/l
Blood glucose	4.1 mmol/l
12-lead ECG	Normal
Echocardiogram	Normal
CT scan brain	Normal
Carotid Doppler studies	Normal
Chest X-ray (**349a**)	

What is the diagnosis?
  a. Bronchial carcinoma.
  b. Polycythaemia rubra vera.
  c. Wegener's granulomatosis.
  d. Hereditary haemorrhagic telangiectasia.
  e. Patent foramen ovale.

Question 350

A 75-year-old male presented with exertional chest pain. On examination he had an ejection systolic murmur consistent with aortic stenosis. The 12-lead ECG revealed voltage criteria for left ventricular hypertrophy. Echocardiography confirmed calcific aortic stenosis with a pressure gradient of 68 mmHg across the aortic valve.

What is the most important prognostic factor in the history?
  a. Presence of left ventricular hypertrophy on 12-lead ECG.
  b. Presence of left ventricular hypertrophy on echocardiography.
  c. Pressure gradient >60 mmHg across the aortic valve.
  d. Presence of symptoms.
  e. Calcified aortic valve.

Answer 349

> d. Hereditary haemorrhagic telangiectasia.

This young patient presents with a stroke in the absence of any of the conventional risk factors for atherosclerosis. He has a long history of epistaxis. He also has haemoptysis, and his chest X-ray reveals a well-defined round opacity adjacent to the right heart border that has a linear shadow at the 1 o'clock position, consistent with a feeding vessel indicating a pulmonary arterio-venous malformation. There is a family history of anaemia and gastrointestinal haemorrhage and visible telangiectasia in the left nostril. The most likely underlying diagnosis is hereditary haemorrhagic telangiectasia. The increased haemoglobin concentration in this patient reflects physiological polycythaemia due to chronic hypoxaemia.

HHT, also known as Osler–Weber–Rendu syndrome, is a genetic disorder resulting in arterio-venous malformations in various parts of the body including the skin, liver, respiratory system, GI tract and the brain. Abnormalities in the genes encoding the angiogenesis factors endoglin and activin receptor-like kinase 1 have been identified on chromosome 9 and 12 respectively.

The commonest manifestation of the disorder is spontaneous epistaxis, which may be severe. Up to 70% of patients with HHT have pulmonary arterio-venous malformations, which may be asymptomatic but can be associated with haemoptysis, exercise intolerance, hypoxaemia, pulmonary hypertension and paradoxical emboli. The latter may be complicated by migraines, transient ischaemic attacks, stroke and cerebral abscess. Telangiectasia may occur anywhere in the GI tract and grow with age. GI haemorrhage occurs in older patients (aged 60 years or over).

Cutaneous telangiectasia are the commonest physical sign. Bruits over organs with telangiectasias may be heard in a few patients.

Pulmonary arterio-venous malformations are best visualized with contrast CT scan of the thorax (349b). Blood gas analysis may demonstrate hypoxia. Pulmonary function tests reveal a low transfer factor. Some patients with diffuse arterio-venous malformations exhibit orthodeoxia (decrease in oxygen saturation on standing from a supine position), because lying down reduces blood flow through malformations in dependent parts of the lung.

Complications of HHT

- Migraines
- Seizures
- TIA/CVA
- Cerebral abscess
- Cerebral haemorrhage due to cerebral arterio-venous malformation
- Haemothorax
- Massive haemoptysis
- Pulmonary hypertension
- Central cyanosis
- GI haemorrhage
- Anaemia due to blood loss
- Polycythaemia due to chronic hypoxia

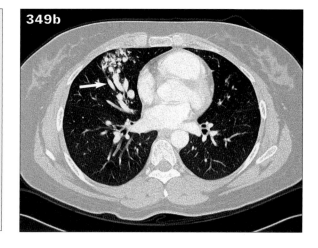

349b

Answer 350

> d. Presence of symptoms.

Indications for surgery in severe aortic stenosis include:

- Presence of symptoms.
- Patients with severe AS undergoing coronary artery bypass surgery.
- Patients with severe AS undergoing surgery on the aorta or other heart valve(s).

Severe left ventricular hypertrophy, a pressure gradient ≥100 mmHg across the aortic valve and systolic dysfunction are indications for surgery in asymptomatic patients. However, most patients in these categories are rarely asymptomatic. Patients with impaired left ventricular function in the context of aortic stenosis have a poor prognosis if untreated.

Question 351

A 36-year-old woman presented with fever and malaise. She had been commenced on carbimazole for symptomatic thyrotoxicosis four weeks previously. On examination her temperature was 39.2°C (102.5°F) and her mouth was red. Examination of all the major systems was normal.

Investigations are shown.

Hb	12 g/dl
WCC	0.8 × 10⁹/l (neutrophils 0.3)
Platelets	190 × 10⁹/l
CRP	240 mg/l
Chest X-ray	Normal
B cultures	No growth
Mouth swabs	No growth
Urine culture	No growth
Stool culture	No pathological organisms

What is the best initial antibiotic combination in this patient?
a. IV cefuroxime and IV clarithromycin.
b. IV benzylpenicillin.
c. IV vancomycin and gentamicin.
d. IV Tazocin and gentamicin.
e. IV acyclovir.

Question 352

A 16-year-old Spanish boy was admitted to hospital with a three-day history of abdominal pain and jaundice. One week before admission he had developed a sore throat, accompanied by fever and myalgia. He had experienced three similar episodes of jaundice and abdominal pain preceded by a sore throat and fever at the ages of 6, 12 and 14, and on each occasion he made an uncomplicated recovery. There was no history of recent travel abroad. He was the only child in the family.

On examination, he had a temperature of 39°C (102.2°F). He was mildly jaundiced and had tender cervical lymphadenopathy. Examination of the throat revealed a purulent exudate. Examination of the lungs was normal. On examination of the abdomen there was a palpable spleen 5 cm below the costal margin.

Investigations are shown.

Hb	9.1 g/dl
WCC	6 × 10⁹/l
Platelets	100 × 10⁹/l
Monospot test	Negative
Bilirubin	33 mmol/l
ALT	23 iu/l
Alkaline phosphatase	120 iu/l
Urinalysis	Urobilinogen ++++
	Nil else

What is the diagnosis?
a. Hereditary spherocytosis.
b. Infectious mononuclueosis.
c. Glucose-6-phosphate dehydrogenase deficiency.
d. Sickle cell anaemia.
e. Gilbert's disease.

Answer 351

> d. IV Tazocin and gentamicin.

The patient has severe neutropenia, presumably secondary to carbimazole therapy (see *Table A* for causes of neutropaenia). Neutropenia is defined as a neutrophil count of $< 1.5 \times 10^9/l$. Many patients with mild neutropenia may remain asymptomatic; however, patients with neutrophil counts $< 0.5 \times 10^9/l$ are at risk of overwhelming sepsis with viral, bacterial and fungal infections, common sites of infection being the skin, gut mucosa and the urinary tract.

All neutropenic patients should have a septic screen (blood cultures, urine culture, mouth nasopharyngeal swabs, culture of any septic focus which is easily visible on examining the patients and chest X-ray) before commencing antibiotic treatment. The antibiotics used to treat severe neutropenia should be broad spectrum and cover both Gram-positive and negative bacteria.

The usual regime is an antipseudomonal beta-lactam penicillin such as azlocillin, tazocillin or aztreonam, or a carbapenem such as meropenem, or a third generation cephalosporin such as ceftazidime, together with an

Table A Causes of neutropenia

Drugs:	Antithyroid (carbimazole)
	Sulphonamides
	Anticonvulsants
	Non-steroidal anti-inflammatory drugs (phenylbutazone)
	Antibiotics (chloramphenicol)
	Phenothiazines
	Any drugs used for chemotherapy
Malignancy:	Lymphomas, leukaemia
Radiotherapy	
Infections:	Tuberculosis
	Viral infections
Megaloblastic anaemia	
Toxins:	Alcohol
	Hypersplenism

Table B Antibiotic use in neutropaenic sepsis

Initial antibiotic therapy
- Monotherapy
  Ceftazidime or imipenem or meropenem
- Dual therapy
  Aminoglycoside plus beta-lactam with anti-pseudomonal action, or a third-generation cephalosporin, or a carbapenem
  Vancomycin should be added to mono or dual therapy if there are indwelling venous catheters, evidence of cardiovascular compromise or severe mucositis

Afebrile within first 3–5 days
- If aetiology identified
Adjust to most appropriate therapy based upon antibiotic sensitivity of organism
- If no aetiology identified
Low risk: Switch to oral antibiotics (usually ciprofloxacin and augmentin)
High risk: Continue with same antibiotics

Persistent fever during the first 3–5 days
- Reassess after 3 days
- If no change: Continue antibiotics. Stop vancomycin if cultures are negative
- If deteriorating: Change antibiotics.
- If febrile after day 5: Consider adding anti-fungal agent

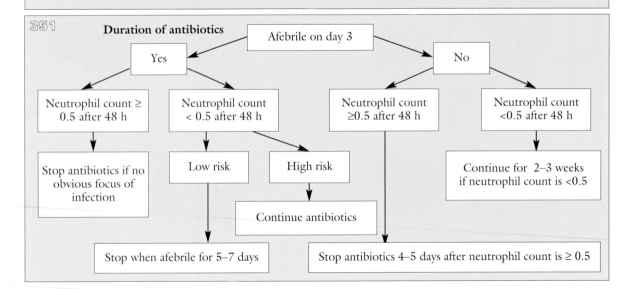

aminoglycoside (*Table B*). Patients may be treated with just one antibiotic instead of dual therapy. Antibiotics used as monotherapy include ceftazidime, imipenem and meropenem. While there is no convincing evidence that monotherapy is inferior to dual therapy (i.e. one of these antibiotics and an aminoglycoside), most authorities choose to treat with dual therapy, as monotherapy may promote antibiotic resistance.

Patients with venous lines or indwelling catheters, evidence of MRSA on skin or nasal swabs should also receive vancomycin.

Fever persisting for over a week on the antibiotics above necessitates the addition of intravenous amphotericin to cover systemic fungal infection.

The duration of antibiotic therapy is outlined in the algorithm (**351**).

Patients with severe neutropenia should receive diligent mouth care and fluconazole lozenges to prevent oral candidiasis.

Answer 352

a. Hereditary spherocytosis.

The history of recurrent episodes of abdominal pain and jaundice precipitated by a sore throat in a young boy with anaemia, splenomegaly and a raised urinary urobilinogen is suggestive of an inherited haemolytic anaemia. There is a family history of splenectomy to treat anaemia in a first-degree relative to support a hereditary anaemia. The most likely diagnosis is HS, although other possible causes of this picture include hereditary elliptocytosis, glucose-6-phosphate dehydrogenase deficiency, pyruvate kinase deficiency. Sickle cell anaemia may be associated with haemolytic crises during infection, however the spleen is impalpable because it has atrophied owing to multiple infarcts. The history of a purulent sore throat and haemolysis could be explained entirely by infectious mononucleosis; however, it would be unusual for a young boy to have three episodes of EBV infection. In this case, the sore throat has been the precipitant for increased haemolysis in an individual with a red cells which are vulnerable to haemolysis. Gilbert's disease is associated with mild jaundice during illness but does not explain the anaemia or haemolysis.

Hereditary spherocytosis (**352**) is an autosomal dominant disorder of red cells. It is due to a defect in the membrane protein spectrin, which results in membrane loss as the cell passes through the spleen. The surface-to-volume ratio is reduced and the cells become spherocytic. Spherocytes are eventually destroyed by the spleen. The disorder may present as neonatal jaundice; however, most

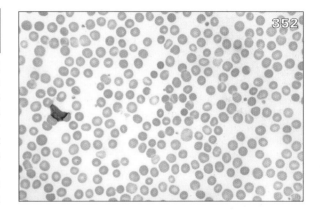

patients have a low-grade haemolysis with an intermittent increase in the rate of haemolysis during infections. During these episodes the patient may become very anaemic and appear jaundiced. Some individuals are asymptomatic and some may present in middle age with complications from gallstones. Aplastic crises may occur following infection with parvovirus, and megaloblastic anaemia may occur owing to folate deficiency. Leg ulcers are well recognized. The blood film will demonstrate at least 50% of spherocytes. When incubated in solutions of increasing hypotonicity or in their own plasma for over 24 hours, the cells demonstrate an increased rate of haemolysis (red cell fragility test). There is evidence of a haemolytic anaemia (raised bilirubin, reduced haptoglobins, increased urinary urobilinogen). Treatment of anaemia is with splenectomy.

Question 353

A 16-year-old boy was found dead in bed by his mother. A detailed post-mortem failed to reveal any obvious cause of death. His father died suddenly aged 30. He had a paternal aunt who was being investigated for syncopal episodes. His sister was diagnosed as having epilepsy aged 11.

What is the most probable cause of death?
  a. Hypertrophic cardiomyopathy.
  b. Ecstasy abuse.
  c. Anomalous coronary arteries.
  d. Commotio cordis.
  e. Long QT syndrome.

Answer 353

> e. Long QT syndrome.

The patient has died suddenly in the absence of previous ill health and the postmortem has failed to reveal any abnormality. By definition this individual is a victim of the sudden adult death syndrome. There are approximately 500 such cases in the UK each year. Most deaths are thought to be secondary to fatal cardiac arrhythmias. Many conditions may be identifiable on 12-lead ECG during life and many may be familial. It is now recommended that all first-degree relatives of victims of SADS undergo cardiovascular evaluation to identify conditions that could potentially cause sudden cardiac death.

In this particular case there is reason to believe that the patient may have died from a familial cardiac disorder since there is a family history of premature sudden death and syncope. Long QT syndrome is a well recognized cause of sudden death in young patients where the post-mortem is normal. The diagnosis can be made ante-mortem with 12-lead ECG. Patients with long QT syndrome may be entirely asymptomatic or experience syncope/sudden death or epileptic seizures due to malignant ventricular arrhythmias. Patients with long QT syndrome are often misdiagnosed as having epilepsy.

Most sudden non-traumatic deaths in young individuals are due to cardiac disease. The causes of sudden cardiac death with normal post-mortem findings are shown below (*Table*).

Brugada's syndrome is a genetic disorder caused by mutations within the sodium ion channel SCN5A. The disorder is inherited as an autosomal dominant trait and characterized by a propensity to fatal ventricular arrhythmias and sudden death in patients with structurally normal hearts. The resting ECG shows a characteristic peculiar pattern consisting of a pseudo-right bundle branch block and persistent ST elevation in leads V1 to V3 (**353**). The widened S-wave in the left lateral leads that usually characterizes RBBB is absent in most patients with Brugada's syndrome, suggesting that there is a high take off of the ST segment in the right precordium (J-wave) rather than true RBBB. The QT interval may be prolonged in leads V1–V3. The prevalence of the Brugada ECG is 0.7–1%. The disorder is much more common in males and in patients from the Far East, e.g. from countries such as Nepal and Thailand. All clinical manifestations of Brugada's syndrome are related to life-threatening ventricular arrhythmias. Sudden death may be the first and only presentation, occurring in up to one-third of patients. Mortality is much more common in males. Arrhythmic events occur between the third and seventh decades. Most arrhythmic events occur during sleep, suggesting that an imbalance between the sympathetic and parasympathetic tone may be important in the pathogenesis of Brugada's syndrome. The diagnosis of Brugada's syndrome is often difficult since the disorder is not well established. ECG and clinical features are important. Brugada's syndrome should be considered in patients who meet one of the following criteria:

Appearance of ECG pattern in more than one right precordial lead (V1–V3) under baseline conditions in the presence or absence of a sodium ion channel blocker, and one of the following:

- Documented ventricular fibrillation.
- Self-terminating polymorphic ventricular tachycardia.
- Family history of sudden cardiac death at <45 years of age.
- Type 1 ECG pattern in family members.
- Electrophysiological inducibility.
- Syncope.
- Nocturnal agonal respiration.

The only effective treatment in the prevention of sudden death in Brugada's syndrome is an implantable cardioverter defibrillator, and it has been proposed that patients with aborted sudden cardiac death or sustained VT should be treated with an ICD.

Commotio cordis is a term used to describe ventricular tachycardia or ventricular fibrillation occurring after being struck in the precordium by a high velocity projectile such as a base ball or an ice hockey puck. The individual may die suddenly on the sports field. The heart appears normal at post-mortem examination. (See Question 368.)

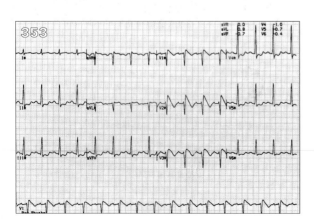

Causes of sudden cardiac death in patients with structurally normal hearts

- Ion channel diseases of the heart such as long QT syndrome or Brugada's syndrome
- Accessory pathways such as Wolff–Parkinson–White syndrome
- Commotio cordis
- Focal myocarditis
- Atypical right ventricular cardiomyopathy that may not be recognized by the pathologist
- Drugs such as amphetamines
- Electrolyte disturbances

Question 354

A 63-year-old male with end-stage renal failure and a 12-month history of dialysis had been on an active renal transplant list for over six months. Over the past few months dialysis therapy had been incomplete owing to poor tolerance, and his general health had started to deteriorate. He had made enquiries about renal transplants and had heard that he could travel to some third-world countries and purchase a kidney at a cheap price. He was married with one son aged 16 years old. He did not have any siblings and both parents had died. His wife was not keen to donate her kidney, however his son was eager to donate to help his father.

What course of action would you advise?
  a. Persuade his wife to donate the kidney.
  b. Encourage him to travel abroad to purchase a kidney.
  c. Advise him to stay patiently on the transplant list.
  d. Advise him to take his son's kidney.
  e. Make an urgent request to the cadaveric transplant co-ordinator to prioritize a transplant for him.

Question 355

A 60-year-old female presented with a dry cough and haemoptysis. She had a past history of tuberculosis. A chest X-ray and CT scan of the thorax are shown in figures **355a** and **b**, respectively.

What is the diagnosis?
  a. Recurrence of tuberculosis.
  b. Bronchogenic carcinoma.
  c. *Staphylococcus aureus* pneumonia.
  d. Aspergilloma.
  e. Aspiration pneumonia.

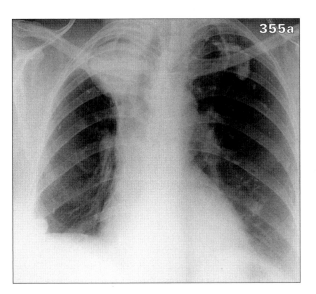

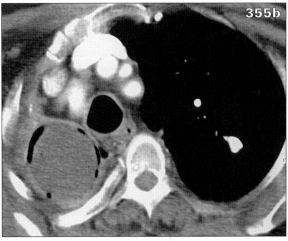

Answer 354

d. Advise him to take his son's kidney.

This question relates to ethical issues around organ donation for transplantation. Availability or renal donors for transplants is a major problem in all developed countries. Most patients receive transplants from cadavers; however, success from live donor transplants is superior to cadaveric transplants even in non-related donors. A blood group match in essential. A HLA match is desirable but not mandatory.

In this particular situation, a first-degree relative is prepared to donate his kidney. The individual in question is above the age of 16 and in a situation where he may sign his own consent to donate his kidney. Absolute contra-indications to organ donation for renal transplantation are tabulated below. The son should undergo routine blood tests, urinalysis, 24-hour urine assessment of protein estimation and creatinine clearance, HLA typing, serology for viral antibodies including CMV and HIV, IVU and renal angiography or equivalent.

It is unethical and potentially dangerous to advise him to purchase a kidney from elsewhere. Attempting to expedite his transplantation via the transplant co-ordinator may be seen as discrimination as there may be other, more stoical individuals with an equal need for a new kidney. Forcing his wife to donate a kidney and asking him to wait patiently for a transplant when there is an ideal option available to him contravenes good medical practice.

Absolute contra-indications to organ donation for renal transplant include:

- Age < 16 years
- Proteinuria or haematuria
- Abnormal creatinine clearance
- HIV infection
- Malignancy
- Psychosis
- Pregnancy
- Chronic illness

Answer 355

d. Aspergilloma.

The plain X-ray reveals a scarring in the left apex consistent with previous tuberculosis. In the right apex there is an opacity surrounded by a crescent of air (Monod's sign). This finding is typical of an aspergilloma (mycetomoa) in an old tuberculous cavity. The CT scan of the thorax demonstrates the mass lesion within the lung cavity (the air around the aspergilloma is black).

Aspergilloma is due to colonization by the species *Aspergillus fumigatus* rather than direct tissue invasion, and is usually not an indicator of an immuno-compromised state. It arises most commonly in old tuberculous cavities but may occur in cavities created by neoplasms, sarcoidosis and other fungal infections such as histoplasmosis (causes of pulmonary cavities are tabulated). The aspergilloma comprises fungal hyphae, inflammatory cells and fibrin. Patients may be asymptomatic but the vast majority experience haemoptysis. Some patients complain of chest pain, wheeze and a fever. The diagnosis is made with radiological tests. The chest X-ray is usually diagnostic but confirmation of the aspergilloma may require a CT scan or MRI scan of the thorax. The identification of *Aspergillus* in the sputum in such patients is highly suggestive of the diagnosis.

Patients with recurrent haemoptysis are treated with surgical resection of the cavity and removal of the aspergilloma.

Causes of cavitating lung lesions

Infections
- *Staphylococcus aureus* pneumonia
- *Klebsiella* pneumonia
- *Pseudomonas* colonization
- Tuberculosis
- Histoplasmosis
- Hydatid disease

Neoplasia
- Benign
- Malignant   Primary
              Secondary

Vascular
- Pulmonary emboli
- Vasculitides

Granulomatous disease
- Sarcoidosis

Question 356

A 26-year-old female with cystic fibrosis wishes to become pregnant. She has never had any previous pregnancies. She was menstruating once or twice every three months. She had been with her partner for six years. She was diagnosed with cystic fibrosis as a neonate after presenting with rectal prolapse. Her condition was relatively satisfactory in childhood. During adolescence she experienced three to four respiratory tract infections per year that were controlled with intravenous antibiotics. Her sputum had cultured *Pseudomonas aeruginosa* for over six years. Her lung function trend showed an FEV_1 of 60–65% predicted over the past four years. Her body mass index was 21.

What advice would you give her?
  a. To avoid pregnancy and consider referral to a gynaecologist for tubal ligation.
  b. To eradicate *Pseudomonas aeruginosa* from the sputum with aggressive antibiotic therapy before conceiving.
  c. To increase her BMI to above 24 with adequate nutrition before conceiving.
  d. To go ahead and become pregnant but explain the risk of her offspring being affected.
  e. To have her partner screened for D508 mutation on chromosome 7 prior to conceiving.

Question 357

A 67-year-old male presented with pain in both groin regions that was worse on walking. He had a long history of diabetes mellitus that was complicated by nephropathy, for which he had a successful renal transplant three years previously. A plain X-ray of the hips is shown (**357**).

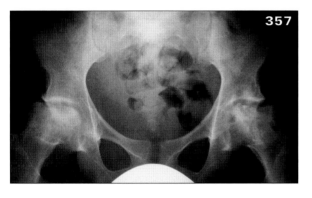

357

What is the diagnosis?
  a. Multiple myeloma.
  b. Avascular necrosis of the femora.
  c. Osteoarthritis.
  d. Osteomalacia.
  e. Paget's disease.

Question 358

Hb	10 g/dl
WCC	10×10^9/l
Platelets	180×10^9/l
MCV	84 fl
ESR	96 mm/h
Sodium	133 mmol/l
Potassium	4.6 mmol/l
Urea	11 mmol/l
Creatinine	180 μmol/l
Calcium	3.2 mmol/l
Phosphate	1.4 mmol/l
Albumin	30 g/l
Total protein	74 g/l
X-ray lumbar spine	Wedge fracture 4th lumbar vertebra

A 78-year-old male was investigated for lower back pain that started suddenly on bending over to pick up a pair of shoes. He had a past medical history of hypertension and had recently been commenced on therapy for depression after presenting with low mood, lethargy and constipation. He was taking bendrofluazidenethi, sennokot, fluoxitene and regular paracetamol

Investigations are shown.

What investigation would you perform next to confirm the diagnosis?
  a. Skeletal survey.
  b. Serum PTH level.
  c. MRI scan lumbar spine.
  d. Bone marrow biopsy.
  e. Chest X-ray.

Answer 356

> d. To go ahead and become pregnant but explain the risk of her offspring being affected.

The patient has stable pulmonary function and normal pulmonary artery pressures, which is the main medical concern with respect to the risk of pregnancy for the female. Females with poor lung reserve may develop respiratory failure once the diaphragm is splinted by the gravid uterus. Patients with pulmonary hypertension are at risk of cardiac failure.

Approximately 20% of females with cystic fibrosis are infertile owing either to malnourishment or to viscid cervical secretions. However, most women are capable of falling pregnant, and advice regarding conception is mainly based on the clinical risk of cardiac or heart failure during gestation. Patients with severe lung disease or significant pulmonary hypertension ($\geq$50 mmHg) should be discouraged from becoming pregnant owing to the high risk of cardio-respiratory failure.

Most women with stable pulmonary function and FEV_1 values $\geq$60% predicted usually tolerate pregnancy without complication. Patients with unstable respiratory function should have treatment optimized to achieve persistent FEV_1 of 60% or more prior to conception. While most adult lungs are colonized with *Pseudomonas* species that are difficult to eradicate completely, patients who harbour *Pseudomonas burkholderia* are at particularly increased risk of pulmonary infections, and efforts should be made to eradicate the organism prior to conception.

All females and their partners should be offered genetic counselling to explain the risks of the offspring being affected. In this respect the partner should be offered genetic screening for the commoner mutations causing cystic fibrosis to predict more accurately the risk of the offspring being affected. However, this is not the main reason for advising against pregnancy.

Following pregnancy, patients should be screened early for gestational diabetes due to underlying insulin deficiency. It is important to ensure that the patient is adequately nourished and gaining weight appropriately.

The anaesthetist should be alerted to the patient prior to delivery. Epidural anaesthesia is advised to reduce the effect of labour on minute ventilation. Supplemental oxygen may be required during the peri-partum period.

Answer 357

> b. Avascular necrosis of the femora.

The patient has increased lucency in both femoral heads below the articular surfaces. The femoral heads have lost their smooth spherical shape, indicating advanced disease. These findings are consistent with the diagnosis of avascular necrosis affecting both femoral heads. Avascular necrosis is a frequent complication following renal transplantation. The aetiology is multi-factorial but steroid therapy for immunosuppression plays an important role. The prevalence of avascular necrosis of bone following transplantation has reduced significantly since the use of ciclosporin. Other causes of avascular necrosis of bone are tabulated below. Patients present with groin or buttock pain that is worse on movement. Treatment may involve conservative measures such as analgesia and reduced movement of the joint concerned, but generally core decompression, osteotomy or joint replacement is required to treat the condition.

Avascular necrosis of bone may complicate deep-sea diving (decompression sickness). It is better known as Caisson's disease. Episodic decompressions can lead to the formation of nitrogen bubbles that occlude arterioles and cause avascular necrosis. The prevalence is related to the frequency of exposure and the depth reached.

> **Causes of avascular necrosis of the head of femur**
> - Congenital dislocation of the hip
> - Perthes' disease
> - Trauma (subcapital fractures of the femur)
> - Steroid therapy
> - SLE
> - Sickle cell anaemia
> - Diabetes mellitus
> - Alcohol abuse
> - Gaucher's disease
> - HIV infection
> - Caisson's disease

Answer 358

> d. Bone marrow biopsy.

Back pain, anaemia, hypercalcaemia, renal impairment and hypergammaglobulinaemia amount to a diagnosis of multiple myeloma. Although a skeletal survey is also useful in the diagnosis of multiple myeloma, bone marrow analysis is the test of choice.

Question 362

A 20-year-old cyclist was seen by a cardiologist after experiencing a sudden syncopal episode while training for a major race. For the past six months he had complained of deteriorating fitness – despite strenuous training – and higher heart rates during training sessions. There was no history of chest pain, palpitation or breathlessness during normal exertion. He was a non-smoker and drank a maximum of 6 units of alcohol per week. He denied all forms of drug abuse.

His father died suddenly at the age of 33 years. The cause of death was not entirely clear but was attributed to a form of 'heart disorder'. His sister had recently seen a cardiologist following a 2-year history of troublesome palpitation and was in the process of having further investigations. The patient had not recently experienced any form of flu-like illness.

On examination he had an athletic build. His heart rate was 60 beats/min and regular and his blood pressure was 110/70 mmHg. The JVP was not raised. The cardiac apical impulse was forceful. On auscultation there was a soft systolic murmur at the left lower sternal edge, which resolved on standing, and a third heart sound.

The patient had the following ECG (**362a**):

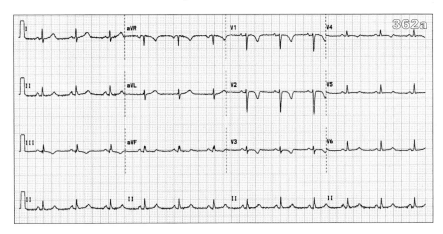

Echocardiography revealed a slightly dilated left ventricle with good systolic function and a dilated right ventricle that was hypokinetic. There was no evidence of any valvular abnormality. He underwent an exercise test following which he experienced dizziness.

An ECG performed while he was symptomatic is shown below (**362b**).

A subsequent 24-hour ECG revealed >5000 ventricular ectopic beats.

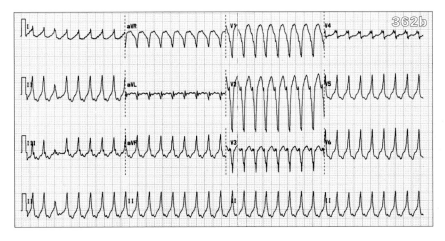

What is the most probable diagnosis?
   a. Right ventricular outflow tract tachycardia.
   b. Hypertrophic cardiomyopathy.
   c. Arrhythmogenic right ventricular cardiomyopathy.
   d. Dilated cardiomyopathy.
   e. Multiple pulmonary emboli.

Answer 362

> c. Arrhythmogenic right ventricular cardiomyopathy.

The combination of T wave inversion in the right ventricular leads (V1–V3), dilated and hypokinetic right ventricle, ventricular tachycardia with left bundle branch morphology and more than 1000 ventricular ectopics with left bundle branch morphology in the context of a family history of premature sudden cardiac death is consistent with the diagnosis of arrhythmogenic right ventricular cardiomyopathy (*Table*).

ARVC is characterized by fibrofatty replacement of the right ventricle, resulting in right ventricular dysfunction and arrhythmias of right ventricular origin (LBBB morphology). The disorder is due to mutations in genes encoding cell adhesion proteins. The two main proteins identified thus far are desmoplakin and plakoglobin. The disorder has a prevalence of 1 in 5000. Over one-third of cases are familial, with an autosomal dominant inheritance pattern. Patients often experience palpitation, presyncope or syncope. Sudden death from ventricular fibrillation may be the first presentation and occurs most commonly during physical exercise.

The ECG is abnormal in 90% of cases with symptoms and usually shows T-wave inversion in the right ventricular leads and depolarization abnormalities after the QRS complex (often termed epsilon waves).

Echocardiography may be normal but in gross cases demonstrates aneurysms of the right ventricular wall.

The MRI scan is more diagnostic, revealing fatty infiltration of the right ventricle.

Right ventricular biopsy is not generally performed to confirm the diagnosis because the free wall of the right ventricle (which is most commonly affected) is the thinnest portion of the right ventricle and is at risk of perforation, the disease is segmental, therefore false-negatives may be generated, and it is impossible to demonstrate transmural fibrofatty infiltration with an endomyocardial biopsy.

The diagnosis relies on family history, electro-cardiography and abnormalities of the right ventricle on imaging (echo, MRI and ventriculography).

Management involves abstinence from strenuous physical exertion and antiarrhythmic therapy in the form of either beta-blockers or amiodarone. Implantation of an ICD is reserved for patients who continue to have syncope or VT despite antiarrhythmic drug therapy.

Causes of VT with LBBB morphology

- ARVC
- Right ventricular outflow tract ventricular tachycardia*
- Dilated cardiomyopathy
- Congenital cyanotic heart disease

* This is an important differential diagnosis but in this case the resting ECG is normal and there are no morphological right ventricular abnormalities on imaging. The condition is benign as opposed to ARVC.

Question 363

This is a chest X-ray from an asymptomatic 50-year-old banker (**363**).

What is the diagnosis?
  a. Cryptogenic fibrosing alveolitis.
  b. Miliary tuberculosis.
  c. Healed chicken pox pneumonia.
  d. Pulmonary metastases.
  e. Histoplasmosis.

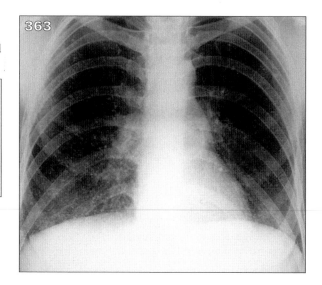

Question 364

A 54-year-old male presented with an acute painful swollen left knee. There was no history of trauma or any systemic features. There was a past history of a bleeding peptic ulcer that was treated 3 months ago. On examination the temperature was 37.8°C (100.0°F). The left knee was tender and erythematous.

Investigations are shown.

Hb	16 g/dl
WCC	13×10^9/l
Platelets	359×10^9/l
ESR	78 mm/h
CRP	92 g/l
Blood cultures	Normal
Joint aspirate	Needle-shaped crystals with strong negative birefringence under polarized light

What is the most appropriate management of the patient?
  a. Diclefenac alone.
  b. Allopurinol.
  c. Indomethacin plus proton pump inhibitor.
  d. Indomethacin plus misoprostol.
  e. Inject joint with steroid.

Question 365

A 77-year-old male was seen in the memory clinic owing to progressive deterioration of cognitive function. According to his daughter he had been diagnosed with Parkinson's disease two years previously, for which he was commenced on L-dopa. Over the past few months he had become intermittently confused and had hallucinations of monkeys in his garden. He had experienced several falls in the house and had been investigated by the cardiologists for recurrent episodes of syncope, but no cause was identified.

On examination he had evidence of bradykinesia, mild tremor and mild cog-wheel rigidity. The mini mental test score was 9. Serial 3 counting was satisfactory. Short-term memory was impaired.

Investigations are shown.

FBC	Normal
ESR	33 mm/h
Serum B_{12}	Normal
Serum folate	Normal
U&E	Normal
Blood sugar	Normal
Thyroid function	Normal
12-lead ECG	SR; left axis deviation
Chest X-ray	Normal
Urinalysis	Normal
CT scan brain	Mild global cerebral atrophy

What is the diagnosis?
  a. Alzheimer's disease.
  b. Pick's disease.
  c. Multi-infarct dementia.
  d. Lewy body dementia.
  e. Side-effect of L-dopa.

Answer 363

> c. Healed chicken pox pneumonia.

There are multiple calcified nodules throughout both lung fields in an otherwise asymptomatic patient. The differential diagnosis of multiple nodular opacities in the lungs is tabulated below. Patients with miliary TB are systemically unwell and complain of fever, cough and night sweats. Although histoplasmosis may present with multiple calcified nodules in the lung, the patient is completely well whereas patients with miliary histoplasmosis usually experience profound respiratory symptoms. Cryptogenic fibrosing alveolitis is associated with diffuse reticulonodular

Causes of diffuse calcified nodules in the lungs	
Infections	TB
	Histoplasmosis
	Coccidiocomycosis
	Chicken pox in adulthood
Occupational dusts	Silicosis
	Caplan's syndrome
Pulmonary metastases	
Alvelolar microlithiasis	

shadowing in both lung bases. Few pulmonary metastases may become calcified but a common example includes follicular adenocarcinoma of the thyroid.

Answer 364

> e. Inject joint with steroid.

The treatment options for acute gout include the use of non-steroidal anti-inflammatory agents, colchicine or injection of the joint with steroids. The most effective method of treating monoarticular gout is aspiration of the joint with intra-articular steroid injection. This method provides rapid relief of symptoms and produces no systemic side-effects. NSAIDs are relatively contraindicated in a patient with a recent history of a bleeding gastric ulcer. Although NSAIDs may be prescribed cautiously with either a proton pump inhibitor or misoprostol, the use of intra-articular steroid is safer and more effective. Colchicine is an alternative to NSAIDs but is also associated with frequent gastrointestinal side-effects and dermatological complications. Allopurinol may exacerbate acute gout but is the drug of choice in preventing further attacks once the acute attack has been treated.

Answer 365

> d. Lewy body dementia.

The presence of hallucinations, falls and syncope in a patient with Parkinson's disease is suggestive of dementia with Lewy bodies, which is the most common form of dementia associated with Parkinson's disease. It is characterized by the presence of Lewy bodies in the brainstem and the cortex. Lewy bodies are intracytoplasmic inclusions composed of alpha-synuclein and ubiquitin. The dementia is slowly progressive. There are fluctuations in cognition in relation to alertness and attentiveness. Memory impairment is mild in the early stages. Patients experience recurrent visual hallucinations of people and animals. Features of parkinsonism are generally mild. Daytime drowsiness and sleepiness, falls, syncope and delusions are well recognized. Patients with Lewy body dementia are particularly sensitive to neuroleptic agents. There is considerable overlap between Parkinson's disease, Lewy body dementia and Alzheimer's disease. Daytime sleepiness or drowsiness appears to be more common in Lewy body dementia than the other two entities.

Picks's disease is a subtype of fronto-temporal dementia that is characterized by Pick bodies in the neocortex and hippocampus. The disorder presents with language and/or behavioural abnormalities. The mean age of onset is the sixth decade. The disorder may occur as early as 35 years but is rare after the age of 75 years. The presence of behavioural or language deficits manifested by early and progressive changes in personality or loss of language function in the absence of another cause, is highly suggestive of Pick's disease. Neuroimaging with CT scan or MRI will reveal atrophy of the anterior temporal and frontal lobes. Extrapyramidal motor symptoms, bulbar and spinal motor neurone disease are recognized manifestations of Pick's disease. There is currently no treatment available for Pick's disease.

Vascular dementias are abrupt in onset followed by step-wise deterioration. Physical examination usually reveals focal abnormalities consistent with previous stroke, and neuroimaging reveals multiple infarcts.

Alzheimer's disease is the commonest cause of dementia and is characterized by gradual and progressive global diminution of cognitive function. Loss of short-term memory is the most prominent feature in the early stages. There is considerable overlap between Alzheimer's disease and the conditions described above. The diagnosis of Alzheimer's disease is clinical.

Question 366

A 68-year-old male with disseminated colonic carcinoma was admitted to hospital having collapsed at home. He had been complaining of severe back pain for 48 hours, for which he was taking two different analgesic agents. He was also taking bronchodilator inhalers for chronic asthma.

On examination he was drowsy and had a Glasgow coma score of 8. The pupils were small and equal and reacted slowly to light. Inspection of the fundi was not possible. The heart rate was 120 beats/min. The blood pressure measured 100/60 mm Hg. The respiratory rate was reduced to 8/min. The tone in the limbs was normal. The lower limb reflexes were brisk and the plantar response was extensor bilaterally.

Investigations are shown.

Sodium	133 mmol/l
Potassium	3.7 mmol/l
Urea	8 mmol/l
Calcium	2.7 mmol/l
Albumin	29 g/l
Arterial blood gases on 60% oxygen:	
pH	7.2
$PaCO_2$	9.6 kPa
PaO_2	28 kPa
HCO_3	28 mmol/l
CT scan brain	Multiple cerebral metastases

What is the most immediate treatment that is required?
  a. Intravenous bicarbonate.
  b. Intravenous naloxone.
  c. Intravenous doxopram.
  d. Intravenous dexamethasone.
  e. Intravenous flumazenil.

Question 367

A 64-year-old male presented with a three-month history of copious diarrhoea associated with lower abdominal cramps and weight loss. The patient moved his bowel up to 20 times per day. There was no blood in the stools. He had a past history of gallstones, for which he underwent a cholecystectomy five years ago. He had not experienced any episodes of biliary colic since surgery. The patient was also in the process of being investigated for intermittent dizziness that usually occurred after meals and was preceded by a burning sensation over the face, neck and chest. According to his wife he developed a red complexion during these episodes, which lasted for 30–60 seconds at a time. On two occasions he had almost lost consciousness when he stood suddenly during these episodes. The patient had not travelled abroad for over eight months. He was not taking any medication. His father had ulcerative colitis and his paternal nephew had gluten sensitive enteropathy.

On examination he had several telangiectasiae on his face, neck and upper trunk. The JVP was raised with prominent V waves. On auscultation of the precordium, there was a soft systolic murmur. The chest was clear. Abdominal examination revealed a palpable liver edge 5 cm below the costal margin that had a firm and irregular consistency. Rectal examination was normal.

Investigations are shown.

Hb	11 g/dl
MCV	80 fl
WCC	12×10^9/l
Platelets	200×10^9/l
ESR	68 mm/h
Sodium	130 mmol/l
Potassium	3.4 mmol/l
Urea	9 mmol/l
AST	40 iu/l
Alkaline phosphatase	320 iu/l
Bilirubin	16 µmol/l
Albumin	29 g/l

What is the diagnosis?
  a. Coeliac disease.
  b. Crohn's disease.
  c. Disseminated colonic carcinoma.
  d. Carcinoma of the head of pancreas.
  e. Carcinoid syndrome.

Answer 366

> b. Intravenous naloxone.

The patient takes analgesia for chronic pain, presumably related to the disseminated carcinoma. He presents with drowsiness, miosis, reduced respiratory rate and a respiratory acidosis. The patient has tachycardia, which is probably due to vasodilatation from the acidosis. The most probable cause of the presentation is opiate overdose, which may be accidental or deliberate. The immediate treatment to reverse the effects is intravenous naloxone. Although benzodiazepine overdose can present in identical fashion, the patient is more likely to have taken excess opiate for his pain rather than a benzodiazepine. Flumazenil, the antidote for benzodiazepine overdose, should be considered only if respiratory depression is not reversed with naloxone.

The patient also has cerebral metastases, which may be causing raised intracranial pressure and may be responsible for the pyramidal tract signs; however, the presentation is more consistent with opiate overdose. Dexamethasone should be instituted if the patient has symptoms of raised intracranial pressure or focal neurology once he is more conscious.

Tricyclic antidepressant overdose also presents with drowsiness, tachycardia, hypotension and upgoing plantars and brisk reflexes. However, acidosis is due to reduced bicarbonate levels rather than retention of carbon dioxide. Patients with tricyclic antidepressant overdose also have antimuscarinic features. In this respect one would expect the patient to have dilated rather than constricted pupils. Intravenous bicarbonate is reserved for managing tricyclic antidepressant overdose.

Doxopram is a respiratory stimulant that is rarely effective and very rarely used in clinical practice nowadays.

Answer 367

> e. Carcinoid syndrome.

The patient has copious diarrhoea and weight loss as well as intermittent dizziness associated with a red complexion, which would be consistent with carcinoid syndrome. The presence of a firm and irregular liver edge is highly suggestive of metastases to the liver which is usually required for the clinical manifestation of carcinoid tumours arising from the gastrointestinal tract.

Crohn's disease and celiac disease rarely cause copious diarrhoea and would not explain the flushing. In ulcerative colitis loose stool is often blood-stained.

Carcinoid syndrome is caused by tumours that have the ability to store and synthesize polypeptides and biogenic amines and prostaglandins. The tumours commonly arise from the gut, notably the small bowel, appendix and rectum, and may arise from the lungs and pancreas. The tumours commonly produce serotonin, a metabolite of the amino acid tryptophan, histamine and kallikrein. These biogenic compounds are inactivated by the liver. After metastasis to the liver, the amines are secreted into hepatic veins and enter the systemic circulation to cause symptoms.

In the vast majority of cases, the symptoms depend largely on the proportion of serotonin, histamine or kallikrein produced by the tumour. In general, hindgut tumours such as those arising from the rectum lack the decarboxylase enzyme that catalyses the conversion of tryptophan to 5-hydroxytryptamine, therefore these tumours are unable to cause the carcinoid syndrome.

Symptoms include flushing, diarrhoea, and bronchospasm. Flushing is the hallmark of carcinoid syndrome and occurs in almost 90% of patients. Flushing is intermittent and affects the upper trunk and face. The patient feels warm during these episodes and may experience palpitation and dizziness due to profound vasodilatation causing a drop in blood pressure. Flushing may be precipitated by eating, defecation, consuming alcohol, emotion, pressure on the liver or general anaesthesia. Diarrhoea is probably the most disabling symptom and may occur up to 30 times per day. It may be explosive and associated with abdominal cramps. Bronchospasm is present in 20% of cases and is exacerbated by beta-agonists.

Cardiac involvement results in a fibrogenic reaction affecting the pericardium and the right heart valves. The left-sided cardiac valves are not affected unless there is bronchial involvement, since the lungs inactivate bioactive amines produced by carcinoid tumours. Cardiac involvement is a very poor prognostic marker.

Patients with carcinoid syndrome are at risk of developing pellagra owing to the utilization of tryptophan to form serotonin rather than nicotinic acid (the active form of niacin).

Treatment is usually with octreotide or alpha-interferon. Resection of hepatic metastases may provide good palliation.

Some tumours may produce polypeptides such as insulin, gastrin, growth hormone, ACTH, vasointestinal peptide and somatostatin.

Question 368

A 16-year-old girl collapsed at school while playing hockey. According to the physical training tutor, she was unconscious for a few seconds and then was completely rousable and did not realize what had happened. The episode occurred without any warning symptoms. There was no history of trauma or head injury during the game, or any ill health before the game. There was no history of epilepsy. She had experienced two previous syncopal episodes at the ages of 8 and 11 years. On the first occasion she had witnessed a road traffic accident, and on the second occasion she collapsed after receiving a hoax telephone call. She had been completely well since the last syncopal episode. She was not taking any medication. She had a younger brother, aged 14, who was well. Her parents were well. Her mother had a past history of syncopal episodes during her adolescence, for which no cause had been found. Her maternal aunt was found dead in her bed at the age of 15, for which no cause was found at post-mortem.

On examination, the patient was 1.55 m tall and weighed 48 kg. Her heart rate was 65 beats/min and irregular. The blood pressure was 110/65 mmHg. Examination of the precordium was completely normal. There were no carotid bruits, and all peripheral pulses were palpable. The chest was clear and abdominal examination was normal. Examination of the central nervous system, including the fundi, was completely normal

Investigations are shown.

The following day, the patient was being seen by the consultant cardiologist and his team on the ward when she had a syncopal episode. The tracing from the ECG monitor is shown (**368b**).

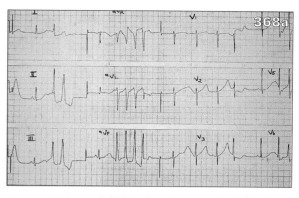

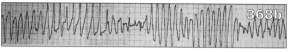

Hb	14 g/dl
WCC	12×10^9/l
Platelets	300×10^9/l
Blood glucose	5 mmol/l
ECG (**368a**)	
Sodium	136 mmol/l
Potassium	3.5 mmol/l
Urea	4 mmol/l

1. What is the diagnosis?
   a. Wolff–Parkinson–White syndrome.
   b. Lown–Ganong–Levine syndrome.
   c. Hypertrophic cardiomyopathy.
   d. Congenital LQTS.
   e. Drug overdose.

2. What is the underlying abnormality in this disorder?
   a. Myocardial disarray.
   b. Accessory conduction pathway.
   c. Abnormal sodium/potassium channels in cardiac myocytes.
   d. Fibrofatty replacement of the myocardium.
   e. Myocardial fibrosis.

3. How would you manage this patient immediately?
   a. Intravenous isoprenaline.
   b. Intravenous atropine.
   c. Intravenous adenosine.
   d. A beta-blocker.
   e. Atrial pacing.

4. What other important investigation would you perform?
   a. Cardiac enzymes.
   b. Echocardiogram.
   c. Electrophysiological studies.
   d. Family screening.
   e. Serum cholesterol.
   f. Serum potassium.
   g. Serum magnesium.

Answer 368

1. d. Congenital LQTS.
2. c. Abnormal sodium/potassium channels in cardiac myocytes.
3. d. A beta-blocker.
4. d. Family screening.

The combination of a family history of premature sudden death, long QT and polymorphic ventricular tachycardia associated with syncope is diagnostic of idiopathic LQTS. The condition is familial in up to 90% of cases, and can be inherited both as an autosomal dominant and recessive trait. The rarer variant (autosomal recessive) is associated with congenital nerve deafness and known as the Jarvell–Lange–Neilsen syndrome. The more common autosomal dominant form is often known as the Romano–Ward syndrome.

In congenital LQTS defects within transmembrane ion channels produce abnormalities in cardiac repolarization, leading to an increased propensity for syncope due to fatal ventricular arrhythmias in situations causing increased sympathetic activity. Syncope may be precipitated by physical exertion, intense emotion and sudden loud auditory stimuli. The classic arrhythmia is a form of polymorphic ventricular tachycardia termed 'torsades de pointes', which may degenerate to ventricular fibrillation, causing sudden death. Thus far, abnormalities have been demonstrated in genes encoding both potassium and sodium ion transport channel proteins which are located on chromosomes 11, 3, 4 and 7 (see below).

Myocardial disarray is a feature of HCM; an accessory conduction pathway would indicate Wolff–Parkinson–White or Lown–Ganong–Levine syndrome; fibrofatty replacement of the myocardium would indicate arrhythmogenic right ventricular cardiomyopathy; and myocardial fibrosis is a finding common to all cardiomyopathies and ischaemic heart disease.

Treatment is aimed at reducing the effects of the sympathetic nervous system on the conduction tissue. The immediate treatment of choice to prevent further ventricular tachycardia is beta-blockers, which may be given intravenously in the first instance. In situations where this produces a profound bradycardia a permanent pacemaker is also implanted. There is some evidence that intravenous magnesium may arrest ventricular arrhythmias in the acute state, even when the serum magnesium level is normal. Patients who continue to have ventricular arrhythmias despite heavy beta-blockade are implanted with an automatic cardioverter defibrillator. It is worth noting that therapy with isoprenaline, a sympathomimetic agent which is useful in acquired LQTS, is contraindicated in congenital LQTS.

Screening of first-degree relatives is very important in this condition. In approximately 60% of cases the diagnosis of idiopathic LQTS is made during screening of first-degree relatives of affected patients. Low serum magnesium and potassium are causes of acquired LQTS which should always be excluded. In this case, there is no obvious cause for an electrolyte deficiency. No marks are awarded for electrophysiological studies because the diagnosis and the potential for VT are obvious.

Acquired causes of LQTS are usually due to drugs and electrolyte disturbances (*Table*). In such cases, treatment involves correction of the electrolyte disturbance and withdrawal of the offending drug. Rectifying serum electrolytes and drug levels can take several days, and prevention of polymorphic VT relies on shortening the QT-interval by atrial pacing at a rate of 60–70 beats/min.

Genetics of LQTS

Congenital LQTS is a recognized but rare cause of sudden death in young adults. Death is due to polymorphic tachycardia (torsades de points) degenerating into ventricular fibrillation. Syncope is common in affected patients, and is due to transient cerebral hypoperfusion from VT. Common stimuli of polymorphic VT include physical exertion, intense emotion and auditory stimuli. Genes encoding sodium and potassium ion channels cause disease. To date, there are four different loci on chromosomes 3, 4, 7 and 11. On chromosome 7, there is a mutation in the HERG gene (potassium channel abnormality). Other mutations include the SCN5A (chromosome 3; sodium ion channels) and KVLQT1 (chromosome 11; potassium ion channels).

(See Question 353.)

Acquired causes of long LQTS

- Drugs
- Class Ia and Ic antiarrhythmic agents
- Tricyclic antidepressants, neuroleptic agents
- Erythromycin
- Ketoconazole
- Certain antihistamines
- Cisapride
- Electrolyte disturbances
- Hypokalaemia
- Hypomagnesaemia
- Hypocalcaemia
- Cardiovascular diseases
- Myocardial infarction
- Complete heart block
- Sick sinus syndrome
- Mitral valve prolapse
- Others
- Subarachnoid haemorrhage
- Liquid protein diet

Question 369

A 44-year-old man presented with recent onset of epigastric burning that was precipitated by hunger or after a heavy meal. His appetite was unchanged and his weight was stable. He consumed 21 units of alcohol per week but was a non-smoker. The patient was not on any medication. There was no family history of carcinoma of the stomach. The urease breath test for *Helicobacter pylori* was positive.

What is the next management step?
a. Reassure.
b. Start omperazole, amoxycillin and clarithromycin for 7–10 days.
c. Start omeprazole, amoxycillin and clarithromycin for one month.
d. Request urgent upper gastrointestinal endoscopy.
e. Cimetidine therapy.

Question 370

A 72-year-old patient with previous admissions for exacerbation of chronic obstructive airways disease was admitted to hospital with a six-day history of cough productive of yellow sputum and dyspnoea. He smoked five cigarettes per day but had previously been a heavy smoker. He had a past medical history of ischaemic heart disease and had had a stent to the right coronary artery following a myocardial infarction two years ago. His medications included inhaled iprotropium bromide, inhaled salbutamol and inhaled pulmicort. His GP had commenced amoxycillin five days previously.

On examination he was cyanosed. The respiratory rate was 30/min. The heart rate was 120 beats/min and regular. The blood pressure measured 150/90 mmHg. Both heart sounds were soft. Auscultation of the lung fields revealed coarse crackles throughout the lungs.

Investigations are shown.

Hb	16 g/dl
WCC	17×10^9/l
Platelets	400×10^9/l
Sodium	138 mmol/l
Potassium	4.0 mmol/l
Urea	7 mmol/l
Creatinine	120 μmol/l
Chest X-ray	Hyperinflated lung markings with reduced vascular markings.
Arterial blood gases (2 l oxygen/min):	
pH	7.1
$PaCO_2$	8.2 kPa
PaO_2	6 kPa
HCO_3	30 mmol/l
12-lead ECG	Atrial fibrillation/RBBB (ventricular rate 120)
Urinalysis	Blood +

What is the most effective management of his presentation?
a. IV aminophylline.
b. Non-invasive positive pressure ventilation.
c. IV doxapram.
d. IV heparin.
e. IV hydrocortisone.

Answer 369

> b. Start omeprazole, amoxycillin and clarithromycin for 7–10 days.

The patient has dyspepsia and a positive urease breath test suggestive of *Helicobacter* infection. Such patients should receive eradication therapy. Recommended eradication therapy for *H. pylori* infection includes a full-dose proton pump inhibitor twice daily, amoxycillin 1 g twice daily and clarithromycin 500 mg twice daily for one week. An alternative regime is full-dose proton pump inhibitor twice daily, metronidazole 400 mg twice daily and clarithromycin 250 mg twice daily for 7–10 days.

The therapeutic recommendations in patients with uncomplicated dyspepsia are as follows:

1. Ensure all ulcerogenic medications have been stopped.
2. Treat dyspepsia with a proton pump inhibitor for a month.
3. If symptoms persist the patient should be tested for *H.pylori* infection with the intent to treat. The most useful test for *H. pylori* is the urease breath test. First-line treatment regimes are described in the first paragraph above. Most duodenal ulcers (more than 90%) respond to eradication therapy.
4. Patients who develop recurrence of symptoms after eradication therapy, particularly those aged over 55 years of age, should be referred for upper gastro-intestinal endoscopy.
5. Upper gastrointestinal endoscopy should also be performed on patients presenting with features of chronic gastrointestinal bleeding, progressive unintentional weight loss, dysphagia, persistent vomiting, iron deficiency anaemia, epigastric mass or suspicious barium meal to exclude a malignant peptic ulcer.
6. In patients noted to have a duodenal ulcer at endoscopy, a urease breath test is performed to check for persistence of *H. pylori* infection (assuming that the patient has already received eradication therapy at initial presentation). In patients with evidence of *H. pylori* infection, second-line eradication therapy is offered (assuming the patient has relapsed on first-line eradication therapy). If the patient becomes asymptomatic after this, no further investigation is necessary. Patients with evidence of persistent *H. pylori* infection on eradication therapy are treated with long-term, low-dose antisecretory therapy with either proton pump inhibitors or H2 receptor blockers. Some patients (5%) have duodenal ulcers in the absence of *H. pylori* infection. These patients are also managed with long-term antisecretory drugs.
7. Patients with gastric ulcers at endoscopy should be biopsed to exclude malignancy. Gastric ulcer patients are treated similarly to patients with duodenal ulcers. Treatment with eradication therapy leads to healing of the vast majority of gastric ulcers. Unlike patients with duodenal ulcers, patients with gastric ulcers should have repeat endoscopy at six weeks, even in the absence of symptoms, to ensure healing of the ulcer, as gastric ulcers are associated with higher complication rates and are often malignant. Failure of a gastric ulcer to heal may be an indication of malignancy and warrants repeat biopsies.

Answer 370

> b. Non-invasive positive pressure ventilation.

The patient has a severe infective exacerbation of chronic obstructive pulmonary disease as evidenced by the marked hypoxia and respiratory acidosis. Early NIPPV is required and has been shown to be as effective as invasive ventilation (without the problems associated with invasive ventilation) in terms of expediting recovery and reducing mortality. Patients who should be considered for NIPPV include those who have a moderate to severe dyspnoea, a respiratory rate of >25/min, an arterial pH <7.35 and a $PaCO_2$ >6 kPa.

There is no place for IV aminophylline in the management of acute exacerbations of COPD. It is not effective and increases the risk of arrhythmias in the hypoxic patient. Similarly doxapram, a respiratory stimulant, is no longer used in the management of acute exacerbations of COPD.

Short-term high-dose steroids (two-week course) have been shown to be effective in the management of exacerbations of COPD (NEJM 1999; **340** (25); 1941–47) (*Table*). Steroids cause a modest increase in FEV_1 and reduce in-hospital stay. Steroid usage for more than two weeks does not have additional benefit. The benefit from systemic steroid therapy does not exceed six months.

> **Management of exacerbations of COPD**
>
> - Oxygen to maintain $PaO_2 \geq 8$ kPa (or O_2 saturation $\geq 90\%$) is essential to prevent tissue hypoxia.
> - Inhaled bronchodilators (beta-agonists and anticholinergic drugs) are the mainstay of treatment. Anticholinergic bronchodilators are most effective. Beta-agonist inhalers have an additive effect.
> - The use of antibiotics remains controversial and is reserved for patients with copious sputum production. Amoxycillin, ampicillin, septrin and tetracyline have been shown to be effective. Newer antibiotics such as the quinolones and the macrolides such as clarithromycin have not been shown to be superior to older antibiotics.
> - Short-term high dose steroids for up to two weeks.
> - Early NIPPV in patients with severe exacerbation associated with respiratory failure.
> - Aminophylline and doxapram are not recommended.

Question 371

A 50-year-old man presented with a 24-hour history of heamatemesis and malena. There was no preceding history of abdominal discomfort. He consumed 80–100 units of alcohol per week.

On examination he was pale. His heart rate was 110 beats/min and blood pressure measured 90/60 mmHg.

Investigations are shown.

Hb	10 g/dl
WCC	16×10^9/l
Platelets	80×10^9/l
PT	22 s
Sodium	131 mmol/l
Potassium	3.2 mmol/l
Urea	14 mmol/l
Creatinine	90 µmol/l
AST	160 iu/l
Bilirubin	32 µmol/l
Albumin	28 g/l

The patient was resuscitated with 2 units of blood and 2 litres of dextrose 5% and underwent urgent endoscopy, which revealed a bleeding oesophageal varix.

What is the best treatment to prevent further bleeding?
   a. Intravenous fresh frozen plasma.
   b. Sclerotherapy of the bleeding varix.
   c. Band ligation of the bleeding varix.
   d. Intravenous octreotide.
   e. Intravenous glypressin.

Questions 372 and 373

A 50-year-old male presented with collapse after a febrile illness. He had been generally unwell for almost two years, complaining of fatigue and listlessness. His GP had commenced him on antidepressant medication after he complained of reduced appetite, constipation and loss of libido. The patient had recently given up his job as a bank clerk owing to inability to cope with the pressure. He had been taking antihypertensive medication that had recently been stopped after the development of postural hypotension.

On examination he was pale. He had sparse axillary hair. The blood pressure on admission was 80/50 mmHg. There was an appendicectomy scar which appeared normal. Both heart sounds were normal. Neurological examination revealed diplopia on lateral gaze on the left side.

Investigations are shown.

Hb	10 g/dl
WCC	7×10^9/l
Platelets	200×10^9/l
MCV	86 fl
Sodium	130 mmol/l
Potassium	4 mmol/l
Urea	5 mmol/l
Glucose	4 mmol/l
TSH	0.3 mu/l
	(NR 0.4–3.6 mu/l)
Chlolesterol	6.9 mmol/l
Chest X-ray	Normal
ECG	Sinus bradycardia rate 60 beats/min

Question 372
What is the full diagnosis?
   a. Primary hypothyroidism.
   b. Addison's disease.
   c. Secondary hypothyroidism.
   d. Herpes encephalitis.
   e. Panhypopituitarism.

Question 373
What treatment is required immediately?
   a. IV saline 0.9%.
   b. IV dextrose 50 ml (50%).
   c. IV tri-iodothyronine.
   d. IV hydrocortisone 100 mg.
   e. IV acyclovir.

Answer 371

c Band ligation of bleeding varix.

The patient has a history of alcohol abuse and presents with a significant oesophageal variceal haemorrhage as defined by a systolic BP <100 mmHg or a pulse >100/min. Varices are a common source of bleeding in patients with cirrhosis of the liver and account for almost one-third of all deaths from this condition. A variceal bleed is associated with a mortality of approximately 50%. Aggressive resuscitation with blood and colloids and achievement of haemostasis saves lives. Following resuscitation, the first method of choice is band ligation of the bleeding varices (see algorithm [371] and *Table* for management).

371 Algorithm for the management of a variceal haemorrhage

Goals in the management of bleeding varices

General
1. Restore circulation to keep systolic blood pressure ≥ 90 mmHg and urine volume ≥ 50 ml/h
2. Maintain Hb >9 g/dl
3. Correct clotting with fresh-frozen plasma in patients with raised prothrombin times
4. Platelet transfusion in patients with platelet count <50 × 10^9/l in the presence of active bleeding. Note large transfusions may produce dilutional thrombocytopenia
5. Prevent aspiration of vomitus by gastric decompression via a nasogastric tube
6. Reduce risk of encephalopathy with lactulose, ensuring the existing hypokalaemia is corrected
7. Antibiotic prophylaxis with cephalosporin or quinolones has been shown to reduce overall mortality from infective complications in patients presenting with variceal haemorrhage

Specific (**371**)
1. Following resuscitation the patient should undergo endoscopy with band ligation of bleeding varices. Band ligation is superior to sclerotherapy and is associated with a lower complication rate. Sclerotherapy should be performed if band ligation is not possible owing to continued bleeding
2. Glypressin and somatostatin (or octreotide) are effective at controlling acute variceal bleeding. Both drugs act by causing mesenteric arteriolar vasoconstriction and reduction of portal pressures. Somatostatin is better tolerated than glypressin. These drugs are usually reserved for situations where endoscopy is not available
3. Gastric varices are not usually amenable to band ligation and are generally treated with injection of fibrin glue or transjugular intrahepatic portosystemic shunt
4. When bleeding is difficult to control (i.e. there is a need to transfuse more than 4 units of blood to achieve an increase in systolic BP of 20 mmHg or to 70 mmHg or more, and/or an inability to achieve a pulse rate reduction to less than 100 beats/min or a reduction of 20/min from baseline), a Sengstaken–Blakemore tube should be inserted until further endoscopic treatment, TIPSS or surgery is instituted

Answers 372 and 373

Answer 372
e. Panhypopituitarism.
Answer 373
d. IV hydrocortisone 100 mg.

The patient presents with collapse following a febrile illness but has been generally unwell with fatigue and depression for almost two years. He has hypotension, sparse body hair, a low sodium and low TSH. The symptoms of fatigue, low affect and loss of libido may be attributed to stress or depression. However, in the context of the overall presentation they are typical of hypopituitarism. Fatigue and loss of libido are early features of gonadotrophin deficiency. Gradual loss of secondary sexual characteristics and reduced muscle bulk follow later. Depression could be explained by deficiency of any of the anterior pituitary hormones. The collapse following a febrile illness and the low sodium almost certainly represent significant cortisol depletion due to low ACTH reserve. The low TSH clinches the diagnosis, as secondary hypothyroidism can only occur as a result of a pituitary disorder. The extra-ocular muscle dysfunction suggests that the most probable cause of the hypopituitarism is a pituitary tumour (see *Table A* for the causes of hypopituitarism). Pituitary tumours cause headache and localized pressure effects. Compression of the optic chiasm causes bitemporal hemianopia and pressure on the cavernous sinus may result in paralysis of the extra-ocular muscle function.

Although the presentation may also be explained by Addison's disease (primary hypoadrenalism) there are two features which favour a low ACTH reserve rather than primary adrenal gland failure. Firstly, the patient has a normal potassium level. Potassium concentrations are governed by aldosterone, which is not influenced by ACTH. Aldosterone levels are normal or increased in panhypopituitarism. The low sodium level in panhypopituitarism is due to SIADH caused by cortisol deficiency. Secondly, patients with low ACTH do not exhibit hyperpigmentation. Hyperpigmentation in Addison's disease is explained by the fact that ACTH is secreted as part of a large hormone precursor pro-opiomelanocortin, which is cleaved to produce both ACTH and melanocyte stimulating hormone. The latter is responsible for hyperpigmentation that is most noticeable in skin creases and scars (*Table B*).

Manifestations of hypopituitary crisis include collapse or coma. The management includes treatment of hypoglycaemia if present followed by urgent administration of intravenous hydrocortisone 100 mg, which should be continued six hourly. Circulation is restored with intravenous saline. The patient should undergo an urgent MRI brain scan to exclude pituitary apoplexy as this is an indication for urgent neurosurgical referral. Thyroid hormone replacement is in the form of intravenous tri-iodothryronine. However, thyroid replacement should only be given after intravenous hydrocortisone has been administered, otherwise the effect of cortisol deficiency becomes even more pronounced.

Table A Causes of panhypopituitarism

Cause	Notes
Pituitary masses	Tumours, cysts
Extra-pituitary tumours	Craniopharyngioma
Pituitary surgery	
Pituitary irradiation	
Sheehan syndrome	Infarction after massive haemorrhage, e.g. during child birth
Pituitary apoplexy	
Infiltrative disorders	Haemochromatosis, lymphocytic hypophysitis
Genetic disorders	Mutation in PROP-1 or Pit-1
Hypothalamic disorders	

Table B Differential diagnosis of Addison's disease and panhypopituitarism

Symptom	Addison's disease	Panhypo-pituitarism
Lassitude, malaise, depression	Common	Common
Loss of body hair	Recognized	Common
Hyperpigmentation	Common	Not part of disorder
Ocular signs	Not present	Dependent on cause*
Collapse	Recognized	Only occurs in severe ACTH depletion
Low sodium	Common	Common
High potassium	Characteristic	Not part of disorder

*Present secondary to tumour

Question 374

A 31-year-old female presented with acute onset of swelling of the neck after attending the funeral of a close friend. On examination she had well-demarcated oedema of the lips, eyes and ear lobes. The heart rate was 100 beats/min. The blood pressure was 90/50 mmHg. The respiratory rate was 24 /min. The chest was clear.

She had previously attended the Accident and Emergency Department with intermittent ankle swelling and abdominal pain. Her father had suffered with similar episodes for many years but had never had to seek medical attention.

What is the most effective immediate management of this patient?
   a. Emergency tracheostomy.
   b. Subcutaneous adrenaline.
   c. Intravenous corticosteroids.
   d. C1 esterase inhibitor concentrate.
   e. Fresh-frozen plasma.

Answer 374

> d. C1 esterase inhibitor concentrate

Hereditary angio-oedema is a genetic disorder inherited as an autosomal dominant trait that results in a deficiency of C1 esterase inhibitor. Deficiencies in this protein allow unchecked activation of the classic complement pathway and other biochemical systems.

Patients can present with any combination of cutaneous angio-oedema, abdominal pain, or acute airway obstruction. Prior to the development of effective therapy, the mortality rate was 20–30%. Typically, presentation is in late childhood or early adolescence following trauma, infection, dental procedures, or emotional stress. There is an increasing frequency and severity of episodes during puberty, menstruation and ovulation. The acquired form typically occurs at an older age and may not be associated with trauma. The symptoms of C1 esterase inhibitor deficiency range in severity from a minor inconvenience to life-threatening oedema.

Although preventable and treatable, the complications of this disease do not respond well to the usual therapies for angio-oedema and are more refractory to the use of intramuscular adrenaline, antihistamines and steroids. Therefore, establishment of the correct diagnosis is critical. The management of hereditary angio-oedema is outlined in *Table*.

Acquired C1 esterase inhibitor deficiency may occur with lymphoproliferative disorders and autoantibodies targeted against C1 esterase inhibitor. The presentation is similar to hereditary angio-oedema. Patients with acquired C1 esterase deficiency also have deficiency in C2 and C4 levels.

Management of hereditary angio-oedema

- Ensure airway is unobstructed (tracheostomy in cases of severe upper airway obstruction)
- Treat circulatory collapse in the event of acute anaphylaxis
- Intramuscular adrenaline 1 in 1000
- C1 esterase inhibitor concentrate is the most effective therapy but it is not readily available. If C1 esterase inhibitor concentrate is unavailable immediately fresh-frozen plasma may be given in the interim. FFP has been given to acutely replete C1 esterase inhibitor and as prophylaxis pre-operatively and before labour. However, this preparation also provides substrate for C1 Inh, which may paradoxically worsen the clinical situation
- Stanozolol and danazol are useful at increasing C1 esterase inhibitor levels acutely and prophylactically and have been shown to be effective in the management of hereditary angio-oedema

(See Question 155.)

Question 375

A 17-year-old female was admitted with a six-week history of malaise and joint pains. She had pain affecting her neck, left shoulder and the small joints of both her hands. She had intermittent fever associated with profuse sweating. She was born in Kenya and travelled to England for further studies two years ago. She had not travelled abroad since. She was well while in Kenya, although she had had two mild attacks of malaria at the ages of 5 years and 12 years. She was a non-smoker and a teetotaller. Two days before coming into hospital she developed some sharp infra-mammary chest pain, which was worsened by movement, deep inspiration and on lying flat. There was no history of cough or sputum production. Her appetite was slightly reduced and she had lost 2 kg in weight.

On examination, she appeared unwell. She had a temperature of 39.2°C (102.6°F) and a widespread rash, shown in (**375a**). The heart rate was 110 beats/min and blood pressure 110/65 mmHg. She had small, non-tender, palpable lymph nodes in the anterior cervical triangle. On examination of the cardiovascular system she had a very soft systolic murmur at the left lower sternal angle, and a soft third heart sound. The chest was clear. Abdominal examination revealed a palpable spleen 3 cm below the costal margin. She had a few shotty lymph nodes in the inguinal region.

Cervical spine movements were slightly limited owing to pain. Her hands were swollen and tender. The left shoulder was painful to abduct, but there was no obvious swelling of the joint. Examination of the central nervous system and fundoscopy were normal.

Investigations are shown – see opposite page.

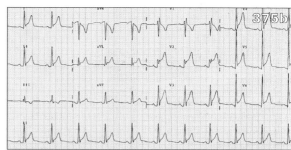

Hb	10 g/dl
WCC	17×10^9/l
Platelets	470×10^9/l
MCV	82 fl
Malaria parasite	Absent
ESR	86 mm/h
CRP	54 g/l
Sodium	134 mmol/l
Potassium	3.8 mmol/l
Urea	5 mmol/l
Creatinine	70 μmol/l
Blood cultures × 3	Negative
Thyroxine	98 nmol/l
TSH	1.1 mu/l
ECG **(375b)**	
Chest X-ray	Normal
Echocardiogram **(375c)**	
Rhesus factor	Absent
Urinalysis	Trace of protein
	No blood

What is the most probable diagnosis?
  a. Adult-onset Still's disease.
  b. Systemic lupus erythematosus.
  c. Brucellosis.
  d. Infective endocarditis.
  e. Lymphoma.

Question 376

An obese woman was diagnosed as having pernicious anaemia when she presented with lethargy and was found to have a raised MCV, low B_{12} level and intrinsic factor antibodies.

A blood count performed at the time was as follows:

She was treated with intramuscular B_{12} injections for a year but continued to complain of lethargy.

Blood results were as follows:

Hb	9.1 g/dl
WCC	7×10^9/l
Platelets	250×10^9/l
MCV	110 fl

Hb	11 g/dl
WCC	7.4×10^9/l
Platelets	260×10^9/l
MCV	105 fl

Which two other coexisting diagnoses should be considered?

  a. Myelodysplasia.
  b. Chronic liver disease.
  c. Folate deficiency.
  d. Orotic aciduria.
  e. Carcinoma of the stomach.
  f. Hypothyroidism.
  g. Chronic renal failure.
  h. Myeloma.
  i. Crohn's disease.
  j. Iron deficiency.

Answer 375

> a. Adult-onset Still's disease.

The characteristics of the chest pain are consistent with acute pericarditis, which is confirmed on the ECG.
The patient has malaise, fever, arthralgia, a rash, lymphadenopathy, arthritis and splenomegaly.

The differential diagnosis is between adult-onset juvenile chronic arthritis or Still's disease, SLE, and lymphoma. The high CRP is against the diagnosis of SLE. While lymphoma is quite possible, the seronegative arthritis, neutrophil leucocytosis, high fever and maculopapular rash are best explained by Still's disease. Adult Still's disease is rare. It affects young adults aged between 16 and 35 years. The characteristics are identical to those of juvenile chronic arthritis in younger patients. The diagnosis is essentially clinical, and the clinical criteria are outlined below (*Table*). Antinuclear factor is negative in Still's disease. Generalized lymphadenopathy is relatively common, and lymph node biopsy shows only reactive changes. If both these tests are negative, then adult Still's disease is the most likely diagnosis.

Infective endocarditis is unlikely with three negative blood cultures. The echocardiogram (**375c**) reveals a normal aortic and mitral valve, and right-sided endocarditis is most unusual in young, previously healthy individuals unless there is a history of intravenous drug abuse. Rheumatic fever may be suspected in a woman living in East Africa with a murmur, fever, arthritis and pericarditis; however, there is no history of streptococcal infection, and her symptoms are relatively long-standing for rheumatic fever. In this case, the murmur is likely to represent hyperdynamic circulation due to the fever; soft systolic murmurs and third heart sounds are relatively common in young individuals with fever. Malaria is unlikely after two years of being completely asymptomatic while in England. While *Plasmodium malariae* infections can be chronic, they do not present with frequent high fever and sweats of sudden onset. Brucellosis partly fits the clinical presentation; however, it is important to remember that it has been eradicated in the UK through pasteurization of milk. Sarcoidosis may mimic Still's disease, but the absence of ocular, respiratory and skin signs make it less probable. Familial Mediterranean fever is most unlikely for two reasons. First, it has a predilection for Jews and Arabs; second, it usually causes a monoarticular arthropathy.

In this case, ANF and lymph node biopsy are necessary to exclude SLE and lymphoma, respectively.

Diagnosis of adult-onset Still's disease

Requires each of:
1. Quotidian fever >39°C (102.2°F)
2. Leucocytosis >15 × 10^9/l
3. Arthralgia/arthritis
4. Macular/maculopapular rash

Plus two of:
(a) Serositis (pleuritic/pericarditic)
(b) Splenomegaly
(c) Generalized lymphadenopathy
(d) Negative rheumatoid factor
(e) Negative anti-nuclear factor

Answer 376

> c. Folate deficiency.
> f. Hypothyroidism.

The patient was diagnosed as having pernicious anaemia on the basis of a large MCV, low B$_{12}$ levels and intrinsic factor antibodies. Indeed, an MCV >110 fl is highly suggestive of a megaloblastic marrow (i.e. B$_{12}$, folate deficiency or treatment with cytotoxic drugs). The patient has responded partly to B$_{12}$ injections as evidenced by the increased haemoglobin and partial improvement in the MCV. However, she continues to remain symptomatic and has subnormal Hb and MCV.

While there are several causes of raised MCV, the two most probable diagnoses in this case include coexisting folate deficiency or hypothyroidism. Coexistent alcohol abuse may also explain the failure to respond completely.

Folate deficiency may coexist with B$_{12}$ deficiency in patients with chronic malabsorption or in patients suffering from alcohol abuse.

Although hypothyroidism is a recognized cause of macrocytosis, approximately 10% of patients with auto-immune hypothyroidism also have pernicious anaemia. Most physicians would normally exclude coexisting auto-immune hypothyroidism in patients with pernicious anaemia. Causes of macrocytosis are tabulated as shown.

Chronic renal impairment causes a normochromic, normocytic anaemia. Carcinoma of the stomach is associated with pernicious anaemia and would normally result in a normocytic or microcytic anaemia (blood loss anaemia). Iron deficiency causes a microcytic anaemia.

Causes of macrocytosis

Cause	Notes
B_{12} or folate deficiency	MCV >110 fl
Cytotoxic drugs	MCV >110 fl
Inherited disorders of DNA synthesis	Orotic aciduria
Hypothyroidism	
Liver disease	
Alcoholism	Even in the absence of established liver disease
Myelodysplastic syndrome	
Haemolysis	Increased reticulocytes in the circulation
Drugs	Zidovudine (increasingly common cause of macrocytosis), azathioprine, methotrexate, hyroxyurea, ddI, ddC
Myeloma	
Hyperlipidaemia	

Question 377

A 58-year-old patient was noted to be in atrial fibrillation prior to ENT surgery. He was asymptomatic. An elective cardioversion was planned to try and restore sinus rhythm. There was no history of hypertension or valve disease. The patient had never experienced a transient ischaemic attack or stroke. On examination the heart rate was 80 beats/min. Both heart sounds were normal and there were no murmurs.

What treatment is most effective at preventing stroke after the restoration of sinus rhythm?
a. Aspirin.
b. Warfarin for two weeks prior to cardioversion and two weeks afterwards.
c. Warfarin for 3–4 weeks prior to cardioversion and four weeks afterwards.
d. Warfarin for four weeks prior to cardioversion only.
e. Lifelong anticoagulation.

Question 378

A 42-year-old woman was rescued from a house fire where she had become unconscious. On admission she was drowsy and had a marked wheeze.

Blood results were as follows:

Arterial blood gases on 28% FiO_2:	
pH	7.2
PO_2	28 kPa
PCO_2	3.4 kPa
Bicarbonate	12 mmol/l
O_2 saturation	100%
Serum lactate	5.6 mmol/l
CarboxyHb level	10%

List two immediate management steps from the following list:
a. 60% oxygen.
b. 40% oxygen.
c. 100% oxygen.
d. Intravenous bicarbonate.
e. Intravenous sodium thiosulphate.
f. Intravenous hydrocortisone.
g. Nebulized salbutamol.
h. Nebulized ipratropium bromide.
i. IV acetylcysteine.
j. IV adrenaline.

Answer 377

> c. Warfarin for 3–4 weeks prior to cardioversion
>   and 4 weeks afterwards.

The three main goals in the management of atrial fibrillation include restoration to sinus rhythm (if possible), control of ventricular rate (if restoration of sinus rhythm is not possible or desirable), and the prevention of systemic thromboembolism. Stagnation of blood in the atrial appendage promotes thrombus formation. Restoration to sinus rhythm from atrial fibrillation increases the probability of thromboembolism (dislodging of the thrombus) since effective atrial contraction is restored. To minimize this risk it is recommended that the patient be anticoagulated for at least three weeks prior to DC cardioversion. Although sinus rhythm is restored after successful DC cardioversion, the atria may remain stunned for a few weeks before they contract properly again, therefore the patient should remain on warfarin for at least four weeks afterwards.

NOTE: Patients with previous TIA or CVA, impaired left ventricular function and mitral valve disease should remain anticoagulated indefinitely irrespective of restoration to sinus rhythm. (See Answer 184.)

Answer 378

> c. 100% oxygen.
> e. Intravenous sodium thiosulphate.

Smoke inhalation is associated with four major consequences (see *Table*).

This question tests the candidate's knowledge of the consequences of inhalation of systemic toxins, which include carbon monoxide and hydrogen cyanide. These substances impair the delivery and/or utilization of oxygen and may result in systemic tissue hypoxia and rapid death.

Carbon monoxide is the main cause of smoke-related fatalities and causes almost 80% of all smoke inhalation deaths. Symptoms and signs include headache, nausea, malaise, altered cognition, dyspnoea, angina, seizures, cardiac arrhythmias, congestive heart failure and/or coma.

Hydrogen cyanide is a highly toxic compound that can be formed in the high temperature combustion of a number of common materials such as polyurethane, nylon, wool and cotton. Cyanide binds to a variety of iron-containing enzymes, the most important of which is the cytochrome a-a3 complex, which is critical for electron transport during oxidative phosphorylation. By binding to this molecule, minute amounts of cyanide can inhibit aerobic metabolism and rapidly result in death.

The typical clinical syndrome due to cyanide poisoning is one of rapidly developing coma, apnoea, cardiac dysfunction and severe lactic acidosis in conjunction with a high mixed venous O_2 and a low arteriovenous O_2 content difference.

The diagnosis of CO poisoning requires estimation of carboxyHb levels, because a pulse oximeter cannot differentiate between HbO_2 and HbCO. The diagnosis of cyanide poisoning is more difficult to make particularly as blood cyanide levels cannot be obtained in a timely fashion but a very high lactate level is an important indicator.

Treatment of CO and hydrogen cyanide poisoning involves inhalation of 100% oxygen to displace both molecules from their protein binding sites. Hyperbaric oxygen at 2 atmospheres decreases the half-life of carboxyHb. It is recommended in unconscious patients and in those with a carboxyHb level of >40%. Specific treatment of hydrogen cyanide is sodium thiosulphate, which converts cyanide to the much less toxic thiocyanate.

The four major consequences of smoke inhalation	
Consequence	*Effect*
1. Thermal injury	
2. Hypoxic gas inhalation	FiO_2 may be as low as 11%
3. Exposure to direct bronchopulmonary toxins (e.g. SO_2, NO, CCl_4, chlorine)	Wheeze, bronchorrhoea
4. Exposure to systemic toxins (e.g. CO and hydrogen cyanide)	Severe hypoxia and acidosis

Question 379

A 58-year-old man presented with a three-month history of lower back pain. He had also noticed weakness in his legs when climbing stairs, and had considerable difficulty in raising himself from a chair. More recently, he was excessively thirsty and was waking frequently at night to pass urine. He had lost over 4 kg in weight since the onset of his illness. Before this he was well. He was married with two children.

He had been smoking over 20 cigarettes per day for more than 30 years. He consumed 3 units of alcohol per day.

On examination, he was thin. The blood pressure was 160/90 mmHg. He had wasting of his thigh muscles. Power in both the arms and legs was slightly diminished, but sensation and reflexes were preserved.

Investigations are shown.

The patient was given 8 mg dexamethasone for three days, and repeat 9.00 am and midnight serum cortisol was over 1,000 nmol/l.

Hb	11 g/dl
WCC	13×10^9/l
Platelets	480×10^9/l
MCV	89 fl
Blood film	Normal
ESR	44 mm/h
Sodium	140 mmol/l
Potassium	3 mmol/l
Urea	8 mmol/l
Bicarbonate	30 mmol/l
Glucose	10 mmol/l
Calcium	2.7 mmol/l
Phosphate	1.5 mmol/l
Albumin	36 g/l
Total protein	60 g/l
LFT	Normal
Serum cortisol at 9.00 am	>1,000 nmol/l
Serum cortisol at midnight	>1,000 nmol/l

1. What is the cause of this patient's lower limb weakness?
   a. Diabetic amyotrophy.
   b. Steroid-induced myopathy.
   c. Hypokalaemia.
   d. Eaton–Lambert syndrome.
   e. Metastatic spinal cord compression.

2. What is the most likely cause of the back pain?
   a. Bone metastases.
   b. Myeloma.
   c. Infiltration of the lower spinal nerves by carcinoma.
   d. Osteoporosis.

3. List two possible diagnoses.
   a. Cushing's disease.
   b. Conn's syndrome.
   c. Cortisol-secreting adenoma.
   d. Ectopic ACTH production from a bronchial carcinoma.
   e. Pseudo Cushing's syndrome secondary to alcohol abuse.
   f. Cortisol secreting adenocarcinoma.
   g. Carcinoma of the pancreas.
   h. Multiple myeloma.
   i. Liddle's syndrome.
   j. Osteoporosis.

4. Which two tests would be most useful in making the diagnosis?
   a. Serum ACTH.
   b. Chest X-ray.
   c. CT scan of the adrenals.
   d. Petrosal venous sampling.
   e. Lying and standing renin and aldosterone levels.
   f. Low-dose dexamethasone suppression test.
   g. High-dose dexamethasone suppression test.
   h. CT scan brain.
   i. Urinary ketosteroid estimation.
   j. Serum gamma GT concentration.

Question 380

A 70-year-old female presented with sudden onset of dyspnoea. There was no preceding history of a cough or chest trauma. She was a smoker. Four weeks previously she had had a right hip replacement.

On examination she was cyanosed. The heart rate was 140 beats/min and irregular. The blood pressure was 70 mmHg systolic. The JVP was raised. Both heart sounds were normal, and auscultation of the lungs revealed decreased air entry at the left lung base. The lower limbs appeared normal.

Investigations were as follows:

Arterial blood gases (air):	
pH	7.21
$PaCO_2$	3.1 kPa
PaO_2	7.1 kPa
HCO_3	11 mmol/l
Chest X-ray	Clear lung fields
ECG	Sinus tachycardia; right ward axis; ST segment depression in leads V2–V4

The patient was treated with 28% oxygen. What other immediate treatment is recommended?
   a. Oral aspirin, oral clopidogrel, subcutaneous heparin, and intravenous tirofiban.
   b. Intravenous alteplase 50 mg.
   c. Subcutaneous fractionated heparin.
   d. Intravenous noradrenaline.
   e. Intravenous unfractionated heparin.

Answer 379

> 1. b. Steroid-induced myopathy.
> 2. a. Bone metastases.
> 3. d. Ectopic ACTH production from a bronchial carcinoma.
>   f. Cortisol secreting adenocarcinoma.
> 4. a. Serum ACTH.
>   b. Chest X-ray.

The patient presented with lower back pain and clinical symptoms of a proximal lower limb myopathy. The latter is confirmed clinically. He is diabetic and hypertensive. Routine blood results demonstrate a low potassium and elevated bicarbonate. The differential diagnosis at this point is between Cushing's disease (ACTH-secreting basophil adenoma from the pituitary), cortisol-secreting adrenal adenoma or ectopic ACTH production. The diagnosis is narrowed down to a cortisol-secreting adrenal adenoma and ectopic ACTH by the failure of suppression of cortisol following high-dose dexamethasone. (See Answer 173.)

The short history of the presenting complaint and history of smoking favour ectopic ACTH production by carcinoma of the bronchus. These patients produce large amounts of ACTH and present primarily with weakness and myopathy associated with hypokalaemia, rather than a Cushingoid appearance.

The proximal myopathy is due to steroid excess, and the accompanying muscle weakness is compounded by the hypokalaemia. The hypokalaemia *per se* does not cause myopathy unless it is very long standing. The diabetes would account for the polydipsia and polyuria, but amyotrophy is unlikely to account for the proximal myopathy in a patient with such a short history and the absence of neuropathy. Eaton–Lambert syndrome may complicate oat cell bronchial carcinoma. It is characterized by proximal myopathy, fatiguability and depressed reflexes or absent reflexes. It is due to a deficient release of acetylcholine from the nerve terminals. The diagnosis does not explain the normal reflexes or the diabetes and hypertension.

The patient has back pain and, in the context of an underlying carcinoma, this may be suggestive of bony metastases to the spine. Further support for this comes from the elevated serum calcium. Spinal cord compression, however, is not plausible in the absence of spasticity in the lower limbs, the absence of a sensory level, and the presence of normal reflexes. In cord compression the reflexes are brisk. Infiltration of the spinal nerves by carcinoma is also unlikely because this would normally cause root pain and weakness of muscles supplied by the nerve affected, as well as altered sensation in the affected dermatomes.

Osteoporosis is a recognized complication of corticosteroid excess, and fractured vertebrae are a recognized complication of osteoporosis; thus, it is possible for either to be the cause of lower back pain in this situation. The bone biochemistry in osteoporosis, however, is normal (with the exception of raised alkaline phosphatase in the presence of a fracture). In this case the calcium and phosphate are elevated. Myeloma would explain the raised ESR, raised calcium and the back pain; however, in the context of the abnormal dexamethasone suppression test this diagnosis is unlikely.

Answer 380

> b. Intravenous alteplase 50 mg.

The patient presents with acute dyspnoea associated with severe circulatory collapse, hypoxia, hypocarbia and metabolic acidosis. In addition her JVP is raised, indicating right heart strain. The ECG shows ST segment depression, which may be part of right heart strain or myocardial ischaemia secondary to severe hypoxia.

Patients with massive pulmonary embolism judged clinically by cardiac arrest, circulatory collapse, severe hypoxia, acidosis or signs of right heart strain are treated with early thrombolysis. The usual treatment is a 50 mg bolus of alteplase followed by a heparin infusion. The diagnosis of massive pulmonary embolism can be confirmed by echocardiography or CT pulmonary angiography; however, the seriousness of the circulatory collapse may not allow time for investigation until thrombolysis has been instituted.

Patients with intermediate or high probability of non-massive pulmonary embolus are treated with heparin until imaging. Low-molecular weight heparin is preferable to unfractionated heparin, as it is equally effective and easier to use. Unfractionated heparin is only considered in situations where rapid reversal of anticoagulation is required.

Once the diagnosis has been confirmed all patients are commenced on warfarin and the heparin is stopped once the INR exceeds 2. Patients remain on warfarin for six weeks if the pulmonary embolus was secondary to a temporary risk factor such as recent lower-limb orthopaedic surgery. In patients with idiopathic pulmonary embolus warfarin is continued for three months. Patients with recurrent pulmonary emboli or permanent risk factor for pulmonary emboli are anticoagulated indefinitely if the risks of pulmonary embolism outweigh the dangers of haemorrhage.

Question 381

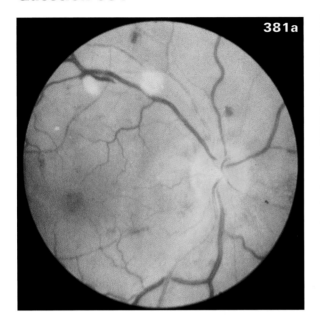

381a

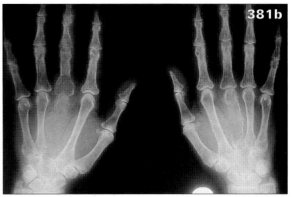

381b

Hb	9 g/dl
WCC	$10 \times 10^9/l$
Platelets	$180 \times 10^9/l$
MCV	82 fl
Sodium	136 mmol/l
Potassium	6 mmol/l
Urea	43 mmol/l
Creatinine	500 µmol/l
Calcium	2.0 mmol/l
Phosphate	1.7 mmol/l
Alkaline phosphatase	305 iu/l
Albumin	35 g/l
Chest X-ray	Slight increase in the cardiothoracic ratio
	Upper lobe venous distension
X-ray of hand (**381b**)	
US kidneys	Bilaterally shrunken kidneys

A 21-year-old male presented with headaches, drowsiness, nausea, lethargy and general malaise. His appetite was reduced, but he had not lost any weight. The only other positive feature in the history was that of troublesome back pain and cramps in the legs over the past 18 months. The past medical history comprised a long history of intermittent lower abdominal pains as a child which were associated with vomiting but had subsided by the age of 15 years. At the age of 17 he was seen by a paediatrician for short stature and delayed puberty, but was then lost to follow-up. He had worked as an assistant in a florist's shop for eight years. He took very occasional analgesia for the back pain. He was single. He was a non-smoker, and did not consume alcohol.

On examination, he was 1.53 m tall and weighed 45 kg. Secondary sexual characteristics were present. The heart rate was 98 beats/min, and regular, and blood pressure was 210/110 mmHg. The jugular venous pulsation was just visible in the neck with the patient recumbent at 45°. On examination of the precordium, the apex was not displaced, but was heaving in nature. The second heart sound was loud. Examination of the respiratory system and the abdomen was normal. On examination of the central nervous system, the patient was slightly drowsy, and the Glasgow coma scale was 13/15. The pupils were both equal in size and reacted to light. The appearances on examination of a fundus is shown (**381a**).

Investigations are shown.

1. List four abnormalities on the fundi.
2. What is the cause of the hypertension?
3. Explain the low calcium.
4. Describe the abnormality on the hand X-ray, and with what is it consistent?
5. Explain the anaemia.
6. What is the best explanation for the tachypnoea?
7. What is the best management of the hypertension in the short term?
8. List five steps in the long-term management of this patient.

Answer 381

1. i. Arteriovenous nipping.
   ii. Flame-shaped haemorrhages.
   iii. Cotton wool spots or retinal infarcts.
   iv. Blurred disc or papilloedema.
2. Chronic renal failure (*Table A*).
3. Failure of 1a-hydroxylation of vitamin D, causing low levels of 1,25-dihydroxycholecalciferol, which is an active vitamin D metabolite.
4. Subperiosteal bone resorption and severe demineralization of the third metacarpals bilaterally. There is also an expansion in the proximal phalanx of the left third digit. Such a cystic appearance is seen in severe hyperparathyroid-related bone disease.
5. Deficiency of erythropoietin.
6. Uraemic acidosis. Pulmonary oedema is less likely, given the relatively clear chest and absence of interstitial shadowing on the chest X-ray (*Table B*).
7. Haemodialysis.
8. i. Regular haemodialysis.
   ii. Control hypertension.
   iii. Erythropoietin for anaemia.
   iv. a-1-calcidol for hypocalcaemia.
   v. Calcium carbonate to bind phosphate and prevent osteodystrophy.

Table A Causes of chronic renal failure

- Chronic glomerulonephritis
- Chronic pyelonephritis
- APCKD
- Diabetes mellitus
- Chronic hypertension
- Renal artery stenosis
- Renal papillary necrosis secondary to chronic analgesia
- Hyperuricaemic nephropathy
- Chronic nephrolithiasis

Table B Complications of renal failure

- Anaemia secondary to erythropoietin deficiency
- Osteomalacia/rickets secondary to deficiency of active vitamin D metabolites
- Hypertension (secondary to salt and water retention) and its complications
- Metabolic acidosis
- Hyperkalaemia
- Osteodystrophy secondary to hyperparathyroidism resulting from chronic hyperphosphataemia
- Fluid overload causing pulmonary and peripheral oedema
- Pruritis secondary to hyperphosphataemia
- Skin pigmentation
- Hyperlipidaemia
- Premature coronary artery disease (combination of hypertension and hyperlipidaemia)
- Neuropathy

Table C Wegener's classification of hypertensive retinopathy

I	Silver wiring of the arterioles
II	Arteriovenous nipping
III	Flame-shaped haemorrhages and cotton wool spots
IV	Papilloedema

The patient presents with hypertension, grossly abnormal renal function, grade IV hypertensive retinopathy (*Table C*) and drowsiness. These features could be explained by primary accelerated hypertension; however, the anaemia, bone biochemistry and X-ray appearance of the hand indicate that the most likely cause of the hypertension is chronic renal failure. It is difficult to be certain about the aetiology of the renal impairment because the past history is vague and the kidneys are shrunken. Renal biopsy in these instances reveals extensive glomerular scarring and is rarely helpful in the management of the patient. The history of intermittent abdominal pain and vomiting and investigation for short stature suggest that the cause may be chronic pyelonephritis. Other causes of chronic renal failure and its complications are shown (*Tables A and B*).

The long- and short-term management of this patient is outlined in 7 and 8 above. It is important to be aware that erythropoietin itself may worsen hypertension; therefore, extra care is required in managing hypertension in an individual taking erythropoietin. Good hypertensive control will reduce the rate of decline in renal function; however, given his weight of just 45 kg, a serum creatinine of 500 μmol/l almost certainly represents end-stage renal failure requiring dialysis. In some patients with chronic renal failure and hypertension, reducing intravascular volume with dialysis is all that is required to control blood pressure.

Question 382

A 42-year-old male was investigated for a three-year history of intermittent abdominal pain. He had suffered four episodes of pyelonephritis in the past four years which were treated by his GP. There was a long history of migraines, for which he took mefenamic acid and paracetamol. Over the past few months he had complained of increasing lethargy. There was no history of diarrhoea, weight loss, urinary hesitancy, nocturia or post-micturition dribble. Four months ago he was noted to have a blood pressure of 180/110 mmHg, which was under review. He was a florist by occupation. He was a non-smoker and consumed very occasional alcohol. His father died suddenly from a subarachnoid haemorrhage at the age of 40 years, but his mother was still alive and well. He had three brothers aged 44, 45 and 46 years respectively; the eldest brother had hypertension.

On examination, he appeared well at rest. There was no clubbing or peripheral oedema. The blood pressure was 180/105 mmHg. Examination of the abdomen revealed tenderness in both loins. Deep palpation of the loins was difficult owing to tenderness. The percussion note throughout the abdomen was resonant and auscultation demonstrated normal bowel sounds. Examination of the cardiovascular and respiratory system was normal. Fundoscopy demonstrated silver wiring and arteriovenous nipping.

Investigations are shown.

Hb	15 g/dl
WCC	5×10^9/l
Platelets	240×10^9/l
ESR	15 mm/h
Sodium	128 mmol/l
Potassium	3.8 mmol/l
Urea	20 mmol/l
Creatinine	400 µmol/l
Calcium	2.1 mmol/l
Phosphate	1.9 mmol/l
Albumin	39 g/l
Serum renin	Elevated
Urinalysis	Protein ++
	Blood ++
	24-hour urinary sodium 89 mmol/l

What is the most likely diagnosis?
a. Bilateral renal artery stenosis.
b. Chronic pyelonephritis.
c. Hypernephroma.
d. Genetic polycystic kidney disease.
e. Analgesic nephropathy.

Question 383

A 16-year-old East African female was admitted with a two-week history of intermittent, sharp, right upper quadrant pain which was worse on inspiration. The pain radiated to the umbilicus and right loin and was most severe on the night of admission. There were no other symptoms. She had just finished menstruating. Her family had very recently immigrated to Britain from Kenya.

On examination, she had shallow respiration. The temperature was 37.5°C (99.5°F). There were tenderness and guarding in the right hypochondrium. The liver was palpable 6 cm below the costal margin, and there was tenderness in the 9th intercostal space in the mid axillary line. The right lung base was dull to percussion with reduced air entry on auscultation.

Investigations are shown.

Hb	13 g/dl
WCC	16×10^9/l (neutrophil leucocytosis)
Platelets	590×10^9/l
ESR	70 mm/h
U&E	Normal
Chest X-ray	Raised right hemidiaphragm
	Clear lung fields
Urinalysis	Normal

1. What is the most likely diagnosis?
2. List at least three investigations you would perform to confirm the diagnosis.

Answer 382

> d. Genetic polycystic kidney disease.

This middle-aged patient presents with abdominal pain and advanced renal failure. All of the options given may cause abdominal pain and renal failure (*Table*). The episodes of pyelonephritis in a middle-aged male should raise suspicion of obstructive uropathy or an anatomical abnormality in the renal tract. In the context of the possibility of the latter, the family history of subarachnoid haemorrhage and hypertension should arouse the suspicion of APCKD. The normal Hb in the presence of chronic renal failure should clinch the diagnosis because APCKD is one of the few causes of chronic renal failure where the Hb is preserved. This is due to inappropriate erythropoietin secretion in some patients with the condition. Hypernephroma may also cause polycythaemia for the same reason but does not cause a salt-losing nephropathy as seen in this case.

APCKD is inherited as an autosomal dominant trait. It is characterized by multiple thin-walled cysts in the kidney, which become progressively larger over the years and cause renal failure by compression of the nephrons. In 90% of patients, the abnormal gene is on the short arm of chromosome 16 (PKD 1) which encodes a transmembrane protein termed polycystin. The exact function of it is unclear but it is thought to be involved in mediating cell-matrix interactions. Of the other 10% of patients, some have abnormalities linked to a locus on

Abdominal pain and renal failure

- Henoch–Schönlein purpura
- Haemolytic uraemic syndrome
- Polyarteritis nodosa
- APCKD
- Nephrolithiasis
- Analgesic nephropathy
- Retroperitoneal fibrosis
- Dissecting aortic aneurysm
- Legionnaire's disease
- Acute pancreatitis
- Ethylene glycol poisoning

chromosome 4 (PKD 2). Clinical symptoms comprise flank pain, haematuria, nocturia and recurrent urinary tract infections. Hypertension develops in 75% of cases. End-stage renal failure may occur at any age. The patients may be anaemic owing to haematuria and uraemia; however, polycythaemia secondary to increased erythropoietin is recognized. Malignant transformation within cysts is also recognized. Associations include berry aneurysms causing intracranial haemorrhage and mitral valve prolapse. Management includes family screening of first-degree relatives, early treatment of urinary tract infections, and meticulous blood pressure control.

Answer 383

> 1. Hepatic abscess secondary to *Entamoeba histolytica* (amoebic liver abscess).
> 2. i. Ultrasound of the liver.
>   ii. Microscopy from liver aspirates.
>   iii. Indirect haemagglutination tests (over 95% with liver abscess are positive, but the test cannot distinguish between past and current infection).

The patient presents with hepatomegaly, a raised right hemidiaphragm, and localized tenderness in the 9th intercostal space. These features are consistent with a hepatic abscess. She has been in East Africa, which makes an amoebic abscess the most probable cause of her signs and symptoms. Some 50% of patients with amoebic abscess have no history of dysentery. Symptoms include right hypochondrial pain, fever, sweating, intermittent fever and rigors. There may also be hepatic enlargement and localized tenderness in the right hypochondrium or intercostal spaces. Enlargement of the liver abscess is usually upwards, and may cause compression of the right hemidiaphragm and atelectasis of the overlying lung. Jaundice and abnormality of LFT are rare. US or CT scan will demonstrate the abscess or abscesses. Aspiration of the pus may demonstrate the organism. Sigmoidoscopy and biopsy for microscopy and stool microscopy have a low yield, but indirect haemagglutination tests have high titres in the presence of a hepatic abscess. The lesions may be as large as 10 cm. Rupture of the abscess into the lung and development of a hepatobronchial fistula is a recognized complication (anchovy-sauce sputum). Peritonitis, pericarditis and cutaneous sinus formation are rare complications.

Treatment is with metronidazole or tinidazole. Diloxanide is also given to eliminate any on-going gastrointestinal infection.

Question 384

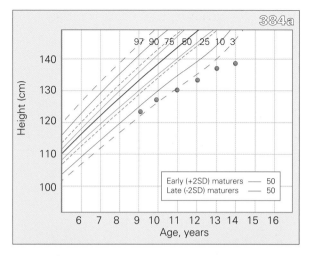

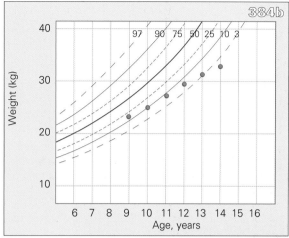

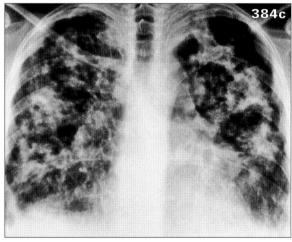

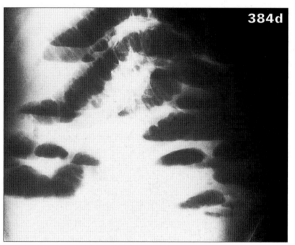

A 14-year-old male was admitted to hospital with a 12-hour history of colicky right-sided abdominal pain and vomiting. He had a past history of recurrent chest infections that had been treated by his GP. He was also thought to be asthmatic, and took a regular bronchodilating inhaler. He had intermittent loose, bulky stool but had never experienced abdominal pain. He had a younger brother and sister who were well. His father was a shop assistant and his mother was a part time GP's receptionist.

On examination, he did not appear acutely unwell. He had mild clubbing. The abdomen was distended. There was generalized tenderness on palpation, as well as a firm mass in the right iliac fossa. Bowel sounds were tinkling. The rectum was empty. Auscultation of the lung fields revealed coarse crackles throughout the lung fields.

Growth charts for height and weight are shown (384a, b). Investigations are shown.

Hb	10 g/dl
WCC	14×10^9/l
Platelets	480×10^9/l
MCV	80 fl
Sodium	135 mmol/l
Potassium	3.2 mmol/l
Urea	9 mmol/l
Total protein	70 g/l
Albumin	34 g/l
Calcium	2.2 mmol/l
Phosphate	0.7 mmol/l
Chest X-ray (384c)	
Abdominal X-ray (384d)	

1. What is the abnormality on the growth chart?
2. Comment on the chest X-ray.
3. Comment on the abdominal X-ray.
4. What is the cause of his presentation problem?
5. What is the management of his current problem?
6. What is the full diagnosis?
7. What test would you request to confirm the diagnosis?

Answer 384

1. This patient has fallen off the third centile for height at the age of 10 years and for weight at the age of 14 years.
2. The chest X-ray is grossly abnormal. There is widespread fibrotic change, patchy consolidation, and bronchiectasis. In the context of this history the findings are consistent with cystic fibrosis.
3. The erect abdominal X-ray reveals dilated loops of small bowel and multiple fluid levels consistent with small bowel obstruction.
4. Meconium ileus equivalent. This is bowel obstruction resulting from a combination of steatorrhoea and viscid intestinal secretions causing faecal impaction in the ascending colon or the ileocaecal junction.
5. The management steps are as follows:
   - Rest the bowel; the patient should be completely restricted from oral solids and fluids and should have intravenous fluid supplements. A nasogastric tube should be placed *in situ* to prevent gastric dilatation and vomiting.
   - Diagnostic and therapeutic manoeuvres: a Gastrografin enema – which is both diagnostic and therapeutic – should be performed. Patients with any form of obstruction should not have barium studies.
   - Other therapeutic steps: acetylcysteine given intravenously or through the nasogastric tube has been shown to be very useful in resolving bowel obstruction.
   - In the long term, the plan is to reduce steatorrhoea, which can be done by increasing pancreatic supplements. There have been recent reports of fibrous colonopathy in association with a high dose of Pancrease pancreatic supplements. The risk of the condition with Creon pancreatic supplements is very small.
6. The full diagnosis is cystic fibrosis. The diagnosis should be suspected in any young child who presents with chronic gastrointestinal and respiratory complaints.
7. The diagnosis of cystic fibrosis can be confirmed by demonstrating a sweat sodium concentration exceeding 60 mmol/l.

Cystic fibrosis is an autosomal recessive condition with a prevalence of 1/2,500 which is characterized by viscid respiratory and gastrointestinal secretions. The abnormality is in the gene encoding a chloride ion channel in the nasal epithelium, lungs, salivary glands, pancreas, intestine and bile ducts. This chloride ion

Table A The clinical manifestations of cystic fibrosis

Respiratory
Nasal polyps
Otitis media
Asthma

Bronchiolitis	Recurrent pneumonia	*Staphylococcus aureus, Haemophilus influenzae, Pseudomonas aeruginosa*
Bronchiectasis	Lung abscess/empyema	
	Haemoptysis	
	Aspergillus infection	
	Lung fibrosis	
	Pneumothorax	
	Cor pulmonale	

Gastrointestinal
Meconium ileus (birth)
Rectal prolapse (neonate)
Steatorrhoea (pancreatic insufficiency)
Meconium ileus equivalent (infancy onwards)
Malabsorption (fat-soluble vitamins due to pancreatic insufficiency usually, or biliary obstruction)
Gall stones
Secondary biliary cirrhosis

Miscellaneous
Non-erosive arthropathy
Infertility in males

Table B Causes of a false-positive sweat
sodium test

- Hypothyroidism
- Familial hypoparathyroidism
- Mucopolysaccharidoses
- α-1 antitrypsin deficiency
- Addison's disease

channel has been termed the CFTR. The gene is located on chromosome 7. Over 200 different mutations have been described within the gene, but by far the most common is a point mutation which results in the deletion of the amino acid phenylalanine on position 508. This mutation accounts for 70–80% of all cases. The clinical manifestations are listed (*Table A*). The differential diagnoses are other causes of recurrent respiratory infections and diarrhoea in young children, which include hypogammaglobulinaemia and intestinal lymphangiectasia. The genetic heterogeneity of the condition means that the diagnosis continues to rely on the demonstration of a sweat sodium >60 mmol/l. However, there are conditions associated with a false-positive sweat sodium test (*Table B*). It is also worth noting that a small proportion of patients with cystic fibrosis do not have a positive sweat sodium test.

Question 385

A 6-year-old female was seen in the Accident and Emergency Department with a two-year history of a painful swollen right knee which developed after she fell at school. Two years previously she had a similar episode affecting the left knee, following which she had persistent swelling and discomfort for several weeks. At that stage she had an FBC which was normal and an X-ray of the left knee which revealed soft tissue swelling. In the interim she had recurrent episodes of painful swelling of the left knee for no obvious reason, which would subside after a few days. At the age of two years she sustained a large haematoma on her forehead after a fall at home. The only other past history of note was a recent review by the ophthalmologist for a left convergent squint.

She had achieved her milestones normally, but had problems with reading which were attributed to her squint. She was one of three siblings. All three were adopted and had come from different families. Her parents appeared very caring. The father was a businessman who spent many days away from home and the mother was a housewife.

On examination, she was below the third centile for height and was on the 50th centile for weight. There was a painful swelling over the left knee consistent with a synovial effusion. The right knee was not swollen, but movement of the knee demonstrated crepitus. There was an obvious convergent squint. The neck was short and the hands, particularly the fourth and fifth digits, appeared small.

Investigations are shown.

Hb	11 g/dl
WCC	6×10^9/l
Platelets	112×10^9/l
Blood film	Normal
PT	12 s
APTT	94 s
BT	8 min
Sodium	136 mmol/l
Potassium	3.8 mmol/l
Urea	6 mmol/l
Creatinine	80 µmol/l
Calcium	2.3 mmol/l
Phosphate	1.0 mmol/l
Albumin	40 g/l
X-ray of left knee	Soft-tissue swelling No bony deformity
X-ray of right knee	Chondrocalcinosis

1. List two different diagnoses.
2. What is the mechanism for the swollen knee?
3. Give two possible underlying causes for the swollen knee.
4. What two investigations would you request to confirm your answer to 1?

Answer 385

> 1. i. Turner's syndrome.
>   ii. Haemophilia A or haemophilia B.
> 2. Haemarthrosis; bleeding into the knee joint.
> 3. i. Haemophilia A.
>   ii. Haemophilia B.
> 4. i. Buccal smear for karyotyping to confirm Turner's syndrome.
>   ii. Factor VIII assay or Factor IX assay to confirm haemophilia A or B respectively.

The patient has several morphological features of Turner's syndrome (*Table C*, Answer 397). All of these morphological features, particularly short metacarpals, may also occur in pseudohypoparathyroidism; however, the normal bone biochemistry is against the diagnosis. Short metacarpals may occur in other conditions (*Table A*).

The patient also has an important clotting abnormality, suggested by the elevated APTT. The swollen knee is most probably due to haemorrhage into the joint. The right knee has features of chondrocalcinosis possibly due to recurrent haemarthroses. The PT is normal, suggesting that the defect is in the intrinsic pathway of the clotting cascade. Causes of a raised APTT include deficiency in any one of the clotting factors in the intrinsic pathway, DIC, or heparin therapy. The normal PT and fibrinogen level make DIC very unlikely. The normal BT excludes von Willebrand's disease (*Table B*). The most likely clotting abnormality here is either Factor VIII (haemophilia A) or Factor IX (haemophilia B; Christmas disease) deficiency. Both are X-linked recessive; thus normal females with two X chromosomes will not exhibit the disease phenotype, even if they have inherited the abnormal gene. However, patients with Turner's syndrome have just one X chromosome and effectively have the same chance of being affected by an X-linked recessive genetic condition as males.

Table A Causes of short metacarpals

- Turner's syndrome
- Noonan's syndrome
- Pseudohypoparathyroidism
- Sickle cell dactylitis
- Juvenile chronic arthritis
- Recurrent hand trauma

Table B Differentiation between haemophilia A, B and von Willebrand's disease

	HA	*HB*	*Von Willebrand's*
PT	Normal	Normal	Normal
APTT	↑	↑	↑
BT	Normal	Normal	↑
Factor VIII$_c$	↓↓	Normal	↓
Factor VIII$_{VWB}$	Normal	Normal	↓
Ristocetin platelet aggregation	Normal	Normal	↓

Question 386

A 48-year-old clerical worker in a large insurance company was admitted with malaise, increasing shortness of breath and confusion. One week before admission he had a dry cough, chills, headaches and generalized aches throughout his body. He saw his GP, who prescribed amoxycillin 500 mg three times daily. Two days later, the patient developed generalized abdominal pain and loose motion. Over the next 24 hours, he had become increasingly confused, and started to hallucinate. His wife became concerned, and brought him to the Accident and Emergency Department. He had been in Spain six weeks before his illness. He smoked 20 cigarettes a day, and consumed 4 units of alcohol a night.

On examination, he appeared unwell and dehydrated. His temperature was 38.7°C (101.7°F). The heart rate was 110 beats/min, and regular, and the blood pressure was 120/70 mmHg. On examination of the respiratory system he was noted to have a respiratory rate of 35/min. On auscultation, there were coarse crackles at the right lung base. Examination of the precordium was normal. Abdominal examination revealed generalized abdominal tenderness, but no guarding or rigidity. Central nervous system examination revealed a Glasgow coma score of 9/15. The patient was disorientated in time and space, but there was no focal neurological abnormality.

Investigations are shown.

Hb	13.5 g/dl		Arterial blood gases:	
WCC	12.1×10^9/l (neutrophils		pH	7.37
	10.2×10^9/l; lymphocytes		PaO_2	7.3 kPa
	1.5×10^9/l)		$PaCO_2$	4 kPa
Platelets	140×10^9/l		Bicarbonate	18 mmol/l
Sodium	128 mmol/l		Oxygen saturation	83%
Potassium	4 mmol/l		Chest X-ray	Right lower lobe
Urea	10 mmol/l			consolidation, and a small
Creatinine	160 µmol/l			associated pleural effusion
Bilirubin	22 µmol/l		ECG	Sinus tachycardia
ALT	75 iu/l		Urinalysis	Trace of blood
Alkaline phosphatase	102 iu/l			Protein ++
Gamma GT	102 iu/l			
Albumin	29 g/l			

1. What is the most probable diagnosis?
2. List three possible causes for the low sodium.
3. List three further investigations you would perform to make a rapid diagnosis.
4. What antibiotic therapy would you institute while awaiting the definitive diagnosis?

5. List three therapeutic interventions you would initiate to manage this condition assuming a definitive diagnosis has already been made.

Question 387

A 34-year-old West African female presented with a three-month history of increasing ankle oedema and abdominal distension. There was no history of cough, exertional dyspnoea or orthopnoea. She was married with a five-year-old daughter. She was a non-smoker, and drank alcohol very occasionally. She had worked as a fish-farm administrator in Nigeria before moving to England three years ago.

On examination, there was no evidence of pallor, jaundice or lymphadenopathy. She had considerable, pitting, lower-limb oedema. The heart rate was 100 beats/min, and irregularly irregular. The blood pressure was 95/75 mmHg. The JVP was elevated to the level of the ear lobes. On examination of the precordium the apex beat was not palpable. The heart sounds were soft. There were no cardiac murmurs. Auscultation of the lung fields was normal. Abdominal examination revealed firm hepatomegaly palpable 6 cm below the costal margin and shifting dullness. The spleen was not palpable. Neurological examination and examination of the skin were normal.

Investigations are shown.

Hb	12 g/dl
WCC	7×10^9/l
	(normal differential)
Platelets	300×10^9/l
Urinalysis	Protein +
Chest X-ray	Normal cardiac size and clear lung fields
ECG	Low QRS voltage and non-specific lateral T-wave changes

1. What investigations would be most useful in making the diagnosis?
2. What is the most probable diagnosis?

Answer 386

1. Legionnaire's disease.
2. i. Syndrome of inappropriate ADH secretion.
   ii. Diarrhoea and vomiting.
   iii. Salt-losing nephritis/acute tubulointerstitial nephritis.
3. i. Urine for *Legionella* antigen.
   ii. Direct immunofluorescent antibody test on sputum, bronchial washings, pleural effusion or blood.
   iii. IgM RMAT for *Legionella*.
4. Intravenous cefotaxime and oral erythromycin.
5. i. Oxygen.
   ii. Intravenous erythromycin or azithromycin and oral rifampicin.
   iii. Intravenous rehydration with CVP monitoring.

This previously fit middle-aged man presents with respiratory problems, abdominal symptoms and confusion. Biochemical tests reveal a low sodium and evidence of renal dysfunction. The full blood count reveals a mildly raised WCC with a relative lymphopenia. The most probable diagnosis which ties all of this together is Legionnaire's disease. The condition is caused by the organism *Legionella pneumophilia*. Epidemic outbreaks can occur among previously fit individuals staying in hotels, institutions or hospitals where the cooling systems have been contaminated with the organism. It can also occur in sporadic cases and in the immunocompromised where the source of infection is unknown. It is spread via the aerosol route. Incubation period is between 2 and 10 days. Males are affected more than females.

Legionnaire's disease is preceded by a prodromal illness similar to a viral infection with headaches, myalgia, anorexia and pyrexia. Approximately 50% have abdominal symptoms (nausea, vomiting and diarrhoea). Neurological symptoms such as confusion, hallucinations, peripheral neuropathy, myelitis and, rarely, a cerebellar syndrome can occur. Patients may develop renal failure, usually secondary to an acute tubulointerstitial nephritis. Liver involvement is usually mild and characterized by abnormal LFT.

Hyponatraemia is common and is usually due to inappropriate ADH secretion; however, loss of sodium from the kidneys (acute tubulointerstitial nephritis) and gastrointestinal tract (diarrhoea and vomiting) may also contribute. Other biochemical features include hypocalcaemia, hypophosphataemia, and raised creatinine kinase (myositis). On the blood film there is a normal or mildly raised WCC with a moderate neutrophilia and relative lymphopenia. A mild coagulopathy can occur. Chest X-ray usually shows a unilateral lobar and then multilobar shadowing, with or without an associated pleural effusion.

Conditions simultaneously involving the lower respiratory tract and central nervous system

Infections
HIV
TB
Legionnaire's disease
Mycoplasma pneumonia
Streptococcal/staphylococcal pneumonia
Malaria
Cysticercosis

Malignancy
Primary or secondary bronchial carcinoma

Granulomatous disease
Sarcoidosis
Histiocytosis X

Vasculitides
Polyarteritis nodosa
Wegener's granulomatosis
SLE

Neuroectodermal syndromes
Neurofibromatosis
Tuberose sclerosis

Sickle cell syndromes

A rapid diagnosis can be made using the tests mentioned above. Urinary *Legionella antigen* has a yield of 90% within the first week of the illness. Serology relies on measuring antibody titres in acute and convalescent serum samples separated by 10–14 days; therefore a reader would not score marks if asked specifically for tests to make a rapid diagnosis. Similarly, culturing this fastidious organism (using buffered charcoal yeast media) may take up to three weeks and has a low yield, and therefore would not score marks.

Treatment involves high-concentration oxygen and antibiotic therapy with intravenous erythromycin or azithromycin plus oral rifampicin. Before the diagnosis of Legionnaire's disease is confirmed, the patient should also receive a cephalosporin to cover the possibility of pneumonia due to *Streptococcus pneumoniae*, which may present similarly. Rehydration would have to be performed with CVP monitoring as the patient has evidence of renal involvement, and the plasma electrolytes should be monitored daily.

Conditions causing lung and brain involvement simultaneously are common in postgraduate examinations in which Legionnaire's disease is commonly tested. Other causes of simultaneous lung and cerebral involvement are tabulated.

Answer 387

> 1. i. Echocardiography.
>   ii. Cardiac MRI.
>   iii. Left and right cardiac catheter.
> 2. i. Pericardial constriction.
>   ii. Restrictive cardiomyopathy.

The patient has signs of severe right-heart failure, but the chest X-ray reveals a normal-sized heart. The differential diagnosis of severe heart failure in the absence of significant cardiac enlargement is between pericardial constriction and a restrictive cardiomyopathy.

If we consider the possibility of restrictive cardiomyopathy (*Table A*), then there is little information in the history to suggest systemic sclerosis, haemochromatosis, carcinoid syndrome or anthracycline therapy. We are left with the possibility of malignancy, amyloidosis, EMF or idiopathic restrictive cardiomyopathy; however, the latter is extremely rare and some cardiologists are unsure if it even exists. There is no real evidence of malignancy. Cardiac amyloidosis is usually associated with myeloma, of which there is no real evidence in this case. Moreover, it is more common in the 6th and 7th decades and more common in males. It is often associated with macroglossia and neuropathy, which appear to be absent here. EMF has two variants: the tropical and temperate forms (*Table B*). The findings in favour of the tropical form of EMF is its insidious presentation and normal eosinophil count. However, tropical EMF is confined to young malnourished, poverty-stricken individuals with a high parasite load, and it is highly unlikely that any of these factors would apply to a fish-farm administrator.

The most probable diagnosis is pericardial constriction. This is usually insidious and presents with signs of severe right-heart failure, but little in the way of left-heart failure. Contrary to popular belief, most cases of pericardial constriction are idiopathic. Other causes of pericardial constriction are listed in *Table C*.

In a tropical country, tuberculous pericarditis would be a possible aetiological candidate; however, there is complete absence of radiological evidence of previous pulmonary TB.

Continued overpage

Table A Causes of restrictive cardiomyopathy

- Idiopathic (extremely rare)
- EMF: temperate
         tropical
- Systemic sclerosis
- Amyloidosis
- Haemochromatosis
- Carcinoid syndrome
- Malignancy
- Anthracycline

Table B Differences between temperate and tropical EMF

	Temperate	*Tropical*
Presentation	Acute	Insidious
Fever	Common	Unusual
Multi-system involvement	Common	Unusual
Previous ill health or malnourishment	Uncommon	Very common
Eosinophil count	High	Normal

Table C Causes of pericardial constriction

Idiopathic	Bacterial pericarditis
TB	Radiotherapy

Table D Echocardiographic features of pericardial constriction and restrictive cardiomyopathy

	Pericardial constriction	Restrictive cardiomyopathy
Left and right atria	Enlarged/normal	Enlarged
Left and right ventricles	Normal	Usually normal/enlarged
Endocardium	Normal	Bright
Myocardial texture	Normal	Normal/bright
Valves	Normal	Affected (mitral and tricuspid regurgitation)
Doppler	Low E/A inspiration High E/A expiration	Large E*, small A**
Pericardium	May be thickened	Normal

* Early or passive left ventricular filling
** Late or active ventricular filling

Echocardiography is useful in differentiating pericardial constriction from a restrictive cardiomyopathy (*Table D*). Restrictive cardiomyopathy has classic echocardiographic features. In pericardial constriction, the pericardium may seem to be thickened. Cardiac MRI may be more useful than echocardiography in demonstrating pericardial thickness.

An unequivocal method of differentiating the two conditions is by performing a left- and right-heart cardiac catheterization. Pericardial constriction encompasses the whole heart, therefore the right and left end-diastolic pressures are equal, as are the atrial pressures. In contrast, restrictive cardiomyopathy is patchy; thus LVEDP is slightly higher than right ventricular end-diastolic pressure (**387**). In addition, there is evidence of mitral and/or tricuspid regurgitation, which is generally absent in pericardial constriction.

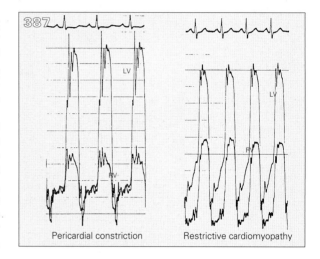

Pericardial constriction   Restrictive cardiomyopathy

Question 388

Hb	13 g/dl
WCC	6×10^9/l
Platelets	310×10^9/l
HIV serology	IgG HIV antibody-positive
CD4 count	510×10^6/l (NR 500–1,300 $\times 10^6$/l)
Viral RNA	20,000 copies/ml
Chest X-ray	Normal

A 23-year-old homosexual requested an HIV test after his partner had been diagnosed as having the condition. Apart from a febrile illness eight weeks previously, he had been relatively well. Physical examination was entirely normal.

Investigations performed in clinic are shown.

1. Does this patient require treatment?
2. Which medication(s) should be considered?

Question 389

A 57-year-old male was admitted with a seven-month history of increasing breathlessness and swollen ankles. Just before admission he had developed paroxysmal nocturnal dyspnoea. He had seen his GP, who had prescribed 80 mg of furosemide, with very slight effect. He had no past medical history of note, and there was no

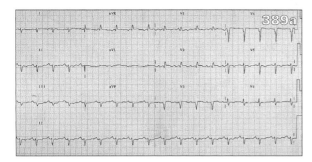

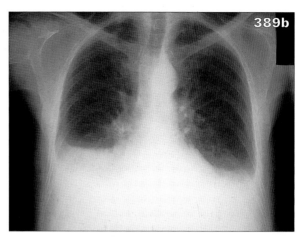

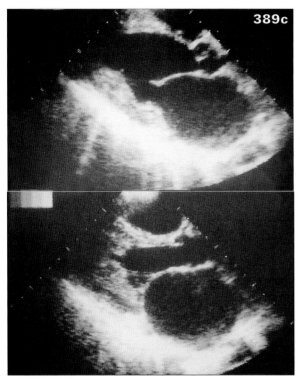

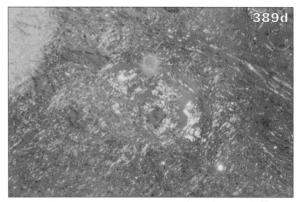

family history of cardiovascular disease. He was a non-smoker and consumed about 7 units of alcohol per week. He had been a patron for a large charity organization for several years.

On examination, he appeared pale and was breathless on very slight exertion. The heart rate was 100 beats/min, and regular; blood pressure was 90/60 mmHg. The JVP was raised 6 cm above the sternal angle and revealed prominent a- and c–v waves. The apex was not palpable, but on auscultation of the precordium there was a loud third heart sound. On examination of the lungs there was reduced air entry bilaterally at both lung bases. Abdominal examination revealed hepatomegaly palpable 7 cm below the costal margin, and some ascites.

Investigations are shown.

Hb	11 g/dl
WCC	6 × 10⁹/l
Platelets	100 × 10⁹/l
MCV	88 fl
ESR	70 mm/h
Sodium	135 mmol/l
Potassium	3.9 mmol/l
Urea	15 mmol/l
Creatinine	110 µmol/l
Bilirubin	33 µmol/l
AST	64 iu/l
Alkaline phosphatase	200 iu/l
Albumin	18 g/l
ECG (**389a**)	
Chest X-ray (**389b**)	
Renal US	Renal size enlarged slightly bilaterally, but no ureteric obstruction
Echocardiogram (**389c**)	
Renal biopsy (**389d**)	

1. Comment on the chest X-ray.
2. Comment on the ECG.
3. What is the renal diagnosis?
4. What is the cause of cardiac failure?

5. What is the overall diagnosis?
6. List two important investigations that you would perform.

Answer 388

> 1. The patient is HIV-positive. His CD4 count is within normal limits, but he has a very heavy viral load, which is generally a poor prognostic marker of disease progression and an indicator for treatment.
> 2. A combination of two nucleoside analogues and a protease inhibitor.

> **AIDS-defining conditions**
>
> *Pneumocystis carinii* pneumonia
> - TB *(Mycobacterium avium intracellulare)*
> - *Cryptococcus neoformans*
> - *Cryptosporidium*
>
> *Isospora belli*
> - Oesophageal or disseminated *Candida* (but not oral)
> - Herpes infection
> - CMV retinitis, colitis, oesophagitis and encephalitis
> - Oral leukoplakia
> - Toxoplasmosis
> - Kaposi's sarcoma

Patients infected with HIV may present following the seroconversion syndrome, with generalized lymphadenopathy or with AIDS-defining opportunistic illnesses (*Table*). The management of HIV infection is dependent on the CD4 count and the viral RNA load. Recommendations for initiating therapy in patients infected with HIV include all patients with a CD4 count of $<500 \times 10^6/l$, as well as asymptomatic patients who have a CD4 count $>500 \times 10^6/l$ but evidence of active viral RNA (>10,000 viral copies per ml). Some experts will initiate treatment in patients with a CD4 count >500 $\times 10^6/l$ in the presence of any detectable level of virus. Patients with AIDS-defining illnesses usually have a CD4 $<200 \times 10^6/l$. Treatment is in the form of triple therapy, comprising combinations of nucleoside analogues that inhibit the viral reverse transcriptase enzyme and a protease inhibitor that inhibits viral protein synthesis.

Examples of nucleoside analogue combinations include AZT and didanosine (AZT/ddI), AZT and zalcitabine (AZT/ddC) and AZT and lamivudine (AZT/3TC). Commonly used protease inhibitors include ritonavir, indinavir and saquinavir.

Answer 389

> 1. i. Bilateral pleural effusions, the right effusion being larger than the left.
>   ii. Prominent pulmonary arteries.
> 2. Small voltage complexes with T-wave inversion in the lateral leads.
> 3. Nephrotic syndrome due to renal amyloidosis.
> 4. Restrictive cardiomyopathy secondary to cardiac amyloid.
> 5. Primary amyloidosis.
> 6. i. Serum immunoglobulins/ immunoelectrophoresis.
>   ii. Urinalysis for Bence-Jones protein estimation.

The combination of nephrotic syndrome and cardiac failure should always raise the suspicion of primary amyloidosis or AL amyloid. Primary amyloid affects approximately 10–15% of all patients with myeloma. In primary amyloidosis, the amyloid is made up of immunoglobulin light chains and glycoprotein. Clinical features include restrictive cardiomyopathy, macroglossia, peripheral neuropathy, nephrotic syndrome, purpura, and isolated clotting Factor X deficiency. Cardiac amyloid has a poor prognosis as it results in a stiff ventricle with poor systolic and diastolic function. It responds poorly to diuretics. Arrhythmias and conduction tissue disease are common. The ECG commonly reveals small complexes, pathological Q-waves and non-specific T-wave changes. Echocardiography demonstrates thickened left and right ventricular walls, which have a ground-glass appearance. The ventricular cavities are small, but the atria are enlarged (as in this case). The interatrial septum is often bright. The definitive diagnosis of amyloidosis rests on tissue diagnosis. Rectal or gingival biopsy is useful; however, the former has a lower yield. Serum amyloid protein scans are useful in identifying tissues infiltrated with amyloid; however, an important exception is cardiac infiltration, which is best identified with cardiac biopsy.

The other important type of amyloidosis for the candidate doing higher specialist examinations in internal medicine includes systemic amyloidosis. In this case, the protein comprising amyloid is protein AA. This occurs in chronic inflammatory conditions or infections. Examples include rheumatoid arthritis, bronchiectasis, inflammatory bowel disease and familial Mediterranean fever. This type of amyloid has a predilection for the kidneys, causing nephrotic syndrome, haematuria and renal failure. Hepatosplenomegaly is present in over 20% of cases.

Question 390

A 28-year-old female presented with a four-week history of progressive difficulty with walking, clumsiness of her hands, and slurring of the speech. Before this she had been relatively well, with the exception of occasional episodes of central chest pain and breathlessness when she was stressed, or on rushing suddenly. In the past four weeks she had fallen twice because she was 'not in control of her lower limbs'. Her hands were clumsy and she was having difficulty washing dishes or holding cups. There was no history of headaches or any family history of neurological disease. She was a non-smoker and consumed 1–2 glasses of wine per week.

On examination, she appeared well at rest. She measured 1.81 m. She had a high-arched palate, kyphoscoliosis and mild bilateral pes cavus. Her speech was mildly dysarthric. On examination of her upper limbs the power was normal. The tone was slightly increased in both forearms. There was clinical evidence of an intention tremor, past pointing, finger nose ataxia and dysdiadochokinesia. The reflexes were brisk bilaterally. On examination of the lower limbs the power was slightly reduced bilaterally. The tone was increased and heel–shin ataxia was present. The knee reflexes were brisk, but the ankle jerks were absent. The plantar response was upgoing bilaterally.

On examination of the cardiovascular system the heart rate was 90 beats/min, and regular; blood pressure was 100/70 mmHg. The apex was not displaced, but was heaving in nature. On auscultation there was a harsh ejection systolic murmur at the left lower sternal edge, which was louder on standing suddenly and softer on squatting. The remainder of the physical examination was normal.

1. What is the diagnosis?
2. What is the cause of the cardiac murmur?
3. List two other associations of the condition.

Question 391

A 44-year-old Nigerian male was investigated for right upper quadrant pain, abdominal distension and ankle swelling:

Chamber	Pressure (mmHg)	Oxygen saturation (%)
Right atrium	19	68
Right ventricle	48/20	68
Pulmonary artery	40/20	68
PCWP	18	
Left ventricle	90/20	96
Aorta	85/65	96

A lateral view chest X-ray is shown (**391a**).

1. What are the abnormalities in the cardiac catheter data?
2. What is the abnormality on the chest X-ray?
3. What is the diagnosis?

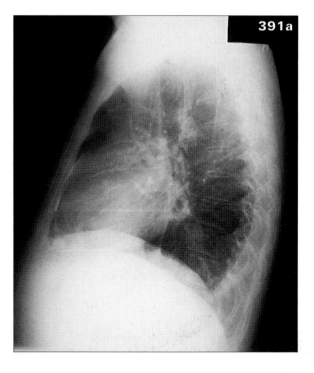
391a

Answer 390

1. Friedreich's ataxia.
2. Hypertrophic cardiomyopathy (hypertrophic obstructive cardiomyopathy).
3. i. Diabetes mellitus.
   ii. Optic atrophy.

The patient has pes cavus and signs of cerebellar and pyramidal tract disease. In addition there is a history of chest pains and breathlessness, suggesting cardiovascular disease, and a cardiac murmur that is compatible with dynamic left ventricular outflow tract obstruction characteristic of hypertrophic obstructive cardiomyopathy. The complete diagnosis is Friedreich's ataxia.

Friedreich's ataxia is an autosomal recessive condition due to a mutation in a gene encoding the protein frataxin on chromosome 9. The mutation comprises unstable expansions of the GAA repeat of variable size (120–1,700) in the first intron. The exact function of frataxin is unknown, but early reports suggest that it is a mitochondrial iron transport protein. The prevalence is 1/50,000. It is the most common example of the hereditary ataxias. There is degeneration of the dorsal spinal column, the spinocerebellar tracts, the pyramidal tracts, and the dorsal root ganglion cells. The syndrome is dominated by progressive ataxia. The usual age of onset is the second decade, but the disease may not appear until as late as the fourth decade. The lower limbs are generally affected before the upper limbs. Difficulty in walking and stumbling regularly are early signs. Cerebellar signs may proceed rapidly and include a coarse intention tremor, ataxia affecting the limbs and the trunk, nystagmus (25%) and dysarthria that may become severe. Involvement of the pyramidal tracts causes weakness of the lower limbs. The tone may be only slightly increased because of the accompanying disturbance affecting the afferent fibres from the muscle spindles. The plantar response is extensor. Dorsal column involvement causes loss of joint position, vibration and two-point discrimination sense. There is a peripheral neuropathy associated with muscle wasting, and depressed or absent reflexes. Optic atrophy is present in approximately 30% of patients. Associated skeletal deformities include kyphoscoliosis, pes cavus, pes equinovarus and high arched palate. Kyphoscoliosis and high arched palates are also present in Marfan's syndrome and homocystinuria, but neither of these conditions is associated with spinocerebellar degeneration.

The condition is associated with HCM in between 50 and 70% of patients. The frequency of HCM increases with the size of the GAA expansion in the first intron. The ECG is abnormal in over 70% of patients and demonstrates widespread T-wave inversion. Diabetes mellitus is present in approximately 10%. A very small proportion of patients may also have sensorineuronal deafness. Death usually occurs in the fourth decade, and is due to cardiac failure

Answer 391

1. i. Elevated and equal right and left atrial pressures.
   ii. Elevated and equal left and right ventricular end-diastolic pressures.
2. Calcification of the pericardium (**391b**, arrowed).
3. The findings are consistent with the diagnosis of pericardial constriction.

(See Interpretation of Cardiac Catheter Data, page 418.)

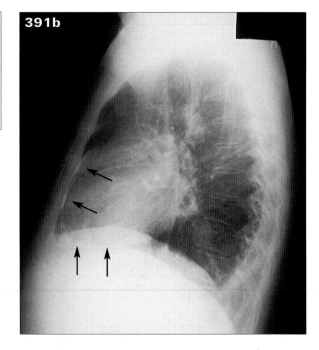

Question 392

Hb	9 g/dl
WCC	$52 \times 10^9/l$
Platelets	$680 \times 10^9/l$
MCV	88 fl
Neutrophils	67%
Myoblasts	8%
Myelocytes	10%
Metamyelocytes	8%
Lymphocytes	2%
Eosinophils	1%
Basophils	2%
Nucleated red cell	2%

A 52-year-old male presented with night sweats and lethargy. On examination, he was pale and had a palpable spleen 7 cm below the costal margin.

Investigations are shown.

1. Suggest two possible diagnoses.
2. Apart from the bone marrow, which two investigations would help differentiate between the two diagnoses?

Question 393

A 59-year-old female presented to the Accident and Emergency Department with sudden onset of retrosternal pain on bending down to get into her car. On examination, she was jaundiced. Her blood pressure was 140/80 mmHg. She was extremely tender over the mid-sternal area, particularly when she attempted deep inspiration. The heart sounds were normal and her chest was entirely clear. Abdominal examination revealed hepatomegaly, which was palpable 4 cm below the costal margin, and a palpable tip of the spleen. Only three days earlier she had seen her GP with a six-week history of malaise and was noted to have jaundice, which was under preliminary investigation. There was no history of abdominal pain or weight loss. She also complained of increasing weakness, with particular difficulty in rising from a sitting position. She had never had any previous hospital admissions, but had seen the GP for troublesome pruritis over the past four years for which she took chlorpheniramine. She was noted to have a serum cholesterol level of 10.5 mmol/l during a routine health check one year ago, for which she had been taking simvastatin. She was widowed two years ago and now lived alone. There was no recent history of travel abroad.

Investigations are shown.

Hb	11 g/dl
WCC	$10 \times 10^9/l$
Platelets	$108 \times 10^9/l$
MCV	90 fl
Sodium	135 mmol/l
Potassium	4.7 mmol/l
Urea	9 mmol/l
Creatinine	125 µmol/l
Bilirubin	90 µmol/l
AST	70 iu/l
Alkaline phosphatase	400 iu/l
Albumin	33 g/l
Protein	80 g/l
Calcium	2.0 mmol/l
Phosphate	0.9 mmol/l
Cholesterol	7 mmol/l
Creatinine kinase	900 u/l
Chest X-ray	Normal-sized heart (PA view)
	Clear lung fields
	Looser's zone right clavicle
ECG	Sinus rhythm
	Partial RBBB

1. What is the most probable explanation for the chest pain?
2. What investigation would you perform to confirm the diagnosis?
3. What is the cause of the failure to rise from a sitting position?
4. Why is the serum cholesterol elevated?
5. How would you account for the raised creatinine kinase?
6. List two steps in the management of her hypercholesterolaemia.
7. What is the cause of her jaundice?
8. List two investigations you would perform to confirm the cause of her jaundice.

Answer 392

1. i. Chronic myeloid leukaemia.
   ii. Myelofibrosis.
2. i. Neutrophil leucocyte alkaline phosphatase.
   ii. Karyotype for Philadelphia chromosome.

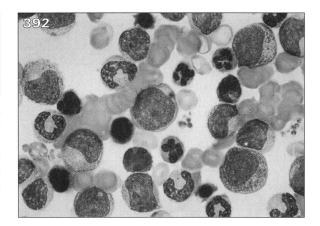

Both chronic myeloid leukaemia and myelofibrosis are myeloproliferative disorders characterized by a high (usually >50 × 10⁹/l) WCC consisting of the granulocyte series. Both may be associated with a large spleen, and therefore the differentiation between the two on clinical grounds alone is difficult. Myelofibrosis is characterized by fibrous replacement of the marrow, and although the white cell and platelet count may be very high, a leucoerthyroblastic blood picture is more characteristic. A list of features which may help distinguish chronic myeloid leukaemia from myelofibrosis is shown (*Table*).

Features which may help distinguish chronic myeloid leukaemia from myelofibrosis

Parameter	Chronic myeloid leukaemia	Myelofibrosis
WCC	>50 × 10⁹/l	>50 × 10⁹/l
Large spleen	Present	Present
Blood film	Numerous granulocytes at varying stages of maturation; may be leucoerythroblastic (**392**)	Leucoerythroblastic Tear drop cells
Neutrophil leucocyte alkaline phosphatase	Low	Normal/high
Philadelphia chromosome	Present in 90%	Absent
Marrow	Numerous granulocytes at varying stages of maturation	Myelofibrosis; stains black with reticulin

Answer 393

1. Fractured sternum due to osteomalacia.
2. Lateral chest X-ray.
3. Proximal myopathy due to osteomalacia.
4. Reduced excretion of cholesterol owing to biliary stasis.
5. Simvastatin-induced myositis/rhabdomyolysis.
6. i. Dietary measures, low-fat diet.
   ii. Cholestyramine.
7. PBC.
8. i. Antimitochondrial antibodies (IgM2).
   ii. Liver biopsy, provided that clotting was not abnormal.

The patient has PBC. There is the classic history of pruritis preceding the onset of jaundice by a few years. The raised serum cholesterol and biochemical and radiological evidence of osteomalacia are suggestive of chronic cholestasis in a jaundiced patient. Hypercholesterolaemia is the result of reduced biliary excretion because bile is the only means for the human body to dispose of cholesterol; thus, many patients with PBC have xanthelasma and palmar xanthomas, which are stigmata of hypercholesterolaemia. Osteomalacia is due to vitamin D deficiency resulting from fat malabsorption. Bile excretion into the small intestine is necessary for fat digestion and absorption. Failure to absorb fats results in failure to absorb fat-soluble vitamins, notably vitamins A, D, E and K. Vitamin D deficiency leads to osteomalacia and pathological fractures. This patient's presentation is almost certainly due to a sternal fracture, which may be detected on a lateral chest X-ray. The raised creatinine kinase is unlikely to represent an acute myocardial infarction, given the chest tenderness. The most likely explanation for the high creatinine kinase level is simvastatin-induced myositis. In liver and/or renal failure, simvastatin may cause frank rhabdomyolysis. Patients also taking fibrates and ciclosporin with the statins are at risk of this complication. In this case, the best method of managing the hypercholesterolaemia is by a low-fat diet and by therapy with cholestyramine, a resin which binds bile and promotes its excretion.

The diagnosis of PBC is confirmed by the demonstration of IgM antimitochondrial antibodies (subtype M2), which are present in over 90% of the patients. A liver biopsy shows a dense infiltration of the portal tract with lymphocytes and plasma cells. There is periportal fibrosis and cholestasis, and granulomas are present around the small bile ducts.

ANF antibodies and rheumatoid factor are present in up to one-third of cases. Associations include CREST (calcinosis, Raynaud's syndrome, oesophageal problems, scleroderma and telangiectasia) syndrome, membranous glomerulonephritis, RTA and Sjögren's syndrome.

There is no specific proven therapy, although ursodeoxycholic acid does retard progression and time to hepatic transplantation. Liver transplantation should be considered when the serum bilirubin exceeds 100 µmol/l.

Question 394

A 35-year-old female with Crohn's disease since the age of 15 years presented with a six-month history of foul-smelling diarrhoea and weight loss.

Investigations are shown.

Hb	10 g/dl
WCC	7×10^9/l
Platelets	199×10^9/l
MCV	106 fl
Serum folate	22 µg/l
Serum B_{12}	65 ng/l
Faecal fat	50 mmol/l
	(NR <20 mmol/l)
Schilling test	Pre-intrinsic factor 2% B_{12} isotope excreted
	Post-intrinsic factor 2% B_{12} isotope excreted

1. List two possible causes for this patient's symptoms.
2. Which investigation would you perform next?

Answer 394

1. i. Primary B_{12} malabsorption.
   ii. Bacterial overgrowth.
2. Repeat Schilling test after a two-week course of antibiotics.

Table A The Schilling test

Part 1
- Give 1 mg ^{58}Co-B_{12} orally to a patient who has fasted overnight, and also give 1 mg of non-radioactive B_{12} by intramuscular injection to saturate B_{12} binding proteins. Collect urine for 24 hours
- Normal subjects excrete >10% of the radioactive dose

If part 1 is abnormal:

Part 2
- Repeat Schilling with oral intrinsic factor
- If excretion becomes normal, the primary abnormality is intrinsic factor deficiency
- If excretion remains abnormal, then the differential is between primary B_{12} malabsorption and bacterial overgrowth

---

Table B Differentiation of primary B_{12} malabsorption from bacterial overgrowth

	1° B_{12} malabsorption	*Bacterial overgrowth*
1. Schilling test after antibiotics	Abnormal	Normal
2. Small bowel meal	Terminal ileal stricture	Fistulae, jejunal strictures
3. Jejunal aspirate	Normal bacteria	High concentration of *Escherichia coli/Bacteroides*
4. ^{14}C-glycocholate breath test	Positive	Positive

The patient has a history of Crohn's disease and now presents with steatorrhoea, B_{12} deficiency and an abnormal Schilling test (*Table A*), with and without intrinsic factor. The two most likely causes for the B_{12} deficiency in Crohn's disease are primary B_{12} malabsorption due to terminal ileal disease, or intestinal destruction of dietary B_{12} by bacterial overgrowth within small bowel strictures (**394**). Both conditions also cause steatorrhoea by impairing fat absorption due to disturbances in bile salt absorption; the former by preventing absorption of bile salts which are required for micelle formation, and the latter by deconjugation and dehydroxylation of bile salts. Repeating the Schilling test after a two-week course of metronidazole and tetracycline may help to differentiate between terminal ileal disease and bacterial overgrowth (*Table B*). Antibiotics destroy the large concentrations of *Escherichia coli* and/or *Bacteroides* which are responsible for bacterial overgrowth, and following this the Schilling test (without intrinsic factor) becomes normal. In terminal ileal disease, the test will remain abnormal. A small-bowel enema may also help in the differentiation by demonstrating a terminal stricture responsible for primary B_{12} malabsorption, and any structural defects which will predispose to bacterial

Table C Causes of B_{12} deficiency

- Low dietary intake (vegans)

Intrinsic factor deficiency
- Congenital
- Pernicious anaemia
- Gastrectomy
- Chronic atrophic gastritis

Primary B_{12} malabsorption
- Terminal ileal disease
- Bacterial overgrowth
- Coeliac and tropical sprue (longstanding)
- Pancreatic insufficiency

Miscellaneous
- Fish tapeworm (*Diphyllobothrium latum*)
- Drug, e.g. colchicine, neomycin

overgrowth. Another method of differentiation is by jejunal aspiration and culture. Although *E. coli* and *Bacteroides* are found in the jejunum, it is unusual to find concentrations exceeding 10^6/ml unless there is

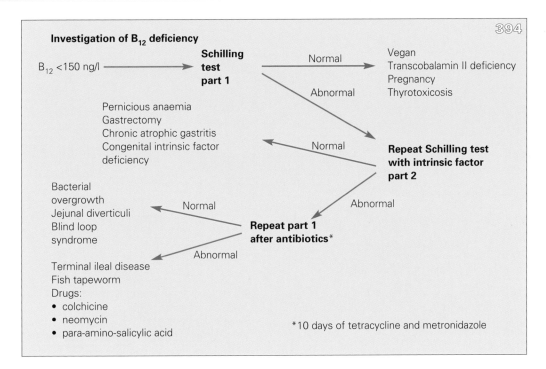

Investigation of B$_{12}$ deficiency

394

B$_{12}$ <150 ng/l ⟶ **Schilling test part 1**

Normal ⟶ Vegan / Transcobalamin II deficiency / Pregnancy / Thyrotoxicosis

Abnormal

Pernicious anaemia
Gastrectomy
Chronic atrophic gastritis
Congenital intrinsic factor deficiency

Normal ⟵ **Repeat Schilling test with intrinsic factor part 2**

Abnormal

Bacterial overgrowth
Jejunal diverticuli
Blind loop syndrome

Normal ⟵ **Repeat part 1 after antibiotics***

Abnormal

Terminal ileal disease
Fish tapeworm
Drugs:
• colchicine
• neomycin
• para-amino-salicylic acid

*10 days of tetracycline and metronidazole

overgrowth. A ^{14}C-glycocholate breath test is characteristically positive in bacterial overgrowth, as bacteria deconjugate bile salts to release ^{14}C-glycine, which is metabolized to $^{14}CO_2$. The radioactivity in the breath is easy to measure; however, it is important to realize that the test may also be positive in terminal ileal disease because unabsorbed radiolabelled bile salts pass into the colon where the concentration of *E. coli* is very high, leading to deconjugation of bile salts and liberation of ^{14}C-glycine. In terminal ileal disease, faecal radioactivity is also high, whereas in bacterial overgrowth the radioactivity level is relatively low. Causes of B$_{12}$ deficiency are tabulated (*Table C*).

Question 395

A 65-year-old male was seen in the out-patient's clinic with a one-year history of dizziness which was worse on getting out of bed, and occasionally associated with collapse. The patient also complained of weakness affecting both legs. On further questioning, he admitted to urinary incontinence and his wife noted that he was generally slow and had an intermittent tremor affecting his right hand.

On examination, he appeared slightly withdrawn. His pulse was 84 beats/min, and blood pressure 155/85 mmHg. The heart sounds were normal. Examination of the respiratory and gastrointestinal systems was normal. On examination of the central nervous system he had sluggish pupillary reflexes and nystagmus. Examination of the fundi was normal. There was a pill-rolling tremor affecting the right hand. There was increased tone in both legs, with the right leg being affected more than the left. Power was slightly reduced (grade 4/5) in all limbs. The reflexes were generally brisk. The plantar response in the left foot was extensor, but was equivocal in the right foot. Sensation was normal. His gait was ataxic.

1. What is the most likely diagnosis?
2. List two further investigations you would pursue to confirm your diagnosis.

Answer 395

1. Multi-system atrophy or Shy–Drager syndrome.
2. i. Lying and standing blood pressure.
   ii. Autonomic nervous system testing (loss of sinus arrhythmias on ECG, loss of reflex bradycardia on carotid sinus massage, absence of a reflex tachycardia after the Valsalva manoeuvre).

Causes of autonomic failure

1. Central (primary)
Progressive autonomic failure (no obvious cause)
Progressive autonomic failure with multi-system atrophy (Shy–Drager syndrome)
Progressive autonomic failure with Parkinson's disease

2. Central (secondary)
Central brain lesions: craniopharyngioma, vascular disease
Encephalitis, tabes dorsalis, Chaga's disease
Spinal cord lesions
Familial dysautonomia

3. Distal autonomic neuropathies
Guillain–Barré syndrome, diabetes mellitus, amyloid, porphyria, rheumatoid arthritis, myaesthenia gravis, Fabry's disease

4. Tricyclic antidepressants, MAOIs, ganglion-blocking drugs

The patient has a pill-rolling tremor and increased muscular tone, indicating an extrapyramidal syndrome such as Parkinson's disease. The presence of additional neurological findings suggests that he has a Parkinson-plus syndrome. There are several Parkinson-plus syndromes in the literature, but the ones which are most commonly tested include multi-system atrophy and the SROS. Multi-system atrophy is the name given to a sporadically occurring condition which begins in adult life, usually in the sixth decade. It is characterized by neuronal cell loss and gliosis changes in:

- The substantia niagra pathways that cause Parkinsonism.
- The olivopontocerebellar tract causing ataxia, dysarthria, nystagmus and pyramidal signs.
- The intermediolateral cell column (pre-ganglionic sympathetic neurones in the lateral horns of the spinal cord) causing autonomic nervous system failure. Other causes of autonomic failure are shown (*Table*).

These changes often overlap and may present as a mixture of neurological abnormalities. When features of Parkinson's disease predominate, the disorder is called striatonigral degeneration. When features of the autonomic failure predominate, the disorder is commonly known as Shy–Drager syndrome, and when cerebellar features predominate it is called olivopontocerebellar atrophy. When all three systems are involved the disorder is known as multi-system atrophy. Unlike Parkinson's disease, there is a shortened life expectancy, with a median survival of 9.3 years.

In Shy–Drager syndrome impotence is often the first symptom. Incontinence is common in both sexes. Speech differs from the hypophonic monotony of Parkinson's disease, incorporating quivering, straining, slurring, and dysarthric components. Patients may develop aphonia, anarthria and dysphagia, which are the same as in Parkinson's disease. Respiratory stridor can occur in about 30% of patients. There is no specific treatment for multi-system atrophy and the associated disorders. The use of compression stockings, fludrocortisone, and pressor agents such as ephedrine have been used for the postural symptoms. The response to L-dopa is usually absent or poor.

Steele–Richardson–Olszewski syndrome
This is another multisystem degeneration syndrome. It is characterized by cell loss and neurofibrillary tangles in the brainstem, globus pallidus, subthalamic and dentate nuclei, and causes the syndrome of progressive supranuclear palsy. It begins in the seventh decade. Patients present with imbalance, particularly falling backwards, a coarse dysarthria, involuntary groans and dysphagia. Perseverance may be obvious in speech with repetition of syllables and words (palilalia) or even of whole phrases (palilogia). Involuntary eye closure is often seen. The brow may be furrowed and the eyebrows raised from frontalis hyperactivity in an attempt to keep the eyes open, resulting in a surprised expression. The characteristic feature in SROS is a supranuclear palsy of voluntary gaze. Voluntary downgaze is slow and incomplete, but when the patient's neck is passively extended while fixing his gaze on the examiner's nose, a downward gaze is obtained. Patients may therefore have problems with reading and eating. Patients with SROS can masquerade as having Parkinson's disease because of axial rigidity and gait disturbances, but lack features of distal Parkinsonism (distal limb akinesia or rigidity). Resting tremor is almost never seen. There is no effective treatment. Median survival is about 6–7 years.

Question 396

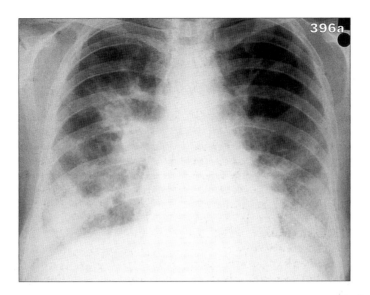

396a

A 31-year-old male was admitted to hospital with a two-week history of progressive dyspnoea on exertion and wheeze. He complained of aches and pains in his arms and legs. He had suffered from ulcerative colitis for four years, and required several courses of high-dose prednisolone until the last two months, when his colitis was relatively quiescent. He also had a past history of hyperthyroidism which was medically treated with carbimazole. He was currently maintained on sulphasalazine 1 g twice daily for the ulcerative colitis.

On examination, he was dyspnoeic, had mild cervical and axillary lymphadenopathy, and a generalized maculopapular rash. He had a fever of 38.5°C (101.3°F). The heart rate was 110 beats/min and regular. The blood pressure was 140/80 mmHg. Heart sounds were normal. Auscultation of the lung fields demonstrated widespread wheeze. His abdomen was very muscular and difficult to examine. All other examinations were essentially normal.

Investigations are shown.

Hb	13 g/dl
WCC	15.3 × 10⁹/l
	(neutrophils 10.1 × 10⁹/l,
	lymphocytes 1.0 × 10⁹/l,
	eosinophils 4.2 × 10⁹/l)
Platelets	308 × 10⁹/l
Sodium	126 mmol/l
Potassium	4.3 mmol/l
Urea	7 mmol/l
Creatinine	100 μmol/l
ESR	98 mm/h
Blood and sputum cultures: Negative	

Arterial blood gases (on air):

pH	7.4
PaCO$_2$	3.3 kPa
PaO$_2$	8.7 kPa
Bicarbonate	21 mmol/l
O$_2$ saturation	92%
Chest X-ray (**396a**)	

What is the diagnosis?
a. Churg–Strauss syndrome.
b. Eosinophilic pneumonitis.
c. Allergic bronchopulmonary aspergillosis.
d. *Pneumocystis jirovecii* pneumonia.
e. Hodgkin's lymphoma.

Answer 396

> b. Eosinophilic pneumonitis.

The patient has a generalized illness consisting of a widespread macular rash, generalized lymphadenopathy, and a very high eosinophil count. He has a wheeze, and his chest X-ray reveals patchy consolidation, which is worse in the right lung. He had been on prednisolone for ulcerative colitis but has recently commenced sulphasalazine. The symptoms and signs appeared after the drug was commenced, and the most likely diagnosis for his respiratory problem is an eosinophilic pneumonia. This question tests the reader's knowledge of causes of eosinophilia (**396b**) of which there are many; however, the most common cause is allergy. An allergic reaction to drugs may precipitate a profound eosinophilia with multi-system involvement, including eosinophilic infiltration into the lungs. Sulphonamides are a well-recognized cause of eosinophilia and subsequent eosinophilic consolidation. Other drugs implicated include erythromycin, nitrofurantoin and imipramine. The most obvious management of a drug-related eosinophilia is to stop the culprit agent. Pulmonary involvement responds well to high-dose steroids, which may be tailed off over a few weeks. However, relapse is not uncommon and some patients require a maintenance dose of 5 mg prednisolone for several months to prevent recurrence.

The differential diagnosis here is the Churg–Strauss syndrome, which is a small-vessel granulomatous vasculitis characterized by skin rash, respiratory involvement giving asthmatic symptoms, neuropathy and eosinophilia. It is a variant of Wegener's granulomatosis, but is a much milder disease and does not usually involve the kidneys. Lymphoma is also associated with eosinophilia; however, it would have to be fairly extensive to involve the cervical and axillary lymph nodes as well as the chest. The normal Hb and lymphocyte count are not consistent with extensive lymphoma.

Although the patient had been on steroids and is currently taking carbimazole, his normal neutrophil count is highly against the development of an opportunistic infection such as TB or *Pneumocystis jirovecii* pneumonia (previously known as *Pneumocystis carinii* pneumonia).

Ulcerative colitis itself is a recognized cause of a mild eosinophilia; however, an eosinophilia as high as in this case and pulmonary involvement cannot be explained by the disease.

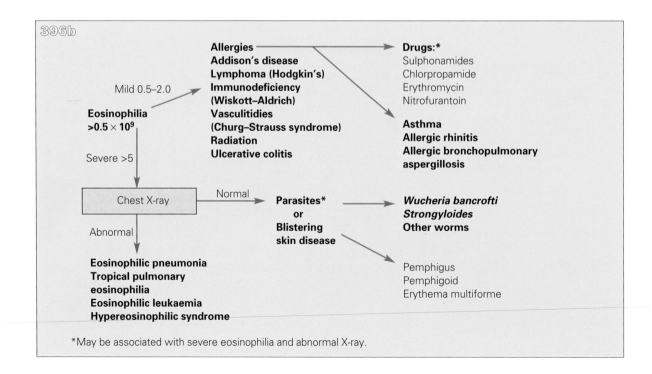

*May be associated with severe eosinophilia and abnormal X-ray.

Question 397

A 16-year-old female is investigated for short stature. The results of a dynamic pituitary function tests following 0.15 iu/kg of insulin, 100 µg of LHRH, and 200 µg of TRH are as follows:

Time (min)	Glucose (mmol/l)	GH mu/l	Cortisol (nmol/l)	TSH mu/l	LH iu/l	FSH iu/l	Oestradiol pmol/l
0	4.0	1.4	400	2.0	29	16	4
20	2.8	12.0	860	5.2	40	24	5
30	1.6	28	1270	-	-	-	–
40	1.5	32	1450	-	-	-	–
60	2.2	20	1120	8	34	20	6

1. The following statements are true with respect to the pituitary function tests above:
   a. There was an inadequate stimulus for GH secretion.
   b. The GH response was abnormal.
   c. The findings are consistent with pituitary Cushing's syndrome.
   d. The patient is hypothyroid.
   e. There is evidence of primary hypogonadism.

2. The following investigations would be useful in confirming the diagnosis:
   a. Buccal smear for karyotyping.
   b. CT scan of the pituitary gland.
   c. Dexamethasone suppression test.
   d. Investigation of other family members.
   e. Thyroid antibodies.

3. The following diagnoses are possible in this patient:
   a. Hypothyroidism.
   b. Turner's syndrome.
   c. PCOS.
   d. Testicular feminization syndrome.
   e. Coeliac disease.

Question 398

A 70-year-old male on treatment for congestive cardiac failure with an angiotensin-converting enzyme inhibitor, spironolactone, digoxin and furosemide was admitted with nausea. An ECG taken on admission is shown (398).

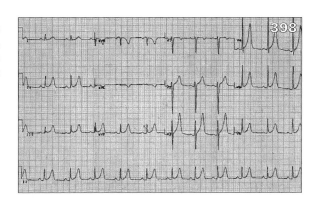

Which investigation would you perform next?
   a. Serum potassium.
   b. Serum magnesium.
   c. Cardiac troponin I.
   d. Echocardiography.
   e. 24-hour ECG.

Answer 397

1. e. There is evidence of primary hypogonadism.
2. a. Buccal smear for karyotyping.
3. b. Turner's syndrome.

In order to answer this question correctly the reader requires knowledge of the normal results of dynamic pituitary function tests and gonadotrophin and sex hormone levels (*Tables A* and *B*).

In this case, there is an adequate stimulus to GH and cortisol secretion. The GH response is normal, and there is no evidence of hypothyroidism. The basal oestradiol is low and the basal LH and FSH are high, suggesting primary hypogonadism. The LHRH test is normal (as is the case) in primary hypogonadism. The most probable diagnosis is Turner's syndrome. Turner's syndrome is characterized by a single X chromosome (karyotype 45 XO). It has an incidence of approximately 1 in 2,500. The main abnormality is gonadal dysgenesis, the consequences of which are primary amenorrhoea and infertility. Oestradiol levels are low, resulting in elevated gonadotrophin levels via the positive feedback on the pituitary. The patients are typically short and have a number of other morphological abnormalities (*Table C*). The diagnosis is confirmed by a buccal smear which reveals an absent Barr body. There are several other causes of hypogonadism in females (*Table D*).

Polycystic ovary syndrome may also cause partial hypogonadism, but in contrast with the other causes of hypogonadism given in *Table D*, the oestradiol levels are only slightly reduced and the FSH level is low (*Table E*). Although coeliac disease is a recognized cause of short stature (and also delayed puberty), the gonadotrophin response to LHRH is entirely normal. The commonly examined causes of short stature in the MRCP and similar examinations are listed (*Table F*).

Testicular feminization syndrome is due to the absence of testosterone receptors on end organs. The patient has male karyotype, but is phenotypically female owing to the absence of the effect of testosterone in the normal development of male gonads. Testicles are present but are usually intra-abdominal or in the hernial orifices. Serum testosterone levels are very high. Lack of testosterone receptors on the pituitary means that there is no negative feedback system to inhibit gonadotrophin secretion, therefore both LH and FSH are very high. Excess stimulation of the testicular remnants leads to excess oestrogen production by the testes, which is comparable with levels found in females. The oestrogen initiates breast development and maintains breasts. Lack of the testosterone effect means that pubic hair may be absent or scanty. These patients are not particularly short. They present with amenorrhoea. The diagnosis can be confirmed by karyotyping.

Pituitary Cushing's is unusual in this age group. It is due to a basophil adenoma within the pituitary which secretes ACTH, causing adrenal hyperplasia and excess cortisol production. The serum cortisol is >900 nmol/l and there is loss of diurnal variation, i.e. the midnight cortisol is also >900 nmol/l (normally 150–750 nmol/l). In the majority of cases high-dose dexamethasone (8 mg per day) suppresses cortisol production (see Answer 173). In some cases the cortisol response to dexamethasone is unaffected and in these instances the main definitive method of diagnosing pituitary Cushing's is to perform inferior petrosal sinus sampling for ACTH.

Table A Normal responses to dynamic pituitary function tests

- Following an insulin tolerance test, the GH level rises to >20 mu/l and the serum cortisol level should rise to ≥550 nmol/l and increase by 180 nmol/l from the basal level. The blood sugar should fall below 2.2 mmol/l to ensure adequate metabolic stress for GH and cortisol secretion. Note: An insulin tolerance test should not be performed if the basal cortisol level is below 180 nmol/l
- Following a TRH test, the TSH should increase by >2 mu/l from the basal level. Basal TSH levels are between 0.5–5 mu/l
- Following an LHRH test, the LH and FSH should double from the basal level

Table B Normal gonadotrophin and sex hormone levels in males and females

Females	*Males*
Follicular phase, FSH 1–10 iu/l and LH 2–20 iu/l	FSH 1–7 iu/l and LH 1–10 iu/l
Oestradiol <110 pmol/l	Testosterone 10–35 nmol/l
Testosterone 0.5–3 nmol/l	

Table C Morphological features of Turner's syndrome

Skeletal
- Short stature
- Cubitus valgus
- Short fourth metacarpals
- High-arched palate*
- Shield chest with widely spaced nipples

Cardiac anomalies
- Septal defects
- Coarctation of the aorta

Renal anomalies
- Horse-shoe kidneys

Miscellaneous abnormalities
- Webbed neck (fused cervical vertebrae)
- Lymphoedema
- Low hair line
- Multiple naevi
- Increased incidence of auto-immune thyroiditis and diabetes

* Also present in Marfan's syndrome, homocystinuria and Friedreich's ataxia.

Table D Causes of primary hypogonadism in females

- Turner's syndrome
- Pure ovarian dysgenesis*
- Swyer's syndrome**
- Auto-immune oophoritis
- Ovariectomy
- Chemotherapy
- Steroid biosynthetic defect
- (17-α-hydroxylase deficiency)

* The pathology is the same as Turner's, but differs in that there is a normal complement of chromosomes and the other morphological features of Turner's syndrome are absent. Some patients may have sensorineuronal deafness.
** Swyer's syndrome is characterized by the XY karyotype and gonadal dysgenesis. Affected individuals are phenotypically female. It is associated with a high incidence of gonadoblastomas.

Table E Characteristics of PCOS (Stein–Levental syndrome)

- Irregular menstruation
- Impaired fertility
- Hursutism
- Acne
- Obesity
- Low oestradiol levels
- Testosterone level slightly higher than 3.0 nmol/l
- High oestrone levels
- Slightly elevated LH level
- Slightly depressed FSH level
- LH/FSH ratio generally exceeds 2

Table F Causes of short stature

- Constitutional delay*
- Familial
- Systemic disorder, e.g. coeliac disease
- Endocrine causes, e.g. hypothyroidism or GH deficiency
- Drugs, particularly steroids
- Emotional deprivation
- Skeletal abnormalities (achondroplasia, vitamin D-resistant rickets)

* Slow growth from the beginning, spontaneous puberty, slight delay in bone maturity, normal LHRH test.

Answer 398

a. Serum potassium.

Tall tented T-waves (>1.25 mV; 12 small squares) is an ECG feature of hyperkalaemia. In this case, the cause of hyperkalaemia is a combination of potassium-sparing drugs and obstructive uropathy. (See *Table B*, Answer 220.)

Question 399

A 65-year-old female was referred to a neurologist with a six-month history of progressive weakness and clumsiness of her left hand. She mentioned having particular difficulty in washing the dishes and using the gear stick while driving her car. Her husband noticed that her gait had been unsteady and she had suffered a few falls in the past year. On systemic enquiry there was no history of headaches, visual disturbance or weight loss, but she had experienced dizziness on turning her head suddenly.

On examination she was thin and had marked kyphoscoliosis. There was evidence of wasting of the small muscles of the hands, which was more prominent on the left side than the right. There was reduced power on flexion and abduction of the arms. The supinator and biceps reflexes on the left side were absent but present on the right. The triceps reflexes were brisk bilaterally. The power in both lower limbs was grade 4 out of 5 in all muscle groups. The tone was increased. The ankle and knee reflexes were brisk bilaterally. The left plantar response was upgoing but the right one was equivocal. Sensation was normal with the exception of vibration sense at both ankle joints.

1. What is the diagnosis?
    a. Motor neurone disease.
    b. Syringomyelia.
    c. Multiple sclerosis.
    d. Cervical myelopathy.
    e. Subacute combined degeneration of the spinal cord.
2. Which investigation would you perform to confirm the diagnosis?
    a. Myelography.
    b. MRI scan cervical spine.
    c. Nerve conduction studies and electromyography.
    d. CSF analysis for oligoclonal bands.
    e. Serum B_{12} level.

Question 400

A young alcoholic who is well known to the local Accident and Emergency Department was admitted to hospital after being found collapsed. On examination, he was unrousable. His temperature was 36.5°C (97.7°F). His heart rate was 120 beats/min, and regular, with a weak pulse volume. The blood pressure was 80/40 mmHg. The heart sounds were normal. Auscultation of the lung fields revealed a few crackles at both lung bases. The abdomen was rigid and bowel sounds were absent. Rectal examination demonstrated soft brown stool. Examination of the fundi was normal.

Investigations are shown.

Hb	7 g/dl
WCC	23×10^9/l
Platelets	50×10^9/l
MCV	102 fl
INR	1.9
Sodium	131 mmol/l
Potassium	5.6 mmol/l
Urea	17 mmol/l
Creatinine	200 µmol/l
Bicarbonate	16 mmol/l
Calcium	1.9 mmol/l
Phosphate	1.0 mmol/l
Albumin	30 g/l
AST	64 iu/l
Bilirubin	53 µmol/l
Alkaline phosphatase	204 iu/l
Gamma GT	190 iu/l
Glucose	21 mmol/l
Urinalysis	Protein +1
	Blood 0
	Ketones +1

1. What is the diagnosis?
    a. Diabetic ketoacidosis.
    b. Perforated duodenal ulcer.
    c. Gastrointestinal haemorrhage secondary to oesophageal varices.
    d. Acute pancreatitis.
    e. Methanol poisoning.
2. List five investigations that you would perform on this patient immediately.

Question 401

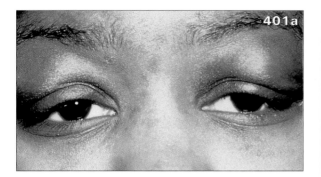

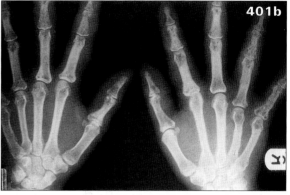

A 44-year-old West Indian male presented with a three-week history of polydipsia, polyuria and nocturia. He was passing copious amounts of urine several times per day, and felt excessively thirsty. According to his wife he was consuming up to five 2-litre bottles of cola per day, and several large (1-litre) flasks of water. His appetite and weight had been normal. He was not taking any medication. For four years he had been intermittently unwell, firstly with chest problems, and then with arthritis affecting his hands and feet. The respiratory problems – which were characterized by a dry cough and accompanied by night sweats, pains in his ankles and tender, raised lesions on his shins – were of relatively sudden onset. The joint pains responded to pain killers prescribed by a doctor whom he saw in the West Indies, but the chest symptoms persisted for several months despite four long courses of antibiotics. The skin lesions on the shins resolved about three months after the onset of his illness. He was eventually referred to a chest physician with breathlessness on exertion, and after respiratory function tests (top panel of results) and a chest X-ray was told he had scarring on the lung, possibly due to several previous chest infections, and was prescribed a steroid inhaler.

The patient's breathing remained stable. He was able to walk for over two miles on the flat, but experienced breathlessness on negotiating inclines. After two years, he developed pain and swelling in his hands and feet, which were controlled to some extent with co-proxamol. His only other complaint was of a gritty feeling in the eyes as the day progressed, and dryness of the mouth for several months before he developed polyuria. He worked as a bus conductor. His brother, aged 58, had rheumatoid arthritis which was complicated with lung fibrosis.

On examination, the patient appeared well at rest, but had mild bilateral parotid gland enlargement. The appearance of the eyes is shown (**401a**). His eyes were red, but the visual acuity, visual fields, pupils and fundi were normal. There was no focal neurological deficit. There was no evidence of a previous BCG scar. There was bone swelling affecting several phalanges in the hands and feet. There was no joint swelling. Cardiovascular examination was normal. Auscultation of the lung fields revealed fine inspiratory crackles in the anterior chest, but auscultation of the posterior aspect of the chest was normal.

Investigations are shown (second panel of results).

	Actual	Predicted
FEV$_1$ (l)	2.2	4.1
FVC (l)	2.5	5.4
TLC (l)	3.3	6.3
KCO (mmol/min/kPa)	0.9	1.40

Sodium	143 mmol/l
Potassium	4.5 mmol/l
Urea	6 mmol/l
Creatinine	90 μmol
Calcium	2.3 mmol/l
Phosphate	1.1 mmol/l
Alkaline phosphatase	120 iu/l
Blood glucose	4.2 mmol/l
X-ray of hands (**401b**)	

Fluid deprivation test:

Time (min)	$P_{mOsm/l}$	$U_{mOsm/l}$
0	303	120
60	310	120
120	318	120
180	328	120
240	335	120
8 h after desmopressin		800

1. What were the painful lesions on the shins?
2. What do the patient's respiratory function tests demonstrate?
3. What does the X-ray of his hands reveal?
4. Why does he have gritty eyes?
5. What is the interpretation of the water deprivation test?
6. What is the overall or underlying diagnosis?
7. What three investigations would you perform to confirm your diagnosis?
8. Give three therapeutic steps in his management.

Answer 399

> 1. d. Cervical myelopathy.
> 2. b. MRI scan cervical spine.

The patient presents with progressive weakness affecting her arms and hands. She has a combination of upper and lower motor neurone signs in the upper limbs and purely upper motor neurone signs in the lower limbs. There is loss of vibration sense at the level of the ankles. This may be a normal finding in patients in their seventh decade but may indicate pathology in the dorsal columns.

The differential diagnosis is between motor neurone disease, cervical cord tumour and cervical myelopathy, and subacute combined degeneration of the spinal cord.

Features against motor neurone disease include her gender (more common in males), the mid-cervical reflex pattern (absent supinator and biceps reflex but exaggerated triceps reflex), which is more suggestive of cervical myelopathy, the association of her symptoms with rigidity in the neck and dizziness on turning suddenly, which again suggests pathology in the cervical cord, and the absence of weight loss, which is usually marked in motor neurone disease.

Subacute combined degeneration of the spinal cord is a remote possibility, but one would want more evidence of a sensory neuropathy in this condition, for example, absence of light touch and proprioception and absent knee or ankle jerks.

Both cervical myelopathy and a cervical cord tumour may present with predominantly upper limb signs, which characteristically produce lower motor neurone disturbances at the level of the lesion and upper motor signs below it. The best investigation to differentiate between the two is an MRI scan of the spinal cord, which has superseded myelography. In this case, the lesion appears to affect the C5 and C6 segments of the cervical cord, hence the absent biceps and supinator reflexes on the left side. This would not explain the weakness and wasting of the muscles of the hand as they are supplied by C8 and T1; however, small muscle wasting in cervical myelopathy appears to be due to reduced blood flow to the lower segments of the cord rather than to direct compression of the C8 and T1 spinal nerves. It is worth noting that sensory disturbance in the upper limbs may be absent or very mild in cervical myelopathy.

Cervical myelopathy is due to bulging or extrusion of the disc material into the cervical canal, which results in pressure atrophy and ischaemia. The main cause is osteoarthritis of the cervical spine. The posterior columns (dorsal tracts carrying proprioception, vibration sense and light-touch fibres) and the lateral columns (pyramidal tracts carrying upper motor neurones) are affected. The 5th–7th cervical segments are most commonly affected. The symptoms are those of lower motor neurone signs at these levels and upper motor neurone signs below. Neck stiffness and upper limb pain may be present. Spasticity of the lower limbs is common and more pronounced than physical examination would suggest. Ataxia may occur owing to dorsal column involvement (sensory ataxia). Lhermitte's sign (electrical shock feeling down the spinal cord and into the legs) is recognized, but may also occur with cervical cord tumours, multiple sclerosis and subacute combined degeneration of the spinal cord.

The presence of lower motor neurone signs and the absence of cerebellar signs is against multiple sclerosis.

The absence of dissociated sensory loss is against syringomyelia.

Answer 400

> 1. d. Acute pancreatitis.
> 2. i. Serum amylase.
>   ii. Arterial blood gases.
>   iii. Full clotting screen.
>   iv. Chest X-ray.
>   v. Ultrasound of the abdomen.

Diagnoses to consider in an unconscious alcoholic

- Hepatic encephalopathy
- Wernicke's encephalopathy
- Methanol poisoning
- Ethylene glycol poisoning
- Alcohol intoxication
- Subdural haemorrhage
- Haemorrhage from peptic ulcer or varices
- Acute haemorrhagic pancreatitis
- Tuberculous meningitis
- Alcohol-induced hypoglycaemia

The clinical scenario is of an alcohol abuser who presents with unconsciousness and a rigid abdomen. The differential diagnosis is between a perforated duodenal ulcer, acute pancreatitis, ethylene glycol poisoning and methanol poisoning, as all four are recognized causes of abdominal pain in alcoholism. The raised gamma GT supports alcohol abuse. The low calcium favours either acute pancreatitis or ethylene glycol poisoning (oxidation of ethylene glycol to oxalic acid results in chelation of calcium). However, the diabetic state is more in keeping with acute pancreatitis, which results in damage to the islets of Langerhans, which produce insulin. Methanol poisoning may also cause hyperglycaemia, but hypocalcaemia is unusual. Furthermore, the acidosis is more severe in methanol poisoning and there is usually evidence of optic atrophy. The anaemia is quite severe, suggesting that there may be ongoing peritoneal bleeding from the pancreatitis. The MCV is high, indicating either alcohol-related marrow toxicity or alcohol-related liver damage. The low platelets indicate either hypersplenism secondary to portal hypertension or a DIC process complicating acute pancreatitis. The raised INR may be due to hepatocellular dysfunction or it may be part of the DIC. Diabetic ketoacidosis would not explain the

unconsciousness in this patient given the fact that the bicarbonate is not very low and the ketonuria is mild. The mild ketonuria in this case is due to reduced dietary intake. Rhabdomyolysis is unlikely because the creatinine is not very high, and there is no evidence of blood in the urine on dipstick testing (remember that myoglobin gives a positive dipstick test for blood).

A very high serum amylase would confirm acute pancreatitis in this case. The most common causes of death in acute pancreatitis are haemorrhage, renal failure and respiratory failure; therefore an FBC, blood gases, chest X-ray and clotting would give important prognostic information.

Answer 401

1. Erythema nodosum. Causes of erythema nodosum are shown (*Table A*).
2. A restrictive lung defect with a low KCO. The differential diagnosis for conditions causing this picture is discussed in Answer 217.
3. The X-ray of the hands demonstrates several lucent lesions at the ends of most phalanges.
4. Bilateral keratoconjunctivitis.
5. The fluid-deprivation test reveals an inability to concentrate urine until the administration of exogenous desmopressin (an ADH analogue), which is indicative of cranial diabetes insipidus. Interpretation of a fluid deprivation test is discussed below. Conditions causing cranial diabetes insipidus and an abnormal chest X-ray include sarcoidosis, TB and histiocytosis X. In rare situations, bronchial carcinoma may metastasize to the hypothalamus or pituitary and cause diabetes insipidus. Other causes of diabetes insipidus are shown (*Table B*).
6. The combination of erythema nodosum, ocular, lung, bone, parotid and lachrymal gland involvement strongly suggests the diagnosis of sarcoidosis.
7. i. Transbronchial lung biopsy to demonstrate non-caseating granulomas.
   ii. MRI scan of the pituitary to demonstrate high-intensity lesions in the mid-brain and hypothalamus.
   iii. Serum ACE level. This is not specific for the diagnosis of sarcoidosis and may be elevated in TB, histoplasmosis, berylliosis, silicosis, lymphoma, diabetes mellitus, chronic liver disease, hyperthyroidism and Gaucher's disease.
8. i. High-dose steroids. Indications for high-dose steroids in sarcoidosis include cerebral involvement, acute diffuse lung disease, uveitis and hypercalcaemia.
   ii. Desmopressin.
   iii. Artificial tears.

Sarcoidosis is a multisystem granulomatous disease of unknown aetiology that usually affects females more commonly than males. It is much more common in black people, and may present acutely with the Lofgren's syndrome, which is characterized by erythema nodosum,

---

Table A Causes of erythema nodosum

Common conditions	*Other conditions*
Streptococcal infections, including rheumatic fever	Behçet's syndrome TB Leprosy
Sarcoidosis	Histoplasmosis
Oral contraceptive pill and pregnancy	*Yersinia* *Neisseria meningitidis* and gonococcal
Inflammatory bowel disease	infections
Sulphonamide drugs	*Pasteurella pestis*

Table B Causes of diabetes insipidus

Cranial	*Nephrogenic*
Familial	X-linked (vasopressin
Autosomal dominant	receptor-2 gene)
DIDMOAD syndrome	Autosomal recessive
Cerebral tumour	(aquaporin receptor
Sarcoidosis	gene)
TB	Hypokalaemia
Histiocytosis X	Hypercalcaemia
Trauma	Lithium
Pituitary haemorrhage	Post-obstructive uropathy
	Sickle cell anaemia
	Glibenclamide
	Aminoglycosides
	Amphotericin

arthralgia, dry cough, bilateral hilar lymphadenopathy on the chest X-ray, and anterior uveitis. Patients with sarcoidosis may have lacrimal and parotid gland involvement, which is characterized by gland enlargement and sometimes referred to as Mikulicz syndrome (causes of parotid gland enlargement are listed in *Table C*). Affected patients may complain of xerostomia and gritty eyes respectively, the latter being due to keratoconjunctivitis resulting from impaired lacrimation. Mikulicz syndrome may also complicate TB, lymphoma and leukaemia. Mikulicz syndrome is relatively common and when it is associated with acute uveitis and facial nerve palsy it is referred to as Heerfordt's syndrome. In most patients the acute illness will resolve, although some will continue to have respiratory symptoms for up to two years, and a small percentage develop a chronic illness characterized by relapses and remissions.

In chronic cases lung parenchyma becomes involved, leading to fibrosis commonly affecting the apices. Ocular involvement is well recognized. Manifestations include anterior and posterior uveitis, which are characteristically associated with visual symptoms and pupillary abnormalities, and episcleritis, scleritis, choroiditis, cataracts and glaucoma. Corneal calcification complicating hypercalcaemia may also occur in sarcoidosis.

Skin infiltration occurs in the chronic form of the illness and comprises papules on the eyelids and around the mouth. Papules affecting the nose may be disfiguring and are referred to as lupus pernio. Arthralgia affecting the hands and feet is common; X-rays demonstrate small lucent cysts in multiple phalanges. Cerebral involvement is rare, but features include cranial nerve lesions, aseptic meningitis, psychosis and a multiple sclerosis-type syndrome. Mononeuritis multiplex is a recognized manifestation of the peripheral nervous system. Hypercalcaemia occurs owing to the presence of excessive production of 1,25-DHCC by granulomatous cells. Other conditions where a similar phenomenon occurs include TB and *Candida* infection.

Water deprivation test

In patients with polyuria and polydipsia and a normal blood glucose, the differential diagnosis is between cranial diabetes insipidus, nephrogenic diabetes insipidus and compulsive water deprivation. The water deprivation test will help differentiate compulsive water drinking from both types of diabetes insipidus (*Table D*). However, the differentiation of cranial diabetes insipidus from nephrogenic diabetes insipidus involves measurement of plasma and urine osmolality following administration of desmopressin. Patients with cranial diabetes insipidus are deficient in ADH and respond dramatically to desmopressin with an increase in urine osmolality, whereas patients with nephrogenic diabetes insipidus are resistant to the effects of ADH and therefore the urine osmolality is not affected by desmopressin.

Table C Causes of parotid gland enlargement

- Mumps
- Sarcoidosis
- Lymphoma
- Leukaemia
- Sjögren's syndrome
- Alcohol abuse
- Bulimia
- Cystic fibrosis
- Haemochromatosis
- Amyloidosis
- Acromegaly
- Malabsorption syndromes
- Drugs; propylthiouracil
- Toxins; lead
- Hyperlipidaemia

Table D After a water deprivation test

	P mOsm/l	U mOsm/l
Normal	300	Over 720 or double the plasma osmolality
Compulsive water drinking	300	Incomplete response, i.e. the U mOsm/l is not quite 720 and does not exceed twice the value of the P mOsm/l. Typical value 600–700 mOsm/l
Cranial diabetes inspidus	>300	<150; over 720 mOsm/l after desmopressin
Nephrogenic diabetes insipidus	>300	<150; remains <150 mOsm/l after desmopressin

Question 402

A 26-year-old female presented with a six-month history of light-headedness on hanging the washing. She was seen by her GP at the onset of her illness and he noted a blood pressure of 80/50 mmHg in both arms but no other abnormality. Over six months she had one episode of weakness and numbness of the right arm and face for almost an hour and two near syncopal episodes. She developed increasing lethargy, night sweats, and aches and pains in her upper limbs. Her appetite had reduced and she had lost almost 3 kg in weight. There was no other past medical history of note. She had smoked 10 cigarettes per day for three years from the age of 17.

On examination she had flushed cheeks but there was no skin rash. The heart rate was 90 beats/min and regular. The systolic blood pressure was 80 mmHg in both upper limbs, but the diastolic blood pressure could not be ascertained. On examination of the precordium, the apex was heaving in nature but not displaced. On auscultation there was an audible fourth heart sound. The radial pulses were absent bilaterally, the brachial pulses were weak bilaterally, the right carotid pulse was absent. The left carotid pulse was prominent. Both femoral pulses were easily palpable. Neurological examination was normal.

Investigations are shown.

Hb	9.4 g/dl
WCC	8×10^9/l
Platelets	430×10^9/l
ESR	112 mm/h
Sodium	135 mmol/l
Potassium	4.5 mmol/l
Urea	6 mmol/l
Creatinine	84 µmol/l
Glucose	4.5 mmol/l
Cholesterol	5.3 mmol/l
Autoantibody screen	Rheumatoid factor absent
	Antinuclear antibodies present in a titre of 1 in 16
Syphilis serology	VDRL and TPHA absent
Chest X-ray	Normal-sized heart
	Clear lung fields
ECG	Voltage criteria for left ventricular hypertrophy
CT scan brain	Normal

1. What is the diagnosis?
   a. Giant cell arteritis.
   b. Polyarteritis nodosa.
   c. Buerger's disease.
   d. Takayasu's arteritis.
   e. Relapsing polychondritis.

2. Which investigation would you request to confirm the diagnosis?
   a. Aortography.
   b. Invasive blood pressure monitoring.
   c. Serum antineutrophil cytoplasmic antibody.
   d. Fluorescent treponemal antibody.
   e. Cardiac biopsy.

3. Which of the three below would best explain the reason for left ventricular hypertrophy on the ECG?
   a. Cardiac amyloid.
   b. Essential hypertension.
   c. Hypertension secondary to renal artery stenosis.
   d. Chronic renal failure.
   e. Fibromuscular dysplasia.
   f. Renal vasculitis.
   g. Acquired co-arctation of the aorta.
   h. Reduced distensibility of the ascending aorta.

Answer 402

1. d. Takayasu's arteritis.
2. a. Aortography.
3. c. Hypertension secondary to renal artery stenosis.
   g. Acquired co-arctation of the aorta.
   h. Reduced distensibility of the ascending aorta.

The absence of pulses in the arms and neck and the associated high ESR value in a young woman should raise the diagnosis of Takayasu's arteritis. Takayasu's arteritis is a rare disorder with a prevalence of 1.5–2 per million. It has a strong female predisposition and is more common in parts of Africa and Asia. The mean age of onset is 29 years, but it can occur from any age between infancy and middle age. It is very uncommon after middle age. The condition is caused by granulomatous vasculitis of large vessels, particularly the aortic arch, which results in obliterative changes in the lumina of the vessels affected. Inflammation may be multi-segmental, interspersed with normal segments. Symptoms comprise a systemic illness (sweats, weight loss, anorexia and myalgia) as well as vascular insufficiency in the limbs affected. Physical signs include pulseless vessels. Hypertension is present in 50% of cases, but was not detected in this case because of disease in both subclavian arteries. The causes of hypertension include renal artery stenosis, acquired co-arctation and reduced distensibility of the aortic arch. Complications are those of long-standing hypertension, aortic regurgitation and congestive cardiac failure. Inflammatory markers are usually raised and there may be an anaemia of chronic disease, but the diagnosis is a clinical one and can be confirmed with aortography. In this case, the patient had an occluded brachiocephalic and left subclavian artery. The differential diagnosis is between other conditions which may produce an aortic arch syndrome, such as syphilitic aortitis and relapsing polychondritis; however, in this case syphilis serology is negative and there are no clinical features of relapsing polychondritis. Treatment is with steroids and vascular stents.

Aortography in this patient demonstrated occluded innominate and left subclavian arteries (**402**). Only the left common carotid artery is patent.

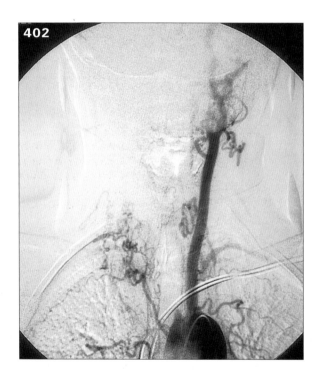

Data Interpretation Tutorials

Calcium Biochemistry

Condition	Ca	PO$_4$	Alkaline phosphatase	Additional
1° and 3° hyperparathyroidism	↑	↓	↑	
2° hyperparathyroidism/CRF	↓/N	↑	↑	
Hypoparathyroidism	↓	↑	N	PTH absent
Pseudohypoparathyroidism	↓	↑	N	PTH elevated
Magnesium deficiency	↓	↑	↑	PTH normal
Pseudopseudohypoparathyroidism	N	N	N	
Osteomalacia/rickets	↓	↓	↑	
Osteoporosis	N	N	N	
Myeloma	↑	N	N*	
Paget's disease	N**	N	↑	↑ urinary hydroxyproline
Malignancy (bony metastases)	↑	N/↑	↑	
Sarcoidosis	N/↑	N	N	
Vitamin D intoxication	↑	↑	N	

* Increased with pathological fractures.   ** Increased after prolonged immobilization.

Genetics

Patterns of inheritance

Autosomal dominant inheritance
- Males and females are equally affected.
- All individuals inheriting the abnormal gene are affected.
- Offspring of affected parents (irrespective of the parental sex) have a 50% chance of inheriting the disease.
- This is in contrast to X-linked conditions where male-to-male transmission of disease does not occur.

Autosomal recessive inheritance
- Males and females are equally affected, but are fewer in number than in autosomal dominant conditions.
- Not all generations will be affected.
- If both parents are carriers for the recessive gene 25% of the offspring will be affected, 50% will become carriers, but will not have the disease and 25% will not have the abnormal gene.
- If an affected individual marries a carrier, then 50% offspring will be affected and 50% offspring will be carriers.
- If an affected individual marries another affected, then all offspring will be affected.

X-linked dominant inheritance
- Males and females are both affected.
- No male-to-male transmission.
- Affected males transmit the disease to 100% of their daughters.
- An affected female will transmit the disease to 50% of all offspring.

X-linked recessive inheritance
- Males are affected.
- Females are carriers.
- No male-to-male transmission.
- Daughters of affected males will be carriers.
- Female carrier will have 50% affected sons and 50% daughters who are carriers.

Inheritance of maternal mitochondrial genetic abnormalities
- During conception, only mitochondria from the ovum are passed on to the zygote.
- Affected females will pass the disease to 100% offspring.
- Affected males will not transmit disease to offspring.
- Examples include Leber's optic atrophy, Kearnes–Sayer syndrome, MELAS (mitochondrial encephalopathy, lactic acidosis and stroke-like syndrome), MERF (mitochondrial encephalopathy and red ragged fibres).

Audiograms

An audiogram of both ears may be presented on the same graph, or there may be a separate audiogram for each ear. A separate suffix will be given to differentiate between air conduction (AC) and bone conduction (BC).

In sensorineuronal deafness, both air and bone conduction are diminished. The air–bone gap is usually narrow, i.e. there is not much difference between air and bone conduction. In conduction deafness, bone conduction is superior to air conduction on the affected side.

Normal hearing can detect sounds of a frequency between 250–8,000 Hz at a sound intensity of 0–10 dB (**1**). The following audiograms are most commonly tested in higher post-graduate examinations.

Sensorineuronal deafness at progressively higher frequencies. In degenerative sensorineuronal loss (presbycusis), deafness is usually bilateral most profound at sounds with high frequencies (**2**). Other causes of bilateral sensorineuronal deafness include congenital rubella infection, mumps infection and drugs such as high dose loop diuretics and aminoglycosides.

Fluctuating low tone deafness (below 4,000 Hz) suggests Ménière's disease. This is bilateral in 10% of cases (**3**) and may progress to sensorineuronal deafness in 25% of patients (**2**).

Sudden and profound hearing loss at a frequency of 4,000 Hz is suggestive of noise-induced hearing loss (**4**).

Unilateral sensorineuronal hearing loss (**5**) may be degenerative or due to unilateral auditory nerve damage as a result of a neuropathic process. It should also raise the suspicion of lesion in the cerebello-pontine angle on the affected side, for example, an acoustic neuroma.

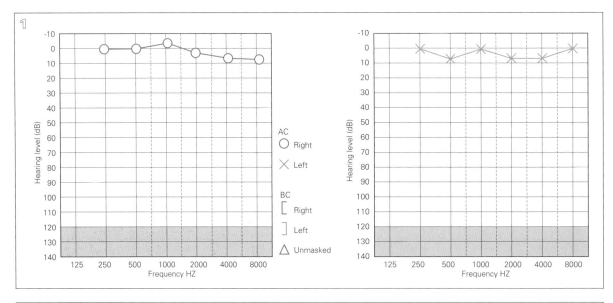

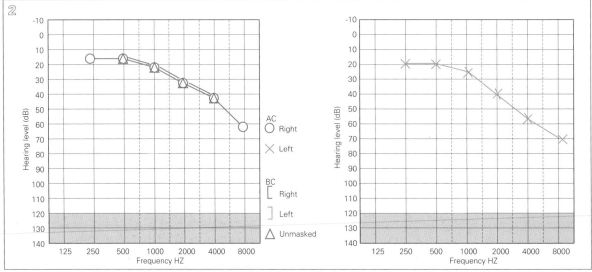

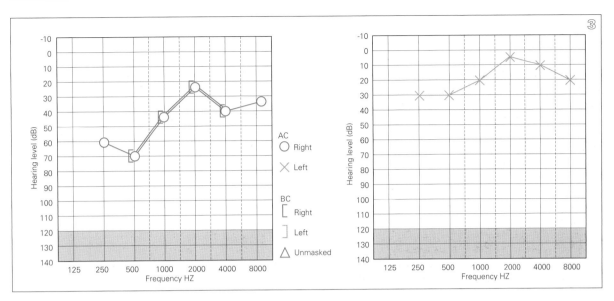

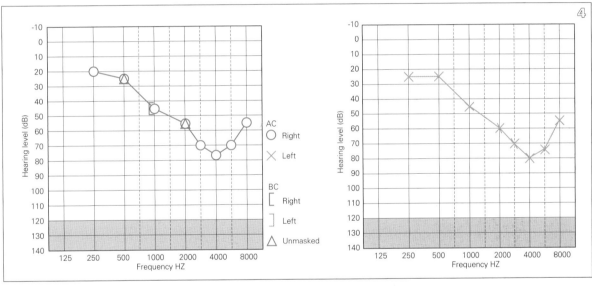

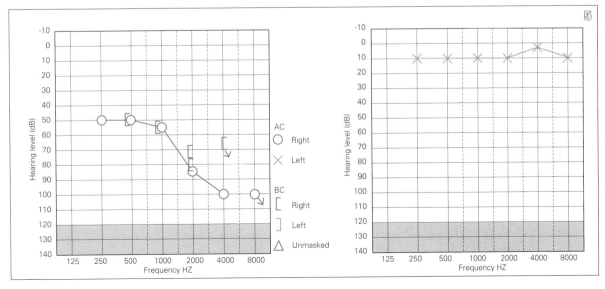

In the example below, bone conduction is superior to air conduction suggesting conduction deafness (**6**). Causes of conduction deafness are shown (*Table*).

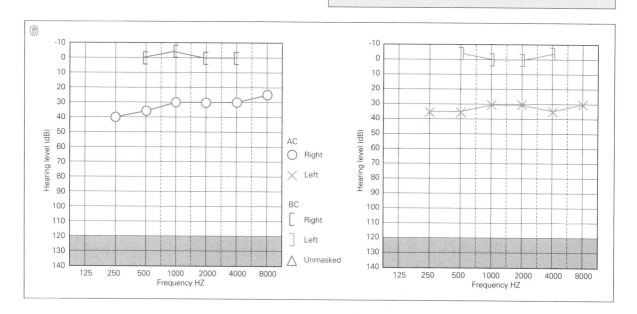

Guidelines for the Interpretation of Cardiac Catheter Data

- Right-heart saturations do not exceed 75%. Saturations more than this are suggestive of a left-to-right shunt.

- Left-heart saturations vary from 96–98%. Saturations less than this are suggestive of a right-to-left shunt.

- In right-to-left shunts, the arterial saturations do not change with inspired high-concentration oxygen.

- A VSD with a right-to-left shunt and pulmonary stenosis can be differentiated from Fallot's tetralogy by examining the oxygen saturation in the left ventricle and the ascending aorta. In the case of a VSD, the saturations in the left ventricle and the aorta will both be low and very similar. In the case of Fallot's tetralogy, the aortic oxygen saturation will be much lower than the oxygen saturation in the left ventricle because the right ventricle pumps most of the deoxygenated blood into the overriding aorta.

- A pulmonary artery pressure exceeding 35 mmHg is suggestive of pulmonary hypertension.

- A pressure drop of more than 10 mmHg across the aortic or pulmonary valve is suggestive of aortic or pulmonary stenosis, respectively.

- The PCWP is equal to the LVEDP. When the PCWP exceeds the LVEDP, the diagnosis of mitral stenosis should be considered.

- The diagnosis of mitral regurgitation cannot be made unless you are given the PCWP 'v-wave'. A v-wave higher than 20 mmHg is highly suggestive of mitral regurgitation.

- Aortic regurgitation is diagnosed by a wide pulse pressure in the aortic pressure.

- The right and LVEDP and the left and right atrial pressures are roughly equal in pericardial constriction.

Respiratory Function Tests

Obstructive lung defect

Examples:
- Chronic bronchitis.
- Emphysema.
- Asthma.
- Bronchiectasis.

Spirometry

FEV$_1$ (l)	↓↓
FVC (l)	↓
FEV$_1$/FVC	<70% (normal 70–80%)
TLC (l)	↑ (gas trapping)
RV	↑
TLCO (l)	↓
KCO (mmol/min/kPa)	↓*

*The KCO is always low in obstructive airways disease, with the very rare exception of a limited number of patients with asthma who may have a high KCO during an attack. The exact mechanism for this is not understood. The KCO is significantly reduced in emphysema, and if a young patient or a non-smoker has a low KCO in the context of an obstructive lung defect, always consider the possibility of α-1 antitrypsin deficiency.

Restrictive lung defect

Examples:
- Interstitial lung disease:
    sarcoidosis,
    fibrotic lung disease
- Pulmonary emboli.
- Pulmonary oedema.
- Neuromuscular disease affecting respiratory muscles.
- Pulmonary haemorrhage.
- Lymphangitis carcinomatosa.
- Thoracic cage defects.

Spirometry

FEV$_1$ (l)	↓
FVC (l)	↓↓
FEV$_1$/FVC	>80%
TLC (l)	↓
RV	↓
TLCO (l)	↓
KCO** (mmol/min/kPa)	↓

** KCO is charcteristically reduced in most cases of restrictive defect, with the exception of pulmonary haemorrhage, where it is increased, and thoracic cage deformities/neuromuscular defects and pneumonectomy where it is unchanged or increased.

KCO

Increased KCO:
- Polycythaemia.
- Left-to-right shunts.
- Pulmonary haemorrhage.
- Asthma (exceptionally rare).
- Thoracic cage deformities (may be normal).

Reduced KCO:
- Interstitial lung disease.
- Primary pulmonary hypertension.
- Multiple pulmonary emboli.
- Pulmonary oedema.
- Lymphangitis carcinomatosa.
- Arteriovenous malformation.
- Anaemia (spirometry normal).
- Obstructive airways disease (rare exception is asthma).

Interpretation of Respiratory Flow Loop Curves

The normal flow loop curve has a triangular expiratory flow limb and a semi-circular inspiratory flow limb (**7**). The explanation for this is as follows: following a full inspiration, the lung's recoil is maximal, as is pleural pressure. The onset of expiratory flow is therefore explosive and reaches its peak within 0.01 s. The expiratory curve decreases its flow gradually as the lung volume drops from TLC to RV. This reflects the gradual drop in the lung's elastic recoil as the lung gets smaller. In contrast to expiration, inspiration does not reach an instant maximal flow. As the respiratory muscles contract, the power increases progressively from the start of the inspiration to achieve a maximal flow. This takes a relatively long time, and the maximal inspiratory flow is only achieved by the mid-point of the vital capacity. The flow then slows again as the maximum inspired volume is reached, giving the inspiratory limb a semi-circular appearance.

Flow loops tested in the examination are those of obstructive airways disease, extrathoracic airways obstruction, intrathoracic airways obstruction, and a restrictive lung defect.

Obstructive airways disease

In obstructive airways disease the amount of elastic recoil in the lung is reduced; therefore the onset of the expiratory limb is not as explosive as in a normal individual and reaches its peak later than usual. As expiration continues the small airways collapse rapidly to produce a very early decline in flow which results in a 'flat' expiratory flow loop curve after the initial peak (**8**).

Extrathoracic airways disease obstruction

Extrathoracic airways may be variable or fixed. In extrathoracic obstruction, the inspiratory loop is reduced significantly compared with the expiratory flow. Normally, during inspiration, the negative intrathoracic pressure pulls the intrathoracic airways open and promotes inspiratory flow. In extrathoracic obstruction this does not happen; therefore the inspiratory flow rate is reduced. In variable extrathoracic obstruction the expiratory flow limb is preserved (**9**). Examples of variable obstruction include tumour in the upper airways, fat, pharyngeal muscle weakness, vocal cord paralysis or enlarged lymph nodes. In fixed extrathoracic obstruction, such as tracheal stenosis, both expiratory flow and inspiratory flow limbs are 'blunted'; however, the inspiratory limb is affected much more than the expiratory limb (**10**).

Intrathoracic airways obstruction

When obstruction is intrathoracic, inspiration is preserved because the large extrathoracic airways are patent; however, the expiratory flow is diminished because an increased intrathoracic pressure is required to overcome the obstruction, which results in closure of the small airways (**11**).

Restrictive lung disease

The flow loop curve has the same shape as the normal curve (**7**), but the lung volume is much smaller.

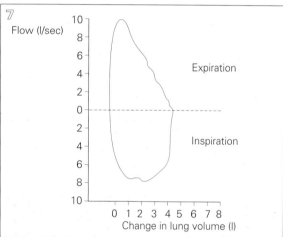

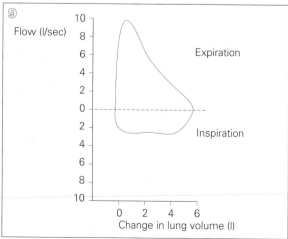

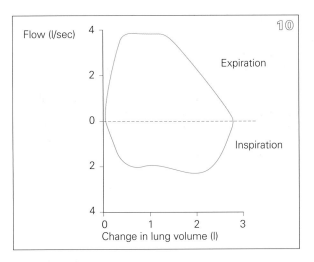

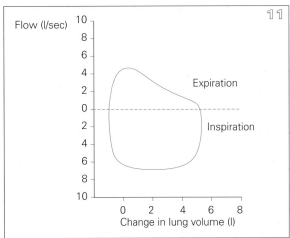

Echocardiography

Echocardiography has featured, and will continue to feature, in postgraduate examinations because it is widely requested, and pictures from 'still frames' are relatively easy to interpret. Both M-mode and two-dimensional (2-D) echocardiography are tested, although the latter is being shown with an increasing frequency because it allows the reader to have a better appreciation of cardiac chambers.

Normal values for cardiac dimensions are shown in the table.

Normal values for cardiac dimensions

Chamber/structure	Measurement
Left atrium	<4.5 cm
Left ventricular diastolic size	<5.5 cm
Interventricular septum	<1.2 cm
Posterior wall	<1.2 cm

2-D echocardiography

The view which is shown most often is the parasternal long-axis view (**12**). In this view it is not always easy to study the right ventricle in detail, and therefore it is unusual to be shown right-sided pathology in the examination. Four-chamber views resemble what the reader envisages the heart to look like, except that the ventricles are at the top and the atria are at the bottom (**13**). Most echocardiograms are accompanied by a scale where each square represents 1 cm.

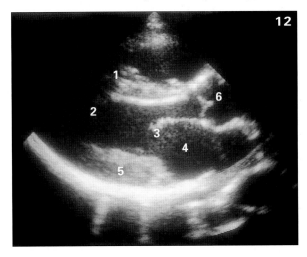

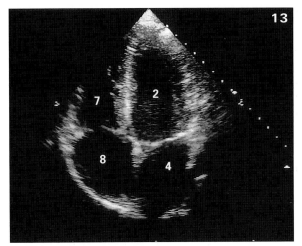

Key:
1 Interventricular septum
2 Left ventricle

3 Mitral valve
4 Left atrium
5 Left ventricular posterior wall

6 Aorta
7 Right ventricle
8 Right atrium

Figures **14** and **15** are diagrammatic representations of a common parasternal long axis and an apical four-chamber view respectively.

Common examples of conditions shown in examinations using 2-D echocardiography:

- Pericardial effusion (**16**, effusion is arrowed).
- Left atrial myxoma (**17**, myxoma is arrowed).
- Mitral stenosis (**18**, stenosed mitral valve is arrowed).
- Vegetation on mitral valve (**19**, vegetation on the anterior mitral valve leaflet is arrowed).

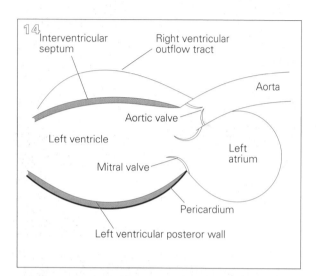

14 — Interventricular septum; Right ventricular outflow tract; Aorta; Aortic valve; Left ventricle; Left atrium; Mitral valve; Pericardium; Left ventricular posteror wall

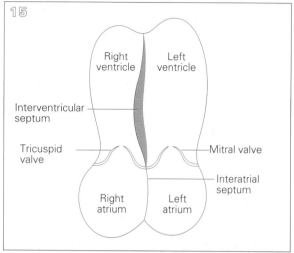

15 — Right ventricle; Left ventricle; Interventricular septum; Tricuspid valve; Mitral valve; Interatrial septum; Right atrium; Left atrium

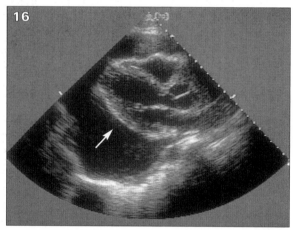

16

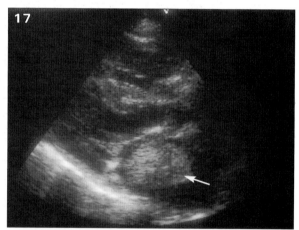

17

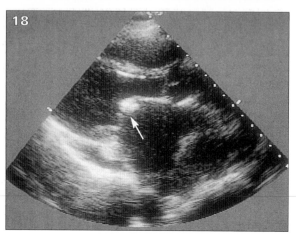

18

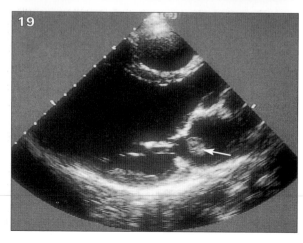

19

- HCM (**20**, gross hypertrophy of the interventricular septum is arrowed).
- Left ventricular thrombus (**21** thrombus at the apex is arrowed; **22** thrombus is arrowed).
- Aortic stenosis (**23**, calcified aortic valve arrowed).
- Vegetation on aortic valve (**24**, echogenic mass on the aortic valve is arrowed).
- Aortic dissection (**25**, aortic dissection flap is arrowed).

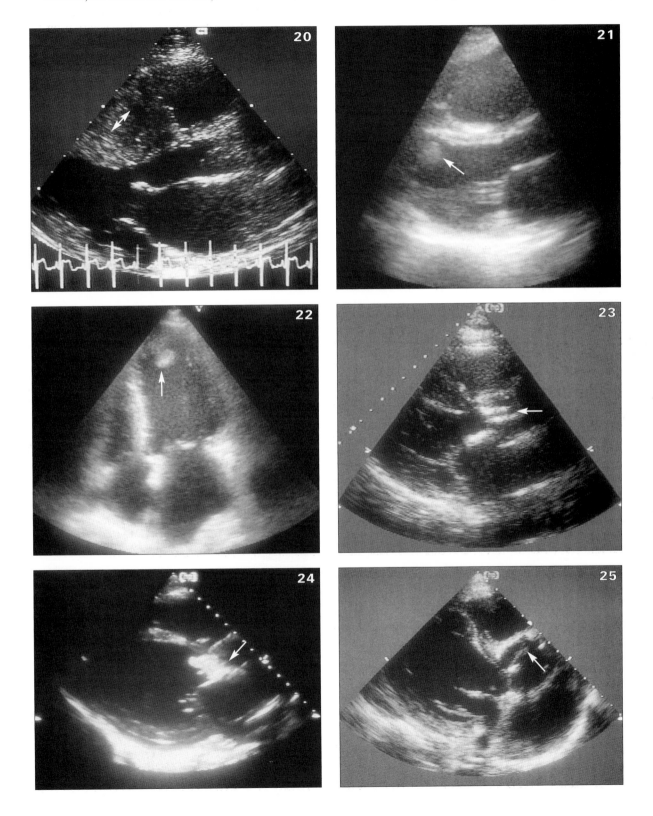

Figure **26** is a diagrammatic representation of common examples shown on parasternal long-axis view. Figure **27** is a diagrammatic representation of common examples shown in the four-chamber view.

M-mode echocardiography

The M-mode picture is derived by taking a cross-sectional view from the 2-D parasternal long-axis view. The three main views include sections at the level of the aortic valve, at the level of the tips of the mitral valve, and at the level of the papillary muscle. The cross-sectional view at the level of the mitral valve tips is by far the most common view which is shown in examinations because it allows the examiners to test the readers on abnormalities on the mitral valve and the left ventricle (**28**).

Examples commonly shown in M-mode echocardiography:
- Pericardial effusion.
- Left atrial myxoma (**29**, echogenic mass prolapsing through the mitral valve orifice in diastole is arrowed).
- Mitral stenosis (**30**, thickened anterior mitral valve leaflet is arrowed; reduced excursion of the mitral valve in diastole is shown [1]).
- Vegetation on mitral valve (**31**, echogenic mass on the posterior mitral valve leaflet is arrowed).
- Mitral valve prolapse (**32**, hammocking of the posterior mitral valve leaflet in diastole is arrowed).
- HCM (**33**, systolic anterior motion of the mitral valve is shown [1]).

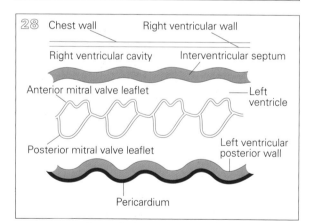

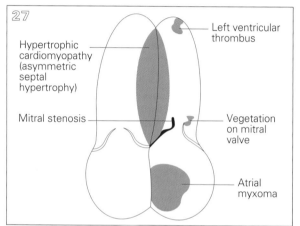

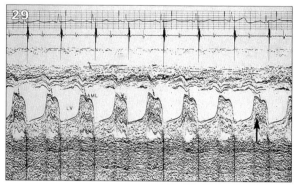

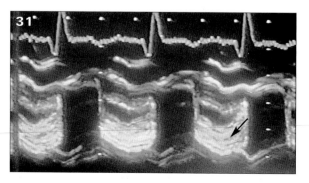

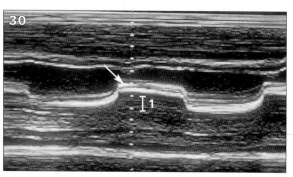

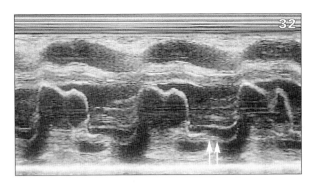

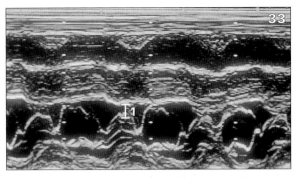

Importance of carefully inspecting mitral valve leaflets to diagnose cardiac abnormalities on the M-mode echocardiogram

On an M-mode echocardiogram, the normal mitral valve has an anterior leaflet which has a characteristic 'M'-shape and a posterior leaflet which has a semi 'U'-shape. In diastole, the anterior leaflet moves forward and the posterior leaflet moves backward, and in systole both leaflets appose. With the exception of pericardial effusion, careful inspection of the mitral valve will enable the reader to diagnose all the abnormalities which are commonly tested (*Table*).

Figure **34** is a diagrammatic representation of the mitral valve in relation to cardiac lesions on the M-mode echocardiogram.

The mitral valve in relation to cardiac lesions on the M-mode echocardiogram

Abnormality	*Mitral valve abnormality*
Mitral valve prolapse	Normal appearance in diastole; however, in mid systole there is prolapse of one or both leaflets
Mitral stenosis	There is loss of the M-shape of the anterior leaflet Mitral valve excursion is reduced and there is anterior movement of the posterior leaflet in diastole
Atrial myxoma	There is obliteration of the mitral valve cavity by an echogenic mass in diastole
Vegetation on mitral valve	Echogenic mass on one or both leaflets
HCM	The mitral valve moves forward towards the septum in systole (a phenomenon termed systolic anterior motion of the mitral valve (SAM). In addition, the left ventricular cavity is small and there is septal hypertrophy
Aortic regurgitation	As the regurgitant jet flows back into the left ventricle it 'tickles' the anterior leaflet, causing a fluttering appearance

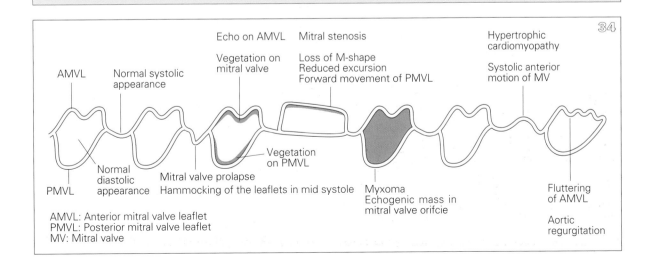

AMVL: Anterior mitral valve leaflet
PMVL: Posterior mitral valve leaflet
MV: Mitral valve

Acid–base Disturbance

Acidosis

The main source of acid (H$^+$ ions) in the body is tissue respiration. Carbon dioxide produced by cellular respiration is converted to carbonic acid, which dissociates to generate H$^+$ (acid) and HCO$_3^-$ ions (buffering base). The retention of CO$_2$, increase in H$^+$ or reduction in HCO$_3^-$ may result in an acidosis.

$$CO_2 + H_2O \leftrightarrow H_2CO_3 \leftrightarrow H^+ + HCO_3^-$$

Three types of acidosis are recognized:
- Respiratory acidosis.
- Metabolic acidosis with a high anion gap.
- Metabolic acidosis with a normal anion gap.

Respiratory acidosis is characterized by a fall in arterial pH (<7.35) due to CO$_2$ retention. Metabolic acidosis may result from the retention of fixed or organic acids causing a reduction in the bicarbonate level (which is the main buffering agent for H$^+$ in the blood) without any change in the chloride situation. In these situations, it is termed metabolic acidosis with a high anion gap. Alternatively, metabolic acidosis may occur as a consequence of bicarbonate loss from the gastrointestinal tract or the kidneys. In these situations, chloride is retained, resulting in a hyperchloraemic acidosis or a metabolic acidosis with a normal anion gap. The anion gap is calculated by subtracting the sum of the sodium and potassium concentrations from the sum of the chloride and bicarbonate concentrations. The normal anion gap is between 10–18 mmol/l. The hallmark of metabolic acidosis of either type is a low arterial pH and a low bicarbonate level.

Regulation of arterial pH is controlled by the kidneys and the lungs. Acidosis can be compensated for either by removing CO$_2$ from the body (lungs) or by retaining bicarbonate ions (kidneys). Respiratory acidosis is compensated for by the kidneys, which retain bicarbonate ions. In compensated respiratory acidosis the pH is normal, or almost normal, and the bicarbonate level is high. In compensated metabolic acidosis the arterial pH is normal, or almost normal, and the pCO$_2$ is low. Respiratory acidosis is compensated by the respiratory system through a centrally mediated mechanism which results in hyperventilation and a consequent reduction in the pCO$_2$. Causes of respiratory and metabolic acidosis are given (*Table*).

Alkalosis

Alkalosis may be respiratory or metabolic in origin. In respiratory alkalosis, there is a high pH due to hyperventilation, causing a low pCO$_2$. Metabolic alkalosis is usually due to increased loss of H$^+$ from the kidney or gastrointestinal tract, or to increased ingestion of alkaline agents. It is characterized by a high bicarbonate and a high pH. Respiratory alkalosis is rare and is usually acute. Chronic cases, usually due to chronic hyperventilation, are compensated for by increasing bicarbonate excretion by the kidneys. Metabolic alkalosis – which is much more common than respiratory alkalosis – is compensated for by respiratory hypoventilation, which results in an increase in pCO$_2$ and hence an increase in H$^+$.

Causes of respiratory and metabolic acidosis

Respiratory acidosis
- Hypoventilation from any cause, e.g. obesity, thoracic cage deformities and neuromuscular disorders
- Obstructive airways disease
- Acute asthma

Metabolic acidosis (high anion gap)
- Diabetic ketoacidosis
- Uraemic acidosis
- Salicylate poisoning
- Lactic acidosis:
  shock
  liver failure
  metformin therapy
  glucose-6-phosphate dehydrogenase deficiency
  leukaemia
- Methylene poisoning
- Ethylene glycol poisoning

Metabolic acidosis (normal anion gap)
- Severe diarrhoea
- Pancreatic fistula
- Ureterosigmoidostomy
- RTA
- Acetazolamide therapy

Causes of respiratory and metabolic alkalosis

Respiratory alkalosis:
- Hyperventilation
- Hysteria
- Encephalitis
- Brainstem lesions
- Aspirin toxicity

Metabolic alkalosis:
- Vomiting
- Diuretics
- Antacids
- Hypokalaemic states (these increase renal loss of H$^+$ by the distal convoluted tubule)

Normal Ranges

		SI units	*Traditional units*
Haematology			
ESR		0–10 mm in 1st h	0–10 mm in 1st h
Hb	male	130–180 g/l	13–18 g/dl
	female	115–150 g/l	11.5–15 g/dl
MCH		27–32 pg	–
MCHC		32–36 g/dl	32–36%
MCV		76–95 fl	76–95 x 10^6/mm^3
PCV (haematocrit)	male	0.40–0.54 l/l	40–54%
	female	0.35–0.47 l/l	35–47%
Platelet count		150–400 x 10^9/l	150–400 x 10^3/mm^3
RBCs	male	4.5–6.5 x 10^{12}/l	4.5–6.5 x 10^6/mm^3
	female	3.9–5.6 x 10^{12}/l	3.9–5.6 x 10^6/mm^3
Reticulocyte count		0.2–2%	0.2–2%
WCC	total	4–11 x 10^9/l	4–11 x 10^3/mm^3
	neutrophils	2–7.5 x 10^9/l	2–7.5 x 10^3/mm^3
	lymphocytes	1.5–4.0 x 10^9/l	1.5–4.0 x 10^3/mm^3
	monocytes	0.2–0.8 x 10^9/l	0.2–0.8 x 10^3/mm^3
	eosinophils	0.04–0.4 x 10^9/l	0.04–0.4 x 10^3/mm^3
	basophils	<0.1 x 10^9/l	<0.1 x 10^3/mm^3
Clotting			
APTT		30–46 s	30–46 s
BT		2–8 min	2–8 min
Fibrinogen		2–4 g/l	0.2–0.4 g/dl
PT		12–14 s	12–14 s
TT		15–19 s	15–19 s
Endocrinology			
Cortisol	09.00 h	170–700 nmol/l	6.1–25.2 μg/dl
	24.00 h	<140 nmol/l	5.0 μg/dl
GH		<10 μg/l	<10 ng/ml
Oestradiol mid-cycle		500–1,100 pmol/l	500–1,100 pmol/l
Prolactin		<360 mu/l	<360 μu/ml
Renin	lying	2–4 μg/l/h	2–4 ng/ml/h
	standing	5–14 μg/l/h	5–14 ng/ml/h
Testosterone	male	10–35 nmol/l	3–10 ng/ml
	female	0.9–3.1 nmol/l	0.3–1.0 ng/ml
Thyroxine		68–174 nmol/l	4.5–13.6 μg/dl
TSH		0.4–3.6 mu/l	0.4–3.6 μu/ml
Biochemistry			
α-fetoprotein		<10 ku/l	<10 u/ml
ALT		5–30 u/l	5–30 mu/ml
Albumin		34–48 g/l	3.4–4.8 g/dl
Alkaline phosphatase		25–100 iu/l	25–100 mu/ml
AST		10–40 iu/l	10–40 mu/ml
B$_{12}$ (serum)		160–900 ng/l	160–900 pg/ml
Bicarbonate		22–30 mmol/l	22–30 mEq/l
Bilirubin		2–17 μmol/l	0.12–1.0 mg/dl

Biochemistry (continued)

		SI units	Traditional units
Calcium		2.2–2.7 mmol/l	8.8–10.8 mg/dl
Cholesterol		3.6–7.8 mmol/l	139–302 mg/dl
Chloride		100–106 mmol/l	100–106 mEq/l
C-reactive protein		0–10 mg/l	0–1.0 mg/dl
Creatinine		50–120 μmol/l	0.57–1.36 mg/dl
Creatinine kinase	males	17–148 iu/l	17–148 mu/ml
	females	10–79 iu/l	10–79 mu/ml
Ferritin		15–250 μg/l	1.5–25.0 μg/dl
Folate	serum	3–20 μg/l	3–20 ng/ml
	red cell	160–460 μg/l	160–460 ng/ml
Gamma GT		5–30 u/l	5–30 u/l
Glucose (blood)		2.5–7.5 mmol/l	45–135 mg/dl
Iron (serum)	males	14–32 μmol/l	78–180 μg/dl
	females	10–30 μmol/l	56–168 μg/dl
Osmolality		280–296 mOsm/kg	280–296 mOsm/kg
Phosphate		0.8–1.5 mmol/l	2.5–4.65 mg/dl
Potassium		3.5–5.0 mmol/l	3.5–5.0 mEq/l
Protein		62–80 g/l	6.2–8.0 g/dl
Sodium		135–146 mmol/l	135–146 mEq/l
TIBC		40–80 μmol/l	224–448 μg/dl
Urate		0.12–0.42	2.0–7.0 mg/dl
Urea		2.5–6.7 mmol/l	15.0–40.2 mg/dl (BUN)

Immunology

	SI units	Traditional units
IgA	0.8–4.0 g/l	80–400 mg/dl
IgG	7.0–18.0 g/l	700–1,800 mg/dl
IgM	0.4–2.5 g/l	40–250 mg/dl

Arterial Blood Gases

	SI units	Traditional units
$PaCO_2$	4.7–6.0 kPa	35–45 mmHg
PaO_2	11.2–14.0 kPa	84–105 mmHg
pH	7.35–7.45	7.35–7.45

Cardiology

		mmHg
Venae cavae	mean	2–8
Right atrium	a-wave	3–6
	v-wave	1–4
	mean	1–5
Right ventricle	systolic	20–30
	end diastolic	2–7
Pulmonary artery	systolic	16–30
	diastolic	4–13
	mean	9–18
PCWP		4.5–12
Left atrium	a-wave	4–14
	v-wave	6–16
	mean	6–11
Left ventricle	systolic	90–140
	end diastolic	6–12
Aorta	systolic	90–140
	diastolic	70–90
	mean	70–110

Index